The Discovery of Hypnosis

The Complete Writings of James Braid, the Father of Hypnotherapy

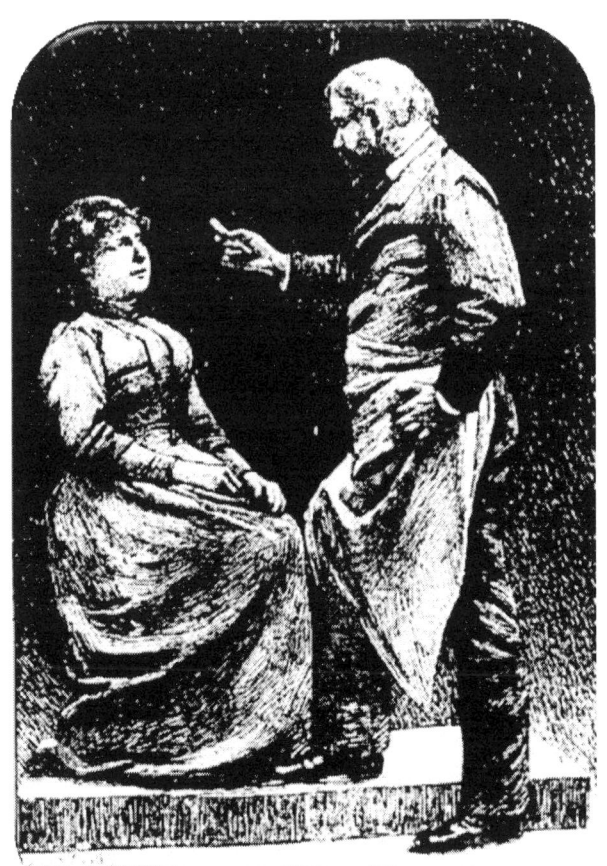

Dr Braid's first attempt to hypnotise

Edited with Commentary by Donald Robertson

Foreword by Dr. Michael Heap

Copyright Notice
Unless otherwise stated, the contents of this volume, including all editorial changes are copyright © the National Council for Hypnotherapy Ltd. (NCH), 2008. All rights reserved. No part of this publication may be reproduced, stored in a retrieval system, or transmitted in any form or by any means, electronic, mechanical, photocopying, recording or otherwise without prior permission of the copyright holder.

Donald Robertson asserts his right under the UK's Copyright, Designs and Patents Act, 1988, and other relevant legislation internationally, to be recognised and clearly identified as the editor and author of this work in this and any future editions.

www.hypnotherapists.org.uk

James Braid's motto:

Possunt, quia posse videntur.

"They can because they believe they can."
– Virgil, *The Aeneid* [1]

"Thus James Braid and his merits are – speaking generally – undeservedly underestimated in his own country.

His portrait ought to be exhibited in all British medical establishments and sanatoria for neurotic and psychopathic patients,

and chiefly on the walls of all psychotherapeutic ordination-institutes.

Yet we do not abandon the hope that at last the time will come when

– like the monument in honour of Emile Coué at Nancy –

ere long the well-deserved monument of James Braid will be erected in England."

– Dr. F.A. Volgyesi [2]

---

[1] This motto from *The Physiology of Fascination* (1850) is quoted in Braid's other writings, and appears in his last manuscript.
[2] Dr. F.A. Volgyesi, 'Discovery of Hypnotism', *The British Journal of Medical Hypnotism*, vol. 7, no. 3, Spring 1956.

Table of Contents

Acknowledgements	20
Editor's Preface by Donald Robertson	0
Foreword by Dr. Michael Heap	2
SECTION I: Articles on Braid	4
James Braid's Life & Work	6
The Original Philosophy of Hypnotism	17
Principal Works by Braid	20
Glossary of Braidism	22
Braid's Hypnotic Induction Technique	26
Braid's Mature Theory of Hypnotism	29
Braid's Theory of Suggestion	33
James Braid's Work & Writings (Bramwell, 1896-1903)	34
Braid's Discovery of Hypnotism (Williamson, 1896)	61
SECTION II: Braid's Collected Works	63
On Hypnotism (1860)	64
The Physiology of Fascination & The Critics Criticised (1855)	78
Hypnotic Therapeutics (1853)	91
"Psycho-Physiology & the Ideo-Motor Reflex" (1853)	117
Magic, Witchcraft, Animal Magnetism, etc. (1852)	128
Lecture on Electro-Biology (1851)	181
Electro-Biological Phenomena Considered Physiologically & Psychologically (1851)	189
Observations on Trance or Human Hybernation (1850)	200
"On Mesmerism & Chemical Anaesthesia": Letter (1849)	226
"On Esdaile & Hypnotic Anaesthetic": Letter to The Medical Times (1847)	229
The Power of the Mind over the Body (1846)	236
"Observations on Mesmeric & Hypnotic Phenomena": Letter to The Medical Times (1844)	252
"On Thomas Wakley & John Elliotson": Letter to The Medical Times (1844)	258
"On Muscular Suggestion": Braid's Letters on Phreno-Hypnotism (1843-1844)	260
Neurypnology: The Rationale of Nervous Sleep (1843)	278
"On Neuro-Hypnotism": Letter to The Medical Times (1842)	372
"The Discovery of Hypnotism": "Satanic Agency & Mesmerism" Reviewed (1842)	374
"On Braid's Hanover Square Talks": Report & Letter in The Medical Times (1842)	382
Bibliography of James Braid's Writings	386

Table of Contents with Section Headings

Acknowledgements	20
Editor's Preface by Donald Robertson	0
Foreword by Dr. Michael Heap	2
SECTION I: Articles on Braid	4
James Braid's Life & Work	6
Sudden Death of Mr. James Braid, Surgeon of Manchester	6
Braid's Biographical Details	6
The Lafontaine Incident (1841)	7
After the Discovery (1841-1843)	7
After Neurypnology (1843-1860)	9
The Discovery of Hypnotism	10
Braid's Change of View	11
"Stage Hypnosis" *versus* Hypnotism	12
Braid as Critic of Complementary Therapies	13
Hypnotism as Early Cognitive-Behavioural Therapy	13
The Future of Braid's Legacy	15
The Original Philosophy of Hypnotism	17
Principal Works by Braid	20
Glossary of Braidism	22
Braid's Hypnotic Induction Technique	26
Braid's Mature Theory of Hypnotism	29
Braid's Theory of Suggestion	33
James Braid's Work & Writings (Bramwell, 1896-1903)	34
Editor's Preface	35
James Braid; His Work and Writings (1896)	36
"Neurypnology"	37
Analogous States	40
General Theory	41
Magnets, etc.	43
Clairvoyance, etc.	46
Phrenology	47
Suggestion, Passes, etc.	48
Dangers	48
Medical & Surgical Cases	50

General Observations	50
Historical	51
[Evaluation of Braid's Work]	52
[Conclusion]	56
[Editor's Addendum]	56
Appendix: Braid's Later Theories (Bramwell, 1903; 1909)	58
Braid's Discovery of Hypnotism (Williamson, 1896)	61
SECTION II: Braid's Collected Works	63
On Hypnotism (1860)	64
Foreword	64
Splitting (Doubling) Of Consciousness	64
Subjective Nature of the Phenomena	65
Initial Supporting Facts	66
Subjective Nature of the Phenomena	66
Baron Reichenbach's Odic Force	67
The Influence of Suggestions	68
Different Stages of Hypnotism	69
Waking Phenomena	71
Suggestion by Tone of Voice	72
The Influence of Suggestions	72
How the (Mesmeric) Passes Work	73
Natural Symptoms, Artificial Symptoms	74
The Influence of Dominant Impressions	74
On Memory, On the Sense of Smell	75
Muscular Sense, Imitation	76
Wilhelm Preyer's Foreword to the German Translation (1881)	77
The Physiology of Fascination & The Critics Criticised (1855)	78
The Physiology of Fascination	79
The Critics Criticised (1855)	84
Appendix: Excerpts from *The Zoist*	89
Hypnotic Therapeutics (1853)	91
Hypnotic Therapeutics	92
[Introduction]	92
[Nature of Hypnosis]	92
[Suggestion & Hypnosis]	92
[Emerging from Hypnosis]	92
[Physical Effect of Suggestion]	93
[Early Placebo Experiments]	93

[Experiments with Suggestion] 94

[Sedative & Stimulating Suggestions in Hypnotic Therapy] 94

[Physiological Theory & Hypnotic Anaesthesia] 95

[Catalepsy & Increased Stimulation] 96

[Suggestion & Passes] 96

[Rejection of Occult Pretensions] 96

[Hypnosis Intensifies Natural Faculties] 97

[Physical Effects of Hypnotic Suggestion] 97

[Hypnosis used as Alterative] 98

[Examples of Cases Treated] 98

[Breaking Down Morbid Dominant Ideas] 100

[Other Conditions Treated by Removing Morbid Ideas] 100

[Most Subjects Remain Conscious in Hypnosis] 101

[Cure of Headache & Loss of Eyesight] 101

[Case of Spinal Irritation] 101

[Rheumatic Pain] 102

[Waking Suggestion & Induced Nausea] 103

[Bitter Laxative Effect] 103

[Overcoming Hallucinatory Odour] 103

[Lactation, Breast Enlargement, Bowel Movement, & Menstruation] 104

[Epilepsy & Waking Suggestion for Menstruation] 105

[Hypnotic Childbirth] 107

[Critique of Homeopathy] 107

[The "Placebo" Power of Dominant Ideas] 108

[Physical Effects of Hypnosis Beyond Suggestion] 108

["Hydro-Hypnotism" for Inducing Sleep] 109

[Concluding Remarks] 109

Appendix 111

"Psycho-Physiology & the Ideo-Motor Reflex" (1853) 117

Editor's Preface 118

Analysis of Dr. Carpenter's Lectures on the Physiology of the Nervous System (1853) 120

[Introduction] 120

[On Sleep & Dreaming] 120

[On Braid & Hypnotism] 121

[On the Ideo-Motor Reflex] 122

[On Hypnotic Somnambulism] 123

    [Muscular Suggestion] 124

    [Concluding Remarks on Hypnotism] 124

  Appendix: "The Psycho-Physiology of Suggestion" (Carpenter, 1874) 126

    The Ideo-Motor Reflex 126

    Monoideism 126

Magic, Witchcraft, Animal Magnetism, etc. (1852) 128

  Editor's Preface 129

  Preface 132

  Observations on J.C. Colquhoun's History of Magic, etc. 133

    [Preliminary Comments] 133

    [Braid Defends Himself Against the Charge of Materialism] 134

    [Colquhoun's Other Criticisms] 135

    [Braid's Critique of Mesmerism] 135

    [Braid's "Discovery" of Hypnotism; its Ancient Precursors] 137

    [Conditioning to the Hypnotic Induction] 138

    [Hypnotism More Credible & Scientific than Mesmerism] 138

    [Hypnotism Developed to Oppose Mesmerism] 138

    [Review of Learned Journals' Reports on Hypnotism] 139

    [Braid Cited as Critic of Pseudoscience in Medicine] 140

    [Mesmerism Struggles to Exclude the Influence of Psychology] 141

    [Effect of Medicine Irreducible to Suggestion or Mesmerism Alone] 142

    [The "Placebo" Effect in Medicine] 143

    [Imagination & Suggestion in Hypnotism & Mesmerism] 144

    [Hypnotic Treatment of Monomania] 144

    [Intelligence & Concentration Required] 145

    [Braid's Stage Demonstration with Fourteen Subjects] 146

    ["Divination" by Intensified Perception & Reasoning] 147

    [Dr. J.J.G. Wilkinson's Account of Braid's Work] 148

    [Prof. William Carpenter's Account of Braid's Work] 148

    [Braid Defines Hypnotism] 149

    [Different Stages of Hypnosis] 150

    [Braid's Hypnotic Induction Technique] 150

    [Effect of Imagination, Belief, & Habit] 150

    [Suggestive Effect of Sympathy & Imitation] 150

    [Suggestive Effect of Voice Tonality] 151

    [Suggestive Effect of Mesmeric Hand Passes] 152

[Positive & Negative Effects of Suggestion] 152
[Tranquilising versus Stimulating Forms of Hypnotism] 152
[The Waking, Partial & Full Hypnotic States] 153
[Effect of "Commanding & Confident" Tone of Voice] 153
[The Subject Rejects Objectionable Suggestions] 154
[Suggestion & the Art of Rhetoric] 154
[Revivification of Memory, Confidence, & Performance] 154
[Categories of Suggestion versus Animal Magnetism] 155
[De-hypnotising Patients] 155
[Alleged Difficulty Arousing from State] 156
[Common Sources of Fallacy in Mesmerism] 156
[Post-Hypnotic Suggestion] 157
[Intelligence is Associated with Hypnotisability] 157
[Critique of Dr. James Esdaile's Mesmerism] 157
[Sympathy & Imitation in Hysterical Dancing Epidemics] 160
[Braid's Special Hypnotic Technique for Insomnia] 162
[Group Experiment on Attention & Spontaneous Sensations] 163
[Experiment on Waking Autosuggestion & Menstruation] 163
[Group Experiment on Self-Hypnosis] 164
[Critique of Baron von Reichenbach's "Odylic Force"] 165
[Critique of Dr. John Elliotson's Mesmerism] 166
[Mesmerism Refuted by Suggestion Experiments] 166
[Conclusion] 167
Appendices 168
  1. Letter of Apology from J.C. Colquhoun (February 1852) 168
  2. Self-Hypnosis & Hindu Yoga Meditation 170
  3. Braid Exposes a Bogus Clairvoyant 172
Additional Appendices 177
  1. Experiments on Mesmerism at Aberdeen University 177
  2. On Newnham's 'Human Magnetism' 179
Lecture on Electro-Biology (1851) 181
Electro-Biological Phenomena Considered Physiologically & Psychologically (1851) 189
    [Introduction] 190
    [Braid's Public Demonstrations of Hypnosis] 191
    [Hypnotic Suggestion Considered] 192
    [Electro-Biology Criticised] 192
    [The Reichenbach Phenomena] 193

- [Braid's Meeting with Mr. Stone] 195
- [The Physical Reality of Suggested Phenomena] 196
- [On Mesmeric Passes] 197
- [Criticism of Paranormal Claims] 198
- [Conclusion] 199

Observations on Trance or Human Hybernation (1850) 200
Preface 201
Observations on Trance or Human Hybernation 202
- [Introductory Remarks] 202
- [The Death-like Trance of Colonel Townsend] 202
- [Sir Claude M. Wade's Account] 203
- [Sir C.E. Trevelyan's Account] 205
- [An Anonymous British Major's Account] 206
- [Self-Hypnosis & Catalepsy] 208
- [The Trance-Like Effects of Cannabis] 209
- [Critique of Paranormal Theories] 210
- [Animal Hibernation] 211
- [Cases of Human Phenomena] 213
- [Three Conclusions Drawn] 215
- [Hypnotic Therapy Restores Menstruation] 215
- [Further Cases of Hypnotic Therapy] 216
- [Braid's use of Self-Hypnosis for Rheumatic Pain] 217
- [Hypnotic Therapy in a Severe Case of Tonic Spasm] 217
- [Concluding Remarks on Hypnotic Therapy] 218

Appendix: On Cannabis 219
Appendix: On Sensory Hyperacuity in Hypnotism 221
Appendix: On Migration & Hybernation 222
Appendix: Hypnotic Therapy for Spinal Distortion 224

"On Mesmerism & Chemical Anaesthesia": Letter (1849) 226
"On Esdaile & Hypnotic Anaesthetic": Letter to The Medical Times (1847) 229
The Power of the Mind over the Body (1846) 236
Editor's Preface 237
The Power of the Mind over the Body 238
- [Introductory Remarks] 238
- [Sensations due to Suggestion not Subtle Energy] 238
- [Braid's Initial Experiments] 238
- [Account of Reichenbach's Theory & Observations] 239
- [Contradictions in Reported Phenomena] 240

- [Braid's Psycho-physiological Explanation] 241
- [Braid's "Placebo" Experiments] 241
- [Considerations on Magnetism] 245
- [Aura Photography Refuted] 246
- [Self-Hypnosis & Yoga] 247
- [Further Experiments with Suggestion] 248
- [Conclusion: The Power of the Mind] 249
- Appendix: On Muscular Suggestion 251

"Observations on Mesmeric & Hypnotic Phenomena": Letter to *The Medical Times* (1844) 252

"On Thomas Wakley & John Elliotson": Letter to *The Medical Times* (1844) 258

"On Muscular Suggestion": Braid's Letters on Phreno-Hypnotism (1843-1844) 260
- Editor's Preface 261
- Observations on the Phenomena of Phreno-Mesmerism (1843) 262
- Letter from Mr. Simpson (1844) 266
- Remarks on Mr. Simpson's Letter on Hypnotism (1844) 272
- Experimental Inquiry (1844) 275

Neurypnology: The Rationale of Nervous Sleep (1843) 278
- Original Dedication 281
- Editor's Preface 282
- Author's Preface 283
  - Introduction 287
    - General Remarks 287
    - Why Hypnotism has been Separated from Animal Magnetism 288
    - How Far Considered useful in the Cure of Disease 288
    - Its Powers on the Animal Functions 288
    - Certain Erroneous Beliefs Refuted 288
    - Opinions and Practice of Bertrand and Abbé Faria, Mr. Brooks, Dr. Prichard 288
    - Its Moral Influence 289
    - Should be used by Professional Men Only 289
    - Definition of Terms 290
  - PART I: The Theory & Practice of Hypnotism 291
    - Chapter 1: The Discovery of Hypnotism 292
      - Introductory Remarks 292
      - Circumstances which Directed to the Investigation 292
      - A Real Phenomenon observed 292
      - Experiments Instituted to Prove the Cause of it 292
      - Opinions and Conclusions Drawn From Them 293
      - Reasons for Separating Hypnotism from Mesmerism 293
      - Hypnotism More Generally Successful than Animal Magnetism 294

    Mr. Herbert Mayo's Testimony on This Point 294

    Proofs of this Referred to 294

    Different Modes by which it can be Induced 295

    Can only be Expected to Succeed by Complying with the Whole Conditions Required ... 295

Chapter 2: On The Hypnotic Induction Process 296

    Mode of Hypnotising 296

    Circumstances Necessary to be Complied with 296

    Peculiar Phenomena which Follow; Excitement first, and Afterwards Depression of Function 296

    How These May be Made to Alternate with Each Other 296

    Extraordinary Influence of a Current of air during Hypnotism 296

    Reasons for Certain Modifications of Original modes of Operating 297

    Hypnotism Proceeds from a Law of the Animal Economy 297

    Arises from the Physical and Psychical Condition of the Patient 297

    Example for Proof 297

    Exhibits no Appreciable Electric or Magnetic Change 297

    Two Patients may Hypnotise each other by Contact 297

    Phenomena arise Spontaneously in Course of Disease 297

    Mr. Wakley's Admission on this Point 298

    Mr. H. Mayo's Testimony as to the Effects of Hypnotism 298

    Effects of Different Positions of the Eyes 298

    Consensual Adjustment of Eyes; Effects on Size of Pupil 298

    Power of Habit and Imagination 298

    Docility of Patients, and Exalted Sensibility, and their Effects 298

    Patient Hypnotised Whilst Operating on Another 299

    Mode of Resisting Influence 299

Chapter 3: On Hypnotism & Natural Sleep 300

    Phenomena of Natural Sleep, Dreaming, and Somnambulism Contrasted 300

    Causes of Common Sleep 300

    Of Dreaming 300

    Effects of Variety and Monotony Compared 300

    Changes Alleged to Take Place in the Structure of the Brain by Exertion 301

    Cause of Hypnotism 301

    M'Nish's article on "Reverie" compared with Mr. Braid's theory of Hypnotism 301

    Mode of Arousing Patients from the State of Hypnotism 301

Chapter 4: On the Nature & Phenomena of Hypnotism 302

    Phenomena of Common Sleep 302

Of Hypnotism 302

Power of Locomotion and Accurate Balancing of Themselves 302

Tendency to Dance on Hearing Appropriate Music; Grace Displayed under its Influence 302

Effects Analogous to Nitrous Oxide in Some 302

In what it Differs from this and Intoxication from Wine and Spirits; Analogous to conium 303

Effects of Monotonous Impressions on any of the Senses 303

Power of Habit and Expectation 303

All the Phenomena Consecutive 303

Power of Hypnotism to Cure Intractable Diseases and Disorders 303

Miss Collins' Case and Miss E. Atkinson's 304

Extent to Which it may be Expected to be Useful 305

Chapter 5: On Hypnotic Sleep Therapy 306

Reasons for Delivering Public Lectures on Hypnotism 306

Mode of Procuring Refreshing Sleep, With Low Pulse and General Flaccidity of Muscle 306

Efficacy of This Plan 306

Chapter 6: On Muscular Suggestion & Phreno-Hypnotism 307

Introductory Remarks 307

Relation between Mind and Matter Illustrated to Disprove Materialism 307

Armstrong, Colton, Brown, Abercrombie, Stewart, Plato 308

General Conclusion, That Mind or Life is the Cause of Organism 309

Power of Conscience 310

The Passions, how Excited 310

Dr. Elliotson's Opinion as to the Efficacy or Non-Efficacy of Volition 311

Modes of Dividing the Brain 312

Causes of Phrenology Being Imperfect 313

Objections to Phreno-Hypnotism 313

Mode of Connection between the Brain and Body 313

First Attempts at Phrenologizing During Hypnotism Were Failures 314

Succeeded by Operating Differently 314

Cases Illustrative 314

A Child Operates Successfully 316

Details of the Case 316

Other Successful Cases 316

Proper Time for Operating 317

Case of an Officer in 1758 318

Inferences as to Its Curative Powers 318

  Opinions of La Roy Sunderland, and Mr. Hall 319
  Presumed Cause of Phenomena Called Cross Magnetism 319
  Return Stolen Property to Proper Owners and Proper Place by Smell and Touch 320
  Power of Hearing Faint Sounds 320
  Additional Cases 320
  Opposite Faculties can be Excited at the Same Time by Acting on the Opposite Hemispheres 320
  Mode of Operating 325
  Concluding Remarks on the Value of Testimony 326

 Chapter 7: Summary & Conclusion 327
  General Résumé 327
  Many Phenomena Admit of Physical and Chemical Proof 327
  Difficulties of Comprehending Many Phenomena 327
  State of the Circulation 327
  Conjectures as to the Cause of the Cataleptiform Condition 328

PART II: Sixty-Six Brief Case Studies 329
 Modes of Operating 329
 Objects of Operations 329
 Cases of Sight Improved 330
 Hearing 333
 Deaf and Dumb 333
 Mr. Curtis' Remarks 335
 James Shelmerdine's Case 336
 Mr. Bingham's Testimony 336
 S. Taylor – Sense of Smell 338
 Touch and Resistance 339
 Tic, Paralysis of Sense and Motion, Cured 339
 Miss E. Atkinson's Case, Voice Recovered 345
 Rheumatism, Ten Cases 347
 Irregular Muscular Action 350
 Headache 351
 Spinal Irritation 352
 Epilepsy 352
 Spinal Curvature 353
 Neuralgia, and Palpitation of the Heart 354
 Surgical Operations without Pain 354
 Diseases of the Skin 355

- Locked Jaw [Tetanus] 356
- Tonic Spasm 356
- Miss Collins 356
- Concluding Remarks 357
- Added Appendices 358
- Appendix: Letter to *The Medical Times* (26th March 1842) with Comments 358
- Appendix On Exercise & Sleep (Müller) 360
- Appendix: On Reverie 361
- Appendix On Monotony Inducing Sleep 363
- Appendix: Some Hypnotic Experiments & Observations 365
- Appendix On Psycho-Physical Dualism 367
- Appendix: Debate on Mesmeric Anaesthesia 368
- Appendix: A Neurological Theory of Hypnotic Catalepsy 370
- Appendix: 'Excerpts from Report on British Association Meeting' 371

"On Neuro-Hypnotism": Letter to *The Medical Times* (1842) 372

"The Discovery of Hypnotism": "Satanic Agency & Mesmerism" Reviewed (1842) 374
- Editor's Preface 375
- "Satanic Agency and Mesmerism" Reviewed 376
  - [McNeile Accuses Braid of Satanism & Deceit] 376
  - [Braid's Statement on his Original Position] 376
  - [Braid Defends Himself] 377
  - [Published Reports of Braid's Hypnotism] 378
  - [Hypnotism Requires the Subject's Compliance] 379
  - [Further Defence of Hypnotism] 379
  - [Cases Treated] 380
  - [Concluding Remarks] 380

"On Braid's Hanover Square Talks": Report & Letter in *The Medical Times* (1842) 382
- Editor's Preface 383

Bibliography of James Braid's Writings 386

Acknowledgements

I would like to express my thanks to the National Council for Hypnotherapy (NCH) for accepting this project and being so helpful in the preparation of the work. Special thanks are due to Jo Goss and subsequently Martin Armstrong Prior from NCH for helping to oversee the whole project.

Thanks also to Su Ricks for her help preparing material, and to Fiona Biddle for helping organise the preparation of *Hypnotic Therapeutics*. Thanks to Sophie Fletcher for her help with the German translation of Braid's unpublished manuscript, to Rae Jenson for her work on the cover design, and to Katy Kendall for proofreading. I am especially grateful to Hilary Norris-Evans for her detailed checking of the translation from French. Thanks also to Rob Woodgate for helping to publicise the book by publishing excerpts in the NCH journal.

Thanks also to the Society for Psychical Research for permission to republish articles by John Milne Bramwell, and to the British Library for their assistance and for permission to reproduce material from their collection. Thanks to Dr. Arreed Barabasz of the *International Journal for Clinical & Experimental Hypnosis* (IJCEH) for permission to reproduce my edition of Braid's 1860 article. Thanks to the Bakken Library and Museum, Minneapolis, for providing us with permission to reproduce a rare copy of Braid's *Electro-Biological Phenomena* (1851). Thanks to Mandy for her moral support and to Daisy Robertson for her special contributions to the manuscript.

And, finally, thanks to James Braid for his courage and perseverance in the face of condemnation, for single-handedly fighting a war on two fronts, against dogmatic Mesmerists like Elliotson, on the one hand, and dogmatic cynics like Wakley, on the other. Thanks to James Braid for putting his quest for scientific truth before material success, and for not being afraid to retaliate against his opponents. Finally, of course, I would like to thank James Braid himself for being so obstinate, argumentative and, ultimately, for being right.

Editor's Preface by Donald Robertson

Selection of Texts

I have tried to include as many of Braid's writings in this collection as possible, and I therefore consider it reasonable to call it *complete*, as it includes all of his major publications and the vast majority of his articles. As far as I am aware, the only omissions are a few articles or letters which are unrelated to hypnotism, which contain passages reproduced elsewhere in this volume, or which contain little of interest to a modern reader. After some consideration, for instance, it was decided not to include Braid's 'On the nature and treatment of certain forms of paralysis', from the *Association Medical Journal* (1855) in this edition. Although a large section of it concerns his later views on hypnotism, almost *all* of the relevant material is reproduced in other texts. Braid's short letter 'On Hypnotism' to *The Lancet* has also been omitted because the key passages have been quoted in full in my prefatory essays.

Some people might object that I have included several sections in other texts where Braid quotes at length from his previous publications, as this leads to several lengthy passages being repeated in this collection. After consideration, I felt that, given the scale of this project, it would be harmless to add a few pages and unnecessarily disruptive to the flow of individual texts to truncate them. Dr. John Milne Bramwell's texts have been included as an introduction because, in my estimation, they are of absolutely indispensable value as commentaries on Braid's work, and deeply valuable in their own right.

Editorial Changes

Certain changes have been made to the original texts. These primarily include the following,

1. I have made several small changes to formatting for the sake of readability, e.g., lengthy quotations have been indented from the main text, according to modern practice.
2. In many places, I have added comments or my own footnotes in square brackets for the sake of clarification, i.e., when an unusual medical term was used, or the name of an individual unlikely to be known to modern readers.
3. Braid had a habit of writing extremely lengthy footnotes; some are virtually small essays in their own right. Most of the longer ones have been added as appendices with new headings clearly denoting their content.
4. Chapter headings and section headings have been inserted into the body of the text. Where possible, e.g., in *Neurypnology*, these have been based directly upon Braid's own table of contents; otherwise they are enclosed in square brackets.
5. Titles of some booklets and letters have been modified because I felt that the original names given were misleading, unhelpful, or simply off-putting to the modern reader. Where this has been done, the new title has been placed in quotation marks and the original title shown in the body of the text.

I intended these changes to be of trivial significance, except insofar as they make Braid's writings more accessible to modern readers.

Foreword by Dr. Michael Heap

It gives me great pleasure to contribute this Foreword to *The Discovery of Hypnosis: The Complete Writings of James Braid, the Father of Hypnotherapy*. My first task is to congratulate its editor, Donald Robertson, on the quality of his work and in particular the fine scholarship displayed in his introductory chapters, of which I am sure all readers will be much appreciative.

When I was first asked to make this contribution I was immediately conscious of how much I have neglected, in my own reading, the original works of key historical figures in the field of hypnosis. I suspect that many of my colleagues would confess likewise. But why should one spend one's time studying such works when (a) their main conclusions have been summarised in up-to-date texts by well-respected authorities and (b) many of the claims and ideas espoused have been contradicted or superseded by advances in research, theory and practice?

As in many other fields of enquiry, the rewards for the time and effort expended in the detailed study of early texts can prove disproportionately small and little more than those gained from reading competent summaries by modern writers. But there are works that stand out and have a timeless quality. They do not merely tell us about the passing fads and fashions of the period in which they were written; they inform us about issues and concerns that we continue to struggle with and about ways that we might resolve them. The report of the Franklin Commission on animal magnetism is a case in point. I am certain that the work of James Braid is another.

Moreover, there are certain periods in the progress of any field of human enquiry when it becomes particularly apposite and instructive to revisit the works of one of the early key figures. For the serious student of hypnosis, now is the time to pay or repay a visit to the writings of James Braid. Let me explain why I believe this to be the case.

There is a consensus that the historical roots of hypnosis can be traced to eighteenth century Europe with the activities of Franz Anton Mesmer. Yet, the methods and ideas of Mesmerism are so different from modern hypnosis. Recall that Mesmer, in his dissertation of 1766 proposed the existence of a universal force that he eventually called 'animal magnetism'. He postulated that illness was associated with disturbances in the natural tidal flow of animal magnetism in the body and that he had the ability to restore this and thus heal the patient. After experimenting with magnets he settled for making slow passes with his hands over the patient's body from the head to the toe. Imagine the scene in one of Mesmer's group healing salons in Paris. Here would be several large *baquets* – tubs filled with water and iron filings, 'magnetised' by Mesmer. Rods protruded from each and the patients sat around and applied them to their afflicted parts. Some of the patients would have crises; they would swoon and go into convulsions, shaking, crying, laughing hysterically, and so on. Finally they would appear to enter some kind of stupor with a glazed look in their eye. Now consider the first part of a modern, and uncontroversial, definition of hypnosis:

> Hypnosis is a process in which one person, designated the hypnotist, offers suggestions to another person, designated the subject, for imaginative experiences entailing alterations in perception, memory and action. (Kihlstrom, 2008: 21)

This part of the definition describes the activity of the hypnotist only, but how different from that of Mesmer! Now consider the response of the hypnotic subject:

> These experiences are associated with a degree of subjective conviction bordering on delusion, and an experienced involuntariness bordering on compulsion. *(Op. cit.)*

…but no histrionics, falling about, going into a stupor and so on.

How the practice of hypnosis today, and the theories that characterise it, evolved from the methodology and theory of Mesmerism is a fascinating and instructive story (see Gauld, 1992, for a comprehensive history). There were a number of key developments. First was the recognition that core aspects of Mesmeric practice, notably the paraphernalia of the *baquet*, the Mesmerist's passes, and the patients' crises, were superfluous for the purposes of treatment. Inactivity and repose became the more typical response of the subject from the start of the procedure. Second was the development of theory grounded in a biological understanding of the nervous system. From this, psychological explanations came to the fore. In particular *verbal suggestion* became the central feature of hypnosis, both procedurally and theoretically. Some of the more ambitious claims made for hypnosis, such as paranormal powers, were rejected and investigators strove to offer parsimonious explanations of how subjects responded to, and experienced, hypnotic suggestions – without reference to unusual or pathological processes. The concept of a 'hypnotic state' was called into question and reformulated in more mundane terms such as 'focused concentration', while the role of the induction procedure was rendered uncertain – neither eye fixation nor relaxation were found to be essential to the hypnotic process and investigators began to talk about 'waking suggestions'. Finally, at quite an early stage it was established that people varied in their responsiveness to hypnosis and only a minority were highly susceptible.

One of the striking features of this evolutionary process is its association with a series of prominent individuals over, let us say, the period of 170 years from Mesmer's original treatise – Mesmer himself, de Puységur, the Abbé de Faria, Elliotson, Esdaile, Braid, Charcot, Bernheim, Janet, and Hull. This clear identification of a particular position on hypnosis (or its forerunner, Mesmerism) with a key individual continued through much of the twentieth century, the latter half of which saw considerable intense, and at times divisive, debate between prominent investigators who held differing opinions about the nature of hypnotic phenomena. Names that are well-known to students of modern hypnosis are Ernest Hilgard, Theodore Barber, Theodore Sarbin, Martin Orne, Nicholas Spanos, Kenneth Bowers, Graham Wagstaff and latterly, Irving Kirsch. Each had his own theory but the main area of contention was whether, in order to account for hypnotic phenomena, it is necessary to posit a 'special state' ('trance') or 'special processes' or whether all can be explained by reference to concepts and processes from mainstream social and cognitive psychology.

This academic debate was neither informative nor inspiring for many people who earned their living by applying hypnosis therapeutically, but one development that did make an impact was the growth in popularity of the approaches of the psychiatrist and psychotherapist Milton Erickson (1901-1980) and his followers. The contribution of this development to our understanding of hypnosis is, in my view, questionable, *but...* time will tell. It is nevertheless true that the interface of theory and clinical practice, something to which Braid himself, as a practising physician, devoted considerable attention, remains much neglected in the modern era.

Through the 1990s, and into the twenty-first century, the theoretical landscape of hypnosis gradually ceased to be dominated by 'heavyweight' individuals with their own coterie of followers. We now have, metaphorically speaking, a more harmonious chorus of highly competent and well-respected authorities who acknowledge the authenticity of hypnotic experiences and the complexity of the processes that determine them, though they may still disagree on which are the key ones. I believe that the study of hypnosis as an academic discipline has now reached the stage where it is unlikely that, once again, one or more Titanic figures will emerge to dominate the field. This, in my opinion is a good thing – a sign of confidence and maturity in the discipline.

So now, with the theoretical storms having abated considerably, it is from this vantage point of greater confidence and maturity that we can profit from a closer study of the works of Braid, his methods, his ideas and, in particular, the ways he set about trying to understand what he observed: a devoted doctor and a humble scholar, who had the courage and honesty to change his mind when the evidence required it. In the context of the history of Mesmerism and hypnosis he emerges as the linchpin around which, not all at once but in the fullness of time, the progress of theory and practice could turn on its course and head towards the position of soundness and strength that it occupies today.

Who is the real father of hypnosis? If we are to make familial analogies I would say that Franz Anton Mesmer was perhaps the 'grandfather'; there is no doubt that the 'father' was James Braid.

References

Gauld, A. (1992) *A History of Hypnotism.* Cambridge: Cambridge University Press.
Kihlstrom J.F. (2008) 'The domain of hypnosis revisited.' In M.R. Nash & A.J. Barnier (eds.) *The Oxford Handbook of Hypnosis: Theory, Research and Practice*, pp. 21-52. Oxford: Oxford University Press.

SECTION I:
Articles on Braid

James Braid's Life & Work

Copyright © Donald Robertson, 2008

Sudden Death of Mr. James Braid, Surgeon of Manchester

'The sudden death of Mr. James Braid, surgeon, of Manchester [aged 65], which took place on Sunday morning, at his residence, Rylaw House, Oxford Street, in that city, is a subject of much regret. He had been in apparently good health all last week, and had made his usual calls upon his patients, displaying the quiet cheerfulness in his interviews with them which generally characterised his demeanour. On Sunday morning he complained of pain up the spine of his back and coldness, and ordered a cup of tea. After partaking of it, he breathed heavily several times, and died almost immediately, it is supposed from disease of the heart. He was best known in the medical world from his theory and practice of hypnotism, as distinguished from Mesmerism – a system of treatment he applied in certain diseases with great effect, and which has recently attracted much attention in Paris. Long before his discovery of hypnotism, however, he had performed some extraordinary cures by operations on contracted muscles, in cases of club-foot and similar contortions, which brought him patients from every part of the kingdom. In addition to a large circle of friends whom his warm-hearted and genial bearing and professional skill attached to him amongst the wealthier classes of society, and amongst the medical profession, he will be much regretted by the humbler classes, whose sufferings under disease he often succeeded in alleviating without recompense.'

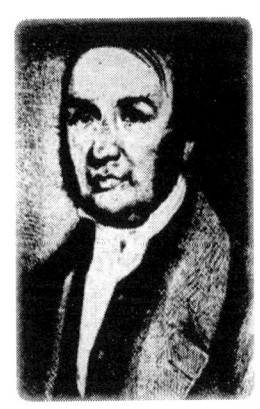

Figure 1. Edward Cocking's lithographed portrait of James Braid in 1854, from Anon., *Mystères des Sciences Occultes (1894)*.

– *The Lancet*, 31st March, 1860.

Braid's Biographical Details

James Braid was born to James Braid (senior), a landowner, and his wife Anne Suttie on 19th June 1795 at Rylaw House in the Portmoak parish of the town of Kinross in Scotland. On 17th November 1813, Braid married Margaret Mason (or Meason). They had a son, James (b. 1822), who also became a doctor, and a daughter.

Braid attended Edinburgh University, from 1812-1814, and graduated at the age of 20 as a Licentiate of the Royal College of Surgeons (L.R.C.S.), subsequently becoming M.R.C.S. Braid was originally apprenticed to the father and son surgeons Charles Anderson in Leith. Anderson was a founding member, and vice-president, of the elite learned society called the Wernerian Natural History Society of Edinburgh. The Wernerian Society was created in 1808 by Robert Jameson, professor of natural history at Edinburgh University, as a break-away group from the Royal Society of Edinburgh. It was dissolved in 1858, a few years before Braid's death.

It seems that Anderson may have provided Braid with access to this learned body; Braid's writings therefore also carry the designation 'C.M.W.S.' or 'M.W.S.', denoting his status as a 'Corresponding Member of the Wernerian Society'. (This little-known fact is supported by his contribution of some early articles, on subjects unrelated to hypnotism, to the society's journal.) Indeed, in *Neurypnology* (1843) Braid emphasises that one of the first people to whom he demonstrated his discovery of hypnotism was Captain Thomas Brown, a fellow Wernerian, respected natural historian, and curator of the Manchester Museum.

In 1816, after his apprenticeship to Anderson, Braid was appointed as a mine physician attached to Lord Hopetoun's silver-lead ore mines in Leadhills, Lanarkshire. Subsequently, in 1825 he opened a private practice working as a surgeon and ophthalmologist in Dumfries. In 1828, however, at the request of a patient named Mr. Petty, he moved to Manchester where he lived and worked for the rest of his life.

Even in his youth, he was a well-respected specialist and published a number of articles in various medical and scientific journals. It is perhaps notable that as a surgeon who treated and published work on *ophthalmology* and *musculoskeletal* conditions, Braid should emphasise the use of eye-fixation and "muscular suggestion" in his method of hypnotism. Certainly, by the time of his death, he had acquired a considerable reputation as a physician and surgeon, apparently specialising mainly in conditions such as strabismus, club-foot, muscular paralysis, and spinal curvature.

> His competence as a surgeon won him a solid practice and his geniality many friends. He was also noted for his compassion towards patients too poor to pay a fee. (*Oxford Dictionary of National Biography*, 'James Braid', 2007)

Braid's charitable nature was demonstrated, e.g., by the fact that he offered *free-of-charge* hypnotic treatment to anyone suffering from hydrophobia (rabies) within travelling distance of Manchester in his 'Author's Preface' to *Neurypnology* (1843).

Given his modest professional status as a provincial surgeon, Braid had a surprising number of friends and supporters among the most distinguished scientists, academics and physicians of his day. To some extent this may be attributed to his early association with the prestigious Wernerian Society. However, his endeavours seem naturally to have attracted the support of the many Victorian empiricists who were keen to disprove "occult" theories such as Mesmerism, and to offer more credible scientific explanations in their stead. Most notable among these was Prof. William B. Carpenter, the distinguished physiologist, whose concept of the "ideo-motor response" became an essential part of Braid's later "mono-ideo-dynamic" theory of hypnotic suggestion.

The Lafontaine Incident (1841)
On 13th November 1841, in Manchester, Braid attended a public stage demonstration of phrenology and animal magnetism, conducted by a Swiss Mesmerist called Charles Lafontaine. This kind of performance – though predating Braid's introduction of hypnotism – is probably the prototype of the modern "stage hypnosis" show. Called the Mesmeric *séance* or *conversazione,* it was a popular form of public lecture or entertainment across Europe at the time. Lafontaine was a well-known and successful Mesmerist who toured his stage show, using two young assistants called Eugen and Mary as his subjects. Curiously, the practice of using one's own assistants for demonstrations was common at the time and did not seem to arouse quite as much suspicion as it might today.

Lafontaine, by all accounts, was an intense-looking man with a heavy accent, and a large beard, who dressed in completely black attire (Forrest, 1999: 193). He spoke very limited English and, somewhat bizarrely, performed with the aid of an interpreter. Braid claims that he was initially a sceptic, believing the whole of Mesmerism to be due to collusion and deception. The letter from Mr. Simpson reporting on Braid's own demonstrations notes, 'It was during a Mesmeric experiment conducted by M. Lafontaine – to which, in his then incredulity and disdain, he was almost dragged by a friend – that this idea occurred to Mr. Braid'. In the first chapter of *Neurypnology* (1843), Braid writes,

> The first exhibition of the kind I ever had an opportunity of attending, was one of M. Lafontaine's conversazione, on the 13th November, 1841. That night I saw nothing to diminish, but rather to confirm, my previous prejudices.

However, for some reason Braid returned.

> At the next conversazione, six nights afterwards [19th November], *one fact, the inability of a patient to open his eyelids,* arrested my attention. I considered that to be a *real phenomenon,* and was anxious to discover the physiological cause of it. Next night, I watched this case when again operated on, with intense interest, and before the termination of the experiment, felt assured I had discovered its cause, but considered it prudent not to announce my opinion publicly, until I had had an opportunity of testing its accuracy, by experiments and observation in private.

One of these lectures was very graphically described by an astute witness, Prof. William Crawford Williamson, a distinguished academic and physician, in his *Reminiscences of a Yorkshire Naturalist* (1896). It seems that, in an attempt to debunk the whole Mesmeric performance, Braid, Williamson, and others, mounted the stage led by a prominent eye surgeon called Mr. Wilson. However, all three were surprised to find, on Williamson raising her eyelids, that the girl's pupils were unusually contracted, an *involuntary* response normally indicative of deep sleep. In his introduction to *Neurypnology*, Braid also remarks that he was impressed by the inability of Lafontaine's subject to open her eyelids, a phenomenon now dubbed "eyelid catalepsy".

With the typical forthrightness of a Victorian physician, Braid proceeded to jam a pin underneath the girl's fingernails but found her completely anaesthetised to what would normally have been an excruciatingly painful injury. He was therefore forced to recognise that a genuine, and noteworthy, transformation had occurred in the subject's state of mind and physiological responses. A week later, Braid returned, this time determined to observe Lafontaine's method more closely and discover a more rational explanation for the phenomena than the supposed power of animal magnetism. For his own part, Lafontaine published his memoirs in 1866, which contain his own rather sensational, and probably somewhat unreliable, report of his time in England and encounter with Braid (*q.v.* Waite's 'Introduction' to *Braid on Hypnotism*, 1899).

After the Discovery (1841-1843)
After attending Lafontaine's show and discovering that he could produce the same results without the need for animal magnetism, Braid appears to have acted very quickly indeed and argued forcefully to establish his views that nervous fatigue, concentration, habit and imagination accounted for the observable results of Mesmerism, without the need for any reference to occult forces or telepathic powers, etc. In the opening chapter of *Neurypnology* he explains,

> In two days afterwards [23rd November?], I developed my views to my friend Captain [Thomas] Brown [a fellow member of the Wernerian Society], as I had also previously done to four other friends; and in his presence, and that of my family, and another friend, the same evening, I instituted a series of experiments to prove the correctness of my theory, namely, that the continued fixed stare, by paralysing nervous centres in the eyes and their appendages, and destroying the equilibrium of the nervous system, thus produced the phenomenon referred to. The experiments were varied so as to convince all present, that they fully bore out the correctness of my theoretical views.

According to his introductory remarks in *Neurypnology*, Braid immediately wrote to the Medical Section of the British Association for the Advancement of Science in order to arrange delivery of a professional report entitled 'Practical Essay on the Curative Agency of Neuro-Hypnotism' before his peers. It seems evident that Braid had therefore already coined the term "neuro-hypnotism" by late 1841.

However, his proposal to the British Association was declined; apparently because of concern over the controversial nature of the subject. Frustrated, Braid advertised his own public reading of the 'Rejected Essay' (as he calls it) on 27th December 1841 which seems to have been attended by many of the British Association members. This was one of five public lectures which he undertook at this time to promote his ideas, and which were reported in detail in the Manchester newspapers. Braid attracted opposition from both Mesmerists and sceptics, but he also immediately drew credible supporters from among his "scientific friends". On 31st December 1841, a *conversazione* on Braid's methods was given by a surgeon, Mr. Duncan, at the Hanover Square Rooms in London, and reported as "A New Theory of Animal Magnetism" in *The Medical Times* (vol. v, 1841-1842, p. 175). This event seems also to have acted as an introduction for Braid who was soon to visit London himself.

On 1st March 1842, Braid travelled to the capital, where he arranged a formal lecture held in the Hanover Square Rooms. In defence of his position, he later recalls,

> [...] I had, at great personal inconvenience as well as pecuniary sacrifice, gone to London, that my views might be subjected "to a rigid examination" of the most learned men in our profession, to propound to them the laws by which I consider it to act, and above all, to prove to them "the uniformity of its action" and its practical applicability and value as a curative agency, by [my] mode of operating. (Braid, *Satanic Agency, etc.*, 1842)

Several eminent scientists and physicians were present, most notably Herbert Mayo, Professor of Physiology & Pathological Anatomy at King's College. Mayo seems initially to have been sceptical but was convinced by his observations. He was himself hypnotised by Braid and also vigorously tested the anaesthesia of a hypnotic subject by pushing a pin straight through the back of the man's hand and out the other side, through the palm. At the same lecture, Braid also hypnotised a group of eighteen people, *en masse*, who were instructed to gaze upon the base of a chandelier. Reportedly, the only ones who did not respond to the satisfaction of the audience were two participants who refused to fully comply with the procedure.

So much interest was generated that it proved necessary to immediately repeat the lecture at the London Tavern the following day to accommodate all those who wished to attend. (The Hanover Square Rooms and London Tavern were venues used for medical and scientific lectures in London.) After this validation, Braid began to report his work in letters and articles in the medical periodicals. On 12th March 1842, *The Medical Times* published an enthusiastic report on Braid's lectures in London, accompanied by a letter by Braid himself on 'Animal Magnetism.' This seems to be his first known publication on the subject, just four months after his encounter with Lafontaine. At this early stage, Braid expresses the essential criticisms of Mesmerism which would become the basis of his theory of hypnotism. He argues that the fixed gaze and "passes" of the animal magnetist were merely monotonous stimuli designed to induce a state of physiological fatigue in which subjects somehow became more liable to respond to their own imagination, and therefore to ideas arising from their own expectations or from external influences, i.e., through suggestion or imitation. The report mentions Braid's introduction of the term "neurypnology" used in distinction from Mesmerism. It was followed on 26th March by another letter on 'Animal Magnetism' in the same publication. In an article entitled 'On Mr. Braid's Experiments' in *The Medical Times* 2nd April 1842, Mayo reported as follows in response to Braid's letter,

> The same cures which you effect have, indeed, before been made by the ordinary process of Mesmerising but that process is so extremely tedious, occupying for the first sittings in general from half to three-quarters of an hour, as, joined to the uncertainty of producing any effect after all, practically to wear out the patience of experimenters, and to prevent the method advancing, either as a subject of inquiry, or its being brought into general use as a curative means. It took up too much time. What you appear to have done is to have found out a method, by which, in five minutes, the susceptibility of any given individual towards the [hypnotic] trance may be determined (or, at all events, by the repetition of the same brief process, a few successive days.)

In the years to follow, Braid would publish many articles and letters in *The Medical Times*, which seemed to welcome his contributions on hypnotism.

At this point, however, he became embroiled in what seems to have been the first of several controversies caused by his views. Reverend Hugh McNeile, one of the most popular and outspoken Anglican preachers in the country at the time, delivered a scathing attack upon Braid in which he appears to accuse him of deceiving his patients, and even of doing the work of Satan. The sermon was given on Sunday 10th April 1842 at St. Jude's Church in Liverpool. Braid immediately wrote to McNeile responding to the accusations, but received no reply. He then held a public lecture on 21st April 1842, in response to the sermon, to which he formally invited McNeile, but he did not attend. In fact, McNeile now responded by publishing the text of his original sermon in his 'Penny Pulpit' review without any acknowledgment of Braid's objections. Frustrated, Braid's hand was forced and he rushed into print on 4th June 1842 with what appears to be the first independent publication on hypnotism, though he had previously penned various letters and his unpublished report. He had this "open letter" printed himself and distributed as a twelve-page booklet expounding and defending his views. As such, this must be the first publication (other than his published letters) in which Braid uses the term "hypnotism".

On 29th June 1842, he delivered a *conversazione* to the British Association in Manchester, which was reported in the *Manchester Times*. Braid seems to have delivered his "rejected" paper on 'The Curative Agency of Neuro-Hypnotism,' once again at this event. He states that he exhibited several patients successfully treated with hypnotism, as discussed in *Neurypnology*, including Sarah Ann Mellor (Case 19), Thomas Morris (Case 21), and Samuel Evans (Case 17). He also exhibited a female subject who seemed able to follow the scent of a rose around, though blindfolded, because of olfactory hyperacuity developed in hypnosis, as discussed in excerpts from the *Manchester Times* quoted in *Neurypnology*. Braid then published another letter entitled 'Neuro-Hypnotism' in *The Medical Times* of 9th July 1842, and then a short case study entitled, 'Account of case of total deafness successfully treated by hypnotism' in *The Manchester Times* of 1st September 1842. As far as I am aware, these were his only publications on the topic of hypnosis prior to *Neurypnology* (1843), which he tended later to refer to simply as his book "on Hypnotism".

Neurypnology was Braid's only full-length book, though it is important to realise that he subsequently published several other small *booklets* on hypnotism, often extended essays based upon previously published articles in medical journals. These smaller books, and his other writings, are essential in order to understand the evolution of Braid's thought, which underwent radical modifications in response to his growing clinical and experimental experience. Indeed, near the end of his life, Braid composed a short essay, summarising the content of his later works and quoting at length from them, which was meant to be included as an appendix to a proposed French translation of *Neurypnology*. It is clear that he felt this was necessary in order to place his earlier views in context.

After Neurypnology (1843-1860)
After publishing *Neurypnology*, only two years after he discovered hypnotism, Braid began to gradually revise his views, shifting emphasis from the physiological state of nervous fatigue onto the psychological state of mental abstraction or "monoideism". This paralleled an increasing recognition of the role of suggestion, a word which itself becomes increasingly common in his writings over time. In *Neurypnology*, Braid had recognised that physical manipulations could evoke certain responses, a phenomenon which he terms "muscular suggestion". He had also recognised the fact that, once induced into nervous sleep, a subject became increasingly susceptible to re-entering the condition as a result of imagination, habit, and expectation. However, the following factors seem to have contributed to his progressive growth of interest in suggestion,

1. Carpenter's "ideo-motor" theory of reflex action, which provided an early neuropsychological framework for understanding the nature and function of suggestion.
2. Braid's own experiments proving that the phenomena attributed by Baron von Reichenbach and the Electro-Biologists to forces such as magnetism, odyl, or electricity, could be reproduced in the "waking state" by a variety of psychological means, such as verbal suggestion, etc.

Even in *Neurypnology*, Braid complains of the misconception that hypnotism should be accompanied by a loss of awareness, resembling sleep. This problem finally led him to argue that the word "hypnotism" should be reserved for those cases in which the subject experiences no recollection afterwards of what happened during the process, though he emphasised that this accounted for only 10% of his subjects. The other 90% of Braid's subjects were in a "sub-hypnotic" state referred to as the "vigilant" or "waking" state, or as "concentration", "abstraction", or "monoideism", meaning focused attention upon a single idea or train of thought to the exclusion of other stimuli. He increasingly recognised, moreover, that hypnotic suggestion and other techniques could be surprisingly effective without any induction whatsoever, in the normal state of mind.

Braid therefore introduced the term "mono-ideo-dynamic", and related expressions, to describe the general theory that focused attention, along with expectation and other psycho-physiological factors, can *enhance* the ideo-motor response and bring about a variety of physiological changes as a result. Braid concluded it was necessary to emphasise the fact that suggestion may be operative in the waking state, and increased even in states of reverie or focused attention which it would be incredibly misleading to describe as "nervous sleep". He carried out many experiments debunking pseudoscientific placebo therapies including "subtle energy" treatments like Mesmerism, magnets, crystals, homeopathy, etc. Ironically, these Victorian "nostrum" (i.e., quack) remedies were the precursors of many of the currently popular complementary therapies with which modern hypnotherapy is frequently associated. However, Braid was perhaps as well-known in his own day as an intelligent and powerful *critic* of pseudoscientific therapies and paranormal claims. In any case, his own observations increasingly forced Braid to recognise that real effects could be produced by various forms of suggestion and autosuggestion in the normal waking state, without any specific induction technique or change in the nervous state.

In his earliest writings, Braid places cardinal emphasis upon the physiological basis of hypnotism, in an obvious attempt to distance himself from those, like Thomas Wakley, the editor of *The Lancet*, who dismissed Mesmerism as mere "imagination" or pretence. Arguably, Braid is somewhat hamstrung in this regard by his Christianity, which biases him against materialism and in favour of a dubious metaphysical theory of mind. In *Neurypnology*, for instance, he enters into a lengthy digression attempting to argue in favour of a Cartesian dualist theory, i.e., that the mind (or immortal soul) and body are two fundamentally distinct entities which causally interact. Later in his career, he introduces the term "psycho-physiology" (we now say "psycho-somatic" or "mind-body") to help clarify the fact that he thinks the psychological and physiological changes in hypnotism causally interact. Physical and mental changes are intertwined. On the one hand, body can affect mind; for instance, changes in physical posture and facial expression can be used to evoke psychological responses – by making a subject frown we evoke feelings of sadness in his mind. On the other hand, mind can affect body; for instance, attention, imagination and expectation may not only make someone believe that he is sleepy, but may actually change his physiological state, and bring about physical phenomena such as lowering of heart rate and dilation of the pupils, usually considered autonomic, or involuntary.

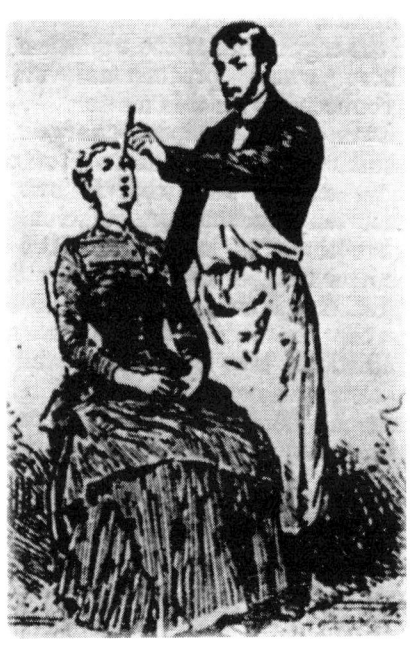

Figure 2. Lithograph portrait of Braid performing his "Eye-Fixation" Induction from Anon., *Mystères des Sciences Occultes (1894)*.

In Braid's writing, therefore, the study of hypnotism, "neuro-hypnology", expands to encompass, more generally, the combined effect of attention and dominant ideas (suggestions) upon the body, termed "mono-ideo-dynamics", and ultimately becomes subsumed within the study of mind-body interaction in the most general sense, or "psycho-physiology". Hypnotism was psycho-physiological therapy, and as Braid repeatedly argued, it conformed to the well-established laws of psychology and physiology. Hence, his later book *Hypnotic Therapeutics* (1853) concludes emphatically,

> I beg farther to remark, if my theory and pretensions, as to the nature, cause, and extent of the phenomena of nervous sleep have none of the fascinations of the transcendental to captivate the lovers of the marvellous, the credulous and enthusiastic, which the pretensions and alleged occult agency of the Mesmerists have, still I hope my views will not be the less acceptable to honest and sober-minded men, because they are all level to our comprehension, and reconcilable with well-known physiological and psychological principles.

Contrary to the popular misconception that confuses Mesmerism and hypnotism with each other, therefore, Braid emphasised from the outset that his theory was intended to oppose the views of the Mesmerists. He wrote in *The Lancet*, 'I adopted the term "hypnotism" to prevent my being confounded with those who entertain these extreme notions, as well as to get rid of the erroneous theory about a magnetic fluid, or esoteric influence of any description being the cause of the sleep'. ('On Hypnotism', *The Lancet*, 1845; vol. 1: 627-628)

The Discovery of Hypnotism
Although the Abbé Faria (1746-1819) and, following him, Dr. Alexandre Bertrand (1795-1831), in France, had proposed psychological interpretations of Mesmerism, Braid was undoubtedly the first person to construct a thorough rational and empirical alternative to Mesmerism. His extensive clinical work, public lectures, repeated publication of his views in medical journals, collaboration with respected physicians and scientists, and many documented experiments contributed enormously to the influence of his work. Braid earned an enviable reputation both as a critic of pseudo-science and as the founder of a rational alternative to Mesmerism.

Braid himself rejects the contention that Faria and Bertrand had pre-empted him in his introduction to *Neurypnology*. There he argues that although they emphasise the subjective nature of Mesmerism, they failed to recognise the physiological factors which might facilitate suggestion, induced by the fixed-gaze method. Braid himself seems to have diminished the emphasis placed on the physiological state of hypnosis in his later writings. He recognised that a variety of physiological states may accompany fixed attention or increased suggestibility. Nevertheless, he does do more than merely explain hypnosis by means of suggestion or imagination, insofar as he continues to emphasise a variety of factors which explain the enhanced effects of suggestion, e.g., double consciousness, monoideism, etc. It is one thing to say that hypnosis operates by means of suggestion, it is another to explain what factors allow hypnosis to utilise suggestion in an especially effective way. As we have seen, Braid saw this as a question of psycho-physiology, of the mind and body reciprocally affecting each other in turn, and therefore not reducible to psychological factors alone.

Did Braid coin the word "hypnotism"? Scholarship has indicated that similar expressions may have been used by the followers of Mesmer in France years before Braid claimed to have invented it. As early as 1821, Baron Etienne Felix d'Henin de Cuvillers had reputedly used various words prefixed with "hypn-" to designate aspects of animal magnetism. Nevertheless, Braid seems to have been unaware of this fact, and he does appear to have been the first writer to use the term in English. He can also claim to have popularised its use far beyond any previous author. There is no doubt that he was regarded by the majority of subsequent hypnotists as being the father of the tradition in which they stood. Even Bernheim, undoubtedly the most influential subsequent authority on hypnosis in the Victorian era, writes,

> Although the doctrine of suggestion had its precursors, it was not until the year 1841 that it was definitely established and demonstrated by James Braid, of Manchester. *To him is due the discovery of hypnotism* [...] a new doctrine which arose in the face of Mesmerism. (Bernheim, 1884: 111, *italics added*)

It is now generally accepted among authorities in the field of hypnosis that Braid merits the title "Father of Modern Hypnotism" (Kroger, 2008: 3).

Braid's Change of View

In the abstract of a lecture on electro-biology (1851) given by Braid to the Royal Institution, we find the following,

> [Mr. Catlow] congratulated Mr. Braid on having come round to a common sense view, well adapted to a popular audience. Mr. Braid started originally with the theory that fixed gazing at some object, until the muscles of the eye were strained, was an absolute necessity in the production of these phenomena, and said nothing about the mind. Dr. Hodgson thought Mr. Braid was not to be disparaged for having changed his views after nine years of study, he was rather to be praised for his candour.

These gentlemen seem to have understood that, recently, Braid had changed in two ways,

1. He had abandoned the practical requirement for fixed gazing and strain of the eye muscles.
2. He had recognised the *mental*, as opposed to merely *physiological*, dimension of hypnotic phenomena.

However, already in *Neurypnology* (1843) and Braid's earliest writings, there is undoubtedly evidence that he entertained both of these positions. Braid had originally resisted the interpretation that hypnotism was due to imagination or suggestion alone. His position was still primarily psychological insofar as he placed central importance upon the deliberate focusing of attention which he found could be aided by eye-fixation, physical stillness, and relaxed breathing. However, he originally felt that the physiological effects of eye-fixation were necessary, at least in most cases, to give the client an *initial* experience of hypnotism.

> Again: my remarks about the influence of imagination are referred to in such a manner as might lead to the belief that I was a supporter of the imagination theory – i.e., that the induction of the sleep in the first instance is merely the result of imagination. My belief is quite the contrary, I attribute it to the induction of a habit of intense abstraction, or concentration of attention, and maintain that it is most readily induced by causing the patient to fix his thoughts and sight on an object, and suppress his respiration. That besides mental influence, the blood is thus inefficiently oxygenated, and this creates a disposition to sleep in the first instance. A repetition of the process renders the subject more and more susceptible, through the well-known law of habit and association coming into play, and thus many become so susceptible as to be liable to be affected entirely through the imagination, sympathy and habit, and will be affected or not affected by the same process, or by no process at all, according to their expectation or belief. However, I have never seen such a result as this take place, unless in patients who had been previously hypnotised or Mesmerised. ('On Hypnotism', *The Lancet*, 1845; vol. 1: 627-628)

Braid's observations on the Reichenbach phenomena and electro-biology soon led him to a growing appreciation of the effects of suggestion upon individuals who had *not* been formally hypnotised, the production of "vigilant phenomena", which later became known as "waking hypnosis".

Perhaps the change in Braid's theory and approach must therefore be understood as a gradual shift in *emphasis* which expands upon the seeds of ideas already present in his early work. Indeed, the change in emphasis from the individual physiological state ("nervous sleep") toward greater recognition of the role of suggestion ("ideo-dynamic" action) can be seen as a precursor of the movement away from "state" theories of hypnosis in the twentieth century, toward socio-cognitive theories which emphasised the role of expectation, imagination, role-modelling, and a complex mixture of inter-acting social, cognitive, behavioural, and physiological factors. The whole "state *versus* nonstate" debate, therefore, appears as a somewhat belated re-enactment of the same broad path followed by Braid in his own evolving understanding of the nature of hypnotism.

"Stage Hypnosis" *versus* **Hypnotism**
Braid's attempt to introduce hypnotism as a rational alternative to Mesmerism has had mixed results. To a large extent, his orientation has won through in relation to medical and psychological research on hypnosis. However, there is an enormous gulf between research and clinical practice in modern hypnotherapy. Many hypnotherapists today have little more than a superficial knowledge of Braid's work, and the origins of hypnotherapy are obscure to them. Consequently, there appears to be considerable confusion among practitioners of hypnotherapy regarding its relation with Mesmerism. This fundamental misconception is fostered by the tendency among professional stage hypnotists to associate their practices with the *mystique* surrounding Mesmerism,

> The modern father of hypnosis was an Austrian physician, Franz Mesmer (1734-1815), from whose name the word 'Mesmerism' is derived. Though much maligned by the medical world of his day, Mesmer was nevertheless a brilliant man. He developed the theory of 'animal magnetism' – the idea that diseases are the result of blockages in the flow of magnetic forces in the body. He believed he could store his animal magnetism in baths of iron filings and transfer it to patients with rods or by 'Mesmeric passes'. (McKenna, *The Hypnotic World of Paul McKenna*, 1993)

However, as Hans Eysenck correctly observed, decades earlier,

> The terms 'Mesmerise' and 'hypnotise' have become quite synonymous, and most people think of Mesmer as the father of hypnosis, or at least as its discoverer and first conscious exponent. Oddly enough, the truth appears to be that while hypnotic phenomena had been known for many thousands of years, *Mesmer did not, in fact, hypnotise his subjects at all*. [...] It is something of a mystery why popular belief should have firmly credited him with a discovery which in fact was made by others. (Eysenck, 1957: 30-31, *italics added*)

To be clear about this, Mesmer believed that he was influencing his patients by means of a *supernatural* ("occult") *energy* called "animal magnetism", a kind of invisible magnetic "fluid", and not by means of normal physical or psychological processes such as concentration, relaxation, or suggestion. His famous *Propositions Concerning Animal Magnetism* (1779), the founding text of Mesmerism, goes so far as to claim that "animal magnetism" resembles ordinary electricity and magnetism, that it is influenced by the planets, and even that it bounces off mirrors and can be stored up and transported in the way that batteries can store electricity, although it seems Mesmerists actually used crystals and bottled water for this purpose.

As can be seen upon close inspection of Braid's writings, modern "stage hypnosis" acts probably evolved out of the public demonstrations of Mesmerism and electro-biology which existed long before the words "hypnosis" or "hypnotism" had even been coined. For instance, Lafontaine's performances in 1841 were probably of this nature. While Braid was developing his ideas, similar stage shows continued to tour Europe and America. He quotes the following from advertisements for the "electro-biology" show of Mr. Stone, which toured England in the early 1850s,

> Persons in a perfectly wakeful state, of well-known character and standing in society, who come forward voluntarily from among the audience, will be experimented upon. They will be deprived of the power of speech, hearing, sight. Their voluntary motions will be completely controlled, so that, they can neither rise up nor sit down, except at the will of the operator; their memory will be taken away, so that they will forget their own name and that of their most intimate friends; they will be made to stammer, and to feel pain in any part of their body at the option of the operator – a walking stick will be made to appear a snake, the taste of water will be changed to vinegar, honey, coffee, milk, brandy, wormwood, lemonade, *etc., etc., etc.* These extraordinary experiments are really and truly performed without the aid of trick, collusion, or deception, in the slightest possible degree.

Performers of this kind appear to have jumped upon the bandwagon of hypnotism in the following decades and rebranded their acts as "stage hypnotism", incorporating hypnotic inductions, though much else remained the same. The use of hypnotic inductions in these stage performances is probably largely for dramatic effect, and of little relevance to the phenomena produced, as illustrated by the fact that Mr. Stone and others already produced similar effects for many decades, in virtually identical shows, without even mentioning hypnosis. Modern-day critics of stage hypnosis, such as the performer known as Kreskin, are able to conduct similar acts without using hypnotic inductions, purely by sleight of hand and carefully chosen suggestions.

It is fair to say, however, that "stage hypnosis" may be something of a misnomer, insofar as such acts typically present themselves to the audience in terms of a mixture of ideas derived from both hypnotism and Mesmerism. For example, Ormond McGill, probably the most popular and influential writer on stage hypnosis, writes in his *New Encyclopaedia of Stage Hypnotism*, that the "master" stage hypnotist combines the *psychological* power of suggestion with the (alleged) *electro-magnetic* power of telepathically projecting thoughts directly into the brain of the subject (1996: 23).

> Some have called this powerful transmission of thought from one person to another "thought projection". The mental energy used appears to be of two types: magnetic energy [...] generated within the body and telepathic energy generated within the mind. [...] The two work together as a unit in applying Power Hypnosis. The operation of the two energies in combination is what Mesmer referred to as "animal magnetism". (1996: 24)

This is not really hypnotism, strictly speaking, but a hybrid of hypnotism and Mesmerism. Moreover, the original theory of hypnotism, as defined by Braid, emphasises the fact that subjects put *themselves* into hypnosis by following instructions to focus on certain dominant ideas, whereas the Mesmerists emphasised their own alleged special power or influence over subjects. Clearly, however, most subsequent stage hypnosis performances follow the *style* of the Mesmerists in this regard, for dramatic effect, using language which seems to attribute responsibility to the "power" of the operator, although they do so under the *name* of hypnotism. For example, 'A hypnotic power resides within you to influence others,' writes McGill (1996: 23).

Braid as Critic of Complementary Therapies

Although there are no modern clinical proponents of Mesmerism *per se*, there are many complementary therapists who espouse essentially quite similar views under more fashionable names. The same criticisms Braid raised against Mesmerism, electro-biology, phrenology, etc., might be raised by him against the current vogue for therapies such as Reiki, EFT, TFT, etc. It would surprise the many modern hypnotherapists who practice "energy therapy" under that heading to know that, as these writings clearly show, Braid would have considered their views and practices fundamentally incompatible with the theory of hypnotism. He dedicated his life to refuting and debunking similar views. Indeed, hypnotherapy is widely considered a branch of "complementary and alternative medicine" (CAM) today, but its founder was one of the most ardent and influential critics of pseudo-science in the history of medicine.

It is notable that Braid repeatedly refers to the fact that he bases hypnotism upon well-established physiological and psychological principles. In doing so, he embraces the scientific principle of parsimony, or Occam's Razor, which requires that established concepts should be tried first as an explanation for observable phenomena before attempting to coin new terms or introduce new hypothetical forces, such as "animal magnetism", etc. The established concepts used by Braid were primarily those of suggestion, association, and imitation, which also constitute what we would now call the "placebo effect". Braid was aware of this and repeatedly refers to the similarity between hypnotic suggestion and the use of bread pills and other placebo remedies, especially in his later writings. However, Braid intended hypnotism to be both *non-deceptive*, insofar as it explicitly claims to employ suggestion, and to provide a means of *amplifying* or *enhancing* the ordinary placebo effect.

Hypnotism as Early Cognitive-Behavioural Therapy

Milton Erickson, perhaps the most influential hypnotic researcher of the 20th century, wrote,

> It was due to the researches of Braid that hypnosis was placed on a scientific basis, and his coining and application of the terms hypnotism and hypnosis to the phenomenon instead of the misnomer of Mesmerism facilitated its acceptance by the medical profession. In the course of his investigations Braid reached the conclusion that hypnotism was wholly a matter of suggestion, which constituted the first attempt at a scientific and psychological explanation. He made a detailed study of the technique of hypnosis and the various phenomena obtained in trances. He was a prolific writer and left extensive treatises which are surprisingly modern in their conceptions. (Erickson, 'Historical Sketch', Medical Record, December 5, 1934).

Moreover, in many respects, Braid's orientation is more compatible with modern cognitive-behavioural and evidence-based approaches to psychotherapy than with New Age or complementary therapies. Indeed, Braid can be seen as pre-empting several of the key concepts employed in cognitive and behavioural therapies. In particular,

1. Counter-Conditioning (Behaviour Therapy)

The central technique of behaviour therapy, systematic desensitisation, was originally a hypnotherapy intervention, referred to as "hypnotic desensitisation" (*q.v.*, Wolpe, 1958; Wolberg, 1948). It is based upon the simple contention that anxiety or nervous arousal is best counteracted by gradually evoking it while simultaneously inducing a competing response, usually relaxation. Wolpe, the founder of behaviour therapy, argues that his approach is distinct from traditional hypnotherapy insofar as it employs the concept of reciprocal inhibition, or counter-conditioning, i.e., the use of competing responses to extinguish maladaptive behaviour and emotion.

> Suggestion, whether or not in the context of hypnotic induction, uses words to elicit desirable responses where undesirable responses are habitual. It may succeed in changing a habit when a suggested response *inhibits* a pre-existing one. If standard hypnotherapy has not had impressive long-term results, it is because it has not usually brought the suggested response into *effective opposition* with the one to be eliminated. (Wolpe, 1990: 5, *my italics*).

However, this basic concept is clearly present in Braid's original writings, and constitutes a central feature of his hypnotic therapy, albeit in a more primitive form. Braid repeatedly asserts that he selectively induces either nervous arousal (by means of intense muscular catalepsy) or nervous sleep (by means of profound muscular relaxation).

> How nervous sleep acts in some such cases it may be difficult or impossible to explain; but it may be reasonably considered to act as an alterative [i.e., a health-restoring medication], producing a new action or counter-impression, during which the morbid action is suspended [...] (Braid, 1853)

Though this was not his only stratagem, Braid usually chose which nervous state to induce deliberately in order to bring it into opposition with the symptoms to be eliminated, i.e., to directly counteract the prevailing symptoms of the client. As pain is usually accompanied by nervous arousal, for instance, Braid treated it primarily by inducing deep "nervous sleep", or relaxation. He seems also to have employed a similar relaxing strategy with hysterical clients suffering from anxiety. However, he also induced states of nervous arousal where he felt that this was more appropriate,

> If tranquillising is the object in view, let the patient remain in a recumbent and easy posture, with all the muscles relaxed to the utmost, and let the mind be sustained by encouraging expressions, and such as shall withdraw attention *from* the part most requiring to be tranquillized. If stimulation is required, then the limbs must be extended, and they will speedily pass into a rigid state, during which the circulation and respiration become much quickened, and by directing the patient's attention and expectation to any organ of sense, its function will naturally be quickened; and so of the function of any other organ or part of the body. [...]
> The first point to be determined, therefore, in this hypnotic mode of treating suitable cases, is the same as is required in any other mode of treatment – viz., to endeavour, by careful examination, to ascertain what is the real nature and cause of the existing symptoms, and whether they require stimulating or depressing [i.e., tranquilising] measures to be adopted, locally or generally; and to what extent, in either direction, the excitement or depression ought to be carried. (Braid, 1852)

Moreover, Braid very frequently employed habitual contracture of antagonistic muscle groups to prevent muscular tics and spasms in a manner which strongly pre-empts the "competing response" approach central to of Azrin & Nunn's (1976) Habit Reversal Therapy, another influential form of behaviour therapy.

2. Countering Negative Cognitions (Cognitive Therapy)
Albert Ellis was the originator of perhaps the earliest modality of modern cognitive therapy, now known as Rational Emotive Behaviour Therapy (REBT). In his seminal *Reason & Emotion in Psychotherapy* (1962), Ellis repeatedly compares the irrational beliefs central to his cognitive theory of emotional disturbance to pre-existing *negative* hypnotic suggestions, i.e., fixed ideas internalised from other people and maintained through persistent, unintentional, negative autosuggestion or self-talk.

> [...] suggestion and autosuggestion are effective in removing neurotic and psychotic symptoms because *they are the very instruments which caused or helped produce these symptoms in the first place*. Virtually all complex and sustained adult human emotions are caused by ideas or attitudes; and these ideas or attitudes are, first, *suggested* by persons and things outside the individual (especially by his parents, teachers, books, etc.); and they are, second, continually *autosuggested* by himself. (Ellis, 1962: 277)

This is hardly a novel view, but is identical to Braid's original theory that hysterical or psychosomatic conditions were due to negative "fixed" or "dominant" ideas in the subject's mind. These negative beliefs became self-fulfilling prophecies. Hence, speaking of the effects of suggestion "for good or for evil", Braid comments,

> And in this way, also, some patients having predicted that certain effects will be manifested in their persons, at a certain time specified, the *predominant idea* will often realise the prophecy. (Braid, 1852: 63, *italics added*)

Nevertheless, Ellis criticised hypnotherapists for "Pollyannaism", by which he meant the attempt to install healthy positive beliefs without first identifying and directly counteracting the clients existing negative and irrational beliefs. However, Braid very clearly recognised that "dominant ideas" were a widespread cause of hysterical illness, i.e., emotional disturbances and psychosomatic disorders. He particularly notes the importance of counteracting negative fixed ideas in cases of hysterical paralysis, which were common in the Victorian era.

> The most striking cases of all, however, for illustrating the value of the hypnotic mode of treatment, are cases of hysterical paralysis, in which, without organic lesion, the patient may have remained for a considerable length of time perfectly powerless of a part, or of a whole body, from a [negative] dominant idea which has paralysed or misdirected his volition. In such cases, by altering the state of the circulation, and breaking down the previous [negative] idea, and substituting a [positive] salutary idea of vigour and self-confidence in its place, *(which can be done by audible suggestions addressed to the patient, in a confident tone of voice, as to what must and shall be realised by the process he has been subjected to)*, on being aroused a few minutes afterwards, with such [positive] dominant idea in their minds, to the astonishment of themselves as well as of others, the patients are found to have acquired vigour and voluntary power over their hitherto paralysed limbs [...].
>
> Assuredly, such cures are as important as they are interesting and surprising, because, such cases may resist ordinary modes of treatment for paralysis, for an indefinite length of time; but still, the rationale is simple enough when viewed according to the principles which I have already explained, of the influence of an expectant dominant idea, either exciting or depressing natural function, according to the faith and confidence of the patient. (Braid, 1853)

These are not the hypothetical "unconscious" complexes later introduced by Freudian psychoanalysts, but rather morbid expectations which involuntarily dominate consciousness. Referring to one such case, he writes,

> It was not, therefore, the induction of the *nervous sleep* alone which effected the cure, but my knowledge of how to *direct the influence* DURING the sleep, so as to break down the pre-existing, involuntary fixed, dominant idea in the patient's mind, and its consequences. (Braid, 1853)

Discussing the treatment of hysterical paralysis in Victorian hypnosis, Aaron Beck, the founder of Cognitive Therapy, wrote that, "These examples suggest that hysteria is the illustration *par excellence* of the phenomenon of cognitive distortion in psychiatric disorders". Beck recognised that, in a manner resembling Cognitive Therapy, hypnosis treated hysterical symptoms by removing a "pathogenic idea".

> When the incorrect belief is modified through suggestion, hypnosis, demonstration, or cognitive therapy, the symptom clears up. (Beck, 1976: 208)

As Beck observed, Freudian psychoanalysis subsequently eclipsed this Victorian theory of psychopathology, replacing it with the dubious notion that hysterical symptoms were the symbolic expression of repressed sexual desires. When Ellis and Beck introduced modern rational and cognitive approaches to psychotherapy, they did so by rehabilitating Braid's original theory of the pathogenic idea or expectation which formed the basis of Victorian hypnotherapy half a century before the advent of Freudian psychoanalysis.

For these reasons, I would argue that Braid has a right to be seen, at least in some respects, as a distant forerunner of modern cognitive-behavioural therapists. In addition to defining hypnotic therapy in terms of specific cognitive-behavioural interventions, he clearly assumed a cognitive theory of psychological disorders and based his whole methodology upon a "rational", "empirical", "scientific" and "common sense" orientation, of the kind espoused in modern CBT. Aaron Beck, in developing modern Cognitive Therapy, also attempted to found it upon a modern "common sense" philosophy, e.g., throughout his chapter 'Common Sense & Beyond' in *Cognitive Therapy & the Emotional Disorders (*1976). Braid's writings provide evidence that he was deliberately fulfilling the agenda set forth by leading Scottish philosophers of the Common Sense realist school of philosophical psychology to re-interpret the observable effects of Mesmerism from a more philosophical and scientific perspective. The concepts Braid employs in explaining hypnotism depend upon the "psycho-physiological" theories of *suggestion*, *association*, and *imitation* which he derived from this psychological school, and supplant the metaphysical "energy" theories of Mesmer and his followers.

The Future of Braid's Legacy
There are many unexplored themes in Braid's writings, including measurable physiological phenomena which he appears to have reproduced many times under the supervision of leading scientists of his day. To pick just one example, Braid's repeated observation that his method of hypnotic catalepsy reliably increased the heart rate to double its normal level, if correct, would have obvious implications for many different forms of modern therapy. As we now move toward a new era of evidence-based practice in the field of psychological therapy, and progressively further away from the introspective excesses and *baroque* speculations of Freudianism, Braid's "common sense" philosophy and empirical orientation have become fashionable once again.

I hope that this new presentation of his writings will allow Braid the opportunity, denied during his lifetime, of having his work appraised as a whole. I have made every attempt to make his previously inaccessible texts more accessible to modern readers by providing as much reorganisation, clarification, and commentary as I felt necessary, while maintaining enough distance to allow Braid to speak for himself. I hope that he will find new readers as a result and that he will, at some future date, receive the recognition due to him as the founder not only of hypnotherapy but, ultimately, of modern *psychotherapy* in general.

References

Beck, A.	(1976)	*Cognitive Therapy & The Emotional Disorders.*
Ellis, A.	(1962)	*Reason & Emotion in Psychotherapy.*
Forrest, D.	(1999)	*Hypnotism: A History.*
Kroger, W.	(2008)	*Clinical & Experimental Hypnosis*, Revised Second Edition.
McGill, O.	(1996)	*The New Encyclopaedia of Stage Hypnotism.*
Waite, A.E. (ed.)	(1899)	*Braid on Hypnotism.*
Williamson, W.C.	(1896)	*Reminiscences of a Yorkshire Naturalist.*
Wolberg, L.	(1948)	*Medical Hypnosis.*
Wolpe, J.	(1958)	*Psychotherapy by Reciprocal Inhibition.*

The Original Philosophy of Hypnotism

Copyright © Donald Robertson, 2008

> 'There is, therefore, both positive and negative proof in favour of my mental and suggestive theory, and in opposition to the magnetic, occult, or electric theories of the Mesmerists and electro-biologists. My theory, moreover, has this additional recommendation, that it is level to our comprehension, and adequate to account for all which is demonstrably true, *without offering any violence to reason and common sense, or being at variance with generally admitted physiological and psychological principles.*'
>
> – Braid, *Electro-Biological Phenomena* (1851).

I am not aware of any author having commented on the fact that Braid seemingly developed his theory and practice of hypnotism out of the conceptual framework provided by a particular philosophical and psychological tradition, the "Scottish School of Common Sense" also known as "Scottish Realism".

Braid was not himself a philosopher in the academic, or any other, sense. However, he was demonstrably influenced by the leading academic philosophers of his time. He makes several explicit references to the Scottish Realist philosophers, especially Prof. Dugald Stewart. Moreover, the broader influence of British "empiricist" philosophy can be seen throughout his writings. Braid developed hypnotism in the wake of the "Scottish Enlightenment", a period in cultural history which, in the latter half of the 18th century, saw an explosion of interest in logic and scientific method. Thomas Reid (1710-1796) founded the Scottish School of Realism or Common Sense, which was continued by his follower Dugald Stewart (1735-1828), and Thomas Brown (1778-1820), and further popularised in Braid's time by the physician John Abercrombie (1780-1844). From them, he absorbed a fiercely pragmatic, rational and empirical attitude toward the field of mental philosophy, or "philosophy of psychology", as it is now known.

Braid wrote, we must remember, during a period in history when psychology was still a branch of academic philosophy. The psychological concepts developed by philosophers of mind, such as "dominant ideas" (akin to the automatic thoughts of Beck's cognitive therapy) "habit and association" (a subjective precursor of Pavlovian conditioning), and "imitation and sympathy" (which we now call "role-modelling" and "empathy"), are repeatedly mentioned by Braid as the theoretical framework upon which his science of hypnotism, "neuro-hypnology", was built. Braid's friend and collaborator, Prof. William B. Carpenter, discusses the theoretical principles of this in his *Principles of Mental Physiology* (1889), especially in the chapter 'Of Common Sense' which concludes by quoting an approving letter from the philosopher John Stuart Mill sent to Carpenter in 1872. Mill agrees with Carpenter's contention that "common sense", by which he means a kind of intellectual intuition analogous to the ancient Greek concept of *nous*, is a combination of innate and acquired judgements, which have a "reflexive" or "automatic" quality and appear to consciousness as "self-evident" truths.

> I have long recognised as a fact that judgements really grounded on a long succession of small experiences mostly forgotten, or perhaps never brought out into very distinct consciousness, often grow into the likeness of intuitive perceptions. [...] When states of Mind in no respect innate or instinctive have been frequently repeated, the Mind acquires, as is proved by the power of Habit, a greatly increased facility of passing into those states and this increased facility must be owing to some change of a physical character, in the organic action of the Brain. (Mill, quoted in Carpenter, 1889)

Carpenter argues that rational judgements may evolve into "common sense" reflex judgements as a result of the law of habit and association, becoming "second nature", a term borrowed from Aristotle. It is, perhaps, possible to interpret Braid as meaning that hypnotic suggestion, or rather focused attention upon a dominant idea ("monoideism"), provides an *artificial* means of acquiring the same sense of conviction.

In his *Elements of the Philosophy of the Human Mind* (1827), Dugald Stewart had specifically discussed the French Royal Commission's report on Mesmerism and speculated that Mesmeric subjects, rather than being influenced by animal magnetism, were reacting to a psychological "law of sympathetic imitation" not yet understood. While rejecting the pseudo-scientific theory of animal magnetism, Stewart recommended that physicians nevertheless take the observable effects of the technique seriously. Braid therefore quotes his remark as the motto to *Neurypnology*, 'Unlimited scepticism is equally the child of imbecility as implicit credulity'. Indeed, Braid toyed with the idea of calling his method "rational Mesmerism" as opposed to "transcendental Mesmerism", though he seems ultimately to have felt that this would obscure the fundamental difference between the competing theories of animal magnetism and the ideo-dynamic reflex.

Stewart claimed that the phenomena of Mesmerism could be salvaged by physicians adopting a more rational and scientific approach, while avoiding the worst excesses of its metaphysical speculations. Moreover, in a discussion of similar ideas propounded by the philosopher Francis Bacon, he specifically recommends that physicians, like Braid, should develop a 'doctrine of the bond between mind and body' (i.e., Braid's "psycho-physiology"). Moreover, Stewart urges enquiry into 'the effect of *fixing and concentrating the attention*, in giving to ideal [i.e., imaginary] objects the power of realities over the belief', adding,

> [Lord Bacon had urged physicians] to ascertain how far it is possible *to fortify and exalt the imagination*, and by what means this may most effectually be done. The class of facts here alluded to, are manifestly of the same description with those to which the attention of philosophers has been lately called by *the pretensions of Mesmer* […]. (Stewart, 1827: 130, *italics added*)

Stewart therefore recommends that medical research should attempt a rational re-appraisal of the effects of Mesmerism, and other "nostrum" or placebo remedies, such as Perkins' tractors,

> I would beg leave […] to recommend warmly to my successors in this branch of study, a careful examination and comparison of the details connected […] with the practice of *animal magnetism*, – as inestimable data for extending our knowledge of the laws which regulate *the connexion between the human mind, and our bodily organization*. The lights, more particularly, which they throw on various *questions relative to the Imagination*, are such, as must for ever entitle Mesmer […] to the gratitude of those who cultivate the Philosophy of the Mind; *whatever the motives* may have been which suggested the experiments of these practitioners, or whatever the *occasional mischiefs* of which they may have been the authors. (Stewart, 1827: 135, *italics added*)

Braid explicitly quotes the following passage from Stewart in *Magic, Witchcraft, etc.* (1852),

> It appears to me, that *the general conclusions established by Mesmer's practice*, with respect to *the physical effects of the principle of imagination* (more particularly in cases where they [i.e., imagination and body] co-operated together), are incomparably *more curious than if he had actually demonstrated the existence of his boasted science*: nor can I see any good reason why a *physician*, who admits the efficacy of the *moral* [i.e., psychological] agents *employed by Mesmer*, should, in the exercise of his profession, scruple to copy whatever processes are necessary for subjecting them to his command, any more than that he should hesitate about employing a new physical agent, such as electricity or galvanism. (Stewart, 1827: 147, *italics added*)

Braid very frequently refers to Stewart's "law of sympathy and imitation" in developing the psycho-physiological theory of hypnotism. It may be worthwhile to clarify the meaning of this term, because Stewart gives it a technical definition,

> The *Imitation* of which I am here to treat, and which I have distinguished by the title of *Sympathetic*, is that chiefly which depends on the mimical powers connected with our *bodily frame*; and which, in certain combinations of circumstances, seems to result, *with little intervention of our will*, from a sympathy *between the bodily organisations* of different individuals. […]
> In general, it may be remarked, that whenever we see, in the countenance of another individual, any sudden change of features; our own countenance has a tendency to assimilate itself to his. (Stewart, 1827: 105-106, *italics added*)

Stewart gives numerous everyday examples, such as the notorious contagion of yawning, melancholy, panic, laughter, etc., as well as more pathological illustrations relating to mass hysteria, etc. Braid's theory of "muscular suggestion" is also clearly pre-empted by Stewart, who writes in the same place,

> As the imitation of any *expression*, strongly marked in the *countenance and gestures of another person*, has a tendency to excite, in some degree, *the corresponding passion in our own minds*, so, on the contrary, the suppression of the external sign has a tendency to compose the passion which it indicates. It is said of Socrates [the Graeco-Roman personification of the composed Sage], that whenever he felt the passion of anger beginning to rise, he became instantly silent; and I have no doubt that by observing this rule, he not only avoided many an occasion of giving offence to others, but actually killed many of the seeds of those malignant affections which are the great bane of human happiness. (Stewart, 1827: 164, *italics added*)

These simple psychological mechanisms are the building blocks which Braid uses to construct a viable "rational" alternative to Mesmerism. Indeed, the basic "laws" of Braid's Common Sense philosophy of psychology can be viewed as broadly corresponding with the certain principles of social, cognitive, and behavioural psychology adopted in modern psychotherapy, *viz.*,

1.   The Law of Habit & Association. Similar to the principle of habit conditioning which underlies the learning theory approach derived from Pavlov, Hull, etc., employed in modern Behaviour Therapy.

2.   The Law of Dominant Ideas. The role of "fixed" or "dominant ideas", and expectation in Braid clearly pre-empts modern Cognitive Therapy's notion of "automatic negative thoughts", etc., and is essentially the forerunner of "autosuggestion", though Braid does not use this term himself.

3.   The Law of Imitation & Sympathy. Braid's emphasis on mimicry also pre-empts the emphasis on "role-modelling" in social learning theory, developed by Bandura and others.

In this way, therefore, Braid's discovery of hypnotism laid the foundation of precisely the rational and empirical alternative to the theories of Mesmer anticipated by Stewart. His work can be seen as the deliberate, practical continuation of the philosophical agenda outlined by the philosophy of psychology predominant among the Edinburgh intellectuals of his day. It is in the Scottish School of Common Sense philosophy, therefore, that we may find the original *philosophy of hypnotism*.

Principal Works by Braid

Copyright © Donald Robertson, 2008

On the Curative Agency of Neuro-Hypnotism (1841, *unpublished*)
Practical Essay on the Curative Agency of Neuro-Hypnotism
Soon after the Lafontaine incident, Braid wrote to the Medical Section of the British Association in order to arrange delivery of a professional report entitled 'Practical Essay on the Curative Agency of Neuro-Hypnotism' (*q.v. Neurypnology*, 1843). However, his offer was declined; apparently because of concern over the controversial nature of the subject. Braid therefore advertised his own public reading of the "Rejected Essay" on 27th December 1841, attended by many of the British Association Members. He seems likely to have repeatedly delivered this report in whole or part at subsequent lectures. It is probable that the material from this essay was largely incorporated into *Neurypnology* (1843). This report precedes his *Satanic Agency, etc., Reviewed* (1842) and probably contained Braid's *first use* of the word "hypnotism".

Neurypnology (1843)
Neurypnology, or the Rationale of Nervous Sleep, Considered in Relation to Animal Magnetism, Illustrated by Numerous Cases of Successful Application in the Relief and Cure of Disease.
Braid's first and most famous work on hypnosis. As Bramwell observes, however, this presents a very primitive picture of views which were to be fundamentally revised as his research progressed. Nevertheless Braid expresses a number of important views in this book which are often overlooked because of his writing style and the lack of descriptive chapter or section headings.

On the Power of the Mind over the Body (1846)
The power of the mind over the body: an experimental inquiry into the nature and cause of the phenomena attributed by Baron Reichenbach and others to a "new imponderable".
A discussion of Braid's experiments on Reichenbach's claims regarding the subjective sensations and muscular responses experienced in response to magnets, etc., which Braid proves to be due to attention, suggestion and imagination. This is perhaps the work to which Braid himself tends to refer back most often in his later writings and seems to have marked a change of emphasis in his writings due to a greater appreciation of the role of suggestion in the waking state.

Observations on Trance (1850)
Observations on Trance, or Human Hybernation.
A discussion of the notion of "human hibernation" in relation to hypnotism and the alleged feats of Indian fakirs who survive entombed for many days without food or water. Not particularly relevant to modern hypnotherapy. It may serve to illustrate the fact that Braid drew parallels between hypnotism and yogic meditation, and that he saw the deepest stages of hypnotic sleep as loosely analogous to coma, hibernation, catatonic disorders, and the trances of fakirs.

Electro-Biological Phenomena (1851)
Electro-Biological Phenomena, Considered Physiologically and Psychologically.
Perhaps the *rarest* of Braid's major works contains his response to J. Stanley Grimes' theory of electro-biology, an American technique, which had been recently exhibited in England and attracted much interest. Braid was rightly concerned that the proponents had copied his eye-fixation technique and turned it into yet another pseudo-scientific "energy therapy", based on the contention that psychological effects were due to the electro-magnetic properties of composite metal discs which were held in the palm of the hand and stared into. This rival theory, nevertheless, further motivated Braid to extend his theory and encompass mind-body interactions in the ordinary waking state as well as "nervous sleep".

Magic, Witchcraft, Animal Magnetism, Hypnotism, and Electro-Biology (1852)
Magic, Witchcraft, Animal Magnetism, Hypnotism, and Electro-Biology; Being a Digest of the Latest Views of the Author on These Subjects.
A detailed defence of hypnotism and critique of Mesmerism by Braid written in response to a book by J.C. Colquhoun in which he is seemingly maligned. Despite the potentially off-putting title, this is one of Braid's most important works, and contains many references to hypnotism and suggestion – and (strangely) none to witchcraft.

Hypnotic Therapeutics (1853)
Hypnotic Therapeutics, Illustrated by Cases, With an Appendix on Table-Turning and Spirit-Rapping.
Undoubtedly one of Braid's most comprehensive and important later works, discussing in detail his mature

views on hypnosis and the ideo-motor theory of suggestion. As the title suggests, this is perhaps the text by Braid which should be considered first in appraising his contribution to modern hypnotherapy, though it has been much neglected in the past.

The Physiology of Fascination (1855)
The Physiology of Fascination and the Critics Criticised.
Two short booklets, published together, the first briefly describing his later theory of monoideism, and the latter a combative response to attacks on Braid and Carpenter published in *The Zoist*.

On Hypnotism (1860, *unpublished*)
This 36-page manuscript, summarising Braid's final views on hypnotism and related phenomena, was written by him in January 1860, according to Bramwell's bibliography. It was sent by the author to Dr. Étienne Eugène Azam, a distinguished French surgeon and psychologist, a few months later in March 1860, just before Braid's death. It was translated into French as *Note sur le sommeil nerveux ou hypnotism* ('Note on nervous sleep, or hypnotism') by Azam and subsequently published as an appendix to Dr. Jules Simon's French translation of *Neurypnology* (1883). A copy was passed to Dr. George Miller Beard, a distinguished American neurologist who then lent it to Wilhelm T. Preyer, professor of physiology at Jena University. Preyer published a German translation entitled *Über den Hypnotismus* ('On Hypnotism') in his *Die Entdeckung des Hypnotismus, etc.*, 1881, but it was never published in English – and it seems the original manuscript is now missing. (I have been unable to trace any subsequent reference to the existence of the original text.)

At this time, following favourable recommendations made to them by Azam, Paul Broca, and others, the French Academy of Sciences, which had established a joint committee to investigate Mesmerism in 1784, formed a new committee to investigate Braid's hypnotism. Braid therefore addressed the foreword to the Academy and it seems Azam was entrusted with the task of conveying his writings to them for their consideration.

This text summarises many points made in Braid's other writings, especially *The Power of the Mind over the Body* (1846) and *Electro-Biological Phenomena* (1851), but nevertheless it provides essentially the last word on his mature views, showing which aspects of his thought he considered most important and highlighting the key aspects of his final theory of hypnotism. As such, it represents a much better introduction to his theory of hypnotism than *Neurypnology*, his best-known publication.

Psycho-Physiology (*Unpublished*)
Psycho-Physiology: embracing Hypnotism, Monoideism, and Mesmerism.
In several of Braid's other writings he comments on his intention to publish another major textbook on hypnotism. It looks as though Braid delayed publication of a revised edition of *Neurypnology*, perhaps because ongoing changes prevented him from settling upon a definitive account of his later theory. In *The Power of the Mind over the Body* (1846), Braid writes,

> It would be inconsistent with the scope of this paper to enter into an elaborate detail of my views as to the philosophical explanation of the modes of exciting and varying certain trains of ideas, and their consequent manifestations during the nervous sleep. The inquiry is not only curious, but also one of great interest, in respect to the power of the mind in controlling physical action, and of physical impressions in reacting on the mind. I have given a pretty ample discussion on these topics in a second edition of my little work on hypnotism [*Neurypnology*, 1843], now preparing for the press, to which I beg leave to refer those who feel desirous of prosecuting the inquiry, and particularly those who desire to do so for curative purposes.

Braid introduced his *Magic, Witchcraft, etc.* (1852) by writing,

> [...] by this means, moreover, I am making up, in some measure, for the delay in the publication of another edition of my work on hypnotism [*Neurypnology*, 1843], which has long been out of print, and so frequently called for. That call I hope shortly to be able to respond to, with fullness of detail as the importance of the subject merits; more particularly as regards its practical application to the relief and cure of some forms of disease, of which numerous interesting examples will be adduced.

In *The Physiology of Fascination* (1855), he then stated, 'It is my intention shortly to publish a volume entitled "Psycho-Physiology: embracing Hypnotism, Monoideism, and Mesmerism".'

It is possible that these comments refer to the same work, and that Braid was planning, or had written, a second, significantly *revised* edition of his major work on hypnotism but felt that the changes in his position were so fundamental as to require a change in the title from *Neurypnology* to the much more general *Psycho-Physiology, etc.* His views seem to have expanded beyond the initial focus upon "nervous sleep" to a wider conception of psycho-physiological ("mind-body") phenomena, encompassing waking suggestion and a variety of interacting and overlapping psycho-physiological states, including nervous sleep (hypnosis), excitation and muscular rigidity (catalepsy) and mental abstraction (monoideism), etc.

Glossary of Braidism

Copyright © Donald Robertson, 2008

Abstraction
A state of intense mental concentration, especially that directed toward a mental representation or idea, without regard to its reality or consistency with other impressions. This implies both an intensification of the dominant idea's vivacity, and also progressive insensibility with regard to other impressions, i.e., in deep abstraction people become oblivious to external distractions, etc. Similar to the concept of "imaginal absorption" in modern cognitive-behavioural theories of hypnosis. Carpenter calls it the automatic mental action of the Reasoner or philosopher, and contrasts it with "reverie" (1874: Chapter XIV). Braid consistently stated that hypnotism was essentially a state of intense abstraction.

"Anatomy of Expression"
A term coined by the physiologist Sir Charles Bell in *Essays on the Anatomy of Expression in Painting* (1806). Used by Braid to refer to the physical expressions of emotion, especially in the facial expression and body posture, etc. Braid argues that by manipulating the facial expression and body posture of hypnotic subjects it is possible, to a surprising degree, to induce the associated emotional state, in what he calls a "reversal" of the ordinary causal relationship. This notion clearly pre-empts the influential "James-Lange" theory of emotion.

Animal Magnetism
Invisible ("occult") force hypothesised by Mesmer and his followers as being channelled from the body of the Mesmerist into that of his subject in order to induce the various phenomena observed. Mesmer believed that animal magnetism could be stored in water and bottled, stored in crystals, or other objects, and that it would bounce off mirrors. It is clear that it was conceived of as a supernatural force imbued with unusual properties, and closely associated with spiritualism and alleged paranormal phenomena. However, Mesmerists were vulnerable to the objection that similar phenomena could be produced when clients merely *believed* that they were being Mesmerised, i.e., due to "placebo" effects.

Catalepsy
A state of muscular seizure, either general or specific to parts of the body. Catalepsy was associated with various medical and psychiatric conditions but it was found that a similar condition could be induced by suggestion, and often appeared spontaneously in certain hypnotic or Mesmeric subjects. Braid made extensive use of catalepsy in *Neurypnology* (1843) as a means of altering the pulse and circulation to specific regions of the body for therapeutic purposes.

Conversazione
A kind of professional symposium or meeting usually consisting of lecturing, demonstrations and discussions. Medical *conversazioni* (the Italian plural) were frequently conducted by Braid and used by him to educate others about hypnotism. At these meetings other professionals would often challenge the speaker to prove his theory and participate in testing his patients, or bring patients of their own to be tested, etc.

Dominant Idea
An idea which somehow becomes the centre of conscious attention or otherwise dominates the mind, tending to bring about physical responses especially when reinforced by belief and expectation. **Nota bene**: The word "idea" (Greek for "form" or "pattern") was originally a *technical* philosophical term derived from Platonic epistemology. In the Victorian era, the word could be used to refer to an abstract concept, but also to a meaningful visual or sensory image or memory. Terms like "monoideism" or the "ideo-dynamic response" can therefore refer to the action of a mental *image* or *memory* upon the body.

Double Consciousness
A state followed by spontaneous, generalised amnesia, which could be reversed by suggestion. Braid stated that 10% of his subjects entered this state in hypnosis. He considered it a defining feature that such amnesia was reversible, and that the subject could remember, either spontaneously or in response to suggestion, everything that had previously occurred when hypnotised for a *second* time. This term is used by Abercrombie (1834), who attributes it to unnamed others; so it does not originate with Braid. The notion of double consciousness is the precursor of subsequent notions of mental "dissociation" or "splitting" in dynamic psychiatry.

Electro-Biology

Theory propounded by the phrenologist J. Stanley Grimes, popularised by John Bovee Dod, and opposed by Braid. The proponents claimed to induce increased suggestibility and other effects following eye-fixation upon a special zinc disc, with a copper spot in the middle, held in the palm of the hand. Though the induction method is clearly similar to, and probably derived from, Braid's eye-fixation method, the electro-biologists claimed that results were due to a peculiar electro-magnetic effect of the metal upon the body. Braid utterly rejected this notion which he viewed as a reversion to the pseudo-scientific notions of the Mesmerists, and attempted to prove that ordinary psycho-physiological factors such as fixed attention and suggestion were the true cause of the phenomena.

Hypnotic Coma
An extremely unusual state of torpor exhibited by some hypnotic subjects, in which amnesia is so profound that it cannot be reversed by subsequent hypnotic suggestions. Braid appears to equate this loosely with animal hibernation, and the medical condition of "trance" or catalepsy (catatonia).

Hypnotism
A state of focused attention and nervous sleep induced by i) suppressed respiration, and ii) fixation of the eyes, or of the mind, upon some unexciting object. Psychologically the opposite of normal sleep, insofar as it consists of a fixed attention upon an unexciting point, e.g., the tip of a lancet case, the top of a bottle, or a cork bound to the forehead.

Ideo-Dynamic Action
Term coined by Dr. Daniel Noble to extend Carpenter's concept of ideo-motor action to encompass not only changes in the skeletal muscles but also sensory and autonomic responses, and other physiological changes throughout the whole body. Braid embraces this term, realising (as Carpenter himself implies) that the mechanism worked on areas of bodily functioning outside normal voluntary control, as well as upon the ordinary muscles of movement.

Ideo-Motor Action
Term coined by Prof. W.B. Carpenter to describe the "reflex action of the cerebrum", and thereby explain how dominant ideas, brought about by verbal suggestion and other means, could cause genuine physical changes. The classic illustration being Michel Eugène Chevreul's demonstration that pendulum dowsing, which was widely assumed to show the effect upon the pendulum of invisible forces, was actually due to unconscious muscular movements in the dowser's hand.

"Law of Association"
The dominant school of psychology in Braid's time was the philosophical theory of the association of ideas. When Braid refers to the laws or principles of association he is alluding to a specific set of theories. Put simply, the British empiricist philosophers following Locke, Stewart, Reid, Mill, etc., typically reduced the laws of association to *three* principles: resemblance, contrast, and contiguity in space or time. Through experience and reflection, ideas tend to become repeatedly associated in the mind such that one may come to habitually evoke the other. The influential 18th century theory of the association of ideas can be seen as a subjective precursor of the physiological model of conditioning developed in the late 19th century by Pavlov, which formed the basis of modern behavioural psychology.

"Law of Sympathy"
The Scottish economist and political philosopher Adam Smith had outlined an influential theory of the laws of sympathy in the opening chapter of *The Theory of Moral Sentiments* (1759). However, an alternative account of sympathy and imitation, specifically in relation to Mesmerism, was developed by Dugald Stewart in *Elements of the Philosophy of the Human Mind* (1827). It is probably Stewart's philosophy of psychology that Braid has in mind on the many occasions when he refers to the laws of sympathy in accounting for the natural tendency to imitation found in hypnotic subjects and in the waking state.

Magnetism
Artificial, metal magnets were invented in 1750 by the English physicist John Canton. The notion of magnetism soon captured the imagination of the public who felt that magnetic forces must somehow have a powerful effect upon the human body. Around 1773, Mesmer was introduced to the notion of using magnets to heal disease by a Jesuit Priest called Father Maximilian Hell. Hell published an article in 1774 describing magnet therapy and leading to a rift with Mesmer over priority. Mesmer immediately abandoned the notion that metallic or "mineral" magnets were required, and argued instead that a universal magnetism ("animal magnetism") existed in nature which could be channelled through the human body and invested in virtually any kind of substance. The popularity of magnetic therapy continued, however, and Braid carried out numerous experiments to prove, once again, that magnets were a placebo. For example, in one influential experiment, Braid placed the key to his medical case in a "sensitive" subject's hand, telling his colleague

within earshot that it was a powerful magnet. Her hand was nevertheless seized with rigid catalepsy, the effect being due to *suggestion* rather than any form of "magnetism" whatsoever.

Mesmerism
The theory and practice of Franz Anton Mesmer which attained widespread popularity, and notoriety, during his lifetime. Braid recognised the physical and psychological effects of Mesmerism as, largely, real – with the exception of the claimed "higher phenomena" or paranormal powers. However, he fiercely rejected and systematically debunked the theory that it was due to an invisible energy ("animal magnetism") communicated by "silent willing" (i.e., quasi-telepathically) and showed the same effects could be produced more reliably by normal psychological and physiological means, using hypnotism and suggestion, etc.

Monoideism
A state of mental concentration ("abstraction") upon a single idea or train of thought, to the exclusion of others, so as for the time being to render the idea dominant and enhance the ideo-dynamic response.

Odylic ("Od" or "Odic") Force
Hypothetical electro-magnetic force postulated by Baron von Reichenbach, named after the Norse god Odin. A similar theory to that of animal magnetism, important merely because Braid undertook a series of informal experiments to show that the effects attributed to it were more likely caused by suggestion. This seems to have contributed to Braid's own growing appreciation of the role of suggestion in hypnotism.

Odometer
Apparently a kind of pendulum used by Herbert Mayo in some obscure experiments upon the odylic force of Reichenbach, but rejected by Braid as another manifestation of the ideo-motor response.

Philosophy of Mind
Braid was not a philosopher but repeatedly makes direct and indirect references to philosophy. At the time he was writing, psychology was still regarded as a branch of philosophy known as epistemology. Hence, the "psychologists" Braid is most influenced by are British philosophers of the European Enlightenment period. Those thinkers mentioned or quoted most by him are Dugald Stewart (1753-1828) and John Abercrombie (1780-1884), both philosophers of the influential "Scottish School of Common Sense" philosophy. (He briefly mentions Thomas Brown, likewise of this school.) These philosophers' ideas on the laws of habit, association and sympathy in psychology appear to have been influential both upon Braid's theory and practice of hypnotism. Most notably, however, it is Dugald Stewart's "common sense" and realist reinterpretation of Mesmerism in terms of the laws of psychology and physiology which Braid seems to be developing into a practical mode of treatment in his theories of neuro-hypnology and psycho-physiology.

Phreno-Hypnotism
Braid originally placed far more emphasis upon "muscular suggestion" than upon verbal suggestion. He experimented with phreno-Mesmerism but soon found that he could create similar effects without attempting to channel any magnetic energy, and that by touching parts of the body other than the scalp various responses could be stimulated. Braid finally came to place increasing emphasis upon his own hypothesis that the effects of touch were due to various forms of suggestion or redirection of attention.

Phrenology
Theory, developed at the start of the 19th century by the German physician Franz Joseph Gall, that different regions of the brain constituted distinct organs which varied in size depending upon their strength of function, leading to the so-called "organology", a specific map of the brain's functions. It was, therefore, assumed that the personality of an individual could be interpreted by reading the bumps on their head, which correlated with the shape of the brain. Phrenology was very popular in the 19th century, and widely combined with Mesmerism. However, both were roundly debunked within a century by sceptical scientists.

Phreno-Mesmerism
A hybrid of phrenology and Mesmerism which found that a variety of emotional responses could be triggered in individuals by touching corresponding areas of the scalp, according to the phrenological organology. It was assumed that this happened by channelling a current of animal magnetism from the body of the Mesmerist through the scalp and into the specific region of the brain to be excited or depressed.

Psycho-Physiology
The study of the reciprocal interaction between body and mind, i.e., the effect of dominant ideas in creating the ideo-motor response, and the effect of "muscular suggestion" in modifying mental and emotional states.

Reverie

A state of spontaneously free-flowing mental absorption, like daydreaming or the modern notion of "free-association". Carpenter called it the automatic mental action of the Poet.

Séance
Demonstrations of Mesmerism were often called *séances*, though this word did not necessarily carry paranormal connotations, merely the literal sense of being a Mesmeric "session" or meeting. Mesmeric *séances* were often large public performances in theatres similar to, and the precursors of, what we now know as "stage hypnosis" shows.

Suggestion
As Bramwell emphasises, a popular misconception arose that Braid did not appreciate the role of suggestion in hypnosis. However, Braid's later works are replete with explicit references to suggestion, and even demonstrate a sophisticated grasp of different forms of suggestion, most notably: autosuggestion (in the form of "expectant ideas"), verbal suggestion, and muscular suggestion.

Tractors (Perkins' Patented Tractors)
Pairs of 3-inch, pointed, metallic (steel and brass) rods which were designed and patented by the US physician Dr. Elisha Perkins (1741-1799) for drawing (i.e., traction) across the surface of the skin. Effects were supposedly due to a peculiar property of the metals used which were meant to remove a kind of electrical charge from the patient's body. Widely ridiculed as a pseudo-scientific remedy ("nostrum") following influential demonstrations by the British physician, Dr. John Haygarth in 1799, that wooden rods (which could not conduct electricity) produced exactly the same effect. Haygarth published an influential book entitled *On the Imagination as a Cause & as a Cure of Disease of the Body* (1800) which contains one of the first detailed discussions of the placebo effect. Braid refers to Haygarth's analysis of the tractors repeatedly and seems to have been greatly influenced by it in developing his own theory of hypnotic suggestion.

Braid's Hypnotic Induction Technique

Copyright © Donald Robertson, 2008

Braid explains the "causes of hypnotism" in *Neurypnology* (1843) as follows,

> It is on this very principle, of over-exerting the attention, by keeping it riveted to one subject or idea which is not of itself of an exciting nature, and, over-exercising one set of muscles, and the state of the strained eyes, with the suppressed respiration, and general repose, which attend such experiments, which excites in the brain and whole nervous system that peculiar state which I call Hypnotism, or nervous sleep. The most striking proofs that it is different from common sleep, are the extraordinary effects produced by it. In deep abstraction of mind, it is well-known, the individual becomes unconscious of surrounding objects, and in some cases, even of severe bodily infliction. During hypnotism, or nervous sleep, the functions in action seem to be so intensely active, as must in a great measure rob the others of that degree of nervous energy necessary for exciting their sensibility. This alone may account for much of the dullness of common feeling during the abnormal quickness and extended range of action of certain other functions.

Elsewhere in the same text, he describes his standard induction technique as follows,

> Take any bright object (I generally use my lancet case) between the thumb and fore and middle fingers of the left hand; hold it from about eight to fifteen inches from the eyes, at such position above the forehead as may be necessary to produce the greatest possible strain upon the eyes and eyelids, and enable the patient to maintain a steady fixed stare at the object.
>
> The patient must be made to understand that he is to keep the eyes steadily fixed on the object, and the mind riveted on the idea of that one object. It will be observed, that owing to the consensual adjustment of the eyes, the pupils will be at first contracted: they will shortly begin to dilate, and after they have done so to a considerable extent, and have assumed a wavy motion, if the fore and middle fingers of the right hand, extended and a little separated, are carried from the object towards the eyes, most probably the eyelids will close involuntarily, with a vibratory motion. If this is not the case, or the patient allows the eyeballs to move, desire him to begin anew, giving him to understand that he is to allow the eyelids to close when the fingers are again carried towards the eyes, but that the eyeballs must be kept fixed, in the same position, and the mind riveted to the one idea of the object held above the eyes. It will generally be found, that the eyelids close with a vibratory motion, or become spasmodically closed. After ten or fifteen seconds have elapsed, by gently elevating the arms and legs, it will be found that the patient has a disposition to retain them in the situation in which they have been placed, if he is intensely affected.
>
> If this is not the case, in a soft tone of voice desire him to retain the limbs in the extended position, and thus the pulse will speedily become greatly accelerated [i.e., doubled], and the limbs, in process of time, will become quite rigid and involuntarily fixed [i.e., cataleptic]. It will also be found, that all the organs of special sense, excepting sight, including heat and cold, and muscular motion, or resistance, and certain mental faculties, are at first prodigiously exalted, such as happens with regard to the primary effects of opium, wine, and spirits. [The "primary" stage, of sensory excitation.] After a certain point, however, this exaltation of function is followed by a state of depression, far greater than the torpor of natural sleep. [The "ulterior" stage, of insensibility.]

Most accounts of Braid's method are based on this passage. However, even in this, his first book on the subject, he described alternative techniques. In a footnote, he adds,

> At an early period of my investigations, I caused the patients to look at a cork bound on the forehead. This was a very efficient plan with those who had the power of converging the eyes so as to keep them both steadily directed on the object. I very soon found, however, that there were many who could not keep both eyes steadily fixed on so near an object, and that the result was, that such patients did not become hypnotised. To obviate this, I caused them to look at a more distant point, which, although scarcely so rapid and intense in its effects, succeeds more generally than the other, and is therefore what I now adopt and recommend.

It is notable that this technique greatly resembles the "eye-roll" induction method popularised in recent decades by Herbert and David Spiegel.

Braid adds the following details in *Neurypnology* (1843), with regard to the specific position of the eyes in the eye-fixation induction and the dilation or contraction of the pupils.

> A patient may be hypnotised by keeping the eyes fixed in *any* direction. It occurs most *slowly* and *feebly* when the eyes are directed straight forward, and most *rapidly* and *intensely* when they can be maintained in the position of a double internal and upward squint.
>
> It is now pretty generally known, that during the effort to look at a very near object, there is produced, according to the direction of the object, a double internal squint, or double internal and downward or upward squint, and the pupils are thereby powerfully contracted. I am not aware, however, that it has been recorded, that by directing the eyes loosely, upwards or downwards, to the right or to the left, as if looking at a very distant

> object, the pupils become very much *dilated,* irrespective of the quantity of light passing to the retina; so that in this manner we can contract or dilate the pupil at will. To those who consider the movement of the iris as the mere effect of irritability, I may observe, in that view, the former position increases, the latter diminishes, the irritability. I may farther remark, if the eyes are much *strained* in ANY direction, I think the pupils will be found to contract as a consequence.

However, following the above passage, he states that he modified his technique to avoid causing excessive strain in the subject's eyes. Braid began simply to make the patient's eyes close once their pupils showed signs of what he calls the "wavy motion" of constriction and dilation. He presumably did so by moving his two extended fingers towards the eyes, as described above, in order to trigger the corneal reflex.

> At first I required the patients to look at an object until the eyelids closed of themselves, involuntarily. I found, however, that in many cases this was followed by pain in the globes of the eyes, and slight inflammation of the conjunctival membrane. In order to avoid this, I now close the eyelids, when the impression on the pupil already referred to has taken place, because I find that the *beneficial* phenomena follow this method, provided the eyeballs are kept fixed, and thus, too, the unpleasant feelings in the globes of the eyes will be prevented. Were the object to produce astonishment in the person operated on, by finding himself unable to open his eyes, the former method is the better; as the eyes once closed it is generally impossible for him to open them; whereas they may be opened for a considerable time after being closed in the other mode I now recommend. However, for curative purposes, I prefer the plan which leaves no pain in the globes of the eyes.

Crucially, Braid also acknowledged at this stage in his career that *expectation* and other psychological factors could produce the same hypnotic state without eye-fixation, or any induction process whatsoever. With some justification, however, he maintained that the physical procedure must usually be carried out at least once for this to be possible. It might be argued that for suggestion or autosuggestion to be completely effective, the client must (typically) be able to imagine the response suggested – a feat which is much easier if they have *previously* experienced it.

> It is important to remark, that the oftener patients are hypnotised, from association of ideas and habit, the more susceptible they become; and in this way they are liable to be affected *entirely through the imagination.* Thus, if they consider or imagine there is something doing, although they do not see it, from which they are to be affected, they *will become affected;* but, on the contrary, the most expert hypnotist in the world may exert all his endeavours in vain, if the party does not expect it, and mentally and bodily comply, and thus yield to it.

Although Braid clearly believed that the process of eye-fixation had certain inherent effects, it seems he thought that these could be enhanced or undermined by the client's expectations and mental attitude. The same is true of many other physical procedures, such as progressive muscle relaxation. In truth, therefore, Braid sees the effect of his eye-fixation induction as a combination of interacting physical and psychological factors, i.e., a genuine physical process of eye-fatigue compounded by verbal suggestion and expectant imagination.

Moreover, in his later writings Braid adds additional details. This may be because he modified his technique over time. However, it also seems likely that the description in *Neurypnology* was incomplete, and did not represent the variations employed by Braid even at an early stage in his work. In *Magic, Witchcraft, etc.* (1852), he writes,

> My usual mode of inducing the sleep is to hold any small bright object about ten or twelve inches above the middle of the forehead, so as to require a slight exertion of the attention to enable the patient to maintain a steady, fixed gaze on the object; the subject being either comfortably seated or standing, stillness being enjoined, and the patient requested to engage his attention, as much as possible, on the simple act of looking at the object, and yield to the tendency to sleep which will steal over him during this apparently simple process. I generally use my lancet case, held between the thumb and first two fingers of the left hand; but any other small bright object will answer the purpose. In the course of about three or four minutes, if the eyelids do not close of themselves, the first two fingers of the right hand, extended and a little separated, may be quickly, or with a tremulous motion, carried towards the eyes, so as to cause the patient involuntarily to close the eyelids, which, if he is highly susceptible, will either remain rigidly closed, or assume a vibratory motion – the eyes being turned up, with, in the latter case, a little of the white of the eyes visible through the partially closed lids. If the patient is not highly susceptible, he will open his eyes, in which case request him to gaze at the object, etc., as at first; and, if they do not remain closed after a second trial, desire him to allow them to remain shut after you have closed them, and then endeavour to fix his attention on muscular effort, by elevating the arms if standing, or both arms and legs if seated, which must be done quietly, as if you wished to suggest the idea of muscular action without breaking the abstraction, or concentrative state of mind, the induction of which is the real origin and essence of all which follows.

It may be that Braid means, in this passage, that he employed what would now be called an "eyelid catalepsy test" or "challenge", i.e., verbally challenging the client to try to open their eyes as a test of responsiveness. Otherwise, it seems unlikely he would claim to know that their eyes were sealed rigidly closed, or that they would open them without being instructed to. At least, modern hypnotherapy clients do not usually do so. He describes the induction of rigid arm catalepsy in a way that resembles his notion of "muscular suggestion", i.e., that the manipulation of the body suggests a certain response to the client's mind. His caution suggests that he may have previously found that carelessly handling the client's arms and legs sometimes broke their concentration and interfered with the technique.

Muscular Suggestion & Hypnotic Induction
I am not aware of any explicit attempt by Braid to interpret his technique of hypnotic induction in terms of his own theory of muscular suggestion. However, it seems tempting to do so. Braid had argued that many phenomena associated with phrenology and Mesmerism can be accounted for in terms of the tendency for muscular movements and body posture to evoke the subjective feelings which typically cause them, thereby reversing the normal causal sequence. For example, Braid observes that when a Christian subject, in hypnosis, is positioned with their hands clasped and head tilted to the heavens, they may experience an intense feeling of spiritual rapture.

Braid could have observed that if a subject is asked to sit motionless, with their eyes tired and closed, and to "suppress" (presumably relax and slow down) their breathing, it might be expected to physically suggest the sense of sleepiness that normally causes these muscular changes to occur, reversing the causal sequence between the feeling and its physical expression. From the perspective of Sarbin's social psychological model, or "role-taking" theory, the subject may begin by adopting the motor expressions of a role, which are more directly under normal voluntary control, in order to gradually evoke the autonomic changes associated with their perception of the role, which are not under their direct voluntary control. This is, of course, analogous to how an actor might approach a role, and even bring himself to tears by acting distraught. Indeed, one can suppose that an actor assuming the external mannerisms of a hypnotic subject may well be able to evoke the subjective experiences also, if he persevered and focused his intention upon doing just that.

Braid's Mature Theory of Hypnotism

> 'The clue to the real nature of this condition [hypnotism], however, having been found by Mr. Braid, in the undisturbed and concentrated operation of that principle of *suggestion*, which has long been well-known to Psychologists, he subsequently, under the guidance of this idea, followed-up the investigation of its varied manifestations with great zeal and intelligence.' (Carpenter, 1874: 617)

Braid's account of hypnotic states in *Neurypnology* (1843) is somewhat difficult to interpret and he never provides a simple outline of it. He may also conceive of the stages differently even in his other "early" writings. He does seem to stress that the states of hypnosis should be seen as consecutive stages (subsequent writers would say "levels"), but that (confusingly) the "deeper" stages can be modified to exhibit the characteristics of the earlier ones, if desired. It also seems likely that Braid thought of these as being loose classifications which merge into one another in graduated steps, i.e., he is describing vaguely *opposite* states, with a range of intermediate stages.

> From overlooking another important fact which I have repeatedly explained, that all the phenomena are consecutive, that is, first increased sensibility, mobility, and docility, and afterwards a subsidence into insensibility and cataleptiform rigidity, this gentleman, by mistaking and exhibiting the *primary* phenomena for the *secondary,* seems to have managed to deceive both himself and some others who are satisfied to look at such matters loosely. (*Neurypnology*, 1843)

He emphasises the varying degrees of responsiveness, but even at this stage stresses that many treatments are conducted with full consciousness, in the first stage of hypnosis,

> Moreover, there is great difference in the susceptibility to the neuro-hypnotic impression, some arriving at the state of rigidity and insensibility in a few minutes, whilst others may readily pass into the *primary* state, but can scarcely be brought into the ulterior, or rigid and torpid state. It is also most important to note, that many instances of remarkable and permanent cures have occurred, where it has never been carried beyond the state of consciousness. (*Neurypnology*, 1843)

Braid originally defined Neuro-Hypnotism as 'a peculiar condition of the nervous system, induced by a fixed and abstracted attention of the mental and visual eye, on one object, not of an exciting nature'. (*Neurypnology*, 1843). In his famous induction technique, the fixed *gaze* ('double inward and upward squint') and 'suppressed respiration' leads through a period of excitation to increasing nervous fatigue, but by the publication of *Neurypnology* Braid had already adopted the view that monotonous fixed *attention* upon an 'unexciting object' was equally important, leading to increasing mental 'abstraction' or absorption in a dominant idea to the increasing neglect of other external distractions or intrusive thoughts, etc. His patient and friend, the author Dr. Wilkinson, puts it in more colourful terms, approved and quoted by Braid,

> The preliminary state (of hypnotism) is that of abstraction, and this abstraction is the logical premise of what follows. Abstraction tends to become more and more abstract, narrower and narrower; it tends to unity, and afterwards to nullity. There, then, the patient is, at the summit of attention, with no object left – a mere statue of attention – a listening, expectant life – a perfectly undistracted faculty, dreaming of a lessening and lessening mathematical point, the end of his mind sharpened away to nothing. (Wilkinson, *The Human Body*, 1851: 396)

To which Braid adds,

> The above is a beautiful description painted in elegant and most felicitous language, of the phenomena manifested by a *certain class of patients*, and *at a certain stage of the sleep*; but at another stage the very opposite state manifests itself: for the abstraction may be so intense as to render the patient unconscious even of inflictions the most severe; and the muscles may be locked in immovable, cataleptic rigidity, or dissolved in the most entire passive flaccidity according to predominant ideas or impressions on the senses, which immediately preceded the full intensity of the all-absorbing abstraction. (Braid, *Magic, Witchcraft, etc.*, 1852)

Shortly after *Neurypnology*, in a series of letters on "phreno-hypnotism" (1843-1844), Braid distinguishes between *three* stages of hypnotism, but in doing so, seems primarily to be equating the first with excitement, the third with torpor, and interposing an intermediating and *transitional* stage (two) between them, which thereby seems to represent the *typical* hypnotic state.

First (Primary) Stage: Muscular Pliancy & Sensory Excitement
State of consciousness, nervous excitation, increased physical mobility, docility and pliancy, hyperacuity of special senses (except vision), especially increased acuteness of hearing, increased "arterialisation" (i.e., oxygenation) of blood. Clear recollection of experience. '[...] from overlooking the fact of the *first* stage of this artificial hypnotism being one of *excitement*, with the possession of *consciousness* and *docility*, many imagine they are *not* affected, whilst the acceleration of pulse, peculiar expression of countenance, and other characteristic symptoms, prove the existence of the condition beyond the possibility of a doubt, *to all who understand the subject.*' (*Neurypnology*, 1843)
Second (Ulterior) Stage: Muscular Catalepsy & Sensory Torpor
State of rigid catalepsy with diminishing sensibility and consciousness, decreased "arterialisation" of blood. Degrees of spontaneous amnesia for experience, or total (but reversible) amnesia in some cases. Braid says that the "second stage" follows naturally from the first with practice, but he also states 'I consider it very imprudent to carry it to the ulterior stage, or that of torpor, at a *first* trial'. (*Neurypnology*, 1843) It is likely that the rigid catalepsy described by Braid was an artefact of his method, which, following eye closure, involved raising the arms and legs (with seated subjects) and physically manipulating them so as to encourage them to be held in a rigid position for roughly 5-10 minutes on average. By the 1950s, at least, he had explicitly recognised that deep hypnosis could be accompanied by intense rigidity or flaccidity of the muscles depending upon the influence of expectation, physical manipulation, and verbal suggestion.

Braid's Later Model (Monoideism)
In *The Physiology of Fascination* (1855), Braid very clearly explains that his views had changed somewhat since the publication of *Neurypnology* (1843), introducing the new term "monoideism" to denote the change of emphasis in his work. In the early 1840s, he had satisfied himself that hypnosis was induced by the reciprocal interaction of internal physiological and psychological causes, stemming from focused attention, rather than by virtue of an invisible force channelled from another person, as the Mesmerists believed. By the 1850s, Braid had grown dissatisfied with the term "hypnotism", however, explaining,

> This term ["hypnotism"] has met with most favourable consideration from many able writers on the subject; still it is liable to this grave objection – that it has been used to comprise not a *single* state, but rather a series of stages or conditions, varying in every conceivable degree, from the slightest reverie, with high exaltation of the functions called into action [the "primary stage"], on the one hand, to intense nervous coma, with entire abolition of consciousness and voluntary power, on the other [the "ulterior stage"]; whilst, from the latter condition, by very simple, but appropriate means, the subject is capable of being speedily partially restored, or entirely roused, to the waking condition. (Braid, *The Physiology of Fascination*, 1855)

Braid's concern, in part, was that the expression "hypnotism" or "nervous sleep", carried the connotation of a loss of consciousness resembling natural sleep, which had been the cause of considerable misunderstanding, as this is not normally the case in hypnosis.

> It is of great importance that it should be clearly understood by patients, that it is by no means generally requisite that they should lapse into the state of *un*consciousness in order to ensure the salutary effects of the nervous sleep. Many imagine, that unless they become torpid and insensible, no beneficial effect can ensue. This is a complete misapprehension, for the happy results of innumerable cases treated with the greatest success by hypnotism, clearly prove that cases which had resisted all ordinary treatment [...] have readily yielded to the impression made on the nervous system by this peculiar influence, even when they were perfectly conscious of all that was done, and could remember, after awakening, every circumstance that had happened during the nervous sleep. (Braid, *Hypnotic Therapeutics*, 1853, *author's italics*)

Braid gradually accepted that in order to circumvent this problem, the terminology would have to be modified,

> I am well aware that, in correct phraseology, the term *hypnotism* ought to be restricted to the phenomena manifested in patients who actually pass into a state of sleep, and who remember nothing on awakening of what transpired during their sleep. All short of this is mere reverie, or dreaming, however provoked, and it, therefore, seems highly desirable to fix upon a terminology capable of accurately characterising these latter modifications which result from hypnotic processes. This is the more requisite from the fact that, of those who may be relieved and cured by hypnotic processes of diseases which obstinately resist ordinary medical treatment, perhaps not more than one in ten ever passes into the state of oblivious sleep, during the processes which they are subjected to. The term *hypnotism,* therefore, is apt to confuse them, and lead them to suspect that, at all events, *they* cannot be benefited by processes which fail to produce the most obvious indication which the name imports. (Braid, *The Physiology of Fascination*, 1855)

Indeed, Braid had argued that, despite his own choice of terminology, "hypnotic sleep" was essentially the *polar opposite* of normal sleep, insofar as it centred upon a state of mental concentration.

> [...] the real origin and essence of the hypnotic condition, is the induction of a habit of abstraction or mental concentration, in which, as in reverie or spontaneous abstraction, the powers of the mind are so much engrossed with a single idea or train of thought, as, for the nonce, to render the individual unconscious of, or indifferently conscious to, all other ideas, impressions, or trains of thought. The hypnotic sleep, therefore, is the very antithesis or opposite mental and physical condition to that which precedes and accompanies common sleep; for the latter arises from a diffusive state of mind, or complete loss of power of fixing the attention, with suspension of voluntary power. (Braid, *Magic, Witchcraft, etc.*, 1852)

Braid's experiments on the Reichenbach phenomena and electro-biology, etc., as well as Carpenter's researches on the ideo-motor reflex had convinced him that many "hypnotic" phenomena could manifest in the "waking state", without the use of any hypnotic induction whatsoever, merely by virtue of focused attention and/or dominant ideas, etc. He therefore proposed a more general term to encompass the whole range of states and phenomena which had arisen in relation to hypnotism – and which are currently considered under the heading of "hypnotism" by modern practitioners.

> And, finally, as a *generic term*, comprising the *whole* of these phenomena which result from the reciprocal actions of mind and matter upon each other, I think no term could be more appropriate than *psycho-physiology*. (Braid, *The Physiology of Fascination*, 1855)

This term is similar to the modern expression "mind-body", and meant to denote an interaction between mind and body, based on an explicitly dualist (Cartesian) theory of mind. It encompasses the full breadth of Braid's researches from the extreme condition of "human hibernation" and the "trances" of the Oriental yoga masters, to the "placebo" effects of phoney magnets exposed in his experiments on the Reichenbach phenomena, etc.

Psycho-Physiology ("Vigilant Phenomena")

In the normal waking state, the ideo-motor reflex, and other forms of ideo-dynamic action, are evoked by means of a wide range of suggestion techniques, to elicit therapeutic responses, without the use of any "induction" technique, or "special state", whatsoever. These are termed the "vigilant" (waking) phenomena of Mesmerism.

In debunking the pseudo-scientific energy therapies of his day – Mesmerism, magnetic therapy, phrenology, electro-biology, etc. – Braid developed a sophisticated theory of suggestion (and autosuggestion) which he soon realised could account for many hypnotic phenomena. However, hypnotism was specifically designed to enhance the effects of suggestion, and so (ironically) rather than falling victim to placebo controlled experiments, as many complementary therapies since have, its rationale was merely strengthened by the discovery of the extent to which expectation and similar factors affect the mind and body.

First Conscious Stage: Monoideism ("Mental Abstraction" or "Reverie")

From the outset, Braid had emphasised the role of "fixed attention", "concentration", "mental abstraction", etc., in hypnotism. By 1855 he had decided to change his terminology to make the centrality of this factor as explicit as possible. If only 10%, or less, of Braid's subjects entered the "double consciousness" state then by far the majority would be better characterised as in a state of mental abstraction or monoideism, being unusually focused on a single dominant idea, image, or train of thought. It should seem obvious that the technique of fixed gaze, which Braid never abandoned, could be seen as a means of narrowing the focus of attention down to a progressively diminishing point.

Braid equivocates about whether to call this "hypnosis" at all, because his subjects complained they did not "feel asleep". In *Magic, Witchcraft, etc.* (1852) he refers to it as the "waking", "vigilant", "sub-hypnotic" or "partial-hypnotic" state. He seems finally to have settled on the new term "monoideism", though retaining the word "hypnotism" to describe the practice in a loose sense, or to specifically designate the double consciousness (amnesic) state.

'Then *monoideism* will indicate the condition resulting from the mind being possessed by a dominant idea.' (Braid, *The Physiology of Fascination*, 1855)

Second Conscious Stage: Hypnotism ("Double Consciousness")

State in which (reversible) amnesia creates a temporary dissociation between the hypnotic and waking states, known by other authors as "hypnotic somnambulism". The subject enters a state superficially resembling sleep but in which the amnesia can be removed by suggestion in subsequent states of hypnosis. Note well, that as Braid observed, this suggests that the "loss of consciousness" attributed to hypnosis, at least in these cases, is illusory, the subject *was* conscious but has forgotten the experience. In *Magic, Witchcraft, etc.* (1852) Braid refers to the "second conscious stage" as the "double consciousness" stage, and as "full hypnosis".

'Let the term *hypnotism* be restricted to those cases alone in which, by certain artificial processes, oblivious sleep takes place, in which the subject has no remembrance on awaking of what occurred during his sleep, but of which he shall have the most perfect recollection on passing into a similar stage of hypnotism thereafter. In this mode, *hypnotism* will comprise those cases only in which what has hitherto been called the double-conscious state occurs.' (Braid, *The Physiology of Fascination*, 1855)

Third Stage: Hypnotic Coma ("Human Hibernation")

The ultimate stage of "torpor" or loss of consciousness. This would be an extremely unusual state insofar as Braid has already stated that only 10% of clients even experience the "double conscious" stage which precedes it. It is possible that Braid has this in mind when he refers to the idea of a state of "human hibernation" induced by Hindu mystics through an extreme form of Oriental "self-hypnotism", as he puts it in *Observations on Trance* (1850) and elsewhere. In Victorian medicine "catalepsy" or "trance" was the name given to a variety of serious medical conditions (including organic disorders and catatonic psychosis) which resulted in a rigid state superficially resembling death. Hence, Braid refers to 'the disease called catalepsy, or trance'. (1850). Unlike other hypnotists, Braid therefore seems to reserve the word "trance" solely for this, extreme, state of hypnosis, which he variously likens to sleep, hibernation, and coma.

'[...] let the term *hypnotic coma* denote that still *deeper* stage of the sleep in which the patient seems to be quite unconscious at the time of all external impressions, and devoid of voluntary power, and in whom no idea of what had been said or done by others during the said state of *hypnotic coma* can be remembered by the patient on awaking, or at *any* stage of *subsequent* hypnotic operations.' (Braid, *The Physiology of Fascination*, 1855)

Braid's Theory of Suggestion

Contrary to common misconception, Braid appreciated and employed the technique of verbal suggestion in hypnosis. Moreover, he considered suggestion essential to the practice of hypnosis and utilised an array of suggestion methods. Braid clearly distinguishes between suggestions given by the hypnotist and those arising from within the subject, e.g., due to expectant ideas, which we would now call "autosuggestion".

In *Magic, Witchcraft, etc.* (1852), Braid acknowledged that in addition to those "fully" hypnotised, many subjects were "partially" hypnotised, and that others did not respond to the induction at all. Nevertheless, they could be influenced by a variety of suggestive factors which he claimed were essential to the production of phenomena even in susceptible hypnotic subjects. In one passage alone, he lists the following six factors, which I have labelled using more contemporary terminology, supplying Braid's description in quotes,

1. **Spoken Verbal Suggestion.** 'The patients *hear the ideas suggested when uttered in a language known to them.*' Braid clearly recognises that changes in voice tonality have a profound effect upon verbal suggestions, and refers to this several times in his later writings.
2. **Written Verbal Suggestion.** 'When they see them written (which is sufficient to affect many).'
3. **Role-Modelling or Imitation.** 'When they can see, by ordinary vision, the movements made in their presence which it is intended they should be forced to imitate, through the power of sympathy and imitation.'
4. **Mental Association.** 'When they feel sensible impressions, associated with certain ideas or previous feelings.' For instance, the subject may hear a piece of music which reminds them of sad feelings; or sense the hand passes of the Mesmerist, and by association, imagine being a child once again, soothed by its mother's touch. Note that the Victorian concept of psychological association was a subjective precursor of the later physiological theory of conditioned responses pioneered by Pavlov's laboratory research.
5. **Muscular Suggestion.** 'When they feel sensible impressions [...] which call subjacent muscles into action.' For instance, when the body posture or facial expression ("Anatomy of Expression") is manipulated so as to evoke the corresponding idea or state of mind. For instance, the hypnotist may firmly grasp and briskly straighten a subject's arm in such a way as to suggest that it should become stiff and cataleptic. Alternatively, by clenching a subject's fist and furrowing his brow, Braid would evoke feelings of aggression, etc. In fact, this was the form of suggestion primarily employed by Braid in *Neurypnology* (1843), and used by him as the basis of his radical re-interpretation of phrenological phenomena. This notion, perhaps surprisingly, has many parallels in modern therapy, e.g., the notion of "acting as if" in George Kelly's work and subsequent cognitive-behavioural therapy.
6. **Focused Attention.** 'Direct attention to the special organs of sense, which excites ideas corresponding with the functions of these different organs, or arouses former ideas arbitrarily or accidentally associated with such and such sensible impressions.' As in the experiments on attention, debunking the Reichenbach phenomena, which show that prolonged or focused attention, can, *by itself,* lead to hyperacuity or create spontaneous hallucinatory sensations. Several modern studies have likewise shown that merely asking subjects to stare at a wall, or even sit with their eyes closed and contemplate their experience, tends to evoke a flow of surprisingly unusual experiences.

At the start of *Hypnotic Therapeutics* (1853), Braid again writes of 'suggestions received through words audibly uttered in his hearing [verbal suggestion], or ideas previously existing in his mind [autosuggestion], or excited by sensible impressions made by touches or passes of the operator [association], which direct the attention of the sleeper to different parts [focused attention], or excite into action certain combinations of muscles [muscular suggestion], and thereby direct his current of thought'. To a large extent, Braid's common sense philosophy of hypnotism and suggestion can be seen as deriving from the three basic laws of psychology adopted in his writings: the law of sympathy and imitation, the law of habit and association, and the ideo-dynamic response, which might be termed the "law of dominant ideas".

James Braid's Work & Writings
(Bramwell, 1896-1903)

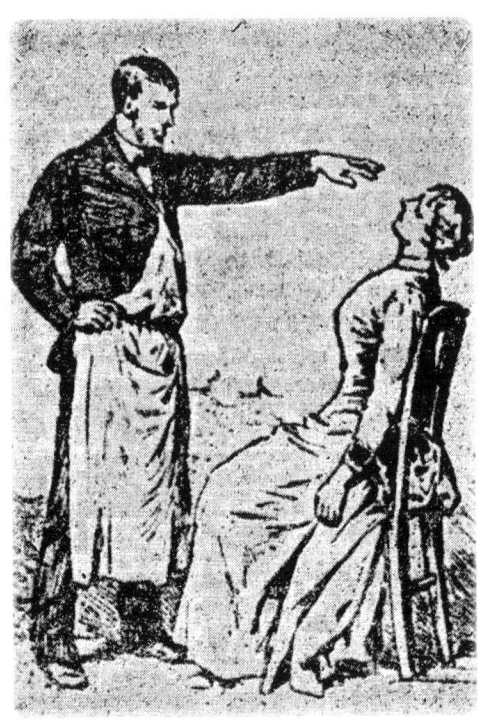

Figure 3. Lithograph portrait of Braid performing his "Two-Finger" Induction from *Anon., Mystères des Sciences Occultes (1894)*.

Editor's Preface
Donald Robertson

Bramwell's admirable summary of Braid's work is a gift to an editor. Over a century after it was written, it still stands up as the ideal introduction to Braid's own writings. John Milne Bramwell (1852-1925) was himself, like Braid, a Scottish physician and hypnotist. It seems he never had the opportunity to meet Braid personally – Bramwell was eight years old when Braid died – but Bramwell became the leading exponent of his views after assembling a personal library of Braid's writings, including several unpublished letters and manuscripts. At the end of the 19th Century, most of Braid's work was unknown in Britain, having fallen into obscurity. His views had been eclipsed in popularity by those of the French "Nancy School" of Liébault and Bernheim. Bramwell rightly highlights the fact that the main innovation attributed to the Nancy School, the shift in emphasis from physiology to psychology and from trance to suggestion, was already pre-figured in Braid's later, and less well-known, writings. Braid, not Liébault, was therefore indubitably the father of the "suggestion" approach to hypnotism.

Modified excerpts from the article were incorporated by Bramwell into *Hypnotism: Its History, Practice, & Theory* (1903), with an updated bibliography of Braid's works. I have included, as appendices to the main article, two short excerpts from Bramwell's later writings which help to illustrate his perception of the fundamental change of emphasis in Braid's later works.

Hypnotism: Its History, Practice & Theory (1903)
In this short excerpt, Bramwell provides a neat summary of the key concepts in Braid's later theory of hypnotism.

Hypnotism & Treatment by Suggestion (1909)
Bramwell's father had an interest in hypnosis, and as a child he had witnessed a number of experiments, including the methods of James Esdaile. Bramwell recounts how, after a demonstration of hypnotic anaesthesia at Leeds, on March 28th, 1890, he attracted a much wider range of clients with different presenting problems. He began to find reliance upon the traditional eye-fixation method insufficient and this led to a deeper investigation of the works of James Braid and further experimentation with hypnotic methods.

After much effort, he was able to hypnotise 75% of patients by trying different methods of inducing sleepiness and persisting throughout repeated sessions, sometimes *hundreds* of sessions. He gradually shifted emphasis, placing far more importance upon the role of verbal suggestion, even with clients who did not enter a sleepy state but remained completely aware. Bramwell realised that this mirrored the apparent movement away from "trance" and toward "suggestion" in Braid's later writings. This passage from Bramwell's *Hypnotism & Treatment by Suggestion* (1909) is important because it clearly illustrates the *re-interpretation* of hypnotism perceived in Braid's later writings by his main British disciple and commentator. Bramwell, like Braid, has become increasingly dissatisfied with the term "hypnosis" and the connotation that the practice *requires* a state resembling sleep.

Editorial Changes
Few changes were required to Bramwell's original text. I have removed his bibliography of Braid's work, because this is dealt with elsewhere in the current volume. I have also removed Bramwell's lengthy list of references. Some minor changes have been made to the formatting of his text in both the article and appendices, and a number of comments have been added in square brackets, where clarifications or additional details seemed necessary.

James Braid; His Work and Writings
(1896)
By Dr. John Milne Bramwell[3]

The name of James Braid is familiar to all students of hypnotism and is rarely mentioned by them without due credit being given to the important part he played in rescuing that science from ignorance and superstition. Regret is usually expressed, however, that he held many erroneous views, which it is claimed the researches of more recent investigators have disproved. The following, as far as I can gather from hypnotic works and from conversation with those interested in hypnotism, are the almost universally adopted opinions in reference to Braid.

(1) He was an English surgeon.
(2) He believed in phrenology.
(3) He was the discoverer or rediscoverer of the subjective origin of hypnotic phenomena.
(4) He knew nothing of suggestion.

In all this, one thing, and one alone, is correct, namely, that Braid was the rediscoverer of the subjective nature of hypnotic phenomena. This estimate of Braid has arisen from imperfect knowledge of his writings. Few seem to be acquainted with any of his works except "Neurypnology" or with the fact that this was only one of a long series on the subject of hypnotism, and that in the later ones his views completely changed. The necessarily limited length of this article will prevent my dealing with each of these separately and in detail. I propose, therefore, first to refer shortly to his earliest publication, then to give an account of the theories which are found in "Neurypnology" alone, and finally to present a general picture of his later opinions.

Meanwhile, a word as to Braid's nationality and to the events which led to his hypnotic researches. The names of Elliotson, Esdaile and Braid stand out prominently in the history of Mesmerism and hypnotism in this country, and it is not without interest to note that all of them studied at Edinburgh University and that both Esdaile and Braid were of Scotch birth and parentage, the latter being born at Rylaw House, Fifeshire, about 1795.

On November 13th, 1841, Braid, for the first time, was present at a Mesmeric séance [as they were known], the operator being [Charles] Lafontaine. At this time Mesmeric phenomena were believed to be due either to mysterious force or fluid, self-deception or trickery. Braid held the latter theory and, on the first occasion, saw nothing to cause him to alter his views. At the next séance, six days later, he noticed that one subject was unable to open his eyes [a phenomenon now known as 'eyelid catalepsy']. Braid regarded this as a real phenomenon and was anxious to discover its physiological cause; and the following evening, when the case was again operated on, he believed he had done so. After making a series of experiments, chiefly on personal friends and relatives, he expressed his conviction that the phenomena he had witnessed were purely subjective, and began almost immediately to place these views before the public, his first lecture being delivered on December 27th, 1841.

In 1842 Braid offered a paper on the subject of hypnotism to the Medical Section of the British Association. This was refused, whereupon he gave a conversazione [a kind of medical symposium or workshop] at which many members of the Association were present, read his paper and showed cases. His first work on Mesmerism was entitled "*Satanic Agency and Mesmerism" Reviewed*, with the lengthy subtitle, 'in a letter to the Rev. H. McNeile, AM., of Liverpool, in Reply to a Sermon preached by him at St. Jude's Church, Liverpool, on Sunday, April 10th, 1842'. McNeile had charged Braid with "refusing to state the laws of nature by the uniform action of which Mesmeric phenomena were produced". [McNeile also insinuated that Braid was doing the Devil's work, hence the peculiar title of his booklet.] To this Braid replied that he had always explained the phenomena on physiological and psychological principles, but that McNeile had refused to attend his lectures or to read any account of them. Braid at this time believed in the physical origin of hypnotic phenomena, and referred to the theory by which he attempted to explain certain changes in the central nervous system, more particularly decreased functional activity, as the result of the exhaustion of other nerve centres from continued monotonous stimulation. "But," he said, "even supposing my theories did not explain the whole of the phenomena, surely, when beneficial application could be made of the extent of the knowledge we had acquired, we ought to be at liberty to do so without being stigmatised from the pulpit as necromancers, or producing our effects by 'Satanic agency'. Supposing a hundred passengers start in one of your packets [a small boat], and 20 or 30 of them become sea-sick, and the others escape, would it be fair to implicate the captain in a charge of acting by Satanic agency because the *whole* were not sick, and because, according to McNeile, 'if it be in nature, it will operate uniformly and not capriciously? (...)

---

[3] [Republished by kind permission from The Society for Psychical Research Proceedings, vol. xii, 1896-1897: 127.]

If it operate capriciously, then there is some mischievous agent at work; and we are not ignorant of the devices of the devil.' Would any man but Mr. McNeile say that, because the captain gave the signal to heave anchor, to spread the sails, and other 'talismanic tokens' for steering the vessel, and because only part of the passengers became sick, he was consequently affecting *them* through Satanic agency – or that it would alter the matter one whit because medical men could not assign the true cause of this, or why anyone should be so affected?"

"Neurypnology"
"Neurypnology, or the Rationale of Nervous Sleep", was published by Braid in 1843, and 800 copies were sold in a few months.

At the séance already referred to, Braid had observed that the Mesmeric condition was induced by fixed staring, and concluded that the inability to open the eyes arose from paralysis of certain nerve centres and exhaustion of the levator muscles [the pair of muscles which raise the upper eyelids]. "I expressed," he said, "my entire conviction that the phenomena of Mesmerism were to be accounted for on the principle of the derangement of the state of the cerebral spinal centres, and of the circulatory, respiratory and muscular systems, induced by a fixed stare, absolute repose of body, fixed attention and suppressed respiration, concomitant with that fixity of attention. That the whole depended on the physical and psychical condition of the patient, arising from the causes referred to, and not at all on the volition, or passes of the operator throwing out magnetic fluid, or exciting to activity some mystical, universal fluid or medium."

Braid induced hypnosis by making the subject look at a bright object, held in such a position above the forehead as was calculated to produce the greatest possible strain upon the eyes and eyelids, while at the same time the mind was to be riveted on the idea of that one object. Braid not only maintained that the condition was a purely subjective one, produced in this mechanical way, but also claimed to have successfully demonstrated that it could be induced in like manner in persons who had never heard of Mesmerism and who were ignorant of what was expected of them. In illustration of this, he mentioned that he had hypnotised one of his servants, who knew nothing of Mesmerism, by giving him such directions as were calculated to impress his mind with the idea that his fixed attention was required merely for the purpose of watching a chemical experiment with which he was already familiar.

After having established the subjective origin of the phenomena, Braid proposed that they should be called hypnotic, instead of Mesmeric, and invented the following terminology:-

Neurypnology, the rationale or doctrine of nervous sleep.
Neuro-hypnotism, or nervous sleep, a peculiar condition of the system produced by artificial contrivance.

Then, for the sake of brevity, suppressing the prefix "neuro", the following terms:–

Hypnotic, the state or condition of nervous sleep.
Hypnotise, to induce nervous sleep.
Hypnotised, put into the condition of nervous sleep.
Hypnotism, nervous sleep.
Dehypnotise, to restore from the state of nervous sleep.
Hypnotist, one who practises neuro-hypnotism.

This terminology is closely followed at the present day, the main difference being that one now speaks of the science of hypnotism, instead of that of neurypnology, applying the term hypnosis to the artificial sleep, and hypnotic both to the phenomena and to the subject in whom they are induced.

Braid at this date came to the following general conclusions:-

1. [Hypnotic Induction.] "That the effect of a continued fixation of the mental and visual eye, in the manner and with the concomitant circumstances pointed out, is to throw the nervous system into a new condition, accompanied with a state of somnolence, and of a tendency, according to the mode of management of exciting a variety of phenomena different from those we obtain either in the ordinary sleep, or during the waking condition.
2. [Stages of Hypnotism.] "That there is at first a state of high excitement of all the organs of that the senses afterwards become torpid in a much greater degree than what occurs in natural sleep.
3. [Nervous Arousal.] "That in this condition we have the power of directing or concentrating nervous energy, raising or depressing it in a remarkable degree at will, locally or generally.
4. [Heart Rate.] "That in this state, we have the power of exciting the force and frequency of the heart's action, and the state of the circulation, locally or generally, in a surprising degree.
5. [Muscle Tone.] "That whilst in this peculiar condition, we have the power of regulating and controlling muscular tone and energy in a remarkable manner and degree.

6. [Physiological Changes.] "That we also acquire the power of producing rapid and important changes in the state of the capillary circulation, and on the whole of the secretions and excretions of the body, as proved by the application of chemical tests.
7. [Hypnotic Therapy.] "That this power can be beneficially directed to the cure of a variety of diseases which were most intractable, or altogether incurable, by ordinary treatment.
8. [Hypnotic Anaesthesia.] "That this agency may be rendered available in moderating, or entirely preventing, the pain incident to patients while undergoing surgical operations.
9. [Muscular Suggestion.] "That during hypnotism, by manipulating the cranium and face, we can excite certain mental and bodily manifestations, according to the part touched."

After hypnotising his patients, Braid manipulated them in various ways [positioning their body, facial expression, etc.], with a view to producing changes in the muscular and circulatory systems, believing that this excited the different hypnotic phenomena and played an important part in the cure of disease. He also held that cures could sometimes be effected by similar methods in the waking condition. From the description of his manner of inducing hypnosis, it is evident that he employed verbal suggestion, but, at this time, this was apparently done unconsciously and in ignorance of its value.

Braid found that he could terminate the hypnotic condition by means of a current of cold air. He also noticed that he could make a rigid limb flexible by blowing on it; that he could restore the sight to one eye by the same means and leave the other insensible; excite one half of the body to action, while the other remained rigid and torpid, or make the patient pass from a general state of inactivity of the organs of special sense and tonic muscular rigidity to the opposite condition of extreme mobility and excited sensibility. He acknowledged that he was unable to explain these extraordinary phenomena, but stated that he had no difficulty in reproducing them, that they were independent of any "rapport" between operator and patient and invariably appeared, no matter whether the current of air came from the lips, a pair of bellows, the motion of the hand, or any inanimate object.

The subjective explanation of the origin of Mesmeric phenomena was not a new one, and had already been given both by the Abbé Faria and [Alexandre] Bertrand. Their views, however, if not entirely forgotten, exercised no practical influence on Mesmeric theory, and Braid evidently was unacquainted with them when he commenced his Mesmeric researches; thus, his conclusions were arrived at independently, and successfully substituted for those universally held in his day. At a later date, when his opponents pointed out the similarity between the theories, Braid asserted that this was more apparent than real, as Faria had attributed everything to the effect of the imagination; on this point they differed, but were alike in asserting that neither contact nor magnetic fluid was necessary.

At this time Braid did not believe that the phenomena of hypnotism were the result of attention, for, in speaking of some articles on animal magnetism which had appeared in the *Medical Gazette* in 1833, he said: "In the writer's opinion, the phenomena are the result of attention strongly directed to different parts of the body, whereas, by my method, the attention is riveted to something outside the body."

In opposition to the theory that hypnotism resembled reverie, Braid said: "Reverie proceeds from an unusual quiescence of the brain, and inability of the mind to direct itself strongly to any one point. There is defect in the attention, which instead of being fixed on one subject, wanders over a thousand, and even on these is feebly and ineffectively directed. This is the very reverse of what is induced by my plan, because I rivet the attention to one idea, and the eyes to one point, as the primary and imperative condition."

Some experiments which Braid made as to the methods of inducing hypnosis appear to have first suggested alterations in his hypnotic theory and shaken his faith in the purely physical explanation of hypnotic phenomena. At first he had required his patients to look for a considerable time at some inanimate object, until the eyelids closed involuntarily. He frequently found, however, that this was followed by pain and slight conjunctivitis, and, in order to avoid this, he closed the patient's eyes at a much earlier stage. Despite this, he was able to hypnotise as easily as before and without subsequent unpleasant sensations. This led to further experiment, when he found he could induce hypnosis as readily in the dark, or with the eyes bandaged, as in the light and with the eyes uncovered; it being only necessary to keep the eyes fixed and the body and mind at absolute rest. He always failed, however, in young children and in persons of weak intellect, or of restless and excitable minds, who were unable to comply with these simple rules. As he succeeded with the blind, Braid concluded that impression was made through the mind and not through the optic nerve. "It is important to remark," he said, "that the oftener patients are hypnotised, from association of ideas and habits, the more susceptible they become; and in this way they are liable to be affected *entirely through the imagination.* Thus if they consider or imagine there is something doing, although they do not see it, from which they are to be affected, they will become affected; but on the contrary, the most expert hypnotist in the world may exert all his efforts in vain, if the party does not expect it, and mentally and bodily comply, and thus yield to it."

Braid at first was inclined to believe in phrenology and considered it possible that the passions, emotions and intellectual faculties could be excited during hypnosis by simple contact or friction over certain sympathetic points of the head and face. He cited 12 cases in which he thought he had observed these phenomena in subjects who were ignorant of phrenology, and who were not influenced by previous training, or by leading questions and suggestions on the part of the operator. He was not satisfied with these results, however, and stated that it was his intention to conduct a new series of experiments on fresh patients in order to ascertain to what extent it might be practicable, by arbitrary associations, to excite the opposite tendencies from the same point. He also thought it probable that errors might have arisen through the remarkable docility of hypnotic subjects, which made them anxious to comply with every suggestion or indication given by the operator. In reference to the proposed further experiments, he said, "There will thus be both positive and negative proof to aid us in determining whether there is any natural and necessary connection existing between the points manipulated and the manifestations excited; whether it may depend entirely upon associations which have originated from some partial knowledge of phrenology, from arbitrary arrangement, or accidental circumstances or causes which have been entirely overlooked or forgotten; and which afterwards produce the result from that ultimate law of the mind which ordains that the repetition of a definite sensation shall be followed by a renovation of the past feelings with which it was before associated. I am inclined to adopt this course, from my anxiety to remove every possible source of error, my object being neither to prove nor disprove the truth of phrenology. That during the nervous sleep, there is a power of exciting patients to manifest the passions and emotions, and certain mental functions in a more striking manner than the same individuals are capable of in the waking condition, no one can doubt who has seen much of these experiments. And it can in no way alter the importance of hypnotism as a curative power and extraordinary means of controlling and directing mental functions in a peculiar manner, by a simple association of impressions, whether we thus act on the brain as a single organ, or as a combination of separate organs; or whether the primary associations have originated from a special organic connection, or from some accidental and unknown cause, or from preconsulted arrangement and arbitrary association."

The following account of some hypnotic phenomena is drawn partly from "Neurypnology", and partly from other sources.

Braid recognised two distinct hypnotic conditions, which correspond practically with the late [English psychologist, and co-founder of the Society for Psychical Research] Mr. Edmund Gurney's "alert" and "deep" stages, also intermediate status between the two, one frequently gliding imperceptibly into the other. The deep stage was characterised by a condition of torpor more profound than that of natural sleep; the alert by exaltation of the special senses, increase in muscular sense and an exaltation of certain mental faculties. By the sense of smell, some patients were able to detect any person known to them, or to find the owner of any glove. They first smelt the glove and then unhesitatingly presented it to its owner, choosing him from amongst a large company. If the nostrils were stopped, however, the apparent clairvoyant faculty instantly disappeared. The sense of touch and the muscular sense were sometimes so remarkably increased that some subjects were able to write with great accuracy during hypnosis, when effectual precautions were taken to prevent their being able to see. They crossed the t's and dotted the i's and could even go back a line, strike out a letter and put it in its proper place. One patient could correct the writing on a whole page of note-paper, but if the relative positions of the table and paper were changed, the alterations ceased to be placed correctly. The following is an interesting account, published in The Medical Times for September, 1847, by an independent observer, of the power possessed by certain somnambules of imitating language and song.

> On Tuesday last, the 3rd [of the month], Mlle. Jenny Lind [a world-renowned *soprano*], accompanied by Mr. and Mrs. Schwabe, and a few of their friends, attended a séance at Mr. Braid's for the purpose of witnessing some of the extraordinary phenomena of hypnotism. There were two girls who work in a warehouse, and who had just come in their working attire. Having thrown them into the sleep, Mr. Braid sat down to the piano, and the moment he began playing, both somnambules arose and approached the instrument, when they joined him in a trio. Having awoke one of the girls Mr. Braid said, although she was ignorant of the grammar of her own language when awake, that when in the sleep she would prove herself competent to accompany anyone in the room in singing songs in any language, giving both notes and words correctly – a feat which she was quite incompetent to perform in the waking condition. He then requested anyone in the room to put her to the test, when Mr. Schwabe sat down to the instrument, and played and sang a German song, in which she accompanied him correctly, giving both notes and words simultaneously with Mr. Schwabe. Another gentleman then tried her with one in Swedish, in which she succeeded.
>
> Next the queen of song, the far-famed Jenny Lind, sat down to the instrument and sang most beautifully a slow air, with Swedish words, which the somnambulist accompanied her in, in the most perfect manner both as regards words and music. Jenny now seemed resolved to test the powers of the somnambulist to the utmost by a continued strain of the most difficult roulades and cadenzas, for which she is so famous, including some of her extraordinary *sostentuto* [sustained] notes, with all their inflections from *pianissimo* to *forte crescendo*, and again diminishing to thread-like *pianissimo*, but in all these fantastic tricks and displays of genius by the Swedish nightingale, even to the shake, she was so closely and accurately tracked by the somnambulist, that several in the room occasionally could not have told, merely by hearing, that there were two individuals singing – so instantaneously did she catch the notes, and so perfectly did their voices blend and accord.
>
> Next, Jenny having been told by Mr. Braid that she might be tested in some other language, this charming songstress commenced '*Casta Diva*,' and the '*A la Bell a mu Ritornella*', in which the fidelity of the somnambulist's performance, both in words and music, was most perfect, and fully justified all Mr. Braid had

alleged regarding her powers. She was also tested by Mlle. Lind in merely imitating language, when she gave most exact imitations; and Mr. Schwabe also tried her by some most difficult combinations of sound, which he said he knew no one was capable of imitating correctly without much practice, but the somnambulist imitated them correctly at once, and that whether spoken slowly or quickly. When the girl was aroused, she had no recollection of anything which had been done by her, or that she had afforded such a high gratification to all present, by proving the wonderful powers of imitation which are acquired by some patients during a state of artificial somnambulism; she said she merely felt somewhat out of breath, as if she had been running.

Despite long perseverance, Braid never succeeded in hypnotising idiots, and he found that one patient, who had been easily hypnotised when well, became refractory during the delirium of fever. With the majority of his patients there was no loss of consciousness; they simply became lethargic and retained complete recollection of all that had occurred; with others many hypnotic phenomena could be produced without their having previously passed through a condition in any way resembling sleep. This state was popularly described as the "electro-biological", a name which Braid justly termed ridiculous. [Two Americans had apparently copied Braid's eye-fixation method but passed it off as a peculiar electro-magnetic effect caused by staring at a metal disc. Their public exhibitions in England had attracted great attention, but Braid rightly dismissed their theory as pseudo-scientific.] In some instances hypnotised patients, even after having undergone surgical operations, remembered nothing, while others, to whom he had taught Greek, Latin, French, and Italian during hypnosis, forgot it all when awake. When re-hypnotised the lost memory frequently returned spontaneously, but if it did not do so, the operator could revive it by placing his hand on any part of the patient's body and thus giving a physical aid to the concentration of attention. [The ability to recover such memories indicates that the patient was probably conscious during hypnosis.] Suggestions made to these patients during hypnosis were fulfilled in the waking state, despite the fact that they had apparently been entirely forgotten.

Analogous States
In hypnotism, Braid found an explanation of the prolonged trance of the fakirs and of the voluntary suspended animation of Colonel Townsend; some instances of the former being remarkably well authenticated by the evidence of English officers of position. On one occasion a fakir was buried at a depth of four feet; it was arranged that the experiment should last nine days and an English officer had the grave constantly watched by sentinels. At the end of the third day, the officer, fearing the fakir might be dead, and that this would be the cause of trouble to himself, insisted on the termination of the experiment. When the man was dug up he was as stiff and cold as a mummy and apparently lifeless; he revived, however, after being manipulated for about a quarter of an hour.

Braid considered that there was a marked resemblance between the condition produced by hashish and certain hypnotic states, and in support of this, quoted the following experiments made by Dr. O'Shaughnessy at Calcutta, and published in Pereira's "Elements of Materia Medica":–

> At 2 p.m. a grain of the resin of hemp was given to a rheumatic patient. At 4 p.m. he was very talkative, sang, called loudly for an extra supply of food and declared himself in perfect health. At 6 p.m. he was asleep. At 8 p.m. he was found insensible, but breathing with perfect regularity, the pulse and skin natural, and the pupils freely contractile on the approach of light. Happening by chance to lift up the patient's arm, the professional reader will judge of my astonishment, when I found it remained in the posture in which I had placed it. The patient had become cataleptic. We raised him to a sitting posture, and placed his arms and limbs in every imaginable attitude. A waxen figure could not be more pliant. He continued in this state till 1 a.m., when consciousness and voluntary motion quickly returned.

A similar experiment was made with another patient with like results.[4]

Before considering the later works, it will be well to examine some of the opinions expressed in reference to Braid, which apparently indicate that the writers were acquainted with "Neurypnology" alone. Dr. Bastian, in his article on Braidism in Quain's *Dictionary of Medicine*, expressed his regret that Braid did not reject all the so-called phenomena of phrenohypnotism. Professor [George John] Romanes [a Victorian psychologist] also appears to have been only acquainted with "Neurypnology", and mentions it alone in his article on "Hypnotism in the *Nineteenth Century*" for September, 1880. He refers to the fact that Heidenhain omits all reference to Braid and maintains that it would be doing scant justice to "Neurypnology" to say that all Heidenhain's results had been anticipated.

> [...] in the vast number of careful experiments which it ["Neurypnology"] records – all undertaken and prosecuted in a manner strictly scientific – it carried the inquiry into various provinces which have not been entered by Heidenhain. No one can read Braid's work without being impressed by the care and candour with which, amid violent opposition from all quarters, his investigations were pursued; and now, when after the lapse of nearly 40 years, his results are beginning to receive the confirmation which they deserve, the physiologists

---

[4] [A "grain" is a minute measure of weight and it is difficult to understand how such a small quantity of cannabis resin could induce any effect, though similar effects might be induced by a much larger quantity of the same substance.]

who yield it ought not to forget the credit that is due to the earliest, the most laborious, and the hitherto most extensive investigator of the phenomena of what he calls hypnotism.

The following passage in "Suggestive Therapeutics", published in 1890, shows that, at that date at all events, Bernheim was unacquainted with Braid's advanced theories:– "Braid made use of suggestion without knowing it. We must come down to 1860 to find the doctrine of suggestion freed from all the elements that falsified it, even in the hands of Braid himself, and applied in the simplest manner to therapeutics. The patient is put to sleep by means of suggestion. He is treated by means of suggestion. The subject being hypnotised, Liébault's method consists in affirming in a loud voice the disappearance of his symptoms. Such is the method of therapeutic suggestion of which M. Liébault is the founder. He was the first to clearly establish that the cures of pain by the old magnetisers, and even by Braid's hypnotic operations, are not the work either of a mysterious fluid or of physiological modifications due to special manipulations, but the work of suggestion alone."

In the *Journal of the Society for Psychical Research* for March, 1896, M. Boirac, in replying to Dr. Walter Leaf's criticism of "L'Hypothèse du Magnétisme Animal", which appeared in the number of the *Proceedings* for December, 1895 (Part XXIX.), states that he associates Braid with the Paris school (hypnotism) and Faria with the Nancy school (suggestion).[5]

General Theory

In the commencement of "Neurypnology", as we have seen, Braid explained hypnotic phenomena mainly from the physical standpoint, and held that they could be induced by fixed staring at an inanimate object, even in persons who had heard nothing of hypnotism or Mesmerism, and who were ignorant of what was required of them. In the later chapters, however, these views were considerably modified and he talks of persons being hypnotised entirely through their imagination, and also of the uselessness of the efforts of the most expert Mesmeriser if the patient were ignorant of his aims. In his other works the physical theory is entirely abandoned in favour of a purely psychical one. After explaining what induced him to adopt the term hypnotism in preference to that of Mesmerism, he stated that the word hypnotism was liable to grave objections, as under it had been comprised, not a single state, but a series of stages or conditions varying in every conceivable degree, and that:–

> "In correct phraseology, the term hypnotism ought to be restricted to the phenomena manifested in patients who actually pass into a state of sleep, and who remember nothing on awakening of what has transpired. Of those who may be relieved or cured by hypnotic processes, perhaps not more than one in ten ever passes into the state of oblivious sleep. The term hypnotism, therefore, is apt to confuse them and lead them to suspect that they cannot be benefited by processes which fail to produce the most obvious indication which their name imports."

Braid, therefore, proposed to alone call hypnotic those cases of artificial sleep followed by amnesia on awakening, but in which there is perfect recollection of what has happened when the patient is again hypnotised. [This form of hypnosis was sometimes called "double consciousness" or "artificial somnambulism".] Hypnotic coma he described as that deeper stage in which the lost memory is not revived in subsequent hypnoses.

> I became satisfied that the hypnotic state was essentially a state of mental concentration, during which the faculties of the mind of the patient were so engrossed with a single idea or train of thought as, for the nonce, to render it dead or indifferent to all other considerations and influences. The consequence of this concentrated attention, again, to the subject in hand, intensified, in a correspondingly greater degree, whatever influence the mind of the individual could produce upon his physical functions during the waking condition, when his attention was so much more diffused and distracted by other impressions. Moreover, inasmuch as words spoken, or various sensible impressions made on the body of an individual by a second party, act as suggestions of thought and action to the person impressed, so as to draw and fix his attention to one part or function of his body, and withdraw it from others – whatever influence suggestions and impressions are capable of producing during the ordinary waking condition, should naturally be expected to act with correspondingly greater effect during the *nervous sleep,* when the attention is so much more concentrated, and the imagination, faith, and expectant ideas in the mind of the patient are so much more intense than in the ordinary waking condition. Now, this is precisely what happens; and I am persuaded that this is the most philosophical mode of viewing the subject; and it renders the whole clear, simple, and intelligible to the apprehension of the unprejudiced person, who may at once perceive that the real object and tendency of the various processes for inducing a state of hypnotism or Mesmerism is obviously to induce a state of abstraction or concentration of attention – that is, a state of monoideism, whether that may be by requesting the subject to look steadfastly at some unexciting, and empty inanimate thing, or ideal object, or inducing him to watch the fixed gaze of the operator's eyes, his pointed fingers, or other manoeuvres of the Mesmeriser. (…)
>
> Then, inasmuch as I feel satisfied that the mental and physical phenomena which flow from the said

---

[5] [Charcot's "Paris" school saw hypnosis primarily as a physiological state, whereas the rival "Nancy" school of Liébault and Bernheim argued that it was primarily a psychological state of heightened suggestibility – the Nancy school effectively won the debate.]

processes result entirely from the mental impressions or dominant ideas, excited thereby in the minds of the subjects, changing or modifying the previously existing physical action, and the peculiar physical action thus superinduced reacting on their minds – and that, whether these dominant expectant ideas existed in the minds of the subjects previously, or were suggested to them after passing into the impressible condition, audible suggestions or sensible impressions excited by manipulations of a second party – under these circumstances, I consider the following terms calculated to realise all the precision which we may desire on this point.

Let Mono-ideology indicate the doctrine of the influence of dominant ideas in controlling mental and physical actions.
Then Monoideism will indicate the condition resulting from the mind being possessed by dominant ideas.
To monoideise will indicate the act of performing processes for inducing the act of monoideism.
Monoideiser will indicate the person who monoideises.
Monoideised will indicate the condition of the person who is in a state of monoideism.
And Monoideo-dynamics will indicate the mental and physical changes, whether of excitement or depression, which result from the influence of Monoideism.
And, finally, as a generic term, comprising the whole of these phenomena which result from the reciprocal actions of mind and matter upon each other, I think no term could be more appropriate than Psycho-Physiology." [*The Physiology of Fascination* (1855)]

This theory was first published by Braid in 1847. The fascination of birds by serpents, the phenomena of electro-biology, of table-turning, the gyrations of the odometer of Dr. Mayo, the magnetometer of Mr. Rutter, the movements of the divining rod, the supposed levity of the human body when lifted on the tips of the fingers of four individuals, were all, according to Braid, examples of unconscious or involuntary muscular action resulting from dominant ideas. When the attention of man or animal, he said, is absorbed by an idea associated with movement, a current of nervous force is sent into the muscles and a corresponding motion produced, not only without conscious effort, but even in many instances in opposition to the volition. The subject loses the power of neutralizing the dominant idea and is irresistibly drawn or spellbound according to the nature of the impression produced, and may, in this way, be brought under the control of others by means of audible, visible, and tangible suggestions.

The mental and physical phenomena, no matter what processes were employed to induce hypnosis, resulted entirely from the mental impressions or dominant ideas, thereby excited in the minds of the subjects. It was a matter of indifference whether these ideas existed in the subject's mind previously, or were afterwards suggested by audible suggestions or sensory impressions created by the manipulations of the operator.

Braid held that the operator acted like an engineer and called into action the forces in the patient's own organism, and controlled and directed them in accordance with the laws which governed the mind upon the body.

In reference to "Electro-Biological Phenomena, considered physiologically and psychologically", published in 1851, Braid stated that its object was to prove the subjectivity of the hypnotic and Mesmeric condition, and to show that the phenomena resulted from the concentrated mental attention of the patient acting on his own physical organism, and of the changed condition of the physical action thus induced reacting on the mind of the patient. That the changed physical condition arose from the action of predominant ideas, and that those ideas might arise in the minds of the patients, and become operative on them, through their own unaided acts – or from the mere remembrance of past feelings, without any co-operation or act of a second party; and that, in certain subjects, they might also be excited by audible, visible, or tangible suggestions from another person, to any extent whatsoever – even before they passed into a state of sleep. Braid stated that he had held and endeavoured to prove this theory *more than five years previously.*[6]

In reply to a writer [J.C. Colquhoun] who had adopted in a modified form the objective theory of Mesmeric phenomena, Braid says [in his book *Magic, Witchcraft, Animal Magnetism*, etc. (1852)]:–

If Mr. Newnham would only condescend to consider the simple subjective theory which I have ventured to propound, I think he might readily comprehend how the new modes of excitement, or depression, or peculiar distribution of the nervous or vital influence *within the patient's own body* might arise through the influence of *his own mind acting on his physical organism,* and might thus account for all which is realised without the transmission of any occult influence from one human being to *another.* I readily grant, however, that the looks, words and actions of a second party may furnish suggestions influential upon others – just as a word of encouragement, spoken or written by a friend, may nerve our arm with greater power, and inspire our tongue with greater eloquence – and that a lively companion, or encouraging expression may excite us; whilst a grave companion or doubtful expression would chill and depress – and that hope and confidence, or the contrary, in the means used, may modify, to a remarkable extent, the results under any mode of treatment. Still, I believe that there is no positive interchange or transference of *nervous* or *vital* force *from* the operator to the patient as the *actual cause* of these results, as has been alleged by the Mesmerists. I do *not* believe that, in such

---

[6] [In other words, Braid claimed to have shifted from a physiological to a psychological theory of hypnotism, emphasising the role of expectation and suggestion, just prior to his publication of The Power of the Mind over the Body (1846).]

instances, *A* loses an amount of power equivalent to what *B* gains. I do *not* believe that a preacher, an orator, or an author loses an amount of vital force in *exact ratio to the numbers* influenced by his spoken or printed ideas, sentiments and illustrations – which would necessarily be the case were the magnetic theory true. On the contrary, *I do believe* that the perusal of a posthumous work might be equally influential as if the book had been printed when the author was alive – and that the simple suggestion of new ideas to the mind of the reader, through the printed symbols of thought, is the real efficient cause of the future results.

In "Neurypnology", Braid stated that he was unable to account for the action of a current of air upon hypnotised subjects; at a later date he gave the following theory. In hypnosis the attention is concentrated upon the particular function called into action, while the others merge into a state of torpor; thus, only one function is active at any one time and hence intensely so. The arousing of any dormant function is equivalent to superseding the one in action, and he explained, therefore, the termination of a state of muscular rigidity when a current of cold air is directed to the skin, by suggesting that this called the attention to the skin, and withdrew it from the muscular sense.

Braid considered the following to be the chief points of difference between spontaneous and induced somnambulism. Spontaneous somnambulists are impelled to certain trains of action by internal impulses, while the induced [i.e., hypnotised] tend to remain at absolute rest and to lapse into a state of profound sleep, unless excited by some impression from without.

Natural and artificial sleep were not regarded by Braid as identical, and the following are further points of contrast in addition to those already mentioned [in the earlier section on *Neurypnology*]. The pupils are dilated in hypnosis and the eyelids either quiver continuously, or are firmly closed by spasmodic contractions. In passing into hypnosis, anything held in the hand is grasped still more firmly. There is an increase of the muscular sense, and hypnotic subjects possess an extraordinary power of balancing themselves. Chronic rigidity of the muscles is not followed by corresponding exhaustion. Sometimes in the hypnotic state there is excitement, similar to that produced by wines and spirits, at others there is muscular quiescence, with acute hearing and dreamy, glowing imagination, closely resembling the condition induced by Conium [i.e., hemlock, a poison used in Victorian medicine as a sedative].

> The principal difference between the hypnotic or nervous sleep and common sleep consists in the state or condition of the mind. In passing into common sleep the mind is diffusive or passive, flitting from one idea to another indifferently, thereby rendering the subject unable to fix his attention on any regular train of thought, or to perform any acts requiring much effort of will. The consequence of this is that a state of passiveness is manifested during the sleep, so that audible suggestions and sensible impressions addressed to the sleeper, if not intense enough to wake him entirely, seldom do more than excite a dream, in which ideas pass through his mind without exciting definite physical acts; but, on the other hand, the active and concentrated state of the mind engendered by the processes of inducing the nervous sleep, are carried into the sleep, and, in many instances, excite the sleeper, without awaking, to speak or to exhibit physical manifestations of the suggestions received through words audibly uttered in his hearing, or ideas previously existing in his mind, or excited by sensible impressions made by touches or passes of the operator, which direct the attention of the sleeper to different parts, or excite into action certain combinations of muscles, and thereby direct his current of thought.

Another difference is the wonderful power of hypnosis in curing many diseases, which had resisted natural sleep and every known agency for years. For instance, a few hypnotic séances of ten minutes each cured a patient who must have had during his long illness at least eight years' sleep. [Hypnotic sleep, therefore, appears to be much more therapeutic than natural sleep.]

Magnets, etc.
In Braid's time the Mesmerists held that magnets, certain metals, crystals, etc., possessed a peculiar power and, with sensitive subjects, were capable of producing attraction and other remarkable phenomena. Some experienced an unpleasant sensation like an aura, others got headache, or attacks of fainting or catalepsy, with spasms so violent that they apparently endangered life. Frequently there was hyperaesthesia of the special senses [i.e., heightened sensory perception]. Many also fancied they saw fiery bundles of light stream from the poles of the magnet. All this was said to happen even when the subjects did not see the magnets and did not know what was being done. Braid performed many experiments in order to test these statements, with the following results:– the phenomena appeared when the patients had preconceived ideas on the subject, or when these were excited by leading questions, but were invariably absent when they were ignorant of what was being done. Pretended magnets also produced the phenomena when the patients knew what was expected to occur. [Baron Karl von] Reichenbach [a distinguished German chemist who postulated an invisible energy, called "odylic", after the Norse god Odin] recorded an instance where, by the mere exposure of a sensitive plate in a box with a magnet, an impression had been made, as if it had been exposed to the full influence of the light. Braid repeated this experiment, and also had similar ones performed for him by an expert photographer and, when all sources of fallacy were guarded against, the results were invariably negative. According to Braid, the mind of the patient alone was sufficient to produce the affects attributed to magnetic or odylic force and suggested ideas were capable of exciting a great variety of physical sensations and mental conditions.

The following is an account of an experiment of Braid's to show that suggestion was the true explanation of the supposed Mesmeric powers of magnets and certain metals:–

> When in London lately I had the pleasure of calling upon an eminent and excellent physician, who is in the habit of using Mesmerism in his practice, in suitable cases, just as he uses any other remedy. He spoke of the extraordinary effects he had experienced from the use of magnets applied during the Mesmeric state, and kindly offered to illustrate the fact on a patient who had been asleep all the time I was in the room, and in that state during which I felt assured she could overhear every word of our conversation. He told me that when he put the magnet into her hands, it would produce catalepsy of the hands and arms, and such was the result. He wafted [air onto] the hands and the catalepsy ceased. He said that the mere touch of a magnet on a limb would stiffen it, and such he proved to be the fact.
>
> I now told him that I had got a little instrument in my pocket, which although far less than his, I felt assured would prove quite as powerful, and I offered to prove this by operating on the same patient, whom I had never seen before, and who was in the Mesmeric state when I entered the room. My instrument was about three inches long, the thickness of a quill, with a ring attached to the end of it. I told him that when put into her hands, he would find it catalepsize both hands and arms, as his had done, and such was the result. Having reduced this by wafting, I took the instrument from her, and again returned it, in another position, and told him it would now have the very reverse effect – that she would not be able to hold it, and that although I closed her hands on it, they would open and that it would drop out of them, and such was the case – to the great surprise of my worthy friend, who now desired to be informed what I had done to the instrument to invest it with such new and opposite power. This I declined doing for the present; but I promised to do so when he had seen some further proofs of its remarkable powers. I now told him that a touch with it, on either extremity, would cause the extremity to rise and become cataleptic, and such was the result; that a second touch on the same part would reduce the rigidity, and cause it to fall, and such again was proved to be the fact. After a variety of other experiments, every one of which proved precisely as I had predicted, she was aroused.
>
> I now applied the ring of my instrument on the third finger of the right hand, from which it was suspended, and told the doctor, when it was so suspended, it would send her to sleep. (To this he replied, 'It never will,' but I again told him that I felt confident that it would send her to sleep.) We then were silent, and very speedily she was once more asleep. Having aroused her, I put the instrument on the second finger of her left hand, and told the doctor it would be found she could not go to sleep when it was placed there. He said he thought she would, and he sat steadily gazing at her, but I said firmly and confidently that she would not. After a considerable time, the doctor asked her if she did not feel sleepy, to which she replied, 'Not at all'. 'Could you rise and walk?' When she told him she could, I then requested her to look at the point of the forefinger of her right hand, which I told the doctor would send her to sleep, and such was the result; after being aroused, I desired her to keep a steady *gaze* at the nail of the thumb of the left hand, which would send her to sleep in like manner, and such proved to be the fact.
>
> Having repaired to another room, I explained to the doctor the real nature and powers of my little and apparently magical instrument, that it was nothing more than my portmanteau key and ring, and that what had imparted to it such apparently varied powers was merely the predictions which the patient had overheard me make to him, acting upon her in the peculiar state of the nervous sleep, as irresistible impulses to be effected, according to the results she had heard me predict. Had I predicted that she would see any flame, or colour, or form, or substance, animate or inanimate, I knew from experience that such would have been realised, and responded to by her; and that, not from any desire on her part to impose upon others, but because she was self-deceived, the vividness of her imagination in that state inducing her to believe, as real, what were only the figments of fancy, suggested to her mind by the remarks of others. The power of suggestions of this sort also in paralysing or energising muscular power is truly astonishing; and may all arise in perfect good faith with almost all patients who have passed into the second conscious state [i.e., "artificial somnambulism"] and with some during the first conscious state.

In 1843, Braid referred to Elliotson's belief in the powers of certain metals, and to Wakley's experiments. The latter, operating with a non-Mesmerising metal, made the patient believe he was using a Mesmerising one, whereupon she fell asleep; and he concluded that all the subjects were imposters. Braid denied this, asserting that the active agent was simply the imagination, and that the metals were neither Mesmeric nor non-Mesmeric. In the same way, he explained the action of the wooden tractors which Dr. [John] Haygarth, in 1799, successfully substituted for the metal ones of Mr. Perkins. The latter consisted of two pieces of metal, one apparently of iron and the other of brass, about three inches long, blunt at one end and pointed at the other. They were invented by Dr. Elisha Perkins of Norwich, Connecticut, who in 1796 took out a patent for them, and were applied by drawing [the pointed ends of] them lightly over the [skin covering the] part affected for about 20 minutes. This method of treatment, which was very fashionable at one time, was termed Perkinism, in honour of its inventor. [Perkinism gradually fell out of fashion, becoming ridiculed as a *nostrum*, or quack remedy.]

According to Braid, it had long been recognised that various anomalous sensations followed the prolonged direction of the attention to any part of the body; but notwithstanding the fact that remarkable cures had occasionally been caused by mental excitement, and severe illness and even death had resulted from fear, it was usually supposed that these anomalous sensations were unaccompanied by physical change. With the exception of Dr. [Henry] Holland, who wrote on the influence of attention on the bodily organs in his "Medical Notes and Reflections" [1839], no one, Braid said, entertained the idea that definite and special physical changes could be excited, regulated, and controlled at will by the voluntary mental efforts of a healthy individual directed towards his own body; or that the same results might be produced involuntarily, by the suggestions of another person conveyed directly, verbally, or indirectly, by means of passes, etc. The following are examples of the power of suggestion in causing alterations in bodily function:–

> I had told a friend that it sufficed to arouse certain ideas as to her condition in the patient's mind in order to produce the corresponding alterations in the functions of the organ or part of the body referred to; as he was not inclined to believe my statement, I told him I could increase the secretion of milk in one of his wife's breasts (she happened to be nursing a child at the time), by calling her attention to the breast during hypnosis. Eight months previously I had hypnotised this lady and cured her of severe headache. She was a good somnambule.

After obtaining the patient's consent, but without telling her of the proposed experiment, Braid hypnotised her and drew her attention to her breast. On being awakened, she remembered nothing of what had been said or done, but complained of a feeling of tightness and tension in the breast. Her husband then told her that Braid had been trying to increase the secretion of milk. She replied, "That would be no light matter, for my child is 14 months old, and I have hardly any milk." Braid asked her to send for the child and to put it to the breast, when it got so much milk that it was nearly choked. A few days later the patient complained that her figure was deformed in consequence of the swelling of the left breast. Braid hypnotised her again and repeated the experiment with the right breast. The result was precisely the same, and both breasts now secreted so much milk that the lady was able to suckle her child for six months longer [until it was aged 1 year and 8 months], whereas before she had always complained of lack of milk.

The value of the hypnotic mode of treatment was best shown, according to Braid, by "cases of hysterical paralysis, in which, without organic lesion, the patient may have remained for a considerable length of time perfectly powerless of a part or of the whole body, from a dominant idea which has paralysed or misdirected his volition. In such cases, by altering the state of the circulation, and breaking down the previous idea and, substituting a salutary idea of vigour and self-confidence in its place, *which can be done by audible suggestions addressed to the patient, in a confident tone of voice, as to what must and shall be realised by the processes he has been subjected to* – on being aroused a few minutes afterwards, with such dominant idea in their minds, to the astonishment of themselves as well as of others, the patients are found to have acquired vigour and voluntary power over their hitherto paralysed limbs, as by a magical spell of witchcraft."

The power of imagination and excited attention, in producing a specific influence in a healthy person, was beautifully illustrated, he said, in the following case:–

> Having heard an account of some extraordinary discovery in America, of certain medicines which could manifest their influence through glass, that is, that by taking hold of a phial in which the medicine was contained, it would impart its peculiar medicinal virtue through the closed phial [a similar assumption is employed today in "applied kinesiology" used for food intolerance testing, etc.] – having read this account, I named it to certain parties, who scouted the idea as preposterous. I told them I did not doubt the fact of such physical effects resulting from such means, but added that I very strongly suspected [i.e., doubted] the correctness of the physiology of the explanation. I was inclined to believe it quite possible that it arose from vivid imagination, attention and expectation, exciting the particular function to be acted upon. This they scouted as equally preposterous, which induced me to repeat my conviction of the possibility of such a result taking place (although I had never tried it), and I also proposed to test it forthwith, in their presence. With this view, I requested an ounce phial to be brought to me, filled with common water, coloured with syrup of poppies which I meant to use for the purpose of acting as an emetic [a drug that stimulates vomiting]. We then repaired to a room, where there was a female friend, who knew nothing of our intentions. I then commenced talking to the gentlemen, but so that she could hear the conversation, about the remarkable discovery of this extraordinary medium, which could act as an emetic through the glass. I then requested this lady to oblige me by trying its effects. She was very unwilling to encounter it, but at length was prevailed upon to do so, by my assuring her it would much oblige me, and we could all place the most implicit confidence in her veracity. She very soon stated that it gave her an unpleasant feeling extending up the arm. I encouraged her to persevere, assuring her it would only make her sick, and added that when it got as high as the shoulder it would suddenly dart across the chest, when it would induce vomiting. When the feeling had extended as far as the elbow, we observed her become as pale as ashes, and from this it speedily mounted to the shoulder and across the chest, and was evidently about to be followed by vomiting had I not suddenly put an end to the experiment. This I did by desiring her to take another phial into the other hand, which would neutralise the effects of the emetic phial. The result was equally successful. The experiment did not last more than two or three minutes. I repeated the experiment a second time with the same patient, with like effect. [...]
>
> A consideration of these facts renders it easy to understand how hypnotism may become available for the relief and cure of various diseases. By various modes of *suggestion,* either by audible language, spoken within the hearing of the patient, or by definite physical impressions, certain ideas are fixed strongly and involuntarily in the mind of the patient. These act as stimulants or sedatives, according to the nature of the expectant idea, and either direct attention to, or withdraw it from, particular organs or functions. Similar results are effected in ordinary practice, by prescribing medicines which stimulate or irritate these organs, thereby directly increasing their functions, or which produce the reverse effect, either by direct sedative action on the

> organs, or by diminishing the heart's action, or by stimulating some distant part, and. thereby producing revulsion. The great object of all treatment is either to excite or to depress function, or to increase or to diminish the existing state of sensibility and circulation locally or generally, with the necessary attendant changes in the general, and more especially in the capillary, circulation. For this purpose I feel convinced that hypnotism may be applied in the cure of some forms of disease, with the same ease and certainty as our most approved methods of treatment.

Braid cited the alteration in the capillary circulation which takes place in the phenomenon of blushing and which may appear immediately as the result of a mental impression.

> Where then is the difficulty in comprehending why a dominant expectant idea in the mind of the patient should be adequate to produce effects equally potent on other parts of the body, and in special organs, when strongly concentrated on such organs or parts? The same effects are produced then by hypnotism as are produced by various drugs which depress or excite the circulation. In other cases hypnotism may be supposed to act as an alterative, producing a new action or counter or counter impression, during which the morbid action is suspended, which affords an opportunity for a natural and healthy action to be resumed when the influence of hypnotism is suspended.

In support of this theory, Braid called attention to the number of recoveries which took place during the use of infinitesimally small doses of medicine in homeopathic practice. These, he said, benefited the patient, not by their physical or chemical qualities, but as suggestions, and quoted Professor Simpson, who had proved that in one homeopathic dilution a patient would have to take a dose every second of time, night and day, for 30,000 years before he consumed one grain of the original drug, while another was so attenuated that it would require a mass of the dilution equal to 61 times the size of the earth, to contain a single grain of the medicine.

While, according to Braid, the action of homoeopathic remedies was a purely subjective one, he also thought that the mental element associated with the administration of drugs in general had been far too much ignored, and said,

> It is worthy of inquiry how much of the benefits derived during ordinary treatment may be due entirely to the effects of the medicine, and how much indirectly by its directing attention to, or withdrawing it from the seat of morbid action. [...] A mental impression is necessarily brought into operation whenever any substance is taken, supposed to be of a medical quality, and it will either excite or depress the functions of the morbid part (to or from which the mind is naturally directed) according to circumstances, independently of the mere physical influence which would otherwise ensue from the particular medicine, supposing the patient had not been aware he had taken any medical substance.

This mental impression, Braid thought, accounted for the remarkable revolutions which have taken place at different times as to the estimate of the virtues and powers of particular medicines.

> At one period a universal favourite appeared to be possessed of every valuable quality; anon, discarded and forgotten as utterly worthless; again, arising into meridian power and splendour, to be followed by another decadence in due course. [In other words, medicines come and go, waxing and waning in faddish popularity.] All this arises very naturally in the following manner. A zealous and sanguine professor prescribes it with high confidence of its potency for good, and patients, who are generally acute physiognomists as regards their medical attendants, catch the inspiration and the results are most propitious.[7]
>
> Every successful result exalts the confidence of the physician and patient; and others, prescribing with confidence, realise equally favourable results, and thus the remedy attains the culminating point of its fame and favour [i.e., its *maximum* placebo effect]. Others, however, follow in their wake, but neither with the same hopes nor desire that they should find the discovery of some rival practitioner deserving such laudation. The patients discern the doubtful omen portrayed in the words, looks and manner of the attendant; the effects are correspondingly less salutary, and every succeeding case makes a decadence in the reputation of the once fashionable and omnipotent remedy. Others espouse this view, and thus, through their combined moral impressions, they subvert the natural tendency of the remedy, and prevent the good which should legitimately have attached to it, independently of either enthusiasm, or envy or caprice. [The scepticism of others thereby creates the *opposite* effect when the remedy is subsequently tested by them.] It thus slumbers for a time in forgetfulness, to give place to another rival, which is now in the ascendant, until some other zealous patron at length takes the former under his special favour, and by a similar process as at first, it once more rises to the highest honours, but only to sink again, in its turn, to unmerited neglect.

Clairvoyance, etc.
In Braid's opinion, much of the reluctance to accept the genuine phenomena of Mesmerism and hypnotism arose from the extravagant assertions of the Mesmerists in reference to clairvoyance – assertions which he described as being opposed to all the known laws of physical science and a mockery of the human

---

[7] [In other words, a positive and enthusiastic professor's confident facial expression is easily read by patients who benefit accordingly from the medicine prescribed by him.]

understanding. As the result of frequent experiments made, not only on his own patients, but also upon many of the renowned clairvoyants of the day, Braid was able to find nothing but hypnotic exaggeration of natural powers. The following sources of error, he said, ought always to be kept in mind:–

1. The hyperaesthesia of the organs of special sense, which enables impressions to be perceived through the ordinary media that would pass unrecognised in the waking condition. [Heightened sensory perception.]
2. The docility and sympathy [i.e., social compliance] of the subjects, which tend to make them [semi-automatically] imitate the actions of others.
3. The extraordinary revival of memory ["hypnotic hypermnesia"] by which they can recall things long forgotten in the waking state.
4. The remarkable effect of contact in arousing memory.
5. The condition of double [i.e., dissociated] consciousness or double [i.e., dissociated] personality.
6. The vivid state of the imagination, which instantly invests every suggested idea, or remembrance of past impressions, with the attributes of present realities.
7. The tendency of the human mind, in those with a great love of the marvellous [i.e., the supernatural], to erroneously interpret the subject's replies in accordance with their own desires. ["Confirmation bias".]
8. Deductions rapidly drawn by the subject from unintentional suggestions given by the operator.

Braid considered that the belief in thought-transference arose from the failure to guard against sources of error similar to those just described, and stated that he had never met with any case where the subjects could correctly interpret his unexpressed desires, without some sensible indication of them. In reference to the alleged intuitive powers of certain Mesmeric subjects, Braid held that, whereas with animals instinct was usually right, with somnambules it was generally wrong.[8] It was true that certain patients could successfully predict their own hysterical attacks, but here the prophecy produced its own fulfilment through self-suggestion.[9]

Phrenology
Braid's increased knowledge of the power of mental influences in provoking the various phenomena of the hypnotic state soon led him to discard even the slightest belief in phrenological phenomena.[10] He complained that the author of an article in the *North British Review* for November, 1854, confounded him with the Phreno-Mesmerists and attributed to him the belief that touching particular parts of the head would make a hypnotised patient laugh, pray, sing, steal, and fight, etc.

> Now the fact is that I never adduced the said manifestations as a proof of the organology of phrenology [i.e., the false neurological theory of the phrenologists]. I exhibited the phenomena and explained how they were to be accounted for upon totally different principles, so that they neither proved nor disproved the doctrine of phrenology, but left that precisely where they found it. These manifestations [the patient responding to the stimulations of phrenological trigger points on their scalp] may arise either from a previous knowledge of phrenology, or from a system of training during the sleep, so that they may come out subsequently as acts of memory, when corresponding points are touched, with which particular ideas have been associated through audible suggestion, which arbitrary association may be equally readily established by touching other parts of the body as by touching different parts of the head – or they may arise from the touch calling into action certain muscles of expression of mental conditions, exciting in the mind of the subject the ideas with which they were usually associated in the waking condition.
>
> This latter mode, I consider the only natural mode of exciting these manifestations, and it is a mere inversion of the sequence which ordinarily obtains between mental and muscular expression; *viz.*, firstly, the touch calls into play the muscles constituting the 'Anatomy of expression' of any given passion or emotion, idea or train of thought; and, secondly, this physical expression suggests or excites in the mind of the subject the corresponding idea, passion or emotion with which it is usually associated in the waking condition; i.e., under ordinary circumstances, the mental impression precedes and acts as the exciting cause of physical manifestations of different mental conditions, but here the physical condition precedes and acts as the exciting cause of the mental condition. [...]
>
> It is well-known, however, that so long ago as December, 1841, I particularly pointed out the remarkable docility of patients during hypnosis, which made them most anxious to comply with every proper request or supposed wish of others. I have, therefore, no doubt that they might be trained to manifest, during hypnotism, the opposite tendencies, in accordance with conventional arrangements.

---

[8] [In other words, even animals have more reliable instincts than alleged psychics, though relying on their senses rather than telepathy.]
[9] [Braid therefore recognised the role of negative autosuggestion, or harmful cognition, in psychopathology over half a century before Emile Coué's New Nancy School, and over a century before Aaron Beck's cognitive therapy.]
[10] [The phrenologists believed that specific areas of the scalp were linked to particular "organs" or regions of the brain, and that stimulating the scalp could evoke certain psychological responses. This theory was proved false, however, when the true neurology of the brain was discovered and failed to correspond with their mapping of it.]

As early as 1843, Braid had adopted the view that the supposed phrenological manifestations were due to muscular expression exciting corresponding mental conditions, and in 1844 he showed that he was able to induce all the phenomena by verbal suggestion, no matter what part of the head was touched.[11]

Suggestion, Passes, etc.
At first Braid employed mechanical methods alone, both for the induction of hypnosis and its phenomena. But when he abandoned his physical theory, his views as to the value of passes, etc., naturally changed, and he soon regarded them as only of secondary importance, and attached most value to suggestion. With certain impressionable subjects, hypnosis might be caused by self-suggestion; if they believed that something was taking place at a distance, capable of putting them to sleep, they would fall asleep even if nothing was happening. Direct verbal suggestion, however, was best both for the production of hypnotic phenomena and for the cure of disease. After hypnotising his patients Braid stated in a confident manner the results he wished to obtain and, in certain subjects, found that these could be varied by simple change in the voice. Thus, if he made a patient see an imaginary sheep, and then asked him in a cheerful manner what colour it was, this tone usually elicited the reply "White," or some light colour. If he then asked "What colour is it *now*?" giving a sad intonation to the word *now,* the reply would usually be "Black". [Bramwell's account is slightly flawed. The only obvious alternative to white, for a sheep, would be black. However, Braid's own account clearly shows that he asked a more satisfactory variety of questions in which alterations in his voice tonality were shown to elicit a range of different responses. This is independently substantiated in the account published by Braid's patient, Dr. Wilkinson, in his own book *The Human Body*.]

The action of passes, etc., is explained by Braid in the following manner. Everything which produces a new impression will modify or change existing functions, whether the new impression be of a mental or physical nature. The brain receives many impressions, which subsequently influence the mind, although they were not perceived when conveyed to it by the organs of sense; and others, too slight ever to become conscious, may nevertheless be sufficient to produce a local influence on the nerves and capillaries. Thus, a person may be engaged in reading, so as not to notice he is sitting in a draught, and yet this may cause rheumatism. Passes may have a mechanical action through the agitation of the air, or by touch, or they may produce changes in temperature and electrical states. They are most powerful, however, when they directly excite mental action, either by fixing the attention on one part or function of the body and withdrawing it from others, or by arousing ideas previously associated with the physical impression. All these effects may be neutralized by direct suggestion, and it is quite possible, by a system of training, to make passes, etc., produce the opposite of the result attributed to them. Thus, "supposing that, with each touch or agitation of the air the operator speaks aloud and predicts what shall happen, the auricular suggestion may be so strong as to cause the predicted manifestation to be realised instead of what otherwise would have been the case; and thus, from this time forward, through the double conscious memory, the like impression on that part or organ of sense will recall the previously associated idea and manifestations". Some sort of material combination may be sufficient to produce hypnosis when it is positively affirmed that it will do so, while a moment later the same method will produce nothing, when it is suggested it will be a failure. "All these phenomena may be realised without the patient intending to play off any deception on others, or having any remembrance of the fact on coming out of the sleep." Braid also stated that the entire value of passes and various other mechanical methods, was altogether a suggestive one and that he used them just as he would use audible suggestion.

Dangers
In passing into the hypnotic state, Braid held that reason and will were the first mental powers to wane; thus the imagination gained the ascendancy, and cerebro-spinal functions became more excitable, as the controlling powers of the will were withdrawn. This interference with the volition, however, had its limits, and in an unpublished letter in my possession, in which he replied to some questions regarding the dangers of hypnotism, Braid stated:–

> [...] that the Almighty would never have delegated to man such a dangerous influence over his fellow-man as to have given him such irresistible power over his volition. [...] While under the hypnotic influence, the patients evince great docility, but there is, however, such a state of the perceptive faculties and judgement that they will be quite as fastidious of correct conduct as when in the natural state. So far as I know, there is no more, or not so much, chance of gaining a knowledge of the thoughts of others than might be attained by giving the patient a glass or two of wine. And I have no experience of any such irresistible influence over individuals for producing those malign effects you refer to. I strongly suspect they only exist in the imagination of the parties operating or operated on. At all events, no such effects result from my operations, although undoubtedly I have been able to produce the most wonderful effects in many instances where ordinary treatment had been unavailing.

Braid also asserted that he could give instructions to those who had been successfully hypnotised, no matter how often, by means of which they could completely resist the influence of anyone afterwards.

---

[11] [Braid thereby appears to pre-empt the use of "trigger points" in subsequent hypnotherapy and conditioned "cues" in behaviour therapy.]

In 1847, Braid contrasted the dangers of ether with those of hypnotism, from a moral point of view, and concluded in favour of hypnotism. He referred to the moral abuse to which ethereal narcotism is capable of being turned by cruel and unprincipled individuals. [The anaesthetic properties of ether had recently been discovered and the drug was widely used and abused for "recreational" purposes in the Victorian era.] The opponents of Mesmerism and hypnotism had asserted that their employment was calculated to excite the animal passions and that virtuous women might be victimised by unprincipled men, even without their consciousness of the fact when restored to the waking state, or their possessing any mode of bringing home to the culprits a charge of their villainy, while there was not a whisper *against* the use of ether as liable to be converted to such unholy purposes. Braid's experience of both ether and hypnotism enabled him to confidently state that ether was much the more dangerous of the two. He had never seen a hypnotised patient who did not strenuously resist any attempt at taking a liberty with her. Such patients could not be induced to take off their stockings, for example, or to give a kiss to a gentleman, even should he be a hallucinatory one. On the contrary, they would repel such suggestions with more energy than in the waking condition.

> What might be achieved by systematic and persevering attempts to corrupt a virtuous person during that state, I do not pretend to tell; I should never condescend to witness such attempts being systematically made; but my present convictions are that the same individual might be more readily demoralised when awake, than when in the second conscious state of nervous sleep, which evidently has a tendency with virtuous people to quicken their perceptions and heighten their notions of what would be immoral or highly indecorous, whilst at the same time it renders them most docile and obliging in all which is reasonable and seemly in their estimation. Thus, while they still indignantly repel the proposal to kiss an imaginary gentleman, they will be quite willing to do so to an imaginary child. A libidinous manifestation I have never seen during hypnotism, but I have witnessed the most intense manifestations of erotism arise spontaneously on several occasions during the primary or exciting state of etherisation, and that even in a patient of high respectability and of the most modest and virtuous conduct and pious disposition in her general deportment when awake.

Again, he said, supposing an unprincipled person were placed in the most favourable circumstances for perpetrating a hypnotic crime and succeeded, after systematic and persevering attempts, in doing so, and that, on awaking, the patient had no remembrance whatever of the injury inflicted on her:–

> Let not the criminal indulge in a delusive hope that he could not possibly be inculpated. From the well-established and most beneficent law of double consciousness, it is quite certain that, however completely the transactions which occurred during the sleep may be forgotten on awaking, she has only to be hypnotised or Mesmerised when put into the witness box, to render her as competent to give accurate testimony of all which occurred in her former state of nervous sleep, as in the waking state she could testify to the facts which occurred in her waking condition. Now, I maintain there is not a like security for the person who might be victimised during ethereal narcotism. By this means patients might be rendered speedily entirely oblivious of what was occurring, and that without the benefit and security of the double-conscious memory to be summoned to the conviction of the perpetrators of their wrongs. [...]
>
> I have proved by experiments, both in public and private, that during the state of excitement the judgment is sufficiently active to make the patient, if possible, even more fastidious, as regards the propriety of conduct, than in the waking condition; and from the state of rigidity and sensibility, they can be aroused to a state of mobility, and exalted sensibility, either by being rudely handled, or even by a breath of air. Nor is it requisite that it should be done by the person who put them in the hypnotic state. It will follow equally from the manipulations of anyone else, or a current of cold air impinging against the body, or from any mechanical contrivance whatever. And, finally, the state cannot be induced, in any stage, unless with the knowledge and consent of the party operated on. In this, hypnotism has an advantage over medicine, for many powerful medicines have been used for criminal purposes and can be administered without the knowledge of the intended victim. I have vindicated hypnotism against the erroneous prejudices cited against it as having an immoral tendency; I did not, and do not, claim for it the power of implanting a principle. I do not say it will make a vicious person virtuous; but I am most confident it will not make a virtuous person vicious. On the contrary, I feel assured that a person of habitually correct feelings will, during the somnambulistic condition, while consciousness lasts, manifest fully as much delicacy and circumspection of conduct as in the waking state. Moreover, I have proved that no one can be affected at all *unless by voluntary* compliance, and consequently it has no right to be held as an agency which could be converted to immoral purposes, as many have supposed.
>
> If anyone would say it may have this tendency, because in a state of torpor, insensibility, and cataleptiform rigidity, the party is unconscious, immovable, and incapable of self-defence, I beg to remind such individuals that the same argument might be urged against the proper use of wine, spirits, or opium, because excess in the use of either might be followed by like results. I am quite certain no one can be affected by it, in any stage of the process, unless by the free will and consent of the patient which is at once sufficient to exonerate the practice from the imputations of being capable of being converted to immoral purposes, which has been so much insisted on to the prejudice of animal magnetism. This has arisen from the Mesmerisers asserting that they have the power of overmastering patients irresistibly, even whilst at a distance, by mere volitions and secret passes.

Braid stated that he had been careful in hypnotic experiments and had neither met with accidents, nor seen a single case which he could not awaken in two minutes.

Medical & Surgical Cases

Braid records a good many minor surgical operations, performed painlessly during hypnosis. He mentions the fact that in some instances general consciousness was unimpaired, and the patients remembered afterwards all that had been done, although they had experienced no pain during or after the operation. He also records an immense number of medical cases which were cured or relieved by hypnotism. The majority of these were functional nervous disorders, but remarkable results were also obtained in many cases of organic illness. The clearing up of a long-standing corneal opacity, in a patient who was being hypnotised for the relief of a rheumatic affection, is one of the most interesting. He also obtained marked improvement in many cases of organic paralysis. In one instance, the patient afterwards died from another apoplectic seizure, and post-mortem examination revealed evidence of the earlier organic mischief. In this case, the symptoms had improved greatly under hypnotic treatment.

> It is of importance beforehand to inform the patient that it is not necessary for him to become unconscious in order to obtain the beneficial effect of the nervous sleep. Many believe that a favourable result can only be obtained if the consciousness has been completely lost, whereas, in numerous cases, where the usual internal and external treatment has been quite in vain, the most favourable results have been obtained by the impression on the nervous system, even if the patient has noticed everything that has taken place and upon awakening from the nervous sleep has remembered everything which occurred during its duration.

Braid stated he had experienced this himself, when, on account of a severe attack of rheumatism, he had hypnotised himself for eight or nine minutes and awoke completely free from pain, although he had not lost consciousness in the least during the so-called sleep.

General Observations

Braid desired to place all his results and methods before his medical brethren; he insisted that they alone ought to use hypnotism, and warned the ignorant against tampering with such a powerful agency, which might produce either good or evil according to the manner in which it was managed and applied.

> Hypnotism is capable of curing many diseases for which hitherto we knew of no remedy; but none but a professional man, well versed in anatomy, physiology and pathology, is competent to apply it with general advantage to the patient, or credit to himself, or the agency he employs. I must beg, however, that it be particularly understood that I by no means hold up this agency as a universal remedy. Whoever talks of a universal remedy, I consider must either be a fool or a knave; for, as diseases arise from totally opposite pathological conditions, all rational treatment ought to be varied accordingly.

In hypnotism, Braid asserted that he could teach any intelligent medical man to do what he had done, and that his object had always been not to mystify but to dispel all mystery. He also claimed that he was able to hypnotise a larger percentage by his mechanical methods, than the Mesmerisers could do with the supposed aid of mysterious agencies. Hypnotism could be applied with the greatest confidence by those who understood it, and benefit might be derived from it, even in incurable cases, neither pain, discomfort, nor dangers being associated with it. In doubtful cases, it was sometimes of service in obtaining a correct diagnosis.

Braid stated that he had taken every care to avoid deception in his experiments, but did not expect, on this account, that his conclusions would be accepted by others. He hoped, however, that his professional brethren would investigate the subject coolly, with an honest desire to arrive at truth.

> Having myself been sceptical, I can make every reasonable allowance for others. Everyone should examine the phenomena for themselves, but at the same time they should know something about them.

In illustration of the importance of this, he referred to the fact that different subjects showed varying susceptibility and that many people, even professional men, expected that all should present uniform hypnotic phenomena.

> It must be borne in mind that the opposite mental conditions may glide into each other by the most imperceptible degrees, or by the most abrupt transitions, according to the modes of management; and thus consciousness or unconsciousness, sound sleep, dreaming, or somnambulism, will result, according as sensations or ideas predominate, or are equally vivid. It is no unusual thing for different parties to be testing, or calling for tests, for the opposite conditions, at the same instant of time.

In many instances, Braid published the written testimony of others in support of his alleged successful treatment of different patients by hypnotism, and explained that he did this because,

> [...] most unwarrantable interferences had been resorted to by several medical men, in order to misrepresent some of them. In one instance, in order to obtain an attested erroneous document, the case was read to the patient, and others present, the very reverse of what was written. However extraordinary such conduct may appear, the fact of its occurrence was publicly proved, and borne testimony to by the patient and other parties present on the occasion when the document was obtained.

He referred again and again to the almost incredible opposition which he had to combat at the hands both of the orthodox medical practitioner and of the Mesmerist, and complained that having been attacked in *The Zoist,* the editors of that journal would not permit him to reply in their pages. He sent his answer to the *Association Medical Journal,* as he considered that the most, natural medium for a member of the Provincial Association to publish his defence in, but it was also refused there.[12]

> Throughout the whole of my inquiries my chief desire has been to arrive at what could be rendered most practically useful for the relief and cure of disease and I hesitate not to say that, in the hands of a skilful medical man, who thoroughly understands the peculiar modes which I have devised for varying the effects in a manner applicable to different cases, hypnotism, besides being the speediest method for inducing the condition is, moreover, capable of achieving *all* the *good* to be attained by the *ordinary Mesmerising processes* and *much more.* [...]
>
> Of course there is one point which renders hypnotism less an object of approbation with a certain class of society, *viz.,* that I lay no claim for it to produce the marvellous or transcendental phenomena; nor do I believe that the phenomena manifested have any relation to a magnetic temperament, or some peculiar or occult power, possessed in an extraordinary degree by the operator. These are all circumstances which appeal powerfully to the feelings of the lovers of the marvellous, and therefore tell in favour of Mesmerism; and, moreover, seeing that, for conducting the hypnotic processes with any degree of certainty and success, I contend that, in many cases, a knowledge of anatomy, physiology, pathology, and therapeutics are all requisite; it is obvious that such requirements must be less calculated to secure the approbation of *non-professional Mesmerists* and amateurs, whose magnetic creed taught them to believe that the mere possession by them of the magnetic temperament – of a surcharge by nature, within their own bodies, of a magnetic fluid or odyle – is quite sufficient to enable them to treat any case as efficiently as the most skilful medical man in the universe, simply by walking up to the patient with the *will* and *good intention* of doing him service, or by adding thereto, occasionally, the efficacy of Mesmeric touches, or manipulations. [...]
>
> Like the originators of all new views, however, hypnotism has subjected me to much contention; for the sceptics, from not perceiving the difference between my method and that of the Mesmerists, and the limited extent of my pretensions, were equally hostile to hypnotism as they had been to Mesmerism; and the Mesmerists, thinking their craft was in danger – that their mystical idol was threatening to be shorn of some of its glory by the advent of a new rival – buckled on their armour, and soon proved that the *odium Mesmericum* was as inveterate as the *odium theologicum* [the notorious hatred of rival theologians for one another].

Historical

Braid died suddenly on March 25th, 1860 [aged 65], according to some accounts from apoplexy [stroke], according to others from heart disease; he left a widow, sons and daughter. He maintained his active interest in hypnotism up to the end, and three days before his death sent his last MS. to Dr. [Étienne Eugène] Azam, with the following inscription:– "Presented to M. Azam, as a mark of esteem and regard, by James Braid, Surgeon, Manchester, March 22nd, 1860." Sympathetic notices of Braid's death appeared in the local papers and different medical journals, all of which bore warm testimony to his professional skill and high personal character. *The Lancet* drew attention to the fact that, though he was best known in the medical world by his theory and practice of hypnotism, he had also obtained wonderfully successful results by operations in cases of club foot and other deformities, which brought him patients from every part of the kingdom. Up to 1841 he had operated on 262 cases of Talipes ["club foot"], 700 cases of Strabismus ["squint"], and 23 cases of spinal curvature [scoliosis].

In 1852, in the Preface to the Third Edition of "Magic, Witchcraft, etc.," Braid stated that he now gave his view of all important hypnotic and Mesmeric theories, and hoped, by this means, to make up in some measure for the delay in the publication of another edition of his work on Hypnotism [*Neurypnology*, 1843], which had long been out of print, and was frequently called for. "That call," he said, "I hope shortly to be able to respond to, with such fullness of detail as the importance of the subject merits; more particularly with regard to its practical application for the relief and cure of some forms of disease, of which numerous interesting examples will be adduced." At the conclusion of "The Physiology of Fascination, etc.," he also said:– "It is my intention shortly to publish a volume entitled, "Psycho-Physiology; embracing Hypnotism, Monoideism and Mesmerism". This work will comprise, in a connected and condensed form, the results of the whole of my researches in this department of science; and it will, moreover, be illustrated by cases in which hypnotism has been proved particularly efficacious in the relief and cure of disease, with special directions how to regulate the processes so as to adapt them to different cases and circumstances." Shortly before his death, Braid contemplated publishing a second edition of "Neurypnology", in France; this was

---

[12] [Braid published more than fifty books, pamphlets, letters, and articles in his life; however, not once was he ever granted publication in The Zoist, the main journal of Mesmerism, edited by his rival John Elliotson.]

never done, nor did the two proposed works above referred to ever see the light. All Braid's books and articles are out of print, and of the former, Nos. 2, 3, 4, 6, and 7 [see Bramwell's bibliography], are alone to be found in the Library of the British Museum. [The British Library, as it is now known, is the UK's national publications library, and normally retains a copy of every published book.] I possess Nos. 1, 2, 4, 5, 6, and 8, as well as most of his articles and two long MS. letters addressed to M. Highfield, Esq., Surgeon, dated respectively October 28th and November 16th, 1842. These letters contain an interesting *résumé* of Braid's views on the subjective nature of hypnotic phenomena; some account of the hyperaesthesia of the special senses and reference to successful medical cases, together with the denial of the alleged dangers of hypnotism and of the supposed automatism of the subject.

In 1859, Dr. Azam, of Bordeaux [a surgeon and psychologist], became acquainted with Braid's hypnotic work, and commenced to investigate the subject for himself; an account of his experiments with much reference to Braid, appeared in the *Archives de Médecine* in 1860. About the same time [Paul] Broca [the distinguished neuro-anatomist], who had obtained marvellous results with Braid's methods, read a paper on Hypnotism before the *Académie des Sciences* [the French Academy of Sciences, one of the world's foremost learned societies], which attracted much attention, and [Prof. Alfred] Velpeau [Chair of Surgery at the University of Paris] presented a copy of "Neurypnology" to the same Society. A commission, composed of members of the four sections of the Institute [of France], was then formed to report on the subject. On hearing of this, Braid wrote to the *Académie* to say how much pleasure Azam's brilliant results, and the action of the Society, had given him.

From this date, the subject of hypnotism was never lost sight of in France; but it was not until 40 years after its original publication that "Neurypnology" was translated by Dr. Jules Simon, who stated that, "Braid's researches procured for him numerous enemies; but despite this he pursued them with the precision of genius, and was able to add artificial somnambulism to the pathology of the nervous system – a chapter which the investigations of the greater number of modern neuro-pathologists have confirmed."

Braid's first translator was [Wilhelm] Preyer, Professor of Physiology at the University of Jena, who in 1881 published "The Discovery of Hypnotism". This was a condensation of "Neurypnology," together with the translation of the [unpublished] pamphlet sent by Braid to Azam in 1860, which had passed into the possession of Dr. [George Miller] Beard of New York, who lent it to Preyer. The same pamphlet is also translated into French and forms an appendix to Dr. Jules Simon's "Neurypnology" published in 1883. In 1882, Preyer published "Hypnotism", which consisted of a translation of all Braid's works, with the exception of "Neurypnology", and "Satanic Agency".

[Evaluation of Braid's Work]

I do not propose in this article to examine Braid's views critically, but desire briefly to compare them with those of later workers in the same field.

At first Braid believed in the purely physical origin of hypnotic phenomena, and held that they could be induced by mechanical means in subjects who were ignorant of hypnotism or Mesmerism. This doctrine is still held by [Rudolf] Heidenhain and by certain members of the Salpêtrière School. The former says:– "People who have heard nothing about hypnotism, and who do not know for what purpose they are being experimented on, can be hypnotised. The hypnotic condition can be brought about without the instrumentality of a living being, simply by certain definite physical stimuli." Charcot and Gilles de la Tourette say, "Hypnotism can be induced by purely physical means, and a person can be hypnotised, so to speak, unknown to himself." Before Braid appreciated the mental influence in hypnosis, he was inclined to believe in phrenology, and the same cause seems to have led the Salpêtrière School into error as to the action of magnets, metals and medicines in sealed tubes. That all these owed their virtue to suggestion was clearly demonstrated by Braid; yet, despite this fact, the metallo-therapeutics of Burq were revived by Charcot and his disciples, and Dr. [Jules Bernard] Luys still plays with his india-rubber dolls and Professor Benedikt with his magnets. An account, by Dr. F. Peterson and others, of Professor Benedikt's theory of the action of magnets, and of the experimental exposure of its fallacious nature, read before the New York Academy of Medicine, closely resembles what was said and done by Braid on the same subject. According to Professor Benedikt, "certain forms of hysteria are better treated by the magnet than by electricity, hydropathy or drugs. When a magnet is applied to the sensitive vertebrae without removal of the dress, the irritable patient soon becomes quiet and even quasi-paralysed, the muscles gradually relax, the respiration becomes sighing, consciousness slowly disappears; the resistance to conduction in motor nerves could easily become absolute. The two poles have different effects, the magnet must be employed with caution; patients may be injured by it." These statements were tested in America; magnets of enormous power were used and experiments made on human subjects and lower animals. A young dog was subjected to magnetic influence for five hours; but, instead of being paralysed from "increased resistance to conduction in motor nerves", on being liberated, it was more lively than before. The experimenters conclude "that the human organism is in no wise appreciably affected by the most powerful magnets known to modern science; that neither direct nor reversed magnetism exerts any perceptible influence upon the iron contained in the blood, upon the circulation, upon ciliary or protoplasmic movements, upon sensory or motor nerves, or upon the brain. The ordinary magnets used in medicine," they say, "have a purely suggestive or psychic effect, and would in all probability be quite as useful if made of wood."

The theories of the School of Nancy closely resemble Braid's later ones, in which he regarded hypnotic phenomena from a psychical standpoint. They are not alike, however, on all points. For, while both attach much importance to "dominant ideas" and "suggestion", Braid regards the latter simply as a method of inducing the phenomena, and lays stress on the preliminary change which must be brought about in the nervous system, while the Nancy School holds that suggestion explains all the phenomena of hypnosis. Bernheim, for example, considers that there is nothing in hypnotism but the name and says, "Hypnotism does not really create a new condition; there is nothing in induced sleep which may not occur in the waking condition." In this Mr. Frederic Myers agrees with Braid, and has clearly pointed out that suggestion does not explain the phenomena of hypnosis, but is merely the artifice used by the operator in order to evoke them.

Braid is in opposition to the Nancy School in reference to suggested crimes and to what has been called the automatism of the hypnotised subject. On this point he is more in accordance with the Salpêtrière School and his position has recently been greatly strengthened by the observations of [Joseph] Delboeuf [a distinguished Belgian philosopher and psychologist] and others. With regard to this question, Mr. Frederic Myers says, "Let us first observe what is the moral tone of the somnambule when left to himself, as far as possible, without suggestion. In some important points it is the precise opposite of the drunken condition. Alcohol, apparently by paralysing first the higher inhibitory centres, makes men boastful, impure, and quarrelsome. Hypnotism, apparently by a tendency to paralyse lower appetitive centres, produces a contrary effect. The increased refinement and increased cheerfulness of the developed somnambule is constantly noticed. It is a moot point whether any sleepwalker has ever told an untruth; and, so far as I know, no angry or impure gesture has ever shown itself spontaneously in the hypnotic state."

My own observations on this question have led me to conclusions even more pronounced than Braid's. For while I am convinced that it is impossible to communicate or suggest crime during the alert stage of hypnosis, nothing that I have seen has afforded me any ground for supposing that a crime could be committed during the deep stage. As early as 1890, in an account of some dental operations, performed during hypnotic anaesthesia, I drew attention to the fact that there was no interference with the volition of the subject.

Braid, as we have seen, drew important distinctions between natural and induced sleep. These are not recognised by the Nancy School. Bernheim says, "In my opinion nothing, absolutely nothing, differentiates natural and artificial sleep." He admits, however, one point of difference, namely, that "in ordinary sleep, as soon as consciousness is lost, the subject is only in relationship with himself. In induced sleep, the subject's mind retains the memory of the person who has put him to sleep, whence the hypnotiser's power of playing upon his imagination, or of suggesting dreams, and of directing the acts which are no longer controlled by the weakened or absent will." With regard to the relationship between hysteria and hypnotism, Braid agrees with the Nancy and is opposed to the Salpêtrière School. [The followers of Charcot at the Salpêtrière believed that hypnosis was a form of hysteria and only manifested in hysterical patients, all of whom were women; the Nancy School ridiculed this notion arguing that hypnosis has little or nothing to do with hysteria, and that it occurs as easily in healthy individuals, a view shared by Braid and almost universally adopted after the demise of Charcot.]

Braid and the Nancy School differ in reference to [Mesmeric] *rapport*. According to [Prof. William] Carpenter who explained Braid's views in an article in the *Quarterly Review*, *rapport* could be entirely explained on the principle of "dominant ideas". The subject believed that the operator alone had power over him, or could communicate with him; this established the *rapport*. *Rapport* was not discovered until long after the practice of Mesmerism had come into vogue, having been unknown to Mesmer and his immediate disciples; and its phenomena only acquired constancy and fixity, in proportion as its laws were announced and received. Mesmerists, ignorant of *rapport,* produced a great variety of remarkable phenomena, and yet never detected this *rapport* although they obtained immediate evidence of it, when once the idea had been put into their own minds and thence transferred to their subjects. In all the experiments Dr. Carpenter witnessed which seemed to indicate its existence, the previous idea had either been present, or had obviously been suggested by the methods employed to induce the Mesmeric somnambulism; whilst in a large number of other cases, in which the subjects were not *habitués* [frequenters] of the Mesmeric séances, their consciousness was not confined to the Mesmeriser, or to those whom he placed *en rapport* with them, but was equally extended to all around.[13]

Braid, as we have already seen, observed that a somnambule, supposed only to be *en rapport* with the hypnotiser, heard and obeyed the predictions made by a third person. At a much later date, Liégeois

---

[13] [The phrase "hypnotic rapport" is widely misinterpreted today through confusion with the English word "rapport", i.e., the degree of mutual communicativeness between two individuals. This has virtually nothing to do with its original, technical meaning in Mesmerism and Hypnotism. Rapport, in this sense, refers to the Mesmeric hypothesis that "deep" subjects typically lose consciousness of everything except the Mesmerist or hypnotist himself, especially his voice. It was therefore (falsely) assumed that such subjects were unaware of, or unresponsive to, other people present. Hull (1933) describes it as the notion of a "selective auditory anaesthesia". It is now widely dismissed, as Braid and Bramwell observed, as an artificial effect of the Mesmerists' indirect suggestions to their subjects, and therefore persists only as an anachronism in the vocabulary of modern hypnotists.]

drew attention to the fact that when you had suggested to a somnambule that he could not hear you, he was still able to do so. "If," he said, "you address him directly, he will neither reply nor carry out your suggestion; but if you speak impersonally, speaking not in your own name, but as if with an internal voice, then the subject will execute the suggestion. Under such circumstances, if I said in reference to Camille, 'Camille is thirsty, Camille will go to the kitchen and ask for a glass of water,' the order was obeyed."

The following is Liébault's view:– "It is observed that nearly all artificial somnambules are in relation by their senses with those who put them to sleep, but only with them. The subject hears everything that the operator says to him, but him only, provided the sleep is sufficiently deep. He only hears the operator when he is addressed directly by him and not when a third person is spoken to. This *rapport* extends to the other senses." According to Liébault, the subject remains *en rapport* with the hypnotiser because he goes to sleep in thinking of him, and this does not differ from what happens in ordinary sleep. A mother who goes to sleep close to the cradle of her child does not cease to watch over him during her sleep, but watches only for him, and while she hears his slightest cry is insensible to other louder sounds. The concentration of the subject's attention upon the operator, and his mental retention of the idea of the one who put him to sleep, is the cause of *rapport.*

From this it is evident that Braid believed *rapport* to be entirely the result of suggestion, while Liébault considers it to be due to a concentration of attention which resulted naturally from the induction of hypnosis. My own observations have led me to conclusions similar to those of Braid. In subjects who did not know what was expected of them, and to whom neither direct nor indirect suggestions of *rapport* were made, this condition did not appear. On the contrary, they heard and obeyed anyone who might address them. In several instances, similar conditions were observed in the subjects experimented on by the Hypnotic Committee of the Society for Psychical Research [in whose journal the current article was originally published]. These facts apparently disprove Bernheim's conclusion that the only difference which exists between natural and induced sleep is the concentration of the subject's mind upon the operator – a condition which, he holds, not only explains *rapport,* but also the power of the operator to influence the subject.

It is interesting to note that Braid, like Esdaile, recognised the analogy between hypnosis and certain states produced by Cannabis Indica. No reference to these observations is to be found in Schrenck-Notzing's monograph, "*Die Bedeutung narcotischer Mittel für den Hypnotismus*". He refers, however, to O'Shaughnessy's experiments. [Braid discusses the relationship between hypnotism and cannabis, *inter alia*, in his Observations on Trance (1950).]

Some slight difference exists between Braid's view of the value of passes, etc., and that of Professor Forel. While Braid believed that their influence was mainly suggestive, he still held that they were capable of producing some physical effect, though this might be destroyed or reversed by direct suggestion. Forel, on the other hand, denies the physical influence of mechanical processes on the ground that suggestion is capable of altering their supposed action. He says, "The action of blowing upon the face no longer awakens any subjects, because I suggested this would remove pain, in place of awakening them." From this he argues that the act of blowing produces no result; but would it not be equally logical to contend that the prick of a pin produced no physical effect, because by suggestion the patient, rendered insensible to pain, had been taught to regard the pin prick as the signal to evoke some other condition?[14]

Braid forestalled Bernheim in discovering the value of hypnotic treatment in organic paralysis and the power of the operator's touch to assist the patient's mental concentration and thus recall lost memory. [A technique subsequently made famous by Sigmund Freud who initially hypnotised patients and pressed on their foreheads to help them concentrate while attempting to recover (supposedly) repressed memories.] Bernheim says, "If necessary, I lay my hand on the subject's forehead to concentrate his attention; he thinks deeply for an instant, without falling asleep, and all the latent memories arise with great precision." [These quotations, incidentally, indicate that Freud's "pressure technique" for recovering memories was learned from Bernheim, with whom he studied hypnotherapy, and not his own invention, as is often assumed.] This, both as to the observed fact and its explanation, is an almost exact reproduction of the words of Braid. Bernheim's views, as to the part played by suggestion in ordinary medicine, were long ago expressed by Braid clearly and at great length. Similar opinions have recently been advanced by Dr. Wilks, the newly-elected President of the Royal College of Physicians, and one of the ablest thinkers in the medical profession. According to him, "To sit down in one's chair daily and write on a piece of paper the name of some drug for every ailment without exception which comes under our observation is in the present state of medicine an absurdity, and simply a pandering to human weakness. I do not say that drugs are not useful in a moral [i.e., practical] sense, I am merely contending that the method is not scientific, as we usually apply this term. I know of no more successful practitioner than the late Sir William Gull, and his treatment was rational, but he did not credit any particular drug with the properties ascribed to it by the patient. His prescription very often consisted of nothing but coloured water." Dr. Wilks describes a "sixpenny doctor", at a cheap dispensary, who saw on an average 70 patients during one evening, and whose almost universal

---

14 [Braid, with some justification, maintained that physical manipulations, touch, breath, passes, etc., served to focus or divert attention as well as evoking ideas by association and through the "anatomy of expression". Slow, monotonous, downward hand passes before the eyes might naturally be experienced as relaxing, soothing, and as inducing eye closure, drawing attention inward, etc. However, suggestion may easily modify, or even reverse, these "natural" reactions if, e.g., it were suggested that the same passes would arouse nervous tension, increase the heart rate, and widen the eyes.]

medicine was a mixture composed of sulphate of magnesia [a mild laxative], burnt sugar and infusion of quassia [a very bitter herbal remedy used to treat hysteria], and who said, "Always give medicines which produce appreciable effects; then also the mixture must taste like medicine, and if it have a bad smell, the patient will be better satisfied." Dr. Wilks objects "to the attempt to treat cases of disease on principle, when we possess no principles; we do not know sufficiently the action of drugs to do this, and we know less of the meaning or significance of symptoms which we treat." With change of the pathological views of disease, he says, the whole method of its treatment is changed again and again, and further chemical knowledge frequently shows that the drugs we employ do not possess the qualities we have been in the habit of attributing to them. "Medicine began as a superstition, covered and surmounted by fancies and crude theories. By getting rid of these, advance has been made; but the fact is not yet sufficiently realised that many of the old fancies still remain in the profession."

Dr. Hack Tuke [a distinguished Victorian psychotherapist, grandson of the York Retreat's founder], in speaking of Sir Andrew Clark said, "His favourite drugs were Bicarbonate of Potash and a vegetable bitter [a bitter herbal tonic, e.g., quassia]; but neither drugs nor diet formed the central factors of his treatment, or explained his success. 'Suggestion' lay at the root of it all. The term, however, is too mild, unless understood in the technical sense in which it has been employed in recent times. In short, Sir Andrew out-Bernheimed Bernheim; he was, in a word, the most successful hypnotist of his day."

In reference to the many important differences between the theories of Braid and those just referred to, my own observations, I may state, accord on most points with those of the earlier investigator. A careful study of all Braid's writings has led me to the conclusion that, while much has been lost by their neglect, little or no advance has been made upon them until quite recent times. Where progress has been made, and made alone, it has been in the development of the views already expressed by Braid as regards the individuality [i.e., autonomy], in opposition to the automatism, of the hypnotised subject, and in a clearer estimate of what he recognised as double-consciousness [i.e., dissociation]. Above everything, it is worthy of note how Braid at once, by his early experiments, exploded the fallacies of the Mesmerists, which, till then, had flourished successfully, despite the abusive and absolutely unscientific attacks of the combined medical press. In the writings of Mr. Frederic Myers, especially in "The Subliminal Consciousness", are to be found the ablest and clearest expression of those later views. In reference to hypnotism, he justly says, "It is something more and other than the mere production of trance that we have to deal with – something more and other than the mere phenomena of fascination, mimicry, rigidity, which are to be seen on every itinerant Mesmeriser's platform. Discussions on cerebral circulation, on inhibition and dynamogenesis, are useful and needful on the outskirts of the problem; they may give precision to our conception of the condition in which the deeper phenomena begin; but they cannot explain the novel powers to which those phenomena introduce us – the increased, the penetrating control of the brain over the organism."

How is it that Braid's later theories have been almost entirely ignored? The answer is a difficult one. It is true that all his works have long been out of print in this country, and are not to be found in the British Museum. On the other hand, his conclusions were largely adopted by the scientists of his day. In illustration of this, it is only necessary to refer to the works of the late Drs. Carpenter and John Hughes Bennett. The former gives a full exposition of Braid's views in his "Principles of Mental Physiology", Sixth Edition, London, 1881, "Mesmerism, Spiritualism, etc." and elsewhere. The following passage, from an article in the *Quarterly Review* for September 1853, shows how thoroughly Dr. Carpenter understood the importance attached by Braid to suggestion. "The clue to the marvel [Mesmerism] was soon found by Mr. Braid, in the concentrated operation of the principle of *suggestion*[15] [...] and under the guidance of this idea, he has subsequently followed up the investigation with great intelligence, making no mystery of his proceedings, but courting investigation in every possible way." Professor [John Hughes] Bennett, in his "Textbook of Physiology", reproduced the explanation of "Braidism", both from the physiological and psychological side, first given by him in 1851. This formed a part of the lecture on hypnotism he gave annually to his students, in which he urged them to investigate a subject destined to revolutionise the theory and practice of medicine.

The only recent English writer, as far as I know, who refers to Braid's later works, is C. W. Sutton in the "Dictionary of National Biography", where he states that some of them have been translated into French and German. Despite Preyer's translations, Braid's advanced theories seem to be little recognised in Germany and, as far as I have observed, Moll alone refers to them, and in the *Zeitschrift für Hypnotismus*, for December, 1892, he warmly acknowledges Germany's indebtedness to Preyer for his translations and states that the later works are a distinct advance upon "Neurypnology", especially in their psychological explanation of hypnotic phenomena. At the same time, he evidently does not realise how entirely Braid had forestalled the "Suggestion" theory of the Nancy School. He admits, however, that "notwithstanding that many researchers have referred to and valued Braid's writings, the modern works are only in the smallest degree a continuation of his".

In France, Braid's later theories are equally ignored, which is still the more surprising when one remembers that a translation of his last MS. was published in 1883 as a supplement to "Neurypnology". It gives many of his advanced views, and clearly states his reasons for substituting them for his earlier ones

---

[15] [The italics are Dr. Carpenter's]

and for changing the term hypnotism into that of monoideism. It also contains numerous references to verbal suggestion. Bernheim refers to it, but has evidently entirely failed to grasp its importance and merely says that he agrees with Brown-Séquard that Braid did not guard sufficiently against suggestion and that "it seems that at the end of his life, Braid felt some doubt about his experiments relative to phreno-hypnotism. In his last memoir [the unpublished MS.], a remarkable *résumé* of his work, addressed to the Academy of Science in 1860, at the time of the experiments of Azam and Broca, he passes by his phreno-hypnotic researches in silence." Bernheim also mentions Braid's work, "The Power of the Mind over the Body", but only in connection with Grimes' "electro-biological researches".

[Conclusion]

While I have tried to show, both as a point of historical interest and in justice to Braid, how he had anticipated many of the most important observations of the School of Nancy, I do not wish to undervalue the services of that School, and more especially those of its founder [Liébault]. Braid's researches were undoubtedly the exciting cause of the hypnotic revival in France, but at that time little or nothing was known of any of his works, except "Neurypnology", and his last MS. was not published in France until 1883. To Liébault we owe practically the entire development of modern hypnotism. Independently he arrived at the conclusion that the mental condition was the important one in hypnosis, and suggestion the main factor in producing its phenomena, and successfully combated the errors of the *Salpêtrière* School [of Charcot]. Another point in reference to their career is worthy of note. Braid's views at once brought him fame. His books sold rapidly, the demand for them exceeding his power of supply. The medical journals were open to him, to an extent which may well excite envy in those interested in the subject at the present day. When Liébault published his classical work, "*Du Sommeil et des États analogues*", [*On Sleep and Analogous States*, 1866] six copies alone were sold. His statements only found sceptics, his methods of treatment were rejected without examination, and he was laughed at and despised by all. For many years he devoted himself entirely to the poor, and long refused to accept a fee, lest he should be regarded as attempting to make money by unrecognised methods. Even in his later days, fortune never came to him, and his services – services, which he himself, with true modesty, described as the contribution of a single brick to the edifice many were trying to build – only began to be appreciated when old age compelled him to retire from active work. Though his researches have been recognised, it is certain that they have not been estimated at their true value, and that members of a younger generation have reaped the reward which his devotion of a lifetime failed to obtain.

[Editor's Addendum]

In *Hypnotism* (1903), Bramwell adds the following comments on Braid's writings,

> In 1890, Preyer brought out another work on the subject of hypnotism. This contained a translation of a MS. of Braid's, entitled "On the Distinctive Conditions of Natural and Nervous Sleep", which now for the first time saw the light. In reference to this, Preyer stated that Braid left his MSS. to his daughter, and that she, on her death, bequeathed them to her brother Dr. James Braid jun., who died on November 22nd, 1882. Preyer visited him at Burgess Hill, Sussex, in August 1881, and received the MS. from him. In addition to the information drawn from Preyer's books, I am personally indebted to him for the gift of various pamphlets by Braid, with some of which I was previously unacquainted.

Bramwell then mentions that around 1896 Bernheim responded to his articles by publishing a reply in which he insisted that Braid was not fully acquainted with the role of suggestion in hypnotherapy. Bramwell responded to this with evidence to the contrary, after which Bernheim appears to have finally recognised Braid as the true father of hypnotherapy by suggestion.

Bramwell bemoans the fact that A.E. Waite, a well-known English occultist and supporter of Mesmerism, was responsible for publishing the only collection of Braid's writings, under the title *Braid on Hypnotism* (1899).

> Apparently, too, Mr. Waite himself believes in animal magnetism, metallo-therapeutics, phrenology, and clairvoyance, but when he attributes to Braid a belief in these things, he shows that he has absolutely failed to grasp the spirit and significance of his teaching.

Braid himself would undoubtedly have been astounded that someone with Waite's obvious bias for Mesmerism and occultism could be entrusted with the job of editing his writings and commenting upon them. Today, Waite is known primarily for being the co-designer of the most popular set of modern *tarot* cards (Rider-Waite, 1909) and the author of numerous books on occultism and "ceremonial magic".

In his supposedly "complete" collection, Waite re-published the full text of *Neurypnology* and reduced the rest of Braid's work to a few short excerpts in the appendices. Yet, unaccountably, Waite writes, 'It is claimed, therefore, that this edition is representative and substantially complete'. (Waite, in Braid, 1899: ix). In doing so, Waite had omitted most of Braid's works which were critical of Mesmeric and occult claims, and instead opens his 'Introduction' to the collection with the words,

> James Braid, the Manchester surgeon, is regarded as "the initiator of the scientific study of Animal Magnetism," and this is a title to distinction which possesses the guarantee of permanence. (Waite, 'Preface' to *Braid on Hypnotism*, 1899)

On the contrary, however, Braid had dedicated his entire career to *debunking* the inherently occult claims of animal magnetism, and substituting an interpretation based on psychological and physiological principles. A few pages further on, in Braid's *own* Introduction to the very same book published by Waite, he writes,

> I have now entirely separated Hypnotism from Animal Magnetism. (Braid, *Neurypnology*, 1843)

In the first chapter of that book, Braid dedicates a section specifically to explaining in detail why he considered hypnotism to be fundamentally distinct from animal magnetism, prominent among which is the fact that the Mesmerists claimed for themselves occult powers of the kind espoused by Waite. In a letter to *The Lancet*, Braid subsequently wrote,

> [...] I adopted the term "hypnotism" to prevent my being confounded with those who entertain these extreme notions, as well as to get rid of the erroneous theory about a magnetic fluid, or *esoteric influence of any description being the cause of the sleep*. (Braid, 'Mr. Braid on Hypnotism: Letter to the Editor of *The Lancet*', 1845, author's italics)

This viewpoint was maintained and strengthened throughout his lifetime. Braid was *not* a Mesmerist, he was a Hypnotist, and, as the works temporarily *expunged* by Waite clearly show, he dedicated considerable effort to both disputing and disproving the pseudoscientific claims of the Mesmerists regarding the existence of animal magnetism and alleged manifestations of occult powers.

Appendix:
Braid's Later Theories (Bramwell, 1903; 1909)

> In his two books, *Hypnotism: Its History, Practice & Theory* (1903) and *Hypnotism & Treatment by Suggestion* (1909), Bramwell expands Braid's later thoughts into a more generally *suggestion*-oriented (sometimes dubbed "socio-cognitive") interpretation of hypnotism, which in many respects pre-empts modern "non-state", or cognitive-behavioural, research on hypnosis. There is a distinct shift in emphasis from the idea of a special physiological *state* of nervous sleep, to a range of (ideo-dynamic) psychological mechanisms and their social context, e.g., the role of expectation, habit, imagination, imitation, verbal suggestion, association, attention, etc., become increasingly central to Braid's approach and the physiology of rigid catalepsy or nervous sleep becomes somewhat less significant.
>
> However, neither Bramwell nor Braid concluded from this that the classical eye-fixation induction should be completely abandoned, because it may have psycho-physiological effects which are helpful, though non-essential. It is also likely that most subjects expect to experience some kind of recognisable induction ritual, and so the eye-fixation technique, or a similar style of working, may itself be a kind of physical suggestion which facilitates subsequent suggestion by satisfying the client's expectations about hypnotism.

Hypnotism: Its History, Practice & Theory (1903)

Braid's theories changed as his knowledge increased, and he held in all three distinct and widely differing ones. In the first, he explained hypnosis from an almost purely physical standpoint; in his second, he considered it to be a condition of involuntary monoideism and concentration of the attention. His third theory differed from both of these. In it he recognised that reason and volition were unimpaired, and that the attention could be simultaneously directed to more points than one. The condition, therefore, was not one of involuntary monoideism. Further, he recognised more and more clearly that the state was essentially a conscious one, and that the losses of memory which followed on awaking could always be restored in subsequent hypnoses. Finally, he described as "double consciousness" the condition which he had first termed "hypnotic", then "monoideistic". [Bramwell probably meant that Braid wished to reserve the terms "hypnotism" and "monoideism" for special states associated with the use of suggestion, but that he came to see neither as *essential* to suggestion therapy.] As already noted, few students of hypnotism are acquainted with any of Braid's theories except the earliest; and his third and latest one, which he promised to put before the public in a more complete form, never saw the light in the manner he intended. [In *The Physiology of Fascination* (1855), for example, Braid had stated, 'It is my intention shortly to publish a volume entitled "Psycho-Physiology: embracing Hypnotism, Monoideism, and Mesmerism."'] My account is drawn from little-known pamphlets, unpublished MS., etc. [Bramwell had acquired most of Braid's works, including several unpublished pieces.]

The following is a summary of Braid's latest theories:-

1. Hypnosis could not be induced by physical means alone.
2. Hypnotic and so-called Mesmeric phenomena were subjective in origin, and both were excited by direct or by indirect suggestion.
3. Hypnosis was characterised by physical as well as by psychical changes.
4. The simultaneous appearance of several phenomena was recognised and much importance was attached to the intelligent action of a secondary consciousness.
5. Volition was unimpaired, moral sense increased, and suggested crime impossible.
6. *Rapport* was a purely artificial condition created by suggestion.
7. The importance of direct verbal suggestion was fully recognised, as also the mental influence of physical methods.
8. Suggestion was regarded as the device used for exciting the phenomena, and not considered as sufficient to explain them.
9. Important differences existed between hypnosis and normal sleep.
10. Hypnotic phenomena might be induced without the subject having passed through any condition resembling sleep.
11. The mentally healthy were the easiest, the hysterical the most difficult, to influence.

In this country, during Braid's lifetime, his earlier views were largely adopted by certain well-known men of science, particularly Professors W.B. Carpenter and J. Hughes Bennett, but they appear to have known little or nothing of his latest theories. [Bramwell, 1903: 293-294]

Hypnotism & Treatment by Suggestion (1909)

Before discussing hypnotic theories, I wish to draw attention to the cases and experiments just cited. In some, the condition termed hypnosis was present. This varied from slight drowsiness or lethargy to apparently profound sleep, followed by amnesia on waking, i.e., the subjects were unable to recall the events of the so-called hypnosis. At first, both Braid and Liébault regarded this as artificially induced sleep, and believed that it must be evoked before patients would respond to suggestions, either curative or experimental. The condition, however, might be more accurately described as "imitation sleep". The deeply hypnotised subject believed he had been asleep, because he could not afterwards recollect what had happened. Various facts, however, show great dissimilarity between imitation and natural sleep [i.e., between so-called "hypnotic sleep" and natural sleep]. When the subject is re-hypnotised and questioned, he can relate all that took place in the previous hypnosis with the exception of any special sensations inhibited by suggestion. Thus, my patients who had undergone painless hypnotic operations could afterwards describe them, and knew what had been said and done by those around them. They were only unable to recall pain, as that sensation had never reached consciousness. Further, in the so-called lethargic state [the deepest stage of hypnosis according to the Salpêtrière school] the subjects, who lie apparently asleep, hear and respond to the operator's suggestions, even if these are whispered so softly that they could not have heard them in the normal condition. [...] In every instance, where I questioned so-called hypnotic somnambules as to their mental condition in previous hypnoses, I found that they knew where they had been and what they had been doing or thinking about. They felt that they were the same persons in the so-called hypnotic state as in the waking one, and were conscious that their reason and volition were unimpaired. [It was not, therefore, an autonomous "unconscious", "subconscious", or "dissociated" mind, but their normal *conscious* mind, that was listening to the hypnotic suggestions and responding.]

Further, subjects in whom hypnosis had been evoked would afterwards pass into the suggestible condition characteristic of it, at any signal to which they had been taught to respond, and without going through any intermediate state even superficially resembling sleep. [...]

In some of the cases nothing even superficially resembling sleep was induced: the patients simply rested in an armchair while suggestions were made. Yet, in many instances, the curative results were as striking as those obtained after the induction of so-called hypnosis.

In both groups increased suggestibility had been developed, and a control of the organism obtained far beyond the will-power of ordinary life. Examples of this are found in the influence of suggestion upon menstruation, perspiration, the secretion of milk, the action of the bowels, etc. [That is, despite the absence of anything remotely resembling a sleep-like "trance", suggestions given in the waking state were found effective and capable of influencing bodily function usually classed as "involuntary", by means of ideo-dynamic reflex action.] (Bramwell, 1909: 133-135)

Braid's method. – Braid took a bright object, generally his lancet case, held it in his right hand about a foot away from the patient's eyes, and at such a distance above the forehead that it could not be seen without straining. The patient was told to look steadily at it and to think of nothing else. The operator then extended and separated the fore and middle fingers of the right hand, and carried them from the object towards the patient's eyes. The lids generally closed involuntarily; if this did not happen the process was repeated, and rarely failed.

Later, as Braid found that fixed gazing was frequently followed by slight conjunctivitis, he changed his methods: prolonged staring was abandoned, and the patient instructed to close his eyes at an early stage of the proceedings. Hypnosis was induced as easily as before and without unpleasant symptoms. If the body and mind were at rest, Braid found he could hypnotise as readily in the dark as in the light, and he also succeeded with the blind; these facts induced him to abandon his physical theory [of eye-fixation leading to nervous fatigue] and to conclude that the influence was exerted through the mind. He observed that repeated hypnoses increased susceptibility; this arose from habit, association of ideas and imagination. In such cases, if the patients believed something was being done which ought to produce hypnosis, the state appeared. On the other hand, the most expert hypnotist would exert his influence in vain if the patient did not know what was expected and, at the same time, voluntarily yield to the demands of the operator. Later, Braid asserted that *direct verbal suggestion* was the best method for inducing hypnosis and its phenomena; physical methods were simply indirect suggestions, their influence depending upon the mental states they excited. [Braid had already emphasised that physical manipulation of the body posture and facial expression were likely to evoke corresponding ideas and feelings in the mind of the subject; rather than having a direct physical effect, eye-fixation might suggest the idea of focused attention and sleepiness by *mental association*.] (Bramwell, 1909: 159-160)

Before describing my later methods, I wish again to draw attention to several points in connection with the so-called hypnotic state. As we have seen, the subject may have his eyes open, and act like a normal individual who is awake. In the lethargic condition, when he appears to be asleep, he still hears all that is said around him. Further, all the phenomena of so-called hypnosis can be induced in the waking state, without the patient having preliminarily passed through any condition resembling sleep. It is to Braid's earlier work that we owe the theory that it was necessary to induce hypnosis before beginning treatment by suggestion. At first he regarded the condition as an artificial sleep, but pointed out later that only one in ten of those he cured passed into a state even superficially resembling [normal] sleep. He proposed, therefore, to abolish his entire terminology, as it misled the public, and made them believe they could not be cured by suggestion unless they had first been put to sleep. With the majority of Braid's patients there was not even an apparent loss of consciousness – they simply became slightly drowsy, and afterwards remembered all that had happened – while, with others, hypnotic phenomena were induced, without any previous stage in any way resembling sleep. Further, in those cases where sleep had apparently been present, it could be proved that the condition was really a conscious one, as the recollection of all that had occurred could be evoked by suggestion.

Braid's later observations passed unnoticed, and, until recent times, nearly all operators proceeded on his earlier lines. They suggested artificial sleep, lethargy or drowsiness, and then began treatment. They did not recognise that the artificial or, more correctly speaking, imitation sleep was only one of the phenomena of increased suggestibility, due to suggestion. Given increased suggestibility, any of the phenomena of hypnosis might be evoked as readily as imitation sleep, and the patient cured just as easily when that state had been omitted.

For many years, [the founder of the Nancy School] Liébault's methods were similar to Braid's earlier ones, and he always tried to induce what he called *sommeil provoqué* ["artificial sleep"]. Gradually the views of the Nancy School were modified till they resembled Braid's later theories. Now, Bernheim [the leader of the Nancy School] states that there is nothing in hypnotism but the name. All is "suggestion", and patients can be cured without the induction of artificial sleep. Bernheim's statement requires some modification: all the phenomena we have been accustomed to call hypnotic are undoubtedly the result of suggestion; but the suggestions must be accepted by the patient before the phenomena can be evoked.

The essence of the whole condition, then, is an increased suggestibility; the production of a preliminary imitation sleep is not necessary, and is simply a waste of time. In some instances, I tried to induce so-called hypnosis [i.e., "artificial sleep"] a hundred times before I succeeded. Now, with the method I shall presently describe, I commence curative treatment at once, and obtain quicker results.

Lest my readers may be confused by my asserting, on the one hand, that the hypnotic state – i.e., a condition of sleep – does not really exist, and, on the other, by my talking of inducing hypnosis, I will summarise my views. Every stage of the so-called hypnotic condition is a conscious one. In some instances the subjects have their eyes open and are obviously wide awake, in others their eyes are closed and they appear to be asleep; but, even in the most profound condition, the sleep is only apparent, not real, as the subjects retain consciousness, volition and intelligence. The condition described as the hypnotic is essentially one of increased suggestibility. The artificial or imitation sleep, suggested by the operator, is only one amongst the many phenomena which can be evoked by suggestion. In what is described as the deepest stage – i.e., hypnotic somnambulism, followed by amnesia – when the state is terminated, the patients believe they have been asleep, because they do not remember what has happened. This is equally true, whether they have been apparently asleep, or seemingly awake with their eyes open in the "alert" stage. The lost memories of both stages can always be recalled in subsequent hypnosis. Further, it is probable that the amnesia is an artificial one due to the suggestions of the operator. When I use the word hypnosis – and it is almost impossible to avoid doing so until this fresh conception of the condition is accepted – I only mean that I have tried to induce *increased suggestibility* [as opposed to a sleep-like state] by methods which I shall presently describe. The condition – i.e., increased suggestibility – is sometimes preceded by drowsiness, but this is often absent, and the patients are voluntarily thinking of some restful monotonous subject during the whole process. Sometimes the patients' minds are filled with the melancholy thoughts of neurasthenia, or obsessional fears; at others their attention is fixed on their hysterical convulsions or other uncontrollable muscular movements; but, despite this, increased suggestibility is frequently induced. Here there has been neither imitation sleep nor restful monotonous thought, but, nevertheless, brilliant therapeutic results are often obtained in such cases.

I will now describe my present methods. In many respects they resemble those I have used for years; the difference between them, more apparent than real, being due to what I believe to be a clearer conception of the so-called hypnotic state. [...]

The first suggestions refer to the conditions which I wish to create while the patient is in the armchair. I tell him that each time he comes he will find it easier to rest, to turn his attention away from me and to concentrate it upon something restful [after simply closing his eyes normally]. I have previously explained that I do not wish him to go to sleep, but that, if he can get into the drowsy condition which precedes sleep, the suggestions are likely to be responded to more quickly. (Bramwell, 1909: 162-168)

Braid's Discovery of Hypnotism
(Williamson, 1896)

> This little vignette, from the memoirs of Dr. Williamson, Professor of Natural History at Owns College, Manchester, is quoted by Bramwell. Dr. Williamson was present in person on 19th November 1841 to observe the incident that inspired James Braid to develop the original theory and practice of hypnotism. In fact, this seems to have been Braid's second time in the audience at Lafontaine's performance.

During the fourth decade of this century the subject of clairvoyance had been much discussed in social circles, and in the early days of my professional life two men who lectured on the subject visited Manchester. The first of these was a Frenchman, who illustrated his lecture by experiments on a young woman. [The Mesmerist, Charles Lafontaine, was actually Swiss and used two assistant-subjects called Eugen and Mary.] At one of his lectures the girl was declared to be in a state of sound [Mesmeric] sleep. A considerable number of medical men were present, including our leading ophthalmist [eye specialist], Mr. Wilson, and one Mr. Braid. The latter gentleman was loud in his denunciation of the whole affair. The audience then called upon Mr. Wilson for his opinion of the exhibition. Of course the question was, 'Is this exhibition an honest one or is it a sham?' 'Is the girl really asleep, or is she only pretending to be so?' In reply to the call of the audience, Mr. Wilson stood up and said: 'The whole affair is as complete a piece of humbug as I have ever witnessed.' The indignant lecturer, not familiar with English slang phrases, excitedly replied: 'The gentleman says it is all *Bog*; I say it is not *Bog*; there is no *Bog* in it at all.' By this time several of us, including Mr. Wilson, had gone upon the platform to examine the girl. I at once raised her eyelids, and found the pupils contracted to two small points. [Braid claims in *Neurypnology* (1843) that the pupils usually *dilate* at first during hypnosis, but subsequently *contract* as the state becomes deeper.] I called Wilson's attention to this evidence of sound sleep, and he at once gave me a look and a low whistle, conscious that he was in a mess. Braid then tested the girl by forcing a pin between one of her nails and the end of her finger. She did not exhibit the slightest indication of feeling pain, and Braid soon arrived at the conclusion that it was not all 'Bog'.

He subsequently commenced a long series of elaborate experiments, which ended in his placing the subject on a more philosophical basis than had been done by any of his predecessors. For the term 'Animal Magnetism' and other popular phrases, Braid substituted 'Hypnotism' and 'Monoideism'.

The hypothesis which he adopted was that the subjects of these experiments required to have their mental faculties concentrated upon one idea; this accomplished, two effects will be produced in a few moments. The first is a state of sound sleep, which he succeeded in obtaining through [monotonously stimulating] either of the several senses, sight, hearing, or touch; but his favourite plan was to seat the individual operated upon in an armchair, whilst he held a bright silver object, usually his lancet case, a few inches above the person's eyebrows, and required him to raise his eyes upwards until he saw the shining metal, soon after doing which, the patient went off into a sound sleep. But a still more remarkable result followed, indicating a condition of mind [called "double consciousness"] not so easily explained as illustrated.

On one occasion I called Braid in to see a young lad who had been suffering fearfully from a succession of epileptic attacks, which had failed to yield to medical treatment. So far as the epilepsy was concerned the hypnotic treatment was a perfect success; the boy, after having long endured numerous daily attacks, was perfectly relieved after the third day's hypnotic operation. For five subsequent years, during which the youth remained under my observation, the epilepsy did not return.

Braid always awoke his subjects from their hypnotic condition by sharply clapping his hands close to the sleepers' ears, which at once aroused them. One day, before doing this, Braid said to me, 'I will now show you another effect of hypnotism. Lend me your pocket-book and pencil.' I did so. He then placed the book in the boy's left hand, which he raised into a convenient position in front of the lad's breast. My pencil was placed in his right hand, which was lifted into such a position that the point of the pencil rested upon one of the pages of the book. This attitude was rigidly maintained until Braid whispered in his ear: 'Write your name and address.' The lad did so: 'John Ellis, Lloyd Street, Manchester.' This done, the book and pencil were restored to my pocket. Braid then awoke the boy and asked, 'John, what were you doing just now?' He looked about rather wildly for a moment, and persistently answered, 'Nothing.' Braid then sent him off to sleep again. The question was again asked: 'John, what were you doing just now?' The lad answered promptly, but in a low voice: 'Writing my name and address.' A succession of similar experiments clearly indicated two things: first, that a Mesmerised individual would do what he was told to do; second, that things done when in that state were remembered only when the same condition was resumed; otherwise they were forgotten, indicating a *dual state of mind*, which, so far as I know, has not yet been satisfactorily explained.

[However, Braid reported spontaneous amnesia in only 10% of his cases.] I cannot learn that Braid's method of experimental inquiry and of philosophical induction has been continued by any person since he died.

Williamson, William Crawford. *Reminiscences of a Yorkshire Naturalist* (1896).

SECTION II:
Braid's Collected Works

On Hypnotism (1860)
De L'Hypnotisme

Translation from the French edition, copyright © Donald Robertson, 2008[16]

Foreword[17]

I was very happy to learn of the brilliant results from the experiments on hypnotism, tried by Monsieur [Étienne Eugène] Azam according to the principles established in my work of 1843. It was at the time of this success that Monsieur [Alfred-Armand-Louis-Marie] Velpeau, an illustrious member of your academy, thought the matter should be brought to the attention of your learned society. I was also happy to see you judge the question worthy of an investigation; you have appointed a commission comprised from four sections of your glorious Institute. To assist it, as far as I am able, I offer to the academy, by way of tribute, a copy of my book published in 1843, comprising the history of all my research until the time of its publication; I attach several articles to it containing my later work, and finally this manuscript wherein there are extracts of all my works from 1843 up to 1860. These documents will be of a great help in the commission's research.

This learned committee will decide, I can say with confidence, between my *subjective* theory [hypnotism] and the *objective* theory of the magnetisers [Mesmerism]. According to the former, it is the power of a dominant idea in the individual that produces the results: only a small number of phenomena can be caused by means of hypnotism. The magnetisers, on the contrary, allot the results to a *magnetic fluid* or a mysterious force, which, emanating from the person of the operator, penetrates into that of the subject and then produces not only all the phenomena of hypnotism, but also many others of a highly transcendent [i.e., paranormal] nature: the alleged "*higher phenomena*".

James Braid.
Rylaw House, Oxford Street, Manchester.
7th January 1860.

Splitting (Doubling) Of Consciousness[18]

It was in November 1841 that I had occasion for the first time to attend Mesmeric experiments. The operator was a Frenchman, Monsieur [Charles] Lafontaine.[19] From all that I had read and heard on this subject, I was frankly sceptical and I considered the practical experiments and all the phenomena which were caused as the result of a secret complicity or as an illusion; I was determined, if it were possible, to discover, to expose the trickery by which the operator imposed on the public. But I realised soon, without difficulty, that certain abnormal phenomena which occurred during the experiments were *real*; however I do not see any reason to concur with Monsieur Lafontaine that it was an influence of his person acting upon the subject, or that of a magnetic or Mesmeric fluid. I therefore began a series of experiments which soon taught to me that the patients could throw themselves into a similar state, by their personal manner of being only; a state, consequently, of subjective nature and independent of any external influence, coming from the person of the operator. By making the patients gaze fixedly at a small shining object, not being by itself of an exciting nature, the object maintained a little above the ordinary direction of the vision, requesting them to concentrate their attention while the remainder of the body was at rest, I noticed that a great number of them fell more or less promptly into a deep sleep, and displayed all the usual phenomena of animal magnetism or of Mesmerism such as one describes them in the traditional books of the genre. With some individuals, a more or less deep state of sleep was accompanied by a loss of consciousness and willpower, to such an extent that the ear was not affected by the loudest noise, that the patient did not realise the presence of very strong ammonia, held under the nostrils, and that piercing and pinching of the skin did not draw his attention. Strong galvanic currents could be passed through his arm without him showing pain; extremely painful surgical operations had even been carried out completely without his knowledge; he did not retain of it the least memory, once out of his abnormal sleep. Surprisingly, thrown into a second sleep, but to a degree a little less pronounced, the patient remembered perfectly what had occurred during the first. These facts were reproduced on several occasions: forgetfulness on awakening, remembrance with the second sleep, it is what I called the "*double consciousness*".[20]

---

[16] [I would like to express many thanks to Hilary Norris-Evans for her invaluable assistance in preparing the 2008 English translation of this manuscript. DR.]
[17] This foreword directly addresses the [French] *Academy of Sciences* which had just named a commission to study the question of hypnotism (French Translator).
[18] [These section headings are also translated from the French edition.]
[19] [According to other sources, Lafontaine appears to have been Swiss.]
[20] [The term *le dédoublement de la consciense* might now be translated "splitting of consciousness" from French, in accord with subsequent psychiatric terminology, but the original English term used by Braid was probably "double consciousness".]

In certain cases, the muscles remained in a state of relaxation, breathing and circulation were peaceful; in others, there was catalepsy with laboured breathing and considerable acceleration of circulation. But, remarkably, a current of air directed on the face or the ears made the catalepsy and the anaesthesia disappear, and returned consciousness and will to the patient; a state of excessive sensitivity of all the sensory organs was established, and if one renewed the current of air, with the hand, by means of bellows or differently, the patient woke up quickly.

The vast majority of patients, however, never reach this level; it is more common to see them remaining within the stage of reverie with the sensory activity more or less lowered or raised, according to their intellectual or physical characteristics; they also preserve, after awakening, complete memory of all that was said or done in their presence, during this artificial sleep. [Braid seems to say below that 10% of his patients attained a degree of hypnosis resembling loss of consciousness or sleep.]

A curious characteristic of the sleep thus caused is the phenomenon which occurs on the side of the eyelids. Whereas, in ordinary sleep, the eyelids are in a state of absolute rest, here they vacillate continuously, in such a manner that we glimpse the sclera [the whites of the eyes]; or else they are closed by a spasm of the orbicular muscles.

Subjective Nature of the Phenomena
I had already worked for three years to define hypnotism, the process which consists in fixing the eyes on a point and concentrating the attention, and I had demonstrated that it was an influence of a subjective nature which caused the sleep, when, in 1844, by carrying out research for a history of magic and witchcraft, as well as Mesmerism and hypnotism, I discovered in *The History of Hindoos* by [William] Ward and in the *Dubistan (History of the religious sects in India)* [*Dabistān-i Mazāhib*, a 17th century Persian religious text] developments which, through the practices of Fakirs and Yogins [Sufi and Hindu mystics], wholly confirmed my subjective theory.

The Fakirs and Yogins have caused ecstatic trance in themselves for 2,400 years, for religious purpose, by a process quite similar to that which I taught my patients so they could hypnotise themselves using, i.e., continual fixation upon the end of the nose or another part of the body or an imaginary object, and with intense attention and while holding or slowing down their breath. I mentioned some of the results obtained by these [religious] enthusiasts in my small work on trance and lethargy (*human hybernation*) [*Observations on Trance*, 1850] as on pages 108-144 of my work *Magic, Witchcraft, etc.* [1852]. Which I herewith send a copy of to the Institute.

I did not know of the practices of Fakirs and Yogins, when I published my method of hypnotising; they confirm, in the most satisfactory manner, my *subjective* theory, at the expense of the objective theory of the magnetisers.[21]

Certain patients with a roving mind, who cannot manage to concentrate their attention, are not affected in a significant way by the hypnotic processes; this is a fact that I could also observe in idiots[22] when I tried to hypnotise them. It is impossible for them to fix their attention long enough to bring about, as with sensitive and impressionable subjects, the necessary modification in their physiological functions. After careful reflection, I adopted the following conclusion: the phenomena in question are of a psychological as well as physiological nature, and the expression which would encompass all the phenomena that we have the power to cause by our processes and our suggestions would be "*psycho-physiological*".[23]

The most variable symptoms can develop during different stages of the hypnotic state, from extreme insensitivity and catalepsy to the most acute sensitivity, and the greatest excitability. Some of these changes can be caused immediately in the desired phase of hypnotism by auditory or tactile suggestions; because the patients show an exaggerated sensitivity or insensitivity, an incredible muscular power, or the complete loss of will, according to the impressions which one creates within them at the time. These impressions occur following auditory suggestions, *i.e., coming from a person in whom the patient has confidence*, or as a result of some physical impression, with which they had previously associated the same idea, or even in consequence of the position, the activity or the repose that one communicated to their person and to certain groups of muscles. [Braid here recognises three classes of suggestion: through *spoken words, habitual association*, and *muscular manipulation*.] Indeed, one can play with similar patients, in the appropriate phase of sleep, *as on a musical instrument* and make them take the dreams of their imagination for present reality. Their judgement and their will are dimmed so much, they are so under their temporary enchantment and their imagination is excited to such an extent, that they see, feel and act as if all the impressions which pass through their head were reality; they are full of these ideas, however absurd they are, they are possessed, and act accordingly.

---

[21] [Braid seems to mean that because the ancient Sufis and yogis induced similar states through breathing exercises and meditation, this proves that the effect was not due to the power of another person being transmitted to them, as the Mesmerists believed.]
[22] [Victorian physicians referred to the mentally handicapped as "idiots." It is of course not meant to be derogatory.]
[23] [Braid's use of the term "psycho-physiological" might be viewed as prefiguring the modern expression "cognitive-behavioural" as, indeed, he appears to refer to the interaction of conscious cognitive factors, such as expectation, with physiological and behavioural processes, such as nervous arousal or relaxation. Moreover, he elsewhere explicitly recognises the role of "dominant ideas" in shaping the perception and effect of physical processes such as the Mesmeric passes, i.e., through what we now call "cognitive mediation".]

There is more: some individuals are so impressionable to suggestions, that they can be dominated and controlled even in the apparent waking state (by an energetic affirmation), as one does with others in hypnotism and at the stage of double consciousness.[24] It is these individuals who give rise to the alleged "waking phenomena", to which the absurd name of "electro-biology" has been given, as I explain in detail later in this work.

Initial Supporting Facts
The first physical fact which drew my attention, as a *real* phenomenon, was the incapacity of a patient of Monsieur Lafontaine to open their eyes after being Mesmerised by him [i.e., the phenomenon now called "eyelid catalepsy"]. The operator attributed this inability to the all-powerful influence of the Mesmeric fluid, which, emanating from his person, passed into that of the patient during the Mesmeric operations, *i.e.*, with contact of the thumbs and the mutual fixation of their eyes. [The Mesmerist, in such cases, would grasp the subject's thumbs and stare into his eyes.] I came to this conclusion: this fact came from the exhaustion of voluntary control over the levator muscles of the eyelids (because the latter were constantly in activity during eye fixation by the operator) and the disorder of the visual field, as well as increased sensitivity of the conjunctivae and their state of dryness (because of prolonged fixing), and finally the increase in the degree of excitability and power of the orbicular muscles (coming from the prolonged rest). I was convinced that one could obtain the same results while looking in the same way, fixedly and continuously, at any inanimate object, and by concentrating in the same manner one's attention during the fixation. My experiments, made with the aim of elucidating this issue, were absolutely conclusive. They proved the correctness of my theoretical views, and, moreover, are confirmed by all that I have noted in my research for eighteen years. My ordinary method of hypnotising and the means of producing the majority of the phenomena are described in the first part of [*Neurypnology*] my work of 1843; I refer the reader there.

Concerning the remarkable cases of cure by hypnotism, I invite the reader to consult my various booklets as well as my book of 1843 in which they are reported. I regarded as sufficient a certain number of notable examples; I could have multiplied them by drawing from my daily practice. On page 8 of my work on *Trance* [*Observations on Trance*, 1850], and on pages 94-97 of my work on *Magic, Witchcraft, etc.*, [1852] a striking example will be found of the *subjective* nature of the influence and the power of the dominant ideas in the waking state.

Subjective Nature of the Phenomena[25]
Since the publication of my first book, I have continued my studies on hypnotism; I am thus able to clarify certain points which have remained obscure until now. I have previously mentioned them in several of my writings, but I propose here to join together the most important of them, so that with this appendix the translation of my work [*Neurypnology*] of 1843, that Mr. Masson will publish, presents a complete and accurate summary of my research on such a remarkable and interesting subject.[26]

We have seen, in what precedes, how some individuals could, by their own concentration of mind alone, throw themselves into a state similar to that which one can be caused by the Mesmeric operations. The fastest and surest method consists in causing the patient to fixate [their mind and gaze] upon any object of an unexciting nature; the object must be held above the face in such a manner as to be perceived distinctly by both eyes, and at the same time the individual must concentrate all of his attention upon the act to be accomplished.

This process proved the subjective nature of the influence brought into play. What confirmed my conclusion was that the variety of objects which they were made to fix their gaze upon did not seem, in any way, to modify the symptoms determined. With certain very impressionable subjects, the results obviously depended on an expectation of some event; also any physical arrangement was enough to bring about the sleep; it took place when their attention was placed in expectation by the positive assertion that they would fall asleep; on the other hand, a moment later, one could subject them to the same conditions without bringing on sleep, if, by suggestion or in any way whatsoever, one persuaded them that the physical conditions were currently ineffective. As I also demonstrated, with very sensitive individuals, the mere assumption that something was happening at a distance which could send them to sleep was enough to produce the sleep, although absolutely nothing actually happened. As for the [Mesmerists'] claim that certain operators can influence subjects nearby or at a distance by the will alone, I can affirm, after a conscientious study of the question, on the basis of my experiments, that I could never exert the least influence on the patients by my will alone. But patients seemed to quickly and subtly understand the mannerisms, the gaze, the voice, and even the gestures themselves of the operator, and became affected in

---

[24] [Braid therefore recognised that hypnotic virtuosos are frequently highly responsive to suggestion even when they are not formally hypnotised.]
[25] [Preyer's German edition contains the heading "Addition - Chapter from Mr. Braid, added in January 1860" at this point. The preceding sections may therefore derive from an earlier draft written in 1859.]
[26] Mr. Masson returned me my book and gave up the idea of a complete translation of that volume: I therefore wrote the following pages as an appendix and sent it to Monsieur Velpeau, for a Report to the Institute; I now address this copy to Dr. Azam. (James Braid.)

the sense that they gave to them. The operator, however, could have willed the complete opposite.[27]

The typical Mesmeric processes are very numerous, but, according to what I have seen on this subject and according to my ordinary manner of hypnotising, the true cause of the phenomena is simply this: the different methods used favour the production of this state of [mental] abstraction or fixation of attention, in which the mind is absorbed by a single idea. Then, the patient falls into indifference, he is closed, so to speak, to all foreign influences or impressions other than those called to his attention. In this state, his imagination becomes so vivid that any agreeable idea, developed spontaneously or suggested by a person to whom he accords, in a particular manner, his attention and confidence, takes on for him all the power of present events, of reality. The more frequently these phenomena are evoked, the easier and more convenient it becomes to evoke them; such is the law of association and habit. Indeed, the mind is in a state close to dreaming; the difference is that the patients not only think, but are still capable of putting their thoughts and desires into action.

In support of the foregoing, I will remind you again of the difficulty in fixing the attention in idiots[28]; all my efforts to hypnotise them remained without results, in spite of long perseverance. I encountered a patient who was very sensitive in a state of health, but entirely refractory to the hypnotic influence during the delirium of a fever.

Baron Reichenbach's Odic Force
After a series of careful experiments, I was able, in a small work entitled *The Power of the Mind over the Body*, published in 1846, to establish the following point: the act of directing the attention in a continual way upon a part of the body brings in a few minutes a change in the function of the organ considered at length; this modification is, in general, an increase in the intensity in function. But, remarkably, with a considerable number of individuals, the opposite took place, because of the pre-existence of a different impression or a capricious interpretation of an auditory suggestion. If the imagination is excited, the attention, so to speak, is riveted, and the faith of the patient is strong then the phenomena inevitably emerge; they can be noted even in some individuals in an ordinary state of wakefulness. Thanks to my method of hypnotising, the physical phenomena can occur in a surer, faster and more intense way, by the concentration of the mind, even if the eyes are held open, than in the ordinary state of wakefulness. [Braid here implies that subjects can be hypnotised with their eyes kept open, so long as their attention is suitably focused.] But when such individuals are thrown into a hypnotic state as profound as that which gives place to the appearance of double consciousness, suggestions of all kinds then become all-powerful. In fact, hypnotism does not comprise a single state, it is rather a series of different stages each one susceptible of infinite variations, from the lightest reverie with heightening in the functions, to profound [hypnotic] coma with complete absence of consciousness and volition; one can, however, by very simple means, quickly recall, partially or completely, the patient to his normal state of mind.

I therefore maintain the view that the operator acts as an engineer[29] who would put into action the forces in the organism itself of the patient, controlling them and directing them according to the laws which govern the interaction of mind and matter during our present existence.

The following extracts from my work *The Power of the Mind over the Body* [1846], will make me better understood by the reader. [Braid published a detailed critique of Reichenbach's claims to have shown that subjects perceived and were affected by an invisible energy, similar to animal magnetism.] I readily admit that the experiments of Baron von Reichenbach [a respected German scientist] were carried out carefully, and that they were well-suited for the demonstration of physical facts, but it seems to me that they erred with regard to the very important role that the mind of the patient plays in such experiments: it exhibits effects or modifications independently of any external influence. The one and only proof of the so-called "new force", are certain phenomena produced on the nervous system of some very sensitive people. As my experiments clearly show, the above-mentioned kind of phenomena, with individuals as highly impressionable as those with which the baron succeeds, can be produced by the concentration of the patient's mind alone, especially when they expect that something will happen. The effect could be notably increased, when the patient saw or felt any object whatsoever passed over any part of the body; the object which he sees or smells aids him further with the most intense concentration of his mind on the part operated upon, and there is no need for a secret emanation or an external influence coming from the object or the operator and acting on the patient.[30] On this matter, there is no doubt possible. I draw the following facts from the above-mentioned writing.

In his experiments, Baron von Reichenbach started by making slow passes of the magnet from the wrist to the end of the fingers, without immediate contact with the skin; thus he learned from certain subjects,

---

[27] [Braid refutes the notion of a telepathic connection between the Mesmerist and subject, finding instead that the subject is affected by their own expectations and perception of events.]
[28] [Braid seeks here to support his view that concentration of attention is essential to hypnotism.]
[29] [Braid seems to mean that the hypnotist resembles the "engineer", or driver, of a steam train insofar as he merely directs the existing psycho-physiological abilities of the client rather than, as the Mesmerists believed, imposing his own supernatural power upon them.]
[30] [Braid emphatically embraces the scientific principle of parsimony, or "Occam's Razor", according to which novel entities or forces should not be introduced to a theory if the observations in question can already be explained by means of well-established scientific concepts.]

that he names "sensitives", that they felt, under the magnetic pole, an impression of coolness, an *aura*; when the magnet was passed in the opposite direction, the *aura* seemed to them hot. If he took, instead of the magnet, a crystal, he produced with these individuals the same phenomena; he still produced them if, instead of the magnet or of the crystal, he used any inert substance. The ends of the fingers were enough to produce the same effect with sensitive individuals.

He requested some of the latter to look at the poles of a strong magnet in the darkness; they said they could see flames of various sizes and different colours which emanated from it and also much smaller flames emanating from other parts of the magnet. Then, they saw glowing lights and flames coming from crystals and other inert objects as well as from the ends of the fingers.

The Influence of Suggestions
These facts seemed to Baron von Reichenbach entirely distinct from the ordinary phenomena of magnetism. He believed himself to have discovered a new force, which was distinguished from all the other known forces; he gave it the name of "Od" or "odic force". [Named after the Norse god Odin.] He was misguided; he did not take account of the considerable influence of the mind with nervous subjects, an influence that one cannot ignore as shall be well understood from the experiments which I shall now discuss.

> "With nearly all the patients I have tried, many of whom had never been hypnotised or Mesmerised, when drawing the magnet or other object slowly from the wrist to the points of the fingers, various effects were realised, such as a change of temperature, tingling, creeping, pricking, spasmodic twitching of muscles, catalepsy of the fingers, or arm, or both; and reversing the motion was generally followed by a change of symptoms, from the altered current of ideas thereby suggested. Moreover, if any idea of what might be expected existed in the mind previously [autosuggestion], or was suggested orally [hetero-suggestion], during the process, it was generally very speedily realised. The above patients being now requested to look aside, or a screen having been interposed, so as to prevent their seeing what was being done, and they were requested to describe their sensations during the repetition of the processes, similar phenomena were stated to be realised, even when there was nothing whatever done, beyond watching them, and noting their responses. They believed the processes were being repeated, and had their minds directed to the part, and thus the physical action was excited, so as actually to lead them to believe and describe their feelings as arising from *external* impressions." [*The Power of the Mind*, 1846]

Following the appearance of my booklet on *The Power of the Mind over the Body* [1846], I received a letter from Sir Henry Holland, a very capable authority in these matters [whose *Medical Notes & Reflections*, 1839, contained similar arguments]; it testified to the satisfaction which my experiments and their interpretation caused him; the speculations of Reichenbach, on the odic force, he added, seemed to him not to require no further refutation. The *British and Foreign Medico-Chirurgical Review*, *Quarterly Review*, *North British Review*, [three important Victorian medical journals] expressed themselves in the same manner, as did a considerable number of well-known authors in the field of physiology and practical medicine. I had shown, without any doubt, that *the mind of the patient alone* was able to produce the effects allotted to the force named "odic" by Reichenbach and that, with such individuals, audible suggestions can also bring about the same phenomena. It is now more than thirteen years since my little work appeared and the objections that I raised against the validity of Reichenbach's discoveries have not yet been satisfactorily answered.

I borrow once more from the same booklet the following facts[31]: A 56-year-old lady, who had been a somnambulist in her youth, but who, for a long time, had experienced no further incidents and whose health was perfect was led into a dark room; she was asked to look at a powerful magnet made up of nine elements, and to describe what she saw. After a rather long time, she declared that she did not see anything. I asked her to look at it again with attention and announced to her that she would see fire leaving the tips of the magnet; she saw sparks at once, subsequently it seemed to her that they issued forth like those of an artificial eruption of the volcano Vesuvius which she had seen in a park. I dropped the lid of the trunk which contained the magnet, without informing her, *but she continued to see the same apparitions and to describe them*. I asked her, still in a suggestive manner, to say what she saw in another part of the room, where there was absolutely only the bare wall; she started to describe sparks and flames, following in her description the questions which I posed in order to modify her initial impressions. These experiments were renewed on several occasions with the same person and she always gave identical results.

More remarkably, this patient was brought into the same closet after the magnet had been removed without her knowledge, and she claimed to still see the same apparitions of light and flames; there was however nothing in the room to cause these phenomena but the bare walls; fourteen days later, when she went into the closet by herself, the simple association of ideas was enough to make her relive the phenomena of light and flames, and it was thus each time that she entered this room.

In like manner, when she was made to touch the poles of the magnet, while she was in the waking state, she did not perceive any phenomenon of attraction of the hand to the magnet; but as soon as I made her believe that the force of attraction of the magnet was going to hold it fast, and that she would not be able

---

[31] [The following few pages appear to contain a slightly modified version of the text found in *The Power of the Mind* (1846) and elsewhere. I have therefore translated the French rather than substituting direct quotations from the English text.]

to separate her hand, such a result was realised; a new suggestion was enough to deliver it. If, then, having suggested to her that the magnet would not exert any more attraction, and she touched it again, this negative phenomenon took place. I am convinced that this lady was incapable of deception; it is rather probable that she was deceiving herself and that she was surprised by the appearance of preconceived phenomena; she was not less astonished by the power of the instrument than the witnesses who attended the scene.

It was the same with other patients that I led in the dark room and who could see nothing there until the moment when they were made to gaze at a certain point fixedly from whence lights and flames would rise. The announced phenomena took place quickly; however, the patients, fully awakened, looked upon only the bare walls. I have moreover been able to convince myself that a strong impression, even in daylight, with certain people whose imagination is vivid and who are capable of a powerful effort of mind, was sufficient to produce such illusions. The following case of it is an outstanding proof.

It concerns a young man aged 24 years, who had suffered epilepsy for eleven years. This patient had been treated for the whole of this period by ordinary remedies without seeing his state improving, but hypnotism had finally succeeded in decreasing the force and the frequency of his attacks. Led into the room, he initially saw nothing there, but when I had drawn his attention on to the lights and the flames, he claimed to see them perfectly, not only where the magnet was located, but also at other parts of the room. This patient, like the two previously mentioned, saw flames and colours in the room each time that he entered there, though the magnet had been removed long ago.

As soon as he was made to look at the end of a piece of brass wire, he could be made to believe that he saw a sort of flame or *colour*; he saw it issue from the wire, *even in broad daylight*; if one made him touch the wire with a finger, by saying to him that it would be impossible for him to withdraw it, imagination was enough to paralyse his volition; the muscles stiffened and he looked upon his own state with astonishment; but the moment I declared *the attraction gone and the withdrawal of the hand possible*, he withdrew it at once. Hardly had the finger been a little withdrawn when I affirmed boldly that he *could* not any more bring it closer to the wire, because it would repel him away; this new impression paralysed his volition and in spite of anxious and repeated attempts, he could not renew the contact. I thus suggested this last influence had just ended, the stiffness of the arm and of the hand ceased at once; then turning towards one of the people who attended the experiment, I told him, loud enough to be overheard, that the patient was going to feel his hand attracted towards the brass wire in an irresistible way; hardly had I spoken than the phenomenon was carried out. Nobody had touched the wire in question for a long time, and it was, after all, only a bent brass wire [brass being *non*-magnetic], which had become detached from the chimneypiece. It is to a similar force that Virgil may have referred in these words:

Possunt, quia posse videntur.
["They can because they believe they can." – *The Aeneid*, V, 231]

I had informed one of my friends of the remarkable vividness of the imagination of this patient, his blind faith and his credulity, which rendered him liable to admit as facts all the impressions that others suggested to him. I thus requested my friend who came in the room with the same patient to agree to look towards the brass wire and to answer me, each time I would ask him for the colour of the flame which he saw, as if, indeed, whatever he saw was something new with each question. The patient took the bait and saw all the phenomena announced without suspecting that he was misled. He left more convinced than ever of the physical reality of all that he had seen and described; and he affirmed seeing similar phenomena each time that he was so tested on this subject.[32]

I gave this observation at so much length, because it provides an excellent example of a class of patients who readily let themselves be taken in by suggestions, without having – as I will show – the least intention to mislead anybody, and without suspecting, in any way, that they themselves are misled. I have, as proof of all that I advance on this subject, unanimous declarations of many patients, whose sincerity is for me beyond question, and who are perfectly competent to render account of their feelings; there exists, for me, no doubt about all these facts.

One can therefore, while acting strongly and with suggestion on the minds of the patients in the waking state, modify the physical activity of the organ or part which is used for the expression of such function, and make them believe that they see various forms and colours, that they have variable mental impressions, that irresistible forces attract them, repel, or paralyse them.

Different Stages of Hypnotism

Moreover, I showed that the same influence can be exerted in relation to sound, the sense of smell, taste, heat or cold; so that mental suggestion and concentration of the mind are enough with some individuals to evoke images not vague, but absolutely precise, to make them perceive distinct odours, to make it possible with the sense of taste to distinguish different substances, as well as that of touch, heat or cold, as if the

---

[32] [An example of what Braid calls "imitation" or "sympathy", i.e., social role-modelling.]

feelings corresponded to positive facts here. As I demonstrated, it is the case with certain people, with impressionable and colourful imaginations during the waking state and without there being any real manifestation of colour, sound or savour; I have demonstrated, in clear manner, that by mere questions, asking patients which song, which odour, which animal, which taste, and finally which object they perceived as *present* (and said emphatically in order to cause a change in their minds), I could develop impressions in their minds totally different from those which existed in my own at the same time.[33]

The people on whom I carried out these experiments were safe from any suspicion from the point of view of their veracity, uprightness, and capacity to describe their feelings and their thoughts; all these remarkable results must therefore be attributed to the mutual interaction of the mind and the body ["psycho-physiology"]; a reaction which I have so often mentioned. One of the most beautiful examples of these "vigilant phenomena" or "electro-biological" phenomena, as they were later wrongly named [by Grimes & Dodds], an example relevant to *all* the senses, was provided to me by a person endowed with great literary, scientific and philosophical knowledge. He had never attended any experiment of this nature before submitting himself to it. After I had finished with the various phenomena that I wanted to provoke in him, he asked me for the explanation of what had occurred. I requested him to read my writings. He told me, after having read them carefully, that he was entirely satisfied and that he believed that I had discovered the true solution of the problem, as in the preceding remarks. One can formulate it as follows: the true cause of these waking phenomena (*vigilant phenomena*) is not a physical external influence, it is an internal and intellectual illusion, which often occurs following positive assertions that another person makes. This other person has, according to the conviction of the patients, a certain mysterious and all-powerful force. This belief suspends their judgement and volition, and over-excites the imagination to such an extent that, during the charm, they are no more, so to speak, than puppets in the hands of their enchanter at that moment, and he controls them in an irresistible way. They cannot then but see, hear, taste, feel, touch, act, in unison with the expressed will and intentions of an absolute power which for them exists in fact; all their attention being concentrated on what this person *orders* or *says*.

Thus the *mono-ideo-dynamic* influence, that I will presently describe, exhibits its power with every mental and physical function. Some individuals may let themselves be deceived by the *compelling* words of other individuals, but a much more significant number falls into the same state after being hypnotised by continuous eye-fixation upon an object and concentration of mind. This state can even be established before the eyelids are closed or a pronounced tendency to sleep has been felt. Suggestibility can also be increased by the sight of other patients in the experiment, and that by virtue of the laws of sympathy and imitation.

Strictly speaking, the word hypnotism should be reserved only for those patients who actually fall into a state of sleep, and who forget upon awakening all that occurred during this state. When this is lacking, it is a question merely of reverie or dreaming. It would therefore be apposite to establish a terminology, characterising these modifications which result from the hypnotic process; indeed, with regard to those conditions resistant to ordinary medication and suitable for cure by hypnotism, hardly one patient in ten arrives at the unconscious stage of sleep (at least for the whole duration of the process). The word "hypnotism" can then lead them into error and make them believe that they do not benefit in any way from a process of which the characteristic and obvious effects do not appear to be those that the name [i.e., "hypnotic sleep"] indicates. After careful consideration, I estimate that one can fill this gap in the following way:

I will give the name of "*hypnotism*" to the production of the artificial sleep, where there is loss of memory, so that upon awakening, the patient does not have any memory of what occurred during the sleep, but which he remembers, however, when he is again thrown into the same degree of hypnotism. This expression encompasses, consequently, what I have called the double consciousness. There is perhaps no better established fact than the existence of this kind of case; moreover, specific facts, from long years hence, and always forgotten during the waking state, returned to the memory, in a completely precise way, during the hypnotic state.[34]

The name "*hypnotic coma*" will be given to this phase of more advanced sleep, in which the patient has no awareness of external impressions, where he has lost all volition, and where the suggestions of others made either by word, or by action, cannot[35] be recalled to his mind on awakening or in any stage of *subsequent* hypnotisation. The individuals of this kind, and they are relatively small in number [Braid implies they number far fewer than 10%], are the only ones which one can say with certainty are able to endure surgical operations without pain nor any complaint. There are, however, patients who are in a less advanced degree of hypnotism and being aware of the operation of which they are the object, do not feel an intense pain, especially if they are persuaded that it must be so. But in this case, the precise assertion of one of the

---

[33] [Braid means to assert that the effects were due to congruently delivered suggestions, etc., and not telepathic influence as the Mesmerists claimed.]

[34] [This concept of recovering memories from previous episodes of hypnosis appears to resemble Freud & Breuer's (1895) notion of recovering memories of "hypnoid" states through regression.]

[35] [The French text actually says '*can* be recalled' but this must be a mistake. In *The Physiology of Fascination* (1855), which this passage seems to derive from, Braid clearly says that 'no idea of what had been said or done by others during the said state of hypnotic coma can be remembered by the patient on awakening'. I am advised *that* version is also more consistent with the German translation of the current article.]

assistants, *contending* that now they will feel pain, or a draught from a door or a window or any direction and coming to strike the patient on the part operated upon, is enough to break the spell; then the patient feels the pain in the most acute way. It will be understood, on the other hand, under the name of:

Mono-ideology, the science of the influence of predominant ideas on mental and physical activity;
Mono-ideism, the state of mind under the influence of a dominant impression;
Mono-ideise, the act of inducing the state of *mono-ideism*;
Mono-ideised, the state of the person in the stage of *mono-ideism*;
Mono-ideo-dynamics, the mental and physical changes, excitement as well as depression [of the nervous system], which result from the influence of *mono-ideism*.

Dr. [William] B. Carpenter had proposed, a few years ago, the name of "*ideo-motor*" to qualify the reflex or automatic muscular movements which only occur under the influence of impressions associated with these movements alone, without the will having taken any role in the development of these phenomena. In 1853, Dr. [Daniel] Noble pointed out that the expression "*ideo-dynamic*"[36] would be preferable, in the sense that it would apply to a greater number of phenomena. I was entirely of his opinion, because I knew that a suggestion could as well *arrest* as *excite* a muscular movement of an automatic nature. My research had also shown that dominant and expectant suggestions can control and modify all the *other* functions of the human body just as with muscular movements; it is for that reason that I had adopted the expression of "*mono-ideo-dynamic*" which indicated in the most general and most characteristic way the relations between the mental modifications and reactions on the one hand, and the same dynamic phenomena, on the other hand; and this applies to all the functions of the body under the influence of ideas and dominant suggestions, especially during the abnormal state that the hypnotic procedure induces, more particularly with those people who arrive at the double conscious stage.

Waking Phenomena
With the majority of patients, while they remain in the state which allows them to remember upon awakening all that was said and done during the sleep, there exists a certain degree of judgement and will which makes them capable of distinguishing true impressions from false and which gives them the power to resist any unreasonable action. There are, however, individuals who, *even during this state*, are strongly dominated and blinded by the imagination, whose credulity and passive obedience to the will of others are considerable, to such an extent that one can govern and control them as if they were in the state of double consciousness in which the patients take the successive suggestions of others for positive facts and act accordingly; there are even large numbers, who can be thus influenced and controlled during the waking state and in full consciousness of themselves. It is with the latter that the magnetisers produce the "vigilant phenomena", whereby they draw the proof of the existence of a Mesmeric special force, emanating from the person of the operator, controlling the intellectual and physical forces of the patient; it was the individuals of such a nature that were exhibited publicly in America, in England, and other places to explain what has been named "electro-biology", ten years later [than Braid had done]. But I had shown in my work *The Power of the Mind over the Body*, published in 1846, that these effects occurred under the influence of suggestion among certain patients; an influence which can excite or depress the function of any organ of sense. The impression suggested seized the mind of the patient to such an extent, that under its influence one could suspend the function of sight, make him blind to an object placed in front of him, or induce the thought that this object is transformed into another, such that its shape, its colour, are changed; and the fictions of his imagination are too vivid for an appeal to the ordinary function of the eyes to be able to correct them. The same errors can occur for all the other senses, as I could make patients believe that they heard music when there was none, and a moment after I made them deaf for sounds that everyone heard distinctly. The same goes for the sense of smell, taste, and touch; sensation is in accord with the suggestion, instead of with reality, as it should be in a normal state, when the mind of these individuals acts without foreign influence.

As I long ago remarked, neither the action of the will, neither sympathy, nor imitation alone can explain how patients (like individuals in good health) have feelings of unbearable heat or cold; whether with them the organs of sight, hearing, the sense of smell, or taste are paralysed or modified, in order to make them perceive impressions other than those which things should usually produce, were it not for the suggestions of the experimenter. It is known however that a strongly impressed image, and a lively imagination are able to produce the above-mentioned impressions, such cases arising in monomania, in *delirium tremens*, alcoholism, the narcoses produced by opium, hashisch, and other similar causes, as in various other pathological states. The impressions in these various states can develop in a powerful manner, consequently they have for the patient all the force of reality; the latter certainly retains, to a certain degree, the consciousness of all that occurs around him, but it is impossible for him to be freed from the

---

[36] [The ideo-motor, or ideo-dynamic, theory of suggestion was therefore the original neuro-psychological model of hypnosis, though these terms are now widely *misappropriated* by contemporary writers on hypnosis, such as Cheek & Rossi (1988), etc., who seem to use them without acknowledgement of their original meaning in Braid's writings.]

erroneous impression which controls him. The impression can even dominate him so as to make him indifferent to any other impression.

Suggestion by Tone of Voice
To induce images or erroneous impressions among patients, while they have their eyes open and they seem in the ordinary waking state, there is no better way than to say aloud, in an imperious and convincing manner, the thought that one wants to awaken in them. But the patients who are in a high degree of hypnotism, especially at the stage of double consciousness, can be affected in different ways, for example as a result of a simple change in intonation. If they are asked what they see, their answer will be, perhaps, a sheep, a dog or a bird.

"What colour is it?" said in a light-hearted tone, may lead to the answer: "White" or some other light colour. If we then asked: "What colour is it *now*?" giving a sad intonation to the word *now*, the answer may then be "brown" or "black", according to the shade of melancholy that is applied to the word "*now*".

The same applies to the form, substance, taste, sense of smell, sound, and regardless of whether it concerns a true or supposed impression, communicated by speech or song. The question or the word "now" evokes the impression of a lighter or darker shade of colour, a change in the form or quality, according to the inflection of the voice and the emphatic tone which is employed.

The Influence of Suggestions
Here is another way of modifying the primary impression: let us suppose our patient on his knees and consumed with religious sentiments; he is asked what he sees; perhaps he will answer: "Heaven." The skin of his forehead is wrinkled, by drawing it down with the fingers an inch, towards the bridge of the nose; the voice is not changed, but the answer, accompanied by a shivering, will perhaps then be: "Hell." One can repeat these experiments and obtain the same results at will. [Elsewhere, Braid refers to this technique, comparable to the James-Lange theory of emotion, as "muscular suggestion".]

The wrinkling of the skin in the middle region of the forehead evokes sad images, whatever the main impression of the movement, whatever the [so-called phrenological] organ concerned. In the same way, raising his head, the patient being on his knees, brings him to think of heaven and light; lowering the head makes him, on the contrary, think of hell, darkness and sad things; thus one can cause and modify at will ideas in the individuals "possessed". One can lead them from grave to gentle, pleasant to severe. Their manner of being changes, they feel, they see, as if all in question were reality. They act and speak without the least sign of personal volition, while they are subjected to a foreign will in such a categorical way.

As we said, the position of the body significantly influences the emotions and sensations during the desired stage of hypnotism; also, whatever the passion which one wants to express by the attitude of the patient, when the muscles necessary to this expression are brought into play, the passion itself bursts forth suddenly and the whole organism responds accordingly. The upright body, the expanded chest, the contracted extensors, all that suggests the feeling of self-esteem, self-determination, resolve and unconquerable pride. As soon as one decreases the contraction of these muscles, that gives to the patient a depressed attitude, with sunken chest, the expression of the features changes in a very manifest way, the voice and the whole manner of being of the individual now express humility, abasement and pity.

I shall go into some detail about the increase and decrease in muscular movements under the influence of suggestion. This will involve interesting facts which have not thus far attracted attention.

Voluntary movements occur, because the will directs nerve impulse; the muscles which should naturally bring about the intended movement come into play, while the antagonistic ones remain passive.

In experiments designed to prove the paralysis of muscular strength by means of suggested impressions, the suggestion develops, for the muscles which should produce the desired movement, a nervous excitation stronger than that which the patient is in a position to produce for the opposing muscle groups. The two types of muscles are thus put vigorously into action, but as the impression *suggested is much stronger*, the voluntary movements cannot be carried out, in spite of the considerable nervous force that the patient deploys, which one recognises by his rapid exhaustion. I made a patient seize a cane despite himself; he could no longer drop it; I then said aloud: "I will make it so heavy that it will be impossible for him to support the weight of it"; he heard this simple suggestive remark and it was too much for his energetic, but misdirected, muscular efforts; he endeavoured in vain to support this imaginary burden and finally dropped it to the ground exhausted.

After the experiment, the patient said he firmly believed that he had seen at each end of the cane, and he showed the precise location, a fifty pound weight, and that he had felt the weight increase and finally overpower him. It was obvious that the efforts which he had made to support the imaginary weight had tired him, just as much as if he had supported a genuine burden. This feeling and its result are rather common in nightmares during ordinary sleep. The effort and exhaustion are similar in both cases. On the other hand, when the impression that was suggested to him and the firm belief that it establishes agree with his own intention, the effort which the patient can make is enhanced to the extent that it allows him to raise a weight which would be too heavy for him in his ordinary state. History offers to us examples of panic in the armed forces, of acts of audacity and valour, which are accomplished in one moment of enthusiasm, and which, for the most part, are brought together within the subject treated here.

How the (Mesmeric) Passes Work[37]

I will now explain my views on the so-called "Mesmeric passes". We can distinguish between passes with contact, where the fingers of the operator gently glide over the organ to be affected, and passes without contact, which are done by passing the hand, fingers extended and separated, above that part of the body; the fingers have a certain tremor which must communicate to the air a light movement which is just right to influence the part on which one operates.

My experiments led me to attribute the effects of this process to the capacity which the mind of the patient has to bring about changes in the physical activity of the part on which he is inclined to dwell too long, either by external tactile impressions, or by the efforts of his own will (as in the concentration of the attention), especially when he is persuaded that a modification which he expects is in the process of being accomplished. If, at a favourable stage of the sleep, one directs the impressions on the organs of the senses, it causes mental images which act in connection with the specific function of these organs; if one directs them over a part [of the skin] covering the muscles, the muscles begin to act; also, at the same moment, they probably develop other impressions which are usually the cause of, or precede, the physical process. [Braid is probably alluding here to his concept of muscular suggestion, once again.]

Among the most problematic phenomena that I have been fortunate enough to observe, I will mention the *contrary* effects which seemed to be the cause of similar mental impressions. For example: passes with contact or the agitation of the air along an arm or a leg put the muscles into action and brought about raising of the extremities [i.e., the arms and legs]. The magnetisers called these passes: "Mesmerising passes". If the raised extremities were fanned, they fell down, and the process received the name of "de-Mesmerising passes". If a side of the head were fanned, it followed the hand of the operator, first on one side, then the other; or the fast passage of the hand on that of the patient, then the sudden withdrawal of the hand and the repetition of this process brought the patient's hand to rise and made it cataleptic.

This fact was given by the magnetisers as decisive evidence in favour of an attraction between the hand of the operator and that of the patient; one attracted the other like a magnet attracts iron. I soon noticed that during the first transitional stage, of the waking sleep [i.e., the "first conscious stage" of hypnosis], patients preserved enough irritability and sensitivity to be affected by certain impressions and they moved closer or moved away according to whether the quality or the intensity of these impressions were pleasant or unpleasant for them.

Thus, soft music charmed them; they drew near, while noisy and discordant music affected them differently and they moved away. It was the same for odours and feelings of cold and heat. I also observed that ticklings or the agitation of the air above the skin acted upon the subjacent muscles; thus the hand could be bent or the arm raised, then while acting on the antagonistic muscles make the hand and fingers extend and the arm fall. It was an apparently simple and rather comprehensible fact; but I finally discovered finally that a group of muscles put in action by a given impression, and which had preserved the given position for some time, did not contract any more by the repetition of the same mental impression, caused at the same place as previously; *the same apparently exciting cause* produced an absolutely contrary effect, whether one had employed the passes with contact, or the simple current of air. I continued to observe that my will was foreign to this fact, because the results took place in absolutely the same way, though during my operation, I had desired the opposite. These contrary results coming from an apparently similar cause were for me an enigma which intrigued me for a long time; but I finally arrived at a seemingly quite simple solution of this apparently mysterious fact. I concluded that the consciousness and will of the patient are dimmed, that his movements are instinctive and automatic and that consequently the mental impression provides only a tendency to movement; the movements are conducted, however, in the direction and manner *most natural under the present circumstances*. For example: if a muscle is at rest, it becomes active; on the other hand, if it is moving, it becomes inactive, and this occurs from the same stimulus.

If one acts on the hand or the arm, which rests on the knees, as lowering of it can no longer occur, the arm rises and becomes rigid. If after having left the arm in the new position for some time, one reproduces the same stimulus, this brings about a tendency to carry out the most natural movement, and in this case, the arm drops. Whereas when raising or lowering of the arm is prevented in any way, and the experiment is repeated, one will see the limb move sideways.

This process can also be applied to isolated muscles. In this way, we influence the muscles of physiognomy [facial expression] and it is possible for us to arouse any passion or sentiment whatsoever; the contraction of the interconnected muscles, constituting "the anatomy of expression", evokes in the brain of the hypnotised person certain impressions just as these, in the waking state, determine the whole facial expression. It is thus merely a reversal of the usual order [of causation] between the emotions and their

---

[37] [The following paragraphs seem to derive from Braid's *Electro-Biological Phenomena* (1851).]

physical manifestations.[38] It is obvious that there is nothing occult [i.e., paranormal] nor specific [i.e., inherently effective] in the passes made with the hands; indeed a draught produced by bellows gives the same effects as a hand moving, as I so often showed before a host of intelligent observers.

The passes, as visible or sensible impressions, assist the patient in the concentration of his mind upon a particular organ, and influence at the same time the function of this part; they impress a special direction upon the power which modifies the patient himself; but one should no more suppose an occult force in the passes (a force emanating from the operator) than is it befitting to attribute to the lens the creation of the light and heat that it makes perceptible by the concentration of the light rays, and by its concentrating on a focal point the rays of energy. The passes, in the same way as the lens, *assist* the concentration and the manifestation of the influences concerned; but neither the operator nor the lens are causes of the power manifested.

Natural Symptoms, Artificial Symptoms
The foregoing passages provide an explanation of what one can naturally obtain with individuals who have not received any preliminary education on this point, and without making use of auditory [i.e., verbal] suggestions. It is however possible, by education, to entirely invert the order of these natural phenomena: suppose that the operator speaks, with each pass or with each movement that he executes, and that he says in advance what will happen, then what he said in advance can take place instead of what would have occurred naturally.

From this moment and in virtue of the double consciousness, the same impression on the same part or the same organ of sense can cause a phenomenon or an expression similar to the first. We can thus have a series of *natural* symptoms and a series of *artificial* ones, according to the manner of operating of the experimenter, and the goal which he pursues.

It is necessary also to note this point: some individuals in the state of [hypnotic] sleep see through their half-shut eyelids. When, with such subjects, the operator firmly looks at a part of the body, a leg, for example, or an arm, the patient immediately believes that he wishes the movement of the limb thus looked at and his docility pushes him to yield without delay to the suggestion, just as if passes with contact, or some other immediate stimulus had been applied. One thus sees the lowered arm rise, what was raised drops or, if this is prevented, it moves sideways; in the same way, the remarkable tendency to sympathy and imitation among these patients leads them to observe and imitate all the gestures of the operator or those of any other person to whom the operator especially draws their attention. But if one puts a screen between the operator and the one operated upon and one moves the body or the limbs, the subject sticks to hearing instead of sight and proceeds to accurately imitate *only from time to time*. In the first case, he therefore saw through partly closed eyelids and it was generally possible for him to give a *correct* imitation.

All these phenomena can take place without the patient intending to mislead, nor any recollection on awakening of anything that was said or done.

I never yet saw (either in the hypnotic or Mesmeric sleep, or in the state which gives rise to the "vigilant phenomena", which some called the electro-biological phenomena) phenomena which were not in conformity with the generally accepted laws of physiology and psychology. The senses, the mental and muscular forces can be over-stimulated or reduced to an extraordinary extent, according to dominant impressions, suggested or pre-existent, but I have never observed anything which would allow me to believe that individuals had received the gift to read through absolutely opaque bodies, to understand – either during the waking state, or during the state of double consciousness – languages that they had never learned, or to give place to the development of other transcendent phenomena, the so-called [Mesmeric] "higher phenomena". However, the acute sensitivity of hearing, and the mobility of the muscles, as well as the influence of concentrated attention and, applied to the point in question, excited imagination and confidence in oneself, allow certain patients, during the desired stage of hypnotism, to produce remarkable phenomena, for example: phonetic imitation, writing and drawing without the help of sight, discovery of the owners and bearers of certain objects (by means of the exalted sense of smell), *perception* of remarks made in a distant room when moved away, that one could not have heard during the waking state, the memory of circumstances for a long time forgotten during the waking state [hypnotic hypermnesia], finally the deduction of consequences (which indicates an extraordinary finesse of judgement) from assumptions made in the form of suggestion, or occurring spontaneously following memories of old impressions to which they had applied their full attention.

These facts recall the wonders which are reported about the [ancient] Celtic seers, or of the man of "second sight" in Scotland.[39]

The Influence of Dominant Impressions
One draws several important conclusions from the consideration of the phenomena which take place in

---
[38] [Braid is alluding to the eminent Scottish philosopher and scientist Sir Charles Bell's *Essays on the Anatomy of Expression in Painting* (1806), and formulating observations which once again pre-empt the influential James-Lange theory of emotion.]
[39] [Certain rural Scots were particularly renowned at this time for possessing the supposed gift of clairvoyance or "the second sight".]

consequence of the power of primary impressions, lively faith, and attention concentrated on dominant ideas, causes which contribute to modifying physical action, so that the new physical state reacts on the mental activity. It is possible for us today not only to understand [as due to suggestion] the cause and treatment of many diseases on which no specific external influence, nor internal drugs had any effect, but also to explain a great number of phenomena which were attributed to demonology and magic, ghosts and enchantments, to the power of witches who abused and killed their gullible victims by means of hexes and their harmful influence, so readily accepted.

Nowadays we grasp the power of the methods of enchantment, magic formulas and amulets, the means of metal traction of Perkins, the effect of the galvanic rings, the breadcrumb [placebo] pills and the infinitesimal [homeopathic] amounts of powerful drugs which cannot affect a living being either for good or ill. [Braid ridicules homeopathy as a placebo in *Hypnotic Therapeutics*, 1853.] We realise as being of this nature, the alleged clairvoyance of young Egyptians looking fixedly at a black orb [of ink] held in their hand. (Lord Prudhoe and Monsieur Lane published articles on this subject.) The revelations of [Edward] Kelly, of Manchester, whom Doctor [John] Dee made famous under the reign of Queen Elisabeth, and that Kelly had obtained from a spirit by looking at the celebrated magic stone that the doctor preserved at his home; predictions of the soothsayers, who make use themselves of a similar process for reading the future, by means of an egg made out of glass; also as the modern revelations of the same kind, for example, those of the angels in the magic crystal [ball] of Lady [Marguerite Gardiner of] Blessington – all these things fall into the same category; they are only the result of questions, or a different excitation of imagination; an effect which is taken for visions, spoken words, or answers written in quite visible letters by the alleged angels. All that produces a strong excitation, all that modifies the preliminary state of the thoughts and the feelings, surely also modifies the mental and physical state of the individual, especially if it occurs with confidence, expectation, and concentration of mind.

My experiments on contact with the scalp and the emotional phenomena that this contact caused led me to conclude that the results obtained did not prove nor disprove phrenological organology; but I maintained that there were relations between the frontal integument [forehead] and the memory.

Indeed, when I interrogated the patients in the state of double consciousness in hushed tones, they were mistaken in their answers about the simplest things and which they were familiar with during the waking state; but if I touched the middle of the forehead, their answers were correct. As soon as I suspended contact, the answers became again false, whatever the questions were; as soon as the contact was renewed on the face of the sleeping patient, the answers became again correct on each reprise. I discovered later that contact with any part of the scalp or any part of the body had the same effect – the restoration of memory. This fact carried me to publish a report rectifying my error, and to give the following explanation of the influence of these tactile impressions: for me, the patient, in an ordinary state of hypnotism is in a state of distraction or concentration of thought which enables him to hear the questions only superficially and to answer them only carelessly; the answers are thus generally erroneous, but the contact is enough to break the order of prevalent thoughts and to prepare our patient to pay sufficient attention to the question to answer it correctly. As soon as contact ceases, the patient drifts off into his reverie or is absorbed again in his preoccupying images and answers then awry, until the distraction is again dissipated by a new contact, or when the questions are repeated with sufficiently loud voice; the answers are then made correctly just like if there were contact with the finger or an inert object.[40]

On Memory, On the Sense of Smell
The following facts will show in a striking way the astonishing increase which occurs in the intellectual power with a certain phase of nervous sleep.

I have often shown that the sense of smell allows a considerable number of patients in hypnotism to immediately recognise people in the middle of a large crowd, and that they can easily identify the owner of a glove, though the latter is unknown to them. The patient sniffs the glove initially, then going around the room, he puts the glove without hesitation and without error on its owner again, without however touching them. If the nostrils were blocked, "clairvoyance" ceased at once, and it was restored as soon as the obstruction was removed.

In the same way, the increase in sensitivity of the muscular sense and the tactile sense in hypnotised subjects allows them, without the assistance of the eyes, to write correctly, even if a large book is held between the eyes and the paper. This fact is much more convincing than the practice of covering the eyes in any way [i.e., bandaging the eyes]. In spite of all these precautions, the patients write well, crossing '*t*'s and dotting '*i*'s; they even return to the preceding line, erasing a word or a letter to insert into its own place the corrected word or the letter. I remember a patient who corrected again with the greatest care a

---

[40] [Braid's technique of pressing the forehead to encourage concentration upon memories clearly resembles Freud's later "pressure technique" in early psychoanalysis.]

whole sheet of writing paper by beginning his work of revision with the bottom of the page. But, if the relative position of the paper on the table were changed, the corrections took place all at erroneous places; however, if compared to the place which the paper occupied initially, they were correctly positioned. If the paper had been pulled upwards, the corrections were made under the lines, if pulled down, the corrections took place above the line; if the disturbance had been made on the right or on the left, then corrections were on the opposite side. It is a remarkable fact, that this patient began the revision sometimes, in the relative position that he had been given, starting from the top left-hand corner of paper; the disturbance which had been made on the paper did not have any more influence; associations of the muscular sense were not constrained any more; he always sought the corner of his paper and put his corrections at the right places: I even saw him, once, put the two points on a vowel in a German word at the bottom of the page – a thing which greatly astonished his German master, who was present.

Despite everything, I have never seen a sleeping patient write without the use of the eyes as ably as with their help and during the waking state. But there are patients who have the use of their eyes during the sleep; they see, as we already said through eyelids partly closed only, and if they are not put to the test, as I have just indicated, such that it is considered sufficient merely to bandage their eyes, they will be tempted to disturb their bandage or their mask, in order to see through the lower part; they will be able then to read and write much better than in the waking state, to the great astonishment of those who do not understand, that it is the natural organ of sight, the eye, which in this case is the genuine instrument of [so-called] "clairvoyance".

Muscular Sense, Imitation
That it is also the finesse of the hearing and the precision of the muscular sense, added to the confidence which they had in themselves and their tendency to sympathy and imitation, which allow to the patients these really astonishing phonetic imitations which are, however, beyond doubt. For example, many patients very accurately repeat all that one says – in *whatever* language; they are even able to sing correctly with another person in a foreign language while following the sounds and the words of a song which they never heard; the words and the melody seem to them as familiar in the accompaniment of other singers as if they had studied them well already. Thus, one of my patients, who with the waking state did not know even the grammar of her own language and hardly knew what the music was, could correctly accompany [the renowned opera singer] Miss Jenny Lind in several songs and in various languages; she repeated the words and the air in an obviously precise manner. Two people present at this experiment did not want for some time to admit that they heard two voices, so perfect was the performance, from the point of view of the harmony and the pronunciation of Swiss, German and Italian songs. This patient accompanied Miss Jenny Lind, with as much success, in the improvisation of a long and difficult chromatic exercise that this great artist carried out to put to the test the capacities of the somnambule. When awakened, the young patient would not have dared to think of carrying out a *similar test*; in short, extraordinary though it was, it was only a phenomenon of *phonetic* imitation, because she understood, neither during the sleep nor in the waking state, the meaning of even one word of the foreign languages which she had pronounced so correctly.

All these phenomena, however extraordinary they are, are only the result of a heightening of the intellectual functions or powers, which we all have to an average degree in the ordinary or waking state. This exaltation does not go as far as a universal clairvoyance, as far as divination, as far as communion of ideas [i.e., telepathy] with the people who are *en rapport* with us [as the Mesmerists claimed]. During the heightening of her natural gift of phonetic imitation, the young somnambule could, indeed, correctly render the words and the melody of Jenny Lind's songs, but she did not understand even one word of the songs that she repeated. It would also have been impossible for her to repeat even one note of what the artist was playing on the piano – in this case, indeed, one needs a deployment of the will, assisted by teaching and study.

James Braid.
Rylaw House, Oxford Street, Manchester.
January 1860.

Wilhelm Preyer's Foreword to the German Translation
(1881)

On the 27th February 1860 Belpau of the Paris Academy of Natural Sciences presented a number of writings and a manuscript by Braid, noted in the *Comptes Rendus* of the Academy of Sciences (Issue 50., pp. 439, 450), which appeared to be a summary of the observations of Broca of the Academy and which were concerned with the curious nervous state.

It would be left to Broca's discretion as to whether he should give an oral address concerning these papers, however perhaps such an address never took place.

Broca's friend, Azam, a Professor in Bordeaux, had in fact undertaken many hypnotic experiments, just as described in Braid's paper, with great success. Braid sent him a second handwritten manuscript, the same as that presented at the Academy by Belpau, describing his discoveries, which was inscribed by Braid, three days before his death, with the words "Presented to M. Azam as a mark of esteem and regard by James Braid, surgeon, Manchester, 22nd March 1860."

This manuscript was later given to Dr. George M. Beard in New York by a relative of Azam, and was entrusted to me by Mr. Beard in August 1880.

When I presented the documents to him, the son, Dr. James Braid, immediately recognised the handwriting of his father. [Braid's son was named after him, and also became a doctor.]

It is published here in a German translation, the accuracy of which I can vouch for as I have compared it with the original.

That the form leaves a lot to be desired is the fault of the original. Braid was not a stylist. The loose and sluggish way in which his ideas come together, the difficulty of the syntax with multi clause relative sentences and exaggerated changes in participial construction, unnecessary repetition and anacolutha have made the assignment harder. However in hindsight nothing has been omitted and nothing added in this translation, to temper or to moderate the original work.

I'll leave you to fight over its academic worth, the historic worth alone justifies its publication.

Wilhelm Preyer.
Jena.
March 1881.

The Physiology of Fascination & The Critics Criticised
(1855)

"Possunt, quia posse videntur." – Virgil
["They can because they believe they can."]

(The following remarks on the "Physiology of Fascination" were written and sent by me to be read before section D of the meetings of the British Association, held at Glasgow last autumn.)

The Physiology of Fascination

The power possessed by serpents to fascinate birds has always been a source of interest and admiration to the curious. That a crawling reptile, such as a serpent, doomed to move pronely on the earth, should possess the craft and power, by the mere fixed gaze of its glaring eyes, irresistibly to draw down from their proud aerial perch the very fowls of heaven, which cleave the air with rapid wing far beyond the reach of the sportsman's tube, seems to proclaim this as one of the most remarkable of nature's laws, which has ordained that extremes should meet. The question therefore arises, by what means is this remarkable result effected? Is there any magnetic attraction in the eye of the serpent by which the bird is drawn? Or is it the result of any poisonous emanation projected by the serpent? Is it a voluntary, or an involuntary process by which the creature approaches and falls an easy prey to its fell destroyer?

Without occupying your time by entering into any elaborate history of the various speculations which have been advanced on this subject by different authors, I shall at once proceed to state what appears to me to be the true explanation of the phenomenon – one which is quite in accordance with nature's laws, and which, moreover, explains, on scientific principles, some remarkable phenomena observed even in man.

From various observations which I have read and heard on the subject, I feel satisfied that the creatures fascinated do not *voluntarily* surrender themselves to their fate; and this, I consider, is proved by the agitation and alarm which many of them display when advancing to meet their fate, *viz.*, their plaintive cries, and the agitation of their bodies, and the instant escape which they make when any circumstance has occurred to avert from their sight the glaring eyes of the serpent. Their ability to escape so speedily, moreover, under such circumstances, proves that the charm had not been the result of any poisonous emanation proceeding from, or projected by, the serpent. **After due consideration, I feel satisfied that the approach and surrender of itself by the bird, or other animal, is just another example of the *monoideo-dynamic,* or unconscious muscular action from a dominant idea possessing the mind, which I was the first to publish as the true cause of "table-turning",** [in the appendix to *Hypnotic Therapeutics*, 1853] and which has since been confirmed by others, and most satisfactorily so by the report of the medical committee published in The Medical Times *and Gazette,* and by Professor [Michael] Faraday, in the London *Times* newspaper, and in the *Athenaeum,* which contained reports of this acute and profound philosopher's ingenious experiments, and unexceptionable physical tests, for determining the question according to this view.

The law upon which these phenomena are to be explained has long been familiar to me, from observations made during my investigation of hypnotic and Mesmeric phenomena, and it is simply this – that when the attention of man or animal is deeply engrossed or absorbed by a given idea, associated with movement, a current of nervous force is sent into the muscles which produce a corresponding motion, not only *without* any conscious effort of volition, but even in opposition to volition, in many instances, and hence they seem to be irresistibly drawn, or spell-bound, according to the purport of the dominant idea or impression in the mind of each at the time. The volition is prostrate; the individual is so completely *monoideised,* or **under the influence of the dominant idea**, as to be incapable of exerting an efficient restraining or opposing power to the dominant idea; and, in the case of the bird and serpent, it is first wonder which arrests the creature's attention, and then fear causes that *monoideo-dynamic* action of the muscles which involuntarily issues in the advance and capture of the unhappy bird. This is the principle, moreover, which accounts for such accidents as are frequently witnessed in the streets of every crowded thoroughfare, where some persons, when crossing the streets amidst a crowd of carriages, not only become spell-bound by a sense of their danger, so that they cannot move from the point of danger, but it even sometimes happens that they seem impelled to advance forward into the greater danger from which they are anxious to escape, and from which a person with more self-possession or presence of mind may be fired, by the very sense of his danger, to escape, by making an incredible bound – his natural powers having become stimulated to unwonted energy, by a lively faith having taken possession of his mind as to his capability to accomplish such a feat. It is this very principle of involuntary muscular action from a dominant idea which has got possession of the mind, and **the suggestions conveyed to the mind by the muscular action which flows from it**, which led so many to be deceived during their experiments in "table-turning", and induced them to believe that the table was drawing them, whilst all the while they were unconsciously drawing or pushing it, by their own muscular force. As already remarked, it is upon this principle that the bird is drawn to its fell destroyer, and that human beings may appear deliberately and intentionally to leap over precipices, and cast themselves from towers, and other situations, not only of danger, but of certain destruction. It is also upon the same principle that some individuals may be brought so much under the control of others, through certain **audible, and visible, and tangible suggestions by another individual,** as is seen in the phenomena exhibited in the waking condition, in what has been so absurdly called "electro-biology". The whole of these phenomena of "electro-biology", of "table turning", the gyrations of the odometer [a kind of pendulum] of Dr. Mayo, of the magnetometer of Mr. Rutter, the movements of the divining-rod, and the supposed levity [i.e., levitation] of the human body lifted on the tips of the fingers of four individuals, as described by Sir David Brewster, the fascination of serpents, the evil eye and witchcraft, and the charm by which a fowl may be fixed and spell-bound by causing it to gaze at a chalk line, or strip of coloured paper, or of white paper on a dark ground – **all come under the same category, namely, the influence of a dominant idea, or fixed act of attention, absorbing, or putting in abeyance for the nonce, the other and great controlling power of the mind – the *will*.**

The following is an interesting example of a person becoming spell-bound through a dominant idea excited through the suggestion of a second party. The anecdote was communicated to me by a highly scientific friend, as an event which occurred in his own family circle. His grandfather resided in the country, and on going into his orchard one Sunday morning, he descried a boy who had climbed up into one of his apple trees, and was then in the attitude of laying hold of an apple. At this moment the gentleman addressed the boy in a *stern manner,* declaring that he would *fix him there in the position he was then in.* Having said so, the gentleman left the orchard and went off to church, not doubting that the boy would soon come down and effect his escape when he knew the master of the orchard was gone. However, it turned out otherwise; for, on going into the orchard on his return from church, he was not a little surprised to find that the boy had been spell-bound by his declaration to that effect – for there he still remained, *in the exact attitude in which he left him, with his arm outstretched, and his hand ready to lay hold of the apple.* By some farther remarks from this gentleman the spell was broken, and the boy allowed to escape without farther punishment.

My investigations have proved, beyond all controversy, that by these means the ordinary mental and physical functions may be changed, so that the subject shall **lose his freedom of action**, and that *all* the natural functions may be **either excited or depressed** with great uniformity, **even in the waking condition**, according to the dominant idea existing in the mind of man or animal at the time, **whether that has arisen spontaneously, has been the result of previous associations, or of the suggestions of others. The whole of the subsequent abnormal phenomena are due entirely to this influence of dominant ideas over physical action, and point to the importance of combining the study of psychology with that of physiology, and *vice versa.*** I believe the attempt made to study these two branches of science so much apart from each other has been a great hindrance to the successful study of either.

With the view of simplifying the study of the reciprocal actions and reactions of mind and matter upon each other, which have hitherto been comprised under the vague terms, reverie, animal magnetism, Mesmerism, hypnotism, electro-biology, *etc.*, I beg leave to suggest the adoption of the following specific terms. After having convinced myself, by numerous experiments and careful observation and reflection, that the phenomena of the so-called animal magnetism, or Mesmerism, did not result from any influence, *ab extra* [from without], of a magnetic fluid or force, projected from the body of the Mesmeriser, and passing into and charging the body of the subject with its peculiar properties and powers, but, on the contrary, **that the condition arose from influences existing within the patient's own body, *viz.*, the influence of concentrated attention, or dominant ideas, in modifying physical action, and these dynamic changes re-acting on the mind of the subject, I adopted the term *hypnotism,* or nervous sleep, in preference to Mesmerism, or animal magnetism. This term has met with most favourable consideration from many able writers on the subject; still it is liable to this grave objection – that it has been used to comprise not a *single* state, but rather a series of stages or conditions, varying in every conceivable degree, from the slightest reverie, with high exaltation of the functions called into action, on the one hand, to intense nervous coma, with entire abolition of consciousness and voluntary power, on the other;** whilst, from the latter condition, by very simple, but appropriate means, the subject is capable of being speedily partially restored, or entirely roused, to the waking condition. By this means, I maintain that the operator does not communicate any surcharge of a magnetic, odylic, electric, or vital fluid or force from his own body to that of the subject, as the real and efficient cause of the phenomena which follow in altering or modifying physical action and curing disease, **but I hold that he acts merely as the engineer, by various modes exciting, controlling, and directing *the vital forces within the patient's own body,* according to the laws which regulate the reciprocal action of mind and matter upon each other, in organised and living beings, in the present state of our existence.**

I am well aware that, in correct phraseology, the term *hypnotism* ought to be restricted to the phenomena manifested in patients who actually pass into a state of sleep, and who remember nothing on awakening of what transpired during their sleep. All short of this is mere reverie, or dreaming, however provoked, and it, therefore, seems highly desirable to fix upon a terminology capable of accurately characterising these latter modifications which result from hypnotic processes. This is the more requisite from the fact that, of those who may be relieved and cured by hypnotic processes of diseases which obstinately resist ordinary medical treatment, perhaps not more than one in ten ever passes into the state of oblivious sleep, during the processes which they

are subjected to. The term *hypnotism,* therefore, is apt to confuse them, and lead them to suspect that, at all events, *they* cannot be benefited by processes which fail to produce the most obvious indication which the name imports. After much reflection on the subject, it has occurred to me that the object in view might be attained, very satisfactorily as follows:–

Let the term *hypnotism* be restricted to those cases alone in which, by certain artificial processes, oblivious sleep takes place, in which the subject has no remembrance on awaking of what occurred during his sleep, but of which he shall have the most perfect recollection on passing into a similar stage of hypnotism thereafter. In this mode, *hypnotism* will comprise those cases only in which what has hitherto been called the double-conscious state occurs [in which reversible amnesia creates a dissociation between the hypnotic and waking states, known as "hypnotic somnambulism"]; and let the term *hypnotic coma* denote that still *deeper* stage of the sleep in which the patient seems to be quite unconscious at the time of all external impressions, and devoid of voluntary power, and in whom no idea of what had been said or done by others during the said state of *hypnotic coma* can be remembered by the patient on awaking, or at *any* stage of *subsequent* hypnotic operations. [Hypnotic coma therefore occurred in *far less* than 10% of Braid's subjects.] Then, inasmuch as I feel satisfied that the mental and physical phenomena which flow from said processes result entirely from the mental impressions, or dominant ideas, excited thereby in the minds of the subjects, changing or modifying the previously existing physical action, and the peculiar physical action thus superinduced re-acting on their minds – and that, whether these dominant, expectant ideas existed in the minds of the subjects previously, or were suggested to them, after passing into the impressible condition, by audible suggestions or sensible impressions excited by manipulations of a second party – under these circumstances, I consider the following terms calculated to realise all the precision which we need desire on this point:–

Let *monoideology* indicate the doctrine of the influence of dominant ideas in controlling mental and physical action.
Then *monoideism* will indicate the condition resulting from the mind being possessed by a dominant idea.
To *monoideise* will indicate the act of performing processes for inducing the state of *monoideism.*
Monoideiser will indicate the person who *monoideises.*
Monoideised will indicate the condition of the person who is in the state of *monoideism.*
And *monoideo-dynamics* will indicate the mental and physical changes, whether of excitement or depression, which result from the influence of *monoideism.*[41]
And, finally, as a *generic term,* comprising the *whole* of these phenomena which result from the reciprocal actions of mind and matter upon each other, I think no term could be more appropriate than *psycho-physiology.*

It must be obvious that these terms would comprehend every conceivable variety of phenomenon, according to the function of the part on which the dominant idea of the subject might be concentrated, and the liveliness of his faith. Thus, let the mind of the subject be engrossed with the notion that he is to be irresistibly drawn, repelled, paralysed, or catalepsed, and the monoideo-dynamic or ideational condition of the muscles corresponding with this idea will take place, without any conscious effort of volition of the subject to that effect. It was, moreover, this very ideational or unconscious muscular action, which was the cause of "table-turning", which so much excited the public mind two years ago [*q.v., Hypnotic Therapeutics,* 1853]. The experimenters perceived the fact that the table moved, but, not being conscious of putting out any voluntary effort, they imagined that the table was drawing them, whilst all the while their own muscles were imparting the requisite impulse to the table, although they were unconscious that they were doing so.

It was in 1841 that I first undertook an experimental investigation for the purpose of determining the nature and cause of Mesmeric phenomena. Hitherto it had been alleged that the Mesmeric condition arose from the transmission of some magnetic fluid, or occult influence, fluid, or force, projected from the body of the operator, impinging upon, and charging the body of the patient. However, I was very soon able to demonstrate the fallacy of this *objective influence* theory, by producing analogous phenomena simply by causing subjects to gaze with fixed attention for a few minutes at inanimate objects. It was thus clearly proved that it was a subjective influence, resulting from some peculiar change which the mind could produce

---

[41] In order that I may do full justice to two esteemed friends, I beg to state, in connection *with* this term *monoideo-dynamics,* that, several years ago, Dr. W. B. Carpenter introduced the term *ideo-motor* to characterise the reflex or automatic muscular motions which arise merely from ideas associated with motion existing in the mind, without any conscious effort of volition. In 1853, in referring to this term, Dr. [Daniel] Noble said, "*Ideo-dynamic* would probably constitute a phraseology more appropriate, as applicable to a wider range of phenomena." In this opinion I quite concurred, because I was well aware that an idea could *arrest* as well as *excite* motion automatically, not only in the muscles of voluntary motion, but also as regards the condition of *every other function of the body.* [Braid had long recognised that hypnosis could either *stimulate* or *depress* nervous functioning in general.] I have, therefore, adopted the term *monoideo-dynamics,* as still more comprehensive and characteristic as regards the true mental relations which subsist during all dynamic changes which take place, in every other function of the body, as well as in the muscles of voluntary motion.

upon the mental and physical functions, when constrained to exercise a prolonged act of fixed attention. I therefore adopted the term *hypnotism,* or nervous sleep, to characterise the phenomena producible by my processes. **I became satisfied that the hypnotic state was essentially a state of mental concentration, during which the faculties of the *mind* of the *patient* were so engrossed with a single idea or train of thought as, for the nonce, to render it dead or indifferent to all other considerations and influences.** The consequence of this concentrated attention, again, to the subject in hand, intensified, in a correspondingly greater degree whatever influence the mind of the individual could produce upon his physical functions during the waking condition, when his attention was so much more diffused and distracted by other impressions. **Moreover, inasmuch as words spoken, or various sensible impressions made on the body of an individual by a second party, act as suggestions of thought and action to the person impressed, so as to draw and fix his attention to one part or function, of his body, and withdraw it from others, whatever influence such suggestions and impressions are capable of producing during the ordinary waking condition, should naturally be expected to act with correspondingly greater effect during the *nervous sleep,* when the attention is so much more concentrated, and the imagination, and faith, and expectant ideas in the mind of the patient are so much more intense than in the ordinary waking condition. Now, this is precisely what happens; and I am persuaded that this is the most philosophical mode of viewing this subject; and it renders the whole clear, simple, and intelligible to the apprehension of any unprejudiced person, who may at once perceive that the real object and tendency of the various processes for inducing the state of *hypnotism* or *Mesmerism* is obviously to induce a state of abstraction or concentration of attention – that is, a state of monoideism – whether that may be by requesting the subject to look steadfastly at some unexciting, and empty inanimate thing, or ideal [i.e., imaginary] object, or inducing him to watch the fixed gaze of the operator's eyes, his pointed fingers, or the passes or other manoeuvres of the Mesmeriser.**

In passing into sleep, moreover, reason and will, **the *highest* powers of the mind, are the *first to wane*** – as is beautifully illustrated in the writings of Dr. W. B. Carpenter, well-known as one of our ablest writers on physiology – and thus the **imagination gains the ascendancy**, and careers in unbridled liberty; and, as **the cerebro-spinal functions or reflex actions become more excitable** at a certain stage of the sleep, just when the controlling power of the *will*, which is a cerebral function, is withdrawn, a very interesting series of phenomena may be elicited in the functions of the patient by those who thoroughly understand the subject, and how to regulate and control them; and thus various diseases may be speedily and safely relieved and cured by judicious and suitable manipulations and suggestions, which are not at all amenable to ordinary medical treatment. In this manner **cases may be cured in a few minutes, or in a few days**, which, by ordinary treatment, by the administration of drugs, prescribed by the ablest members of the profession, or when left to nature, may require not only weeks or months, but years to effect a recovery. It was to such cases as these that I referred in my article on "Hypnotic Therapeutics", which was published in the *Monthly Journal of Medical Science,* for July, 1853, where I said,

> The most striking cases of all, however, for illustrating the value of the hypnotic mode of treatment, are cases of hysteric paralysis, in which, without organic lesion, the patient may have remained for a considerable length of time perfectly powerless of a part, or of the whole body, from a [negative] dominant idea which has paralysed or misdirected his volition. In such cases, by altering the state of the circulation, and breaking down the previous idea, and substituting a salutary idea of vigour and self-confidence in their place (which can be done by audible suggestions addressed to the patient, in a confident tone of voice, as to what *must and shall be realised by the processes he has been subjected to),* on being aroused in a few minutes thereafter, with such dominant idea in their minds, to the astonishment of themselves, as well as of others, the patients are found to have acquired vigour and voluntary power over their hitherto paralysed limbs, as by a magical spell or witchcraft. Assuredly such cures are as important as they are interesting and surprising, because such cases may resist ordinary modes of treatment for paralysis for an indefinite length of time; but still the *rationale* is simple enough when viewed according to the principles which I have already explained, of the influence of an expectant, dominant idea, *either exciting or depressing natural function, according to the faith and confidence of the patient.*

Cases of this sort are by no means rare, and are obviously closely allied to fascination. Is it not an important boon, therefore, which science has achieved in discovering such a simple, safe, speedy, and certain mode of curing such affections; and that **the same principle of a strongly excited dominant idea, which is so fatal to the unhappy fascinated bird, can, by judicious management, be turned to such salutary purposes for the relief and cure of suffering humanity?** [The comments above, regarding the role of dominant ideas in the causation of hysteria, prove conclusively that Braid had pre-empted the modern notion that psychopathology can be interpreted in terms of negative autosuggestions, or cognitions.]

James Braid.
Rylaw House, Oxford Street,
Manchester.
August, 1855.

Note
It is my intention shortly **to publish a volume entitled "Psycho-Physiology: embracing Hypnotism, Monoideism, and Mesmerism".** This volume will comprise, in a connected and condensed form, the results of the whole of my researches in this department of science; and it will, moreover, be illustrated by cases in which hypnotism has been proved peculiarly efficacious in the relief and cure of disease, with special directions how to regulate the processes so as to adapt them to different cases and constitutions.

The Critics Criticised
(1855)

[*The Critics Criticised* is not one of Braid's most relevant works and is included here largely for completeness and for its historical value. It constitutes a rather involved account of some of his arguments with certain Mesmerists including John Elliotson. Modern readers who are mainly interested in the clinical side of Braid's work might be better advised to read his *Hypnotic Therapeutics* first.]

Preface
The following remarks were sent for publication in the *Association Medical Journal*, as that appeared to me to be the most natural medium for a member of the Provincial Association to publish his defence against wrongs inflicted upon him in the pages of such a journal as *The Zoist*, which habitually refuses to publish replies to attacks upon others which have appeared in that journal. The Editor of the *Association Journal*, however, declined to publish my communication, from his unwillingness to have any controversy on the subject in question in the *Journal*, at a time when he thought it contained more controversy than was desirable on Association Polity. Under the circumstances stated, that the Editor of *The Zoist* [John Elliotson] excluded all rejoinders from me to former attacks in his journal, the publication of my remarks in the *Association Journal* would not necessarily have imposed on the Editor any obligation to publish a reply in the *Association Journal*; and, moreover, independently of the controversial style of my communication, I considered that the observations embraced illustrations of a psycho-physiological character which would have proved a useful postscript to my late publication in the *Journal*, "On the Nature and Treatment of Certain Forms of Paralysis", [1855] and with that view they are now published in this separate form, for distribution amongst my professional and other friends who take an interest in the inquiry. Moreover, in order that I may accommodate my fellow-associates, with whom I am not personally acquainted, to the utmost in my power, I have caused a few extra hundred copies to be thrown off, and given instructions to the printer to send copies by post, at cost price, to any member of the Association who may enclose his address, with three postage stamps, to Grant and Co., Printers, Corporation Street, Manchester.

The Critics Criticised
In the *Quarterly Review* for September, 1853, an article appeared on 'Electro-Biology and Mesmerism'. In general estimation the said article was regarded as one of the most able and lucid expositions which had ever been published on this interesting and recondite inquiry.

The Zoist for 1854 contained some furious articles as criticisms on the above article in the *Quarterly*. The work referred to being very little known or read, it may be as well for me here to explain that ***The Zoist* is a small quarterly journal, devoted chiefly to the enthusiastic advocacy of Mesmeric doctrines and practice, and the laudation of Mesmerists, and to the persecution, misrepresentation and abuse, of all who dare to differ from their dogmas.** Whilst theoretically differing from the Mesmerists as to the mode of explaining the curative results which flow from certain processes, and from the general policy of their proceedings, I have great pleasure in thus publicly stating that *The Zoist* has been the medium of recording many splendid cures effected by the *so-called* MESMERIC treatment.

In these articles in *The Zoist* Dr. Carpenter and myself were assailed, in the coarsest terms, as conjoint authors of the said review, in which they represented me, in addition to other charges, as blowing my own trumpet, anonymously, "as a quack advertisement, with a purpose, and with the hope of turning *something* into profit". Now, inasmuch as I never wrote a single line of the said article, nor ever saw a single line of it in manuscript or in proof, I wrote a short notice of this fact, intended for publication, as I was unwilling to appropriate to myself any share of the credit due entirely to Dr. Carpenter, he having been the *sole* author of that very lucid exposition of the subject.

Unwittingly, however, these *Zoisters* have paid me a very high compliment by the said attack, for I cannot feel it otherwise than a great compliment to find that **a gentleman of Dr. Carpenter's mark, who had enjoyed many opportunities of investigating along with me my various opinions, and the practical illustrations as the reasons thereof, had so thoroughly set forth my views in the said article as to have led even the clairvoyant carping critics in *The Zoist* to suppose that certain portions of it must have been written by myself**; "with a purpose, and with the hope of turning *something* into profit"; for it is obvious that Dr. Carpenter must have had too much respect for his own reputation to have published anything merely to serve me, or anyone else, which he believed to be erroneous.

Having read to a mutual friend what I had written for publication as an act of justice to Dr. Carpenter, so that I might not appropriate to myself, through silence, any share of what was his especial property, that friend dissuaded me from publishing it, by assuring me that he *knew* Dr. Carpenter felt quite indifferent regarding any misrepresentation or scurrility which might be published against him in *such* a work as *The Zoist*. That being the case I withheld it, as I had myself so long been accustomed to misrepresentation and abuse in that print; for, with one or two exceptions, my name has never been introduced into *The Zoist* but with the view of misrepresentation and the grossest abuse, whilst they refused to publish a single line from me to correct their misrepresentations – that, personally, I felt quite regardless of their unwarrantable assaults on myself in that instance.[42] Now, however, that the Rev. G. Sandby, vicar of Flixton, Suffolk, a gentleman who had formerly referred to my labours in a kind and liberal spirit, has once more renewed the charge of my being one of the writers of said article – for he writes in the *plural – and* has resorted to very unfair means in order to misrepresent me and my views, I deem it my duty at once distinctly to avow, through the press, that *I* had *no share whatever in the authorship of the said article* in the *Quarterly Review*.

Having recorded the above declaration, I now beg leave to add a *few* remarks on the Rev. Mr. Sandby's strictures. Seizing the occasion of a blind woman having been relieved of severe pain in the breast from a bruise, by passes made over the seat of the pain without contact, and of her having been relieved, on another occasion, of rheumatism of the knees, and an unpleasant heat in the head, by "rapid tractive passes over the feet", and "common down passes, at the distance of three feet, for ten minutes", when, of her own accord, she said, "I feel a fine glow all over me, especially in the knees – most in this one," pointing to the chief offender. Having still further stated that the patient was *blind;* that the pain left her at the time the passes were being made by Mr. Plowman, without her knowledge, or one word having been said to her on the subject; and that a Mr. Neilson produced an impression on the same *blind* woman, on a subsequent occasion, without informing her of his intention, simply "by Mesmerising the *feet*, at the distance of three feet, when he caused a sensation of coldness in the head". Having made these statements, the Rev. Mr. Sandby then triumphantly asks – "Now, in what manner will our opponents explain away the above facts? What is their *rationale?* How does their hypothesis apply? What is the grand physiological principle which is to solve and settle this case?"

Now, in my opinion these are all fair and legitimate queries; and, far from acting according to Mr. Sandby's expectation and prediction, that these gentlemen "will simply say, 'We are mistaken in our facts,'" and so on, as represented in page 289, I readily admit that I have no doubt whatever that the *facts,* as stated in this case, are *quite true in every particular as there set forth;* and I have great pleasure, moreover, in giving my *rationale,* and pointing out what appears to *me* "the grand physiological principle which is to solve and settle this case"; and that this can be done too independently of "Mr. Braid's *staring process,* expectant attention, or dominant ideas", or a Mesmeric fluid or force. Had expectant attention or dominant ideas been excited in the mind of the patient, however, by audible suggestions, I doubt not the satisfactory results would have been still *more speedily* realised.

At page 288 the Rev. Mr. Sandby says: "For instance will Mr. Braid, who contends that the so-called Mesmeric effects are produced by the patient being made to concentrate his vision on some object for a certain time, assert that the *staring process* was the secret of Mr. Plowman's success? Did the gaze of the *blind* woman excite her nervous temperament, and influence her system so potentially?"

Now, I felt extremely sorry – chiefly on his *own* account – to find that the Rev. G. Sandby had made such an attack upon me, as that contained in the above paragraph; because it was quite unworthy of a gentleman of his sacred office, and of his high talents and attainments; indeed it was unworthy of *any* man who wished to act the part of an honourable and fair controversialist, as I shall now proceed to prove; for here, be it observed, **the Rev. gentleman wishes to represent me as contending that fixation of the visual organ, or the "staring process", is the *sole* cause of the phenomena, which result during hypnotic and Mesmeric processes. Now, with what propriety could he do this when he knew that, at page 31 of my work on hypnotism [*Neurypnology*, 1843], which was published *twelve years ago,* I said "As the experiment succeeds with the *blind,* I consider it not so much the optic, as the sentient, motor, and sympathetic nerves, and the *mind* through which the impression is made?" Such were my recorded sentiments and experience *twelve years ago;* and I have published various remarks since tending to confirm them; and proving, moreover, that whatever produces a *new* impression, will modify or change *existing function,* whether that new impression may be of a mental or physical nature, and whether it may have arisen from a sensible impression by fanning or breathing on, or wafting with the natural hand, or with some artificial contrivance, or the gentle blast from a pair of bellows, or from audible suggestions or sensible impressions directing the circulation *to* certain parts, and withdrawing it *from* others – thus stimulating or depressing function – these natural results, however, being greatly influenced by dominant ideas or expectant attention, either originating from audible suggestions of another person present, or from previous convictions and belief on this point in the patient's own mind. Moreover, whatever changes sensation changes also the circulation, secretion, and the capillary circulation and general function of the part so impressed, and, concurrently, the whole of the other functions of the body become modified in a greater or lesser degree, and that whether the primary impression resulted from a mental or from a physical influence. The brain, moreover, receives many impressions which subsequently influence the mind as conscious impressions, although they were not perceived at the moment when they were conveyed to the brain through the organs of sense; and impressions too slight to be conveyed to the brain at all, so as ever to become the objects of consciousness, may nevertheless be adequate to**

---

[42] [See appendix (originally a lengthy footnote) 'Excerpts from *The Zoist'.*]

produce a *local* influence on the organic nerves and capillaries, and thus alter existing normal or morbid function.

As regards the influence of passes, again, I have fully admitted that, independently of the mechanical influence produced thereby, by the agitation of the air or by touch, they may also produce impressions in some cases through the influence of temperature or electric agency, as it is an undoubted fact that a change in the electrical polarity takes place from the mere proximity or contact of every substance in nature, animate or inanimate, independently of any occult, magnetic, or odylic force, such as the Mesmerists contend for. That electricity, however, was not the chief or important agency was obvious, I remarked, from this fact, that I have found similar results to arise from touching a patient with a glass rod, 3½ ft. long, or from making passes with an artificial hand attached to the end of the said glass rod as when doing so with my own hand or any other conductor of electricity.

Now, bearing these facts in mind, will the Rev. G. Sandby presume to say that because the poor woman, Ann Donaldson, was *blind,* and was not expecting any Mesmerising process to take place, that *therefore* she *could not* be influenced in her organic functions and sensations by the agitation of the air by the passes made over the painful part, or over the feet, so as to draw the circulation to the feet, and thus relieve the oppressed brain, unless there was some *occult agency at work,* such as a Mesmeric fluid or force projected from the body of the operator and charging the body of the blind woman? **Is Mr. Sandby not aware, moreover, that feeling, hearing, and smell are generally prodigiously exalted in blind people, to compensate for their loss of sight; and that from *this* cause his notable example, Ann Donaldson, was the more likely to be easily affected by the passes, irrespectively of the transference to her body of any magnetic fluid or force from the body of the operator?**

Again, is Mr. Sandby not aware that very slight impressions may be sufficient to change existing physical action, through their influence on the organic nerves, which preside over nutrition and special function, so slight as not even to excite consciousness? And is he not aware that organic changes may be effected through mental or physical impressions so slight that, although sufficiently intense to excite consciousness slightly at the time, nevertheless are too faint to make a lasting impression on the memory? Is the Rev. Mr. Sandby not aware that he may be seated at an open window, and so engaged in reading or study, or in conversation, as not to perceive that such effect is being produced upon his frame by the cold draught of air to which he is exposed, as may issue in rheumatism, inflammation of his eyes, or ears, or nose, or glands, or throat, or lungs, or any other organ of his body most predisposed to take on morbid action? Is he not aware that kindness and earnestness in his manner of addressing a suffering fellow-mortal, enforced by the *gentle movement* of his hand *the more completely to arrest the patient's attention,* may so withdraw it from his past and present sufferings as to give a turn to *existing* morbid function, and thus effect a crisis, without any magnetic, odylic, or nervous, or vital force, extruded from the body of the operator, and entering into and charging the body of the patient with its peculiar properties and powers?

And again, is the Rev. Mr. Sandby not aware that patients may be affected, even during sleep, from infancy to old age, by passes, or by the mere breath of heaven – as by the gentle zephyr fanning their frames – so as to excite various effects, visible or invisible, which may not be remembered by the sleepers on awaking? And is he not aware, moreover, that a patient may fall asleep with one side of his face exposed to a draught of cold air, and although unconscious of its influence at the time, and during his sleep, have, on awakening, most convincing physical proof of its influence, from his face being drawn to the *opposite* side, through paralysis of the *portio dura*, caused by the continued stream of cold air impinging against the trunk and ramifications of that nerve?

Now, it is just because a *blind* patient is *"not like a piece of sulphate of iron, which we can find at any moment in our laboratory, and heat up in the retort at will, and because it is a material of a far more delicate and sensitive nature"*, that the passes of Mr. Plowman and Mr. Neilson were so effective in changing the organic functions in the frame of Ann Donaldson – and that even independently of any occult agent of the nature alleged by the Rev. Mr. Sandby and other Mesmerists. Such is *my* "verdict, and the reasons thereof".

As to Dr. Esdaile's case with the blind man, I shall leave it in the safe keeping of Dr. E. and the Rev. Mr. Sandby; but as to Dr. Gregory's case, it proves *too much* for Mr. Sandby's purpose; for, as *this* blind man went to sleep when another gentleman was trying, *at some distance, unknown to this blind man,* to put *another* person to sleep, this fact furnishes strong proof that *this* blind man was one of those subjects who are liable to be affected entirely through the imagination, expectant attention, or a dominant idea and habit; and he might just as likely have been affected in this way when Dr. Gregory fixed his silent gaze upon him as in the instance referred to with the other gentleman. Moreover, the other case referred to by Mr. Sandby very probably was a person of the like susceptibility.

I think, by the foregoing remarks, I have fully satisfied the requirements of the Rev. G. Sandby where he says – "We call upon the adherents of the suggestive theory, first to examine our evidence respecting the facts as rigidly as they wish, and then give in their verdict, and their reasons thereof"; and I maintain that the case of "Ann Donaldson, the poor blind Scotch woman of Greenside" has *not* overthrown *my* theory, nor has it established the *Mesmeric* theory; and I further maintain, that it is to the dogmatic Mesmerists and lovers of the marvellous, and not to me and others who have espoused my views, that the Rev. gentleman's strictures in his concluding paragraph properly apply, as aiming at "laying down positive laws for universal application, and yet omit in their calculation an essential part of the argument, and all the most important facts which militate against their conclusions".

I quite concur in the Rev. Mr. Sandby's observations, when he says, "Different minds are of course differently constituted, and observe the same facts after a different fashion. What looks feasible to one man looks preposterous to another." **I have never, however, said that the *whole* results are the products of the imagination, nothing but the fancy of the brain, the staring process, fixed gaze, or dominant ideas; but I have attempted to demonstrate how far these and other influences co-operate toward explaining various phenomena attributed by the Mesmerists to some more mysterious power; and I do maintain that, so far as I have *seen* and *believe,* the whole results can be accounted for upon the principles of the reciprocal action of mind and matter, of the patient's own body, upon each other, modified and directed by external circumstances, sensible impressions, audible suggestions, and dominant ideas, irrespective of any magnetic, odylic, nervous, vital, or occult force passing from the operator to the patient, as the all-efficient cause, as has been contended for by the Mesmerists.**

Having thus disposed of the Rev. Mr. Sandby, I beg leave now to address a few words to another champion of occult Mesmerism. The Mr. T. referred to in the note *ante,* is the Rev. C. H. Townshend, who was so moved by the "heavy blow and great discouragement" inflicted on Mesmerism by the article in the *Quarterly Review,* as induced him forthwith to come to the rescue, by perpetrating a five shilling volume to stem the torrent set in against his Mesmeric notions. Mr. Townshend's main argument was based upon what he deemed an impregnable dogma about the influence of the *personal presence of the operator,* or, as he styles it, of "the man in the room". As it appears to me that a few simple and obvious examples may be adduced, capable of demolishing this all-powerful argument of "the man in the room" – either as operator or sceptic – I shall venture to enter the lists even with this great champion for occult Mesmerism.

Mr. Townshend says – "I cannot see how phenomena that are induced by *any* methods of which a human being is the employer can apply to the present question. Whatever may be their quality they have been originated, and are wielded, by the presence, the commands, the prescriptions of a human being. *There is the man in the room.* You cannot get rid of him. [...] Without the hypnotist or [electro-]biologist the phenomena do *not* occur. Thus have we seen that the reviewer's handle to his theory does not truly fit the occasion, just because of *the man in the room."*

Now, in refutation of these dogmas, I beg leave to state that, at the very first public lecture delivered by me in 1841, in order to prove the *fallacy of such a fancy,* three of my patients put themselves into the hypnotic state in succession, when I was NOT only NOT in the *room,* but when I was actually in *another* room at a considerable distance from that in which they were, and I only came in after it was announced to me that they had gone to sleep by *their own unaided efforts,* as can be testified by at least six hundred witnesses. My proof, however, does not rest upon these cases only, for I have since had innumerable examples of equally successful results with many other subjects; and I can, moreover, readily adduce other cases of the sort *any* day. Will *The Zoist* presume to say that in any of these cases Mr. Braid was "making Mesmeric passes [I made no passes at all] and *looking hard at his patients* as *he always has done, while making them stare"?* I am, therefore, warranted in retorting on the Rev. Mr. Townshend that in *these* instances we *had* got rid of *"the man in the room";* and that *without* the hypnotist the phenomena *did occur;* and consequently that *Mr. Townshend's* handle to his theory does not truly fit the occasion, just because *"the man was"* NOT *"in the room".*

The self-induced trance of the Fakirs in India, in like manner, furnishes ample proof in point. Nor was it the influence of my *will;* for I *purposely* directed my attention to *other* matters, the more satisfactorily to prove that the influence was entirely subjective. But perhaps Mr. T. will wish to argue, that although patients were not influenced by my *presence in the room, my commands and prescriptions,* before leaving the room, had induced the results. However, I am prepared to rebut that argument also, by other examples. Thus, a patient whom I had previously cured, by hypnotism, of rheumatism and opacity of the cornea, when at a distance of five and forty miles from me put herself into the state, *unknown to me,* to convince one that the effect could be produced by her own efforts without my knowledge or any special influence communicated by me to the patient. The following is another example in point. A lady whom I had hypnotised, with great relief to her sufferings, after the failure of some noted Mesmerists by "old established modes of Mesmerising", became curious to know whether the results might not after all arise from *occult* influence projected from my body during my personal attendance; and, in order to satisfy her mind upon this point, she one day repaired to her room alone, and sat down and fixed her attention in all respects as when I used to be present the result of which was that she fell asleep in her chair. She was found fast asleep an hour or two afterwards by friends, who went in search of her, and could not comprehend the cause of her long absence.

I shall only give one more example, embracing the waking phenomena. In October, 1846, I exhibited the power of suggestion and dominant ideas over certain subjects in the state, by requesting a gentleman of high intelligence to lay his hand on the table, when, through my audible suggestion, his hand was instantly so firmly fixed to the table that neither his own volition nor the physical efforts of others could separate them. By blowing on the hand it was instantly set free; and on being now requested to extend his arm above the table, I then told him to put it down *if he could* – so emphasised as to suggest the idea that he could *not.* He now put forth a strong effort to put his

arm down, when the arm became rigidly cataleptic in its extended position, and his other extremities became quite rigid also, notwithstanding he was wide awake, and had undergone no process whatever that day. The Earl of Carlisle was present, and tested him, as well as Professor Gregory, and others. These experiments in the waking state very much astonished most of those present; and Professor Gregory immediately jumped to the conclusion that it resulted from the influence of my extraordinary magnetic force over the said gentleman when I was near to him, or in Mr. Townshend's phraseology – that it was the all-controlling influence of *"the man in the room"*. I repudiated the notion of it having resulted from any such occult agency; but Dr. Gregory insisted so much in favour of the *occult* theory that, some days thereafter, when this gentleman was at his own home, which is thirteen miles from Manchester, he resolved to put the matter to the proof by experimenting upon himself when no one else was in the room with him, and when I could know nothing of his intentions – for he had been led by Dr. Gregory's remarks to suppose that it was just *possible,* after all, that, when present, I *might* have some *occult* power over him. Well, in his solitary apartment this gentleman laid his hand on the table, as in the former instance, and instantly his arm became firmly and involuntarily fixed in that position. However, his other hand and arm being free, he applied the other hand to rub the cataleptic arm, and thus set himself at liberty; and then he felt satisfied that my explanation was correct, that it was merely the result of a dominant idea and habit, and that Professor Gregory's opinion was erroneous in alleging that, on the former occasion, he had been affected through some *occult* agency emanating from me as *"the man in the room"*.

I have long felt convinced that the *odium Mesmericum* was as inveterate as the *odium theologicum;* what then must be my perilous position, when so hardly and inveterately assailed by the *odium Mesmericum* and *theologicum* combined? Still, however, I entertain a confident hope that time, which is the great reformer, will ultimately give in her verdict in favour of my psycho-physiological theory.

James Braid.
Rylaw House,
Manchester.
23rd October, 1855.

Note
The North British Review for November, 1854, contained a very able article on "Mental Philosophy, Mesmerism, Electro-Biology, etc." The author of the said article merits my best thanks for the very lucid exposition which he gave of my views, and for the handsome terms in which he expressed himself regarding my labours in this department of science. Curiously enough, however, on *one* point he had quite misunderstood me, and laid the lash upon my back very smartly, for sins which I never committed. He had confounded me with the *phreno-Mesmerists* in the following paragraph: "That touching particular parts of the head will make a hypnotised patient laugh, pray, sing, steal, and fight, is a doctrine which we do not scruple to rank among the wildest and most dangerous that have ever been propounded, and we cannot but express our astonishment that it should be maintained by Dr. Braid, who has shown so much sagacity in rejecting the less extravagant pretensions of the Mesmerists." Now the fact is that I never adduced the said manifestations as a *proof* of the *organology of phrenologists.* I exhibited the phenomena, and explained how they were to be accounted for upon *totally different principles,* so that they *neither proved nor disproved the doctrine of phrenology,* but left that precisely where they found it. **These manifestations may arise either from a previous knowledge of phrenology, or from a system of training *during the sleep,* so that they come out subsequently, as acts of memory, when corresponding points are touched, with which particular ideas had been associated through audible suggestion – which arbitrary associations may be equally, readily established by touching other parts of the body as by touching different parts of the head – or they may arise from the touch calling into action certain muscles of expression of mental conditions exciting in the mind of the subject the ideas with which they are usually associated in the waking condition.** This latter mode I consider the *only* NATURAL mode of exciting these manifestations, and it is a mere **inversion of the sequence which ordinarily obtains between mental and muscular excitation – *viz*., firstly, the touch calls into play the muscles constituting the *"anatomy, of expression"* of any given passion or emotion, idea or train of thought; and, secondly, this *physical* expression suggests or excites in the mind of the subject the corresponding idea, passion, or emotion with which it is usually associated in the waking condition;** *i.e.,* **under ordinary circumstances the *mental* impression *precedes* and acts as the *exciting* cause of the *physical* manifestations of different *mental* conditions, but here the *physical* condition *precedes* and acts as the exciting cause of the *mental condition*.**

Appendix:
Excerpts from *The Zoist*

The following are a *few* additional illustrations of the dignity of diction, meekness, modesty, and love of truth, displayed by these *Zoist* reviewers.

> The author, or rather authors, stand forth confessed by their very mannerisms. The materials tell us by their quality what handicraftsmen have been employed. A fancy Carpenter, who well understands the knack of dovetailing his own semi-scientific views into the discoveries of others, and of then overlaying them with a smooth veneer, and a practical embroiderer, who contrives on every occasion to Braid and twist his one-sided facts into consequences, *which he knows are not true,* would seem to have been at work upon the fabric.

This base imputation upon my veracity I repel as the mere invention of this unscrupulous and malicious anonymous slanderer, and I can confidently appeal to all who know me that I am ever most scrupulous in adhering to what *I believe* to be true. Again,

> These humble – most humble, highly informed – very highly informed, far sighted – very far sighted, modest – very modest writers – *par nobile* – *each alter idem,* two writers in one, of the article in the *Quarterly Review.*

Again,

> Oh, the modesty of these youths who, as though those who had studied the subject long, laboriously, and conscientiously, wanted the help of the ignorant, conceited and unscrupulous.[43]

Again,

> Mr. T. castigates and ridicules (the *Quarterly* reviewer) charmingly – though, perhaps, the sin is not ignorance, but wilful and most unprincipled ignoring, which arises from the lowest and worst of feelings.

And again,

> Mr. T. has no mercy upon the conceit of the superficial, flimsy reviewer, for his refusal to be taught by those who are only qualified to teach him, and ridicules him in a way calculated to make him feel, did not his conceit – his enormous development of self esteem – render him as insensible to the exquisite ridicule as the thickness of the skin of the sagacious rhinoceros to a bullet from a Minié *rifle. – Page* 19.

Nothing could be more unwarrantable than for the editor of *The Zoist* to assume that I was one of the writers of the article in the *Quarterly Review,* and charge me with wilfully withholding all allusion to communications published in *The Zoist,* for he well knew that, four or five months previously, to wit in 1853, I sent him a copy of my "Hypnotic Therapeutics", in the appendix to which I criticised and controverted opinions of its leading contributors on "table-turning", and the Od force, *viz.,* the Rev. Mr. Sandby, the Rev. Mr. Townshend, Dr. Elliotson, and Dr. Ashburner, but neither the editor nor any of these gentlemen have yet attempted to refute my arguments in opposition to their dogmas. I was the first to publish the unconscious muscular action [i.e., "ideo-motor"] theory of *table-turning,* and I still maintain that *that* is the true explanation of the phenomenon; and I moreover contend that nothing short of my opponents performing successfully the crucial experiments which I proposed – *viz.,* lifting a small weight, such as an ounce of lead, copper, wood, or marble, from the centre of a table, and holding it suspended in the air, say twelve inches above the table, by the force of the will alone of ten or twenty efficient table-turners, when no human hand is near it, nor any mechanical contrivance has been had recourse to for lifting it – can reasonably satisfy any candid inquirer after truth. Nothing but the *non-contact* plan can, *with certainty,* guard against the fallacy of unconscious muscular action.

Some misrepresentations as to the results of my processes in the hands of Mesmerists are mere repetitions of charges, all of which I long ago proved to be caused by their *mismanagement of my processes,* and then blaming hypnotism for the results of their own blunders, or *intended misdirections.*

The following extracts are avowedly from the pen of Dr. Elliotson, contrasting himself with Sir James Clark, Bart., and they occur in the very next article to that in which the attack was made upon Dr. Carpenter and myself. Dr. Elliotson says – for his name is appended to the article –

> [...] me, who stand quite as high, I trust, as a physician as himself, though neither a baronet nor a royal physician. [...] I have examined hundreds of abdominal enlargements, and never once made a mistake; and could not, I think, by any possibility make a mistake, when the size was not trifling.

---

[43] [Braid and Carpenter, incidentally, had been closely studying Mesmerism for over fifteen years by this date.]

> Let Sir James Clark remember that he is only a lucky man. His rise and progress have not been from hard work in hospitals, for he has never, like me, been physician to any hospital, nor from teaching successfully, for he has never, like me, been a lecturer in a large medical school, or a lecturer at all; whereas, I raised the Medical School of St. Thomas's from nothing to a high condition, and that of University College from a fallen state to a very high condition, from which each fell as soon as I left it. Nor has he risen from writing anything worth reading. (…) He has only been a lucky man.
>
> I never considered it an honour to meet Sir James Clark. I never gained an idea, or heard a sagacious remark from him. [...] When a young man, he went out a very awkward Scotch body to take care of the son of a gentleman of rank and fortune.[44]

When such is the style and manner of attacking a man like Sir James Clark adopted by Dr. Elliotson, the *Magnus Apollo* of *The Zoist,* what is to be expected from his associates and devotees, who attack each other and fight Mesmeric battles under the leadership of such a commander-in-chief?

---

[44] [Clark was originally a naval surgeon who became a successful physician and attendant to Queen Victoria and Prince Albert. He was the author of several books and articles, and specialised in the treatment of tuberculosis. His biographical details suggest that Elliotson's remarks are expressions of professional jealousy, or at least one-sided, as, though subject to some criticism, he held several influential positions, and others specifically commended his wisdom as a physician.]

Hypnotic Therapeutics
(1853)

Illustrated by Cases

With an Appendix on

Table-Moving and Spirit-Rapping

By
James Braid
M.R.C.S., Edin., M W.S., etc., etc.

Reprinted from the Monthly Journal Of Medical Science for July 1853

Hypnotic Therapeutics

[Introduction]
From a paper published by me in the "Monthly Journal" for June 1851, and various works published at different times, my views of hypnotic and Mesmeric phenomena are now pretty generally known, namely, that the influence is subjective or personal, and *not objective* or the effect of any mysterious influence, *ab extra* [from without], communicated from the operator to the patient, during the Mesmerising processes, as has been alleged by the Mesmerists to be the case. In proof of this, it may suffice to state that, at one public lecture, fourteen male adults, who were entire strangers to me, and had never been operated upon before, were desired to stand up together in a row, and maintain a steady gaze and fixed act of attention whilst gazing at inanimate objects, and within ten minutes, ten out of the fourteen [71%] passed into the hypnotic state in various degrees, while I never touched anyone of them until after their eyelids closed involuntarily. Three more of the audience likewise sent themselves into the condition at the same time, unknown to me, by fixing their gaze and attention upon different points of the room. Again, at a conversazione in London [at the Hanover Square rooms in 1842], sixteen out of eighteen [89%] (twelve of whom had never been tried before) went into the condition at the same time, by gazing fixedly and abstractedly on the root of a chandelier. At another public lecture, five deaf and dumb patients, and a paralytic patient, all put themselves into the state at the same time, by gazing at inanimate objects. I have also endeavoured to prove that all the phenomena, interesting and wonderful as some of them undoubtedly are, so far as I have been able to ascertain, never transcend what is reconcilable with generally admitted physiological and psychological principles.

[Nature of Hypnosis]
My researches have led me to conclude that the hypnotic state, which may be induced by various processes described elsewhere, is **essentially a state of mental concentration**, in which the faculties of the mind *of the patient* are so engrossed with a single idea or train of thought, as for the nonce, to be dead or indifferent to all other considerations and influences. The consequence of this concentrated attention to the subject in hand, therefore, intensifies, in a correspondingly greater degree, whatever influence the mind of the individual can produce upon his physical functions during the waking condition, when his attention is so much more diffused and distracted by other impressions. Moreover, inasmuch as words spoken, or other sensible impressions made on the body of an individual by a second party, act as **suggestions** of thought and action to the person impressed, so as to draw and fix his attention to one part or function of his body, and withdraw it from others, whatever influence such suggestions and impressions are capable of producing during the ordinary waking condition, should naturally be expected to act with correspondingly greater effect during the *nervous sleep*, when the attention is so much more concentrated, and the imagination and faith, or expectant idea in the mind of the patient, are so much more intense than in the ordinary waking condition.

I am persuaded that this is the most philosophical mode of viewing this subject, and it renders the whole clear, simple, and intelligible to the apprehension of any unprejudiced person.

The real object of the various processes for inducing the state of *hypnotism* or *Mesmerism* is obviously to induce a state of abstraction or concentration of attention, whether that may be by requesting the subject to look steadfastly at some unexciting and empty inanimate thing or ideal object, or inducing him to watch the fixed gaze of the operator's eyes, his pointed fingers, or the passes and other manoeuvres of the Mesmeriser.

[Suggestion & Hypnosis]
So far as I have seen, the principal difference between the *hypnotic* or *nervous sleep* and common sleep consists in the state or condition of the mind. In passing into common sleep the mind is diffusive or passive, flitting from one idea to another indifferently, thereby rendering the subject unable to fix his attention effectively on any regular train of thought, or to perform any acts requiring much effort of the will. The consequence is this, that a state of passiveness is manifested during the sleep, so that audible suggestions and sensible impressions addressed to the sleeper, if not intense enough to awake him entirely, seldom do more than excite a dream, in which ideas pass through his mind without exciting definite physical acts; but, on the other hand, the active and concentrated state of mind engendered by the processes for inducing the *nervous sleep* are carried *into* the sleep, and, in many instances, excite the sleeper, without awaking, to speak or exhibit physical manifestations of the suggestions received through words audibly uttered in his hearing, or ideas previously existing in his mind, or excited by sensible impressions made by touches or passes of the operator, which direct the attention of the sleeper *to* different parts, or excite into action certain combinations of muscles, and thereby direct his current of thought.

[Emerging from Hypnosis]
Nor must I omit to remark that much depends upon the mode of arousing the patient from the sleep as

respects the results which follow. If I wish any predominant idea, or any physical change which has been induced, to be carried strongly into the waking condition, **I arouse the patient abruptly,** by a clap of my hands near to his ear, when he is in the full height of the desired condition; but if tranquillising is the object in view, then he had better be aroused slowly and softly, such as by gently wafting the face of the patient with the hand, or with a fan, or an open handkerchief; or by placing the balls of the thumbs gently on the eyes of the patient, or on his eyebrows, and then carrying them laterally a few times so as to produce gentle friction, to which may be added gentle fanning when required. If the patient is in the sub or half-waking condition, favourable for manifesting the vigilant phenomena, or "Electro Biological" phenomena, as they have so absurdly been called, a new suggestion, by a word spoken, or a visible movement of any sort being made, calculated to break the previous abstraction, which had been excited temporarily by a former suggestion, will suffice to set the captive free.

[Physical Effect of Suggestion]
It had long been known that keeping the attention of the mind steadily directed to any part of the body was apt to produce various anomalous feelings in the mind of the subject so engaged, especially if such individual was expecting something to happen. Hitherto, however, these phenomena had had reference principally to common sensation [i.e., touch], and were considered to be the effects of a vivid imagination, and that the results were of an illusory nature, rather than being accompanied with positive physical changes. True, it had long been known that some remarkable physical changes and cures occurred, occasionally, from causes of great mental excitement; and that some individuals, moreover, through preconcerted plots, had been frightened into serious illness, or even to death, through mental impressions excited by the systematic suggestion of others. It was also known that excessive joy or sorrow had sometimes effected astonishing cures, and in other cases had induced disease or death with the rapidity of the lightning's flash. Other emotional effects and the power of sympathy and imitation were also pretty well-known, and generally acknowledged. Thus far, however, with the exception of Dr. [Henry] Holland's interesting remarks on the influence of attention on the bodily organs, "Medical Notes and Reflections", [1839] a work which I had not the benefit of seeing until after completing my experiments "On the Power of the Mind", [1846] there seemed to have been no notion entertained that definite and special physical changes could be excited, and regulated, and controlled at will, by the voluntary mental efforts of a healthy individual directed towards his *own body*, or involuntarily, according to the suggestions of another person, by words spoken, or by sensible signs or physical impressions made by him, such as by passes or touches, as is now fully admitted by all physiologists who have carefully and candidly investigated this curious and important branch of inquiry.

[Early Placebo Experiments]
In 1844, I performed some experiments to determine the probable nature and cause of certain effects said to have been realised in America, as *physical* results of medicines manifested on patients *through glass* – viz., that by touching, smelling at, or tasting the outside of a bottle containing such medicines, would be sufficient to manifest their respective powers on patients, whilst the bottles were securely closed and sealed. I published the results of my experiments at the time, which clearly proved that the effects realised were due entirely to the power of an expectant idea in the mind of the patient over his own physical functions, as I made a little coloured water act on a patient as an emetic, when wide awake, by simply assuring the patient, in a confident manner, that it would produce such an effect; and, by removing from the hand the phial containing the coloured water, and putting another phial in the opposite hand, which I predicted would suspend the sickness, the nausea immediately subsided, notwithstanding the contents of said anti-emetic phial had no *physical* property calculated to have done so, more than the other hand to have produced the sickness.

In the year 1845, Baron [Karl] von Reichenbach, a great authority in chemistry and on meteoric stones, published his researches on magnetism and the allied sciences, in which he set forth, with laborious minuteness, a series of experiments conducted by him and others on certain nervous and cataleptic patients, whom he denominated *sensitives*; and he adduced what was described as seen and felt, and manifested in various ways by said patients, as satisfactory proof of the existence of "a new imponderable" force, differing from all the other known imponderables, to which new force the Baron applied the term "od", or the "od force". To this Baron Reichenbach attributed a vast variety of the phenomena in nature, and amongst others the phenomena of Mesmerism. In the spring of 1846, Professor Gregory published "an abstract" of the Baron's views in an English dress. On perusing this abstract, I at once perceived a grave source of fallacy, as the only proof which they had to adduce of the existence of this new physical force, were the declarations and manifestations of these nervous, cataleptic subjects, of what they alleged they saw and felt under such and such circumstances. Some apparently healthy and vigorous and most intelligent individuals, who profess great power of abstraction, or of fixing their attention, with a vivid imagination, are also susceptible of experiencing the like results from mere fixity of attention on any part, or on any function of their minds or bodies, and are especially prone to be led by suggestions of others into particular trains of thought, as will be explained presently. Whatever credit was justly due to the great zeal and industry and honesty of purpose of the Baron and his patients, and his learned translator, and however high Baron Reichenbach and Professor Gregory were entitled to stand as authorities in chemical and physical science, it appeared to me that they were by no means equally well acquainted with physiology and psychology, otherwise I could not have imagined it possible that they should so entirely have overlooked or undervalued the important part which the mind and nervous system of the instruments they were operating with were calculated to play in such an inquiry; and I therefore considered that the whole of their inductions must necessarily be unsatisfactory from this circumstance.

[Experiments with Suggestion]
In order to correct what appeared to me such a grave and palpable source of error, I undertook a laborious course of experiments on patients in the waking condition, as well as on others when in the hypnotic state, from which I was enabled to demonstrate, not only that an act of fixed attention, on the part of a patient, directed to any organ or part of his body, was adequate to change the normal condition of the organ or part, both as regarded sensation and function, even during the *waking* condition; but **I was, moreover, enabled farther to prove that, through audible suggestions, the function of any organ or part might either be excited or depressed in its function with great uniformity, or varied according to the suggestions of a second party, conveyed in an energetic and engrossing manner to the minds of subjects of great fixity of attention, especially if also possessed of a vivid imagination, and lively faith in the fulfilment of the prediction.** Mere fixity of attention clearly brought out an exalted manifestation of the *naturally predominant* susceptibility of the organ or function upon which his attention was fixed; but fixity of attention, together with *an expectant idea as to the peculiar result to be anticipated*, was generally followed by a result corresponding *precisely* with the dominant expectant idea in the mind of the patient during his fixed act of attention. All this was clearly proved by examples given in detail in my little brochure on "The Power of the Mind over the Body", which was published in July 1846. I believe this was the first systematic and *extended* course of experiments published, in which satisfactory proof had been adduced that a fixed dominant expectant idea in the mind of the patient might either *excite* or *depress*, or *temporarily suspend* the function of any one or of all of the special senses, or even the function of any organ or part of the human body; and that an audible suggestion from another person, and the dominant expectant idea excited thereby in the mind of the subject would become so engrossing with some subjects, that they could not avoid realising the *expected* result as regarded all the organs of special sense, and some of the mental faculties; and that all the secretions and excretions might be increased or diminished in a remarkable degree, merely as the result of dominant, sustained, expectant ideas in the minds of such subjects. Here, then, was the *rationale* of the phenomena attributed by Baron Reichenbach to his "new imponderable", which proved at least that his alleged "new imponderable", or "od force", was *unnecessary* for their production; and here, likewise, we had not only the *rationale*, but also many examples in point, of phenomena which, four or five years after the publication of my little brochure, were alleged to have been a new discovery; and imported into this country from America, under the designation of "Electro-Biology". The only novelties, therefore, of this alleged importation were the name and theory or explanation; and in respect to the name, it was absurd, and as to the theory, it was obviously erroneous. It is certain that there was no electricity in the matter more than in any other operation in nature, and that the patients were merely *partially hypnotised* by the fixed gaze at the discs.

In patients, again, who passed into what is called the double-conscious state of the nervous sleep [also called by Braid the "full" hypnotic stage, accompanied by spontaneous amnesia], these results of expectant ideas and fixed attention came out still more promptly and pronounced, but apparently, merely from their attention being still more concentrated, their imaginations and expectant ideas more vigorous, and the counteracting influence of reason being more in abeyance during the complete nervous sleep. Again, when the limbs were extended and rendered cataleptic, and the circulation thereby excited, the influence was still more intense and remarkable in some respects.

[Sedative & Stimulating Suggestions in Hypnotic Therapy]
With due attention to these facts, there need be no difficulty in comprehending how hypnotism may be rendered available for the relief and cure of various maladies, when skilfully directed and controlled. **By our various modes of suggestion, through influencing the mind by audible language, spoken within the hearing of the patient, or by definite physical impressions, we fix certain ideas, strongly and involuntarily on the mind of the patient, which thereby act as stimulants, or as sedatives, according to the purport of the expectant ideas, and the direction of the current of thought in the mind of the patient, either drawing it to, or withdrawing it from, particular organs or functions; which results are effected in ordinary practice, by prescribing such medicines as experience has proved stimulate or irritate these organs, thereby directly increasing their functions, or which produce the reverse effect, either by direct sedative action on the organs, or by diminishing the heart's action, or by stimulating some distant part, and thereby producing revulsion.**

The great object of all treatment is, either to excite or to depress function, or to increase or to diminish the existing state of sensibility and circulation, locally or generally, with the necessary

attendant changes in the general, and more especially in the capillary, circulation. For this purpose I feel convinced that hypnotism may be applied in the cure of some forms of disease with the same ease and certainty as our most simple and approved methods of treatment; and I therefore wish to direct attention to it as a valuable *adjunct* to other treatment, and as one particularly useful in many nervous affections, which resist all ordinary treatment by the exhibition of medicines. I wish it to be distinctly understood, however, that I by no means desire to hold up hypnotism as a panacea or universal remedy; indeed, I do not believe in the existence of *any* universal remedy. Diseases differ in their nature and causes, and the peculiarities of the constitutions of individuals who may be the subjects of disease; and, consequently, they require treatment to be varied accordingly. It is indeed well-known that I use hypnotism *alone*, only in a certain class of cases, to which I have ascertained, by experience, that it is peculiarly adapted; and, that I use it in other cases *in conjunction with medicines*; whilst, *in the great majority of cases I do not use hypnotism at all,* but depend entirely upon the exhibition of medicines, which I administer in such doses as are calculated to produce obvious and sensible effects.

Again, inasmuch as the only rational mode of treating disease is, first of all, to ascertain the pathological condition, and whether the indication is to stimulate or to depress, and to what extent, in either respect, it is obviously equally necessary that a person shall have such professional knowledge as shall qualify him to do this, in order to prepare him for treating cases with general success by hypnotism, as by the ordinary modes of treatment. In proof of this I may state the following facts:– In cases which had been treated Mesmerically by others, with the low circulation, not only without benefit, but with an aggravation of symptoms, so soon as they were subjected by me to the hypnotic process, with the high circulation or stimulating plan, relief and cure were effected immediately. In like manner, at a period when I was much less acquainted with the hypnotic mode of treatment, this same fact was strikingly manifested during my treatment of a severe case of epilepsy. After this case had resisted energetic treatment under medical means, the patient was brought to me to be hypnotised. Being a chronic case, I adopted hypnotism alone, *with the excited circulation, without benefit*, and then I combined this method with the exhibition of medicines, but still without benefit. I then recommended a residence in the country, with fresh air and moderate exercise in the open air, suitable medicines being also used in the meantime, but all to no purpose, as the patient returned as bad as ever. I now hypnotised him daily, *with the low circulation*, and from that day he had but *one fit* subsequently, and has now remained quite well for eight years. I have also had many other examples proving the same doctrine, of how much of our success depends upon proper management *after the hypnotic state is induced*. [Mesmerists, by contrast, had placed most emphasis on simply inducing the state; Braid recognises that the state is a means to an end and must normally be supplemented with suggestion, etc.]

[Physiological Theory & Hypnotic Anaesthesia]
During the nervous sleep, by inducing the low circulation and suppressed respiration, as explained elsewhere in my writings, the blood, from being thus insufficiently arterialised, acts as a narcotic, and depresses all the powers of life below that of natural sleep; and if the attention has also been fixed in some particular train of thought, every other function becomes deadened in an extraordinary degree, so that severe inflictions and operations may be borne in that state without the patient evincing any apparent consciousness of pain, nor, if questioned when he awakes, will he remember having felt any pain. The patient seems to have been reduced to a state of temporary nervous coma, during which anaesthesia was complete. In other cases, a patient who is highly sensible to pain when awake, may be rendered quite tolerant of, or indifferent to, an operation, even when only so partially under the influence as to be quite conscious that the operation is being performed. The following case is a good example in point. I had been attending a lady for affection of the brain, complicated with monomania. At length a tumour formed, burrowing under the upper part of the orbit, which pointed near the inner canthus. From the progress of the case, I suspected that this abscess communicated with the anterior lobe and base of the brain, and I therefore determined to evacuate its contents by a very small puncture, and close the wound, so as to exclude the air from the sac. This I had occasion to do repeatedly, and on every occasion the patient evinced symptoms of intense suffering. I therefore at length proposed to try the effect of hypnotising her, and operating whilst she was in that condition. To this she readily consented, and notwithstanding she was so partially affected as to be quite conscious of what I was doing, she was now enabled to bear the operation without the slightest complaint or apparent suffering. On one occasion I thought it would be interesting, for the sake of contrast, to operate without hypnotising the patient, but the consequence was most distressing and alarming. The operation was precisely similar, and not accompanied by a greater discharge than usual, but now she experienced such exquisite pain and suffering, with prolonged fainting and prostration, that immediate death seemed impending, and it was more than two hours before I durst leave her room. I had frequent occasion to repeat the operation subsequently, but I always preceded it by my hypnotising process, and then all went on satisfactorily.

I have myself performed a number of minor surgical operations on patients in the hypnotic condition without pain, and some capital operations have been recorded as having been performed by others entirely without pain, even in this country. Mesmerism seems peculiarly adapted for this

purpose amongst the natives of India, as Dr. Esdaile's experience proved, seeing he performed 300 important and capital operations, some of them of the most formidable nature, on natives in an hospital in Calcutta, and without pain to the patients, the recoveries, moreover, being far beyond the average success. Still, I suspect, with the European constitution, and in this country in particular, it will be found, that Mesmerism or hypnotism are far less available for inducing anaesthesia for surgical and midwifery purposes, than chloroform and ether, as the latter are more certain and speedy in their results, and are perfectly safe when judiciously and skilfully used. However, from a pretty extensive experience of both methods, I am warranted in saying, that hypnotism is far more useful for the relief and cure of certain forms of disease, than either ether or chloroform are ever likely to become.

[Catalepsy & Increased Stimulation]
Let the circulation and respiration, however, be both increased, by elevating the limbs and rendering them cataleptic, so that the brain and nervous system are excited by an increased activity of circulation of inordinately stimulating and highly arterialised blood, and we thus induce a condition as remarkable for exaltation of function and excitement, as the former was remarkable for depression. Moreover, from the habit of abstraction or concentration of attention, superinduced by the original processes, there seems not only to result a general state of quickness of perception, but also a tendency to absolute concentration of attention on whatever idea the mind is directed to. In consequence of this, by directing the attention of the patient to any particular function or action, mental or physical, the whole or the greater part of the force of the *vis nervosa* or powers of life, seems to be concentrated on that function or action, and hence it is manifested with correspondingly exalted energy; or the function may be suspended or temporarily reduced in force, by suggesting audibly to the patient, what will thereby become with him a dominant idea – for *excitement or depression of function will equally result from a fixed and sustained dominant idea.*

[Suggestion & Passes]
Whilst I do not believe in the reality of any magnetic or occult influence, or nervous or vital fluid or force, passing from the operator to the patient, as has been alleged by the Mesmerists to take place during their making movements with their hands, or agitating the air, called passes and touches – contact or non-contact passes; I readily admit a certain amount of influence to result from them, and with this idea alone I resort to passes, manipulations, and audible suggestions, for their mechanical impression, or that of heat and cold, from the agitation of the air, calling the attention of the subject *to* certain parts, and withdrawing it *from* others, and thus modifying physical action, sensation, and circulation, according to the mental direction and dominant ideas in the mind of the patient. Thus, general wafting whilst the muscles are limber will excite the cuticular and muscular systems, the latter slightly, and leave the internal organs in a state of quiescence or of diminished function; or by calling the patient's attention to any particular organ or function, as already stated, we thereby *excite* or *depress* the function of that organ or part, according to the *expectant idea in the mind of the patient at the time.*

[Rejection of Occult Pretensions]
It is highly probable, that additional mental impressions might be made upon some patients, by investing the subject in mystery, and leading the patients to believe that there is some occult or special influence at work, regulated by particular manoeuvres; but, as I do not believe in the existence of any such occult influence as the true cause of the phenomena manifested, I could not honestly do so. I therefore content myself by acting according to my own notion of producing curative effects by exciting dominant and persistent ideas in the minds of the patients, with the physical results which flow therefrom, and altering the quality and quantity of the blood circulating through a part in a given time, which can be regulated by certain circumstances and modes of management, as already pointed out. This seems to have been overlooked or under-valued by the Mesmerists, but there can be no doubt whatever, that by these means we can produce powerful and positive physical impressions, independently of any occult, magnetic, odylic, or special, or nervous or vital influence or force being transmitted from the body of the operator to that of the patient, as has been alleged by the Mesmerists as the true cause of the phenomena realised during their processes.

It is quite possible that some influence of an electrical nature may be brought into play during the processes of the Mesmeriser, and still farther heighten the effects; for it is a well-established fact, that a change in the electrical polarity necessarily takes place from the simple proximity or contact of all bodies, whether animate or inanimate. However, that this electrical effect is not the chief or important agency is obvious from this fact, that I have found similar results arise from touching a patient with a glass rod 3 ½ feet long, or making passes with an artificial hand attached to the end of said rod, as when doing so with my own hand or any conductor of electricity.

[Hypnosis Intensifies Natural Faculties]

Now, inasmuch as the nervous system is the immediate link in the chain between the soul and the body, between sensation and perception; and since it cannot be doubted that the soul and the body can mutually act and react upon each other, it should follow, as a natural consequence, that if we can attain to any mode of intensifying the *mental* power, we should thus realise, in a corresponding degree, greater control over physical action. Now, this is precisely what my processes do – **they create no new faculties; but they give us greater control over the natural functions than we possess during the ordinary waking condition**, and particularly in intensifying mental influence, or the power of the mind of the patient over his own physical functions; and of a fixed dominant idea and physical state of the organs over the other faculties of the mind during the dominance of such fixed ideas.

[Physical Effects of Hypnotic Suggestion]

In the excited state of the system induced by my processes, therefore, if the object be to stimulate a sluggish function, excite the quickened circulation and respiration, and then, by directing the attention of the patient to the particular organ or function, a greatly excited condition of the function of the respective organ will be the result, **more especially if an audible suggestion to that effect has been made within the hearing of the patient, so as to excite in his mind such a dominate idea.** On the contrary, if the object be to allay over excitement, we must first produce the general depressing condition, and then also direct the patient's attention to some *other function*, or *part*, from that which we wish to depress, and moreover, predict, in audible language, uttered within the patient's hearing, the certainty of the expected or wished for result being realised by such processes. **For example, if we wish to stimulate the skin *moderately*, simply induce the sleep, and by then gently drawing the tips of the fingers over various parts, or by agitating the air by passing the hands over various parts, with a tremulous motion without actual contact, the attention of the subject being thus called to the surface, it will cause increased activity of the sensation and circulation of the parts thus acted upon. If *intense* cuticular excitement be desired, make the fanning and manipulations over the parts requiring high excitement, *whilst the limbs are extended and rendered rigid or cataleptic*; and also suggest, in audible language, the wished for result. By this means you may not only increase the action of the skin, and excite increased perspiration, but the quality of the perspiration and of the saliva and urine may be so changed in chemical constitution, in a quarter of an hour, as to be made manifest by the use of test paper, and other chemical agents. This I have proved repeatedly to be the case with highly susceptible subjects, especially when kept for some time in the cataleptic condition. This is a fact too apparent to admit of any possibility of mistake.**

In proof that the increased frequency and force of the heart's action during the cataleptic state is due to internal congestion, from obstruction to free transmission of blood along the extremities, through the *arteries*, from their trunks being compressed between the rigid muscles and the bones, whilst no such obstruction is offered to its free return through the subcutaneous veins, I may state the following facts:- The mere muscular effort required simply to support the extremities for four or five minutes in a given position in the waking condition, would only excite the pulse about *twenty percent* [e.g., from 70 to 84 bpm], whereas, in *intense* catalepsy, it would cause it to rise a *hundred percent* [e.g., from 70 to 140 bpm], or to any intermediate degree according to the intensity of the rigidity – the pulse becoming less and less developed at the wrist, and more rapid as the rigidity increases, and the impulse of the heart's action increasing as the volume of the pulse at the wrist diminishes. To prove this still farther, about ten years ago, having occasion to bleed a patient who had large veins, I first hypnotised him and rendered his arm cataleptic, in which state I made a free opening into the vein, when the blood came away only in drops. I then blew upon the arm, and thereby reduced the rigidity, when instantly the blood sprang out in a copious stream, which shortly began to diminish as the cataleptic state returned, until it again flowed only in drops. Blowing on the arm, and thereby reducing the rigidity, caused it again to flow in full stream, and it again diminished as the rigidity returned, and by these means I went on increasing the rate of flow, or diminishing it alternately, until I had taken a pint of blood from my patient during the sleep, which was the quantity required.

If you wish to excite the feeling of nausea or vomiting, give the patient a mouthful of cold water, or draw the hand over the stomach, predicting aloud that he must necessarily vomit, as he had taken an emetic, or that the mere touch will be sufficient to produce the like effect; and if the patient is one of those subjects who has passed into the double-conscious ["full" hypnotic] state, or who is liable to manifest the power of suggestion during the waking condition, the desired effect was quite certain to follow. **With all other patients a similar effect, but in a minor degree, may be realised, provided they can fix their thoughts steadfastly, and for a length of time, on the idea suggested.** The same will be the result in respect to the action of the bowels, the tendency to void urine, exciting the secretion of milk in the nurse by directing the attention of the subject to the mammae, or talking within her hearing about her child; and the same of other functions, according to the mental direction and ideas suggested to the mind of the patient by words spoken aloud in his hearing, or otherwise. There is evidently an immediate increased determination of blood, and of increased sensibility, to whatever organ or function, or part, the mind of the patient is directed under such circumstances, especially if he is fully persuaded in his own mind, and expects such exciting results. **Let anyone only reflect for a moment on the physiological phenomena of blushing.** In this case the capillary circulation of the cheeks, or of the whole face and neck in some subjects, immediately assumes such a remarkable change as to paint the cheeks, face, and neck of a scarlet hue, even in those who have a pale complexion generally, from red globules crowding through vessels which, in their ordinary condition, admit chiefly the colourless part of the blood, or red globules in single file only. **All this remarkable physical change is entirely due to mental emotion, and yet it is effected with a rapidity which could scarcely be equalled by the application to the parts so affected of the most violent mechanical or chemical stimuli. Again, pallor from mental emotion is the reverse of blushing, and is equally prompt in its response. Where, then, is the difficulty in comprehending why a dominant expectant idea in the mind of a patient should be adequate to produce effects equally potent on other parts of the body, and on special organs, when strongly concentrated on such organs or parts?**

Upon the same principle, **weakened muscles may be permanently energised by being called into strong or cataleptiform action during the general excitement; or they may be improved by being kept limber, and an inordinate quantity of blood forced to circulate through them, whilst the other muscles are kept rigid**. To manage this with precision and due advantage, however, professional skill is requisite in the operator, to enable him to determine what the indication of cure is, and to what extent it should be carried in each particular case.[45]

From the impossibility of fixing the mental attention of an idiot for any length of time, I have never been able to *hypnotise* any decidedly idiotic patient – which I consider to be an important fact, and one which is strongly confirmatory of my theory of the nature and cause of the hypnotic condition.[46]

[Hypnosis used as Alterative]

In ordinary practice we aim, by different means, at attaining the same ends as those pointed out as producible by my hypnotic processes. Thus, we give digitalis, tartrite of antimony, and aconite, *etc.*, to lower the force of the circulation, and we bleed also for the same purpose, and likewise to render the blood less stimulating, by diminishing the blood globules or carriers of oxygen, and thus we reduce over-excited function. We likewise exhibit stimulants to rouse languid action, general or local, as the case may be. By inducing the nervous sleep, however, we can attain the same ends in many cases more pleasantly, speedily, and safely, than can be accomplished by those other means; and moreover, as already remarked, hypnotism is strikingly successful in a class of painful nervous disorders, in which ordinary treatment is of little or no avail. How nervous sleep acts in some such cases it may be difficult or impossible to explain; but **it may be reasonably considered to act as an alterative, producing a new action or counter-impression, during which the morbid action is suspended, which affords an opportunity for a natural and healthy action to be resumed when the influence of hypnotism is suspended, and that without any marked physical operation or evacuation. This is all which can be said as to the curative operation of most medicines denominated alteratives.** [Braid seems to pre-empt the behaviour therapy notion of "reciprocal inhibition" of nervous functioning by inducing an opposing ("alterative") state.]

[Examples of Cases Treated]

I shall now briefly detail a few of the variety of cases in which I have found hypnotism most successful as a therapeutic agent.

In some affections of the eyes, as loss of nervous power, hypnotism has proved eminently successful, after other means had failed. Also in scrofulous ophthalmia, in which the eyelids are glued together in the morning, hypnotism has produced most satisfactory results. It has also been most successful in some cases of opacity of the cornea of long standing. I have seen it cause an absorption of opacity of the cornea, which had existed for many years, in defiance of all ordinary treatment, and which was a personal disfigurement, as well as an obstruction to vision, and yet this opacity was absorbed in a very short time under the use of hypnotism alone, so as to restore useful vision, as well as to remove the personal blemish. In these chronic cases I had recourse to the quickened circulation, and calling the attention of the patient to the eyes by touches and passes. Acute cases require the low circulation.

In some cases of nervous deafness, in like manner, hypnotism is most successful. It seems speedily to rouse nervous action, and produces **an increase in the secretion of wax in the ears**, the want of which is so often both a cause and accompaniment of deafness.

I had one case of a girl who had been deaf and dumb from birth. At nine and a half years of age she came under my care. Up to that period she was never known to have heard sound, even when a person standing close behind her was calling to her at the top of his voice. I hypnotised this girl, directing her attention to her ears during the quickened circulation, and, in a very short time thereafter, her hearing became so acute, that she could readily hear words spoken in a moderate tone of voice, and imitate them

---

[45] Undoubtedly non-professional persons might be trained to act under the special direction of medical men, as to the mode and extent of management in each particular case. But, from the length of time required for prolonging the processes in some cases, this could not be accorded personally by medical men generally. Until assistants are trained, therefore, for the purpose, hypnotism never can be applied in general practice so much as it otherwise would be.

[46] [Braid appears to mean that hypnosis is primarily a state of mental focus on an appropriate idea and that "idiots", by which Victorian physicians meant the mentally handicapped, lack the ability to concentrate suitably.]

after repeated trials, *without her seeing the motion of the lips of the speaker*. In a short time more her progress was such, that she was sent to school to learn to read and speak in the usual way, in which she made very good progress; and since she left school, she has been many years acting as a domestic servant, receiving her instructions and giving her replies in the usual manner, *by speech only*. Curiously enough there are some sounds, such as the high notes of the pianoforte, which she cannot hear at all, although she hears all within the compass of her voice, so as to be able to imitate them correctly by singing, and the notes at the *extreme* top of the instrument are also heard by her. In like manner she cannot hear the sound of a high-toned bell, but she can hear a low-toned bell, a knock at the door, or a gentle rap on a table.

I had considerable success with some other congenital deaf mutes, but I found them and their friends so unreasonable as to expect, that a miracle ought to be wrought for them, by which they should not only be made to hear, and thus be enabled to *learn to pronounce words, and understand the meaning of them*, but they seemed to be disappointed because they required to be taught to speak, and were not instantly invested with the gift of tongues, and the knowledge of the meaning of language, the moment they had acquired the use of hearing, so as to be able to imitate words spoken behind them, when they could not see the motions of the lips of the speaker. This was obviously too much to be expected by reasonable people; but I found that, amongst the poor, they would not take the trouble of teaching their deaf and dumb relatives, after they had been restored to such a degree of hearing as fitted them for profiting by such instructions. Both patients and their friends preferred the old mode of using signs, as being *immediately* more convenient for both, than the toil of teaching and learning ordinary language, the value of which would have been experienced by them only at a future day, and after much labour both to teacher and scholar. I was compelled, therefore, to leave them to their fate, because, without exercise, the faculty of hearing was likely to lose its power, rather than to advance in acuteness.

The following fact regarding a deaf and dumb boy is interesting in several respects:– After I had attained what I considered an important point with him, I exhibited the lad at a public lecture in London. The audience wished to have him tested by a professional gentleman present, who considered himself very competent to do so. He applied his tests, and then pronounced that the boy had *no* hearing whatever. I proved, however, that he possessed hearing in a limited degree, which enabled him to hear me speak to him in a rather loud tone of voice, whilst my lips were six or eight inches from his ears, when he made a good attempt at imitating a number of words, whilst he could not see the motion of my lips. I went on hypnotising this boy daily, and exercising him in imitation words spoken when he could not see the motion of my lips, and the result was, that on exhibiting the same boy at a public lecture at Liverpool, given a few weeks thereafter, the lad was proved capable of imitating so perfectly words spoken, both by myself and by the head master of the Liverpool Deaf and Dumb School, that many of the audience were inclined to deny the *possibility that this boy could ever have been deaf and dumb*. Could any greater proof than this be wanted to convince anyone that this lad must have improved greatly in quickness of hearing, from the time when he was tested by a medical man in London a few weeks before, and when he was pronounced by that gentleman to have NO hearing at all?

The influence of hypnotism, in curing many cases of tic douloureux, nervous headache, paralysis, rheumatism, chronic gout, epilepsy, tonic spasm, St Vitus' dance, hysteria, spinal irritation, and distortion, natural somnambulism and catalepsy, *etc. etc.*, is most marked, even in cases which have long resisted every other known method of cure. The reader must not mistake me, however, and suppose that I wish it to be believed that by hypnotism I can cure *every* case of *any one* of these classes of diseases. Some of these cases arise occasionally from organic cases, which necessarily forbid the hope of remedy *from any means whatever*; but, in such cases as are curable, in general it can be achieved more speedily, certainly, and pleasantly, by hypnotism, than by any other method of treatment at present known. For example, I have been enabled, *in a few minutes*, to open the jaws with ease, in cases in which they had been locked for a considerable time, and would not yield to violent mechanical force, nor to ordinary treatment; and, with equal celerity, a patient was enabled to swallow, who, from hysteric spasm of the oesophagus, had been for *thirteen months* unable to swallow any thing but liquids, and these with great difficulty. One patient, whose hand and arm were spasmodically locked, so that no force applied in the ordinary way was able to move them from their fixed position, was equally speedily relieved by hypnotism, and continued well from such affection ever after; and another similar case, which had persisted in the same cataleptic condition for seventeen weeks, in defiance of treatment by eminent medical men, was unlocked in a few days, and speedily cured, by hypnotism alone, and has remained well now for years.

I may also mention a most interesting case of a young lady of sixteen years of age. Her head had been immovably drawn close to her shoulder for six and twenty weeks, and had resisted most energetic treatment under an experienced physician, *viz.*, bleeding, blistering, purgatives, mercury, opiates, anti-spasmodics, and galvanism, *etc*. – all of which were pushed to the utmost limits which prudence could sanction. This patient had even been sent to London with a written statement of her case, in order that she might have the benefit of the advice of one of the most eminent practitioners in the metropolis, but all to no purpose – for the spasm had never relaxed either by night or by day, although she was watched with the view of ascertaining whether it abated during sleep. When I examined the patient at my first visit, I ascertained that the utmost force which I could exert was quite inadequate to separate the head and shoulder of the patient in the slightest degree. However, after being hypnotised for a few minutes, with the quickened circulation, I was enabled, with the greatest ease, to change the position of the head from the left to the right shoulder, **by calling the attention of the patient into the muscles antagonistic** to those which were holding the head fixed cataleptically to the left shoulder, and after allowing her to remain a few minutes in the sleep, with her head inclined towards the right shoulder, I awoke her by a clap of my hands near to the right ear, when she was perfectly straight.

[Breaking Down Morbid Dominant Ideas]
The above case may no doubt seem very marvellous to those unacquainted with the hypnotic mode of treatment, and yet, with my views and mode of explaining the nature, cause, and cure of such affections, nothing could be more simple, or more naturally to be expected. **A dominant idea, calling certain muscles into strong action, had become involuntarily fixed in the patient's mind, until cataleptiform rigidity, which is an involuntary power, had locked the muscles in permanent tonic spasm. The patient's own volition was paralysed, or inadequate to overcome this morbid action, and mechanical force only tended to excite these muscles, automatically, into still more vigorous action; but, by stimulating the** *antagonist* **muscles on the** *opposite side of the neck into action***, by slight titillation over them, after I had subjected the brain and the spinal cord to the stimulus of the quickened circulation of a highly arterialised blood – by extending the extremities, and rendering them rigid during the nervous sleep – the previous morbid dominant idea was broken, by the attention being withdrawn** *from the spasmodic muscles, to their antagonists* **on the opposite side, and thus** *by art* **and NOT BY FORCE, I was enabled to move the head of the patient from the left to the right side, with as much ease as a mother can move the head of her sleeping infant. It was not, therefore, the mere induction of the** *nervous sleep* **alone which effected the cure, but my knowledge of how to** *direct the influence* **DURING the sleep, so as to break down the pre-existing, involuntarily fixed, dominant idea in the patient's mind, and its consequences.** In proof of this, I may state the following fact:– This patient was enabled to return home quite straight after *two* hypnotic operations, each being only of eight or ten minutes duration. Several years subsequently, the same patient had a similar seizure in one foot, for which she went to consult an eminent London physician [John Elliotson], who is a sturdy champion for "the old established modes of Mesmerising," and the magnetic and odylic theories for explaining the nature and cause of the phenomena. Well, this gentleman recommended Mesmerism as the remedy, and operated on her daily for about *three months* before she was fit to return home, his operations sometimes being prolonged to *six, eight, or nine hours a day*. Three weeks elapsed of these prolonged operations – from depending entirely upon the general Mesmerising operations – before the patient could stir her foot in bed, which shows a striking contrast with my general hypnotising and manipulating processes, by which the spasm of the neck was removed with so much ease in a *few minutes*. I hesitate not to say that I could have hypnotised this patient, and manipulated so as to have unlocked the foot as speedily as I did the head and neck in the first instance.[47]

[Other Conditions Treated by Removing Morbid Ideas]
In some cases of affection of the larynx, also, with loss of voice, hypnotism has been most rapidly and permanently successful after all other treatment had failed. In nervous palpitation of the heart, hypnotism has also proved of great value, as likewise in dyspepsia and constipation of the bowels, and in some disease of the skin. Moreover, as might be expected, hypnotism may be rendered most useful for procuring sleep without the use of opiates, which is an invaluable boon to many a sufferer, for it frequently happens that sleep procured by the use of opiates can only be obtained with the certain damage of some of the other most important functions of the human body.

In some cases of insanity, especially monomania and delirium tremens, I have found hypnotism most successful. Thus, in a case in which the patient was haunted with the idea of the personal presence of a departed relative, I hypnotised her, and **then excited a different idea in her mind, under the dominance of which idea I awoke her, and the unwelcome apparition never again made its appearance**. In like manner, in a case of delirium tremens from excessive drinking, during which the patient imagined that a menagerie had been let loose, and the wild animals had got into his room, so that he could point out the exact place where each animal was standing in his cage, after I had exhausted all my usual resources in vain, and the patient had become so excited as to imagine the house was on fire, and that the animals would be let loose upon him, which induced him to jump from his bed, and run along the streets in his night dress, in order to escape from the assaults of the animals, as I durst not try the effects of opium administered in greater quantity, and which in the doses given had never been adequate to induce sleep, in the presence of my son, Dr. Braid, I resolved to try the effect of hypnotism; and, having reduced the patient by this means to sound sleep for twenty minutes, I awoke him, and then again reduced him to the somnolent condition, and left him to remain in that condition until he should awake spontaneously. The result of my operation was this, that on awaking, my patient was quite rational, and convalesced from that hour, and he has remained

---

[47] [This case was the cause of some controversy between Braid and Elliotson, and is cited in Braid's letters to The Medical Times.]

well from attacks of the sort ever since, which is now many years.

In the case of another patient who, from excessive drinking, had got into a state of maniacal excitement, on two separate attacks of the sort, I got him to be down on a sofa, and then, in a few minutes I succeeded in reducing him to sleep, in which state he remained for four hours each time, and then awoke perfectly rational on each occasion.

The most striking cases of all, however, for illustrating the value of the hypnotic mode of treatment, are cases of hysteric paralysis, in which, without organic lesion, the patient may have remained for a considerable length of time perfectly powerless of a part, or of the whole of the body, **from a dominant idea which has paralysed or misdirected his volition.** In such cases, by altering the circulation, and **breaking down the previous idea, and substituting a salutary idea of vigour and self-confidence in their place, (which can be done by audible suggestions addressed to the patient in a confident tone of voice as to what** *must* **and** *shall* **be realised by the processes he has been subjected to), on being aroused in a few minutes thereafter with such dominant idea in their minds, to the astonishment of themselves as well as of others, the patients are found to have acquired vigour and voluntary power over their hitherto paralysed limbs, as if by a magical spell or witchcraft.** Assuredly, such cures are as important as they are interesting and surprising, because, such cases may resist ordinary modes of treatment for paralysis, for an indefinite length of time; but still, the *rationale* is simple enough when viewed according to the principles which I have already explained, of the influence of an expectant dominant idea, *either exciting or depressing natural function, according to the faith and confidence of the patient.*

The most interesting part of all, however, is this, that in the hands of those who thoroughly understand it, hypnotism may be tried with the utmost confidence; that, even in cases which it cannot cure, the trial may be made without pain, or the slightest danger or inconvenience to the patient. It is therefore useful in many cases in aiding us in forming correct diagnosis in obscure cases.

[Most Subjects Remain Conscious in Hypnosis]

It is of great importance that it should be clearly understood by patients, that it is by no means generally requisite that they should lapse into the state of *unconsciousness* **in order to ensure the salutary effects of the nervous sleep. Many imagine, that unless they become torpid and insensible, no beneficial effect can ensue. This is a complete misapprehension, for the happy results of innumerable cases treated with the greatest success by hypnotism, clearly prove, that cases which had resisted all ordinary treatment by the exhibition of medicines and external applications, have readily yielded to the impression made on the nervous system by this peculiar influence, even when they were perfectly conscious of all that was done, and could remember, after awaking, every circumstance that had happened during the nervous sleep. This was strikingly verified in my own case, when I cured myself of a violent rheumatic attack by throwing myself into the nervous sleep for eight or nine minutes, from which I was aroused perfectly free from pain, although I had been perfectly** *conscious all the while*.[48]

[Cure of Headache & Loss of Eyesight]

The following is an interesting case of cure of headache of long standing, as also of impaired vision, by the use of hypnotism alone.

In 1849, I was called to attend a severe case of epilepsy of four years standing, in which the parents were anxious to try the influence of hypnotism, as all ordinary treatment of the case had utterly failed in affording relief. During my first visit, the mother of the patient, age 54 years, told me she had been severely afflicted with headache, to such an extent, that she had not known what it was to have lived without headache, when awake, for fourteen years, and that her eyesight had become so impaired, that she could with difficulty manage to read a sign-board when in the street. I offered to try the effect of hypnotism, and on arousing her from the first sleep, which had not been longer than ten minutes, she expressed herself agreeably surprised to find herself free from headache *for the first time for fourteen years*. Next day she had a slight return of headache, which was again removed by another dose of hypnotism. She was less and less afflicted with her headache every day, and by repeating the operations for about ten minutes daily within a week, the headache was gone, and has never recurred since, unless for a short time occasionally, as will occur to anyone. Moreover, a most remarkable improvement in the sight also took place from the hypnotising – an improvement which has been permanent to this date.

[Case of Spinal Irritation]

I could readily adduce many important instances of speedy relief and cure, by hypnotism, of spinal irritation, which had resisted ordinary modes of treatment. I shall allow the following, however, to suffice, which also illustrates the beneficial effect of hypnotism on the action of the skin and bowels. I was consulted in the case of the late Lady S.G., who was then upwards of 64 years of age. She had suffered much from the state of

---

[48] [Elsewhere, Braid suggests that only 10% of his subjects experienced amnesia or apparent loss of consciousness during hypnosis.]

her spine for 45 years, but for some years previous to consulting me it had become so much worse, that, notwithstanding her carriage had double springs, she dreaded riding in it even for two or three miles, from the intense aggravation of pain in the back caused thereby. The state of her skin was dry and harsh, and unpleasantly hot, the bowels obstinately constipated, requiring tremendous doses of cathartic medicines to procure sufficient alvine [i.e., bowel] evacuations, her sleep was most disturbed and unrefreshing, and the appetite capricious. Having hypnotised her ladyship, **notwithstanding she did not become unconscious**, it was found, on arousing her, that the skin was moist, and she slept comfortably all night for the *first time for many months*. I went on hypnotising her ladyship night and morning with the happiest results, and soon had the satisfaction of enabling her to keep her bowels sufficiently active, by the assistance of about one-sixth part the doses of aperient [laxative] medicine required when she came under my care; her headache and feverish state of the skin was gone; her general health and strength became quite renovated, and the spinal irritation so much relieved, that she could bear carriage exercise with comfort, and walk much farther and firmer than for many years.

Some years after, I was summoned to attend this patient for an attack of gout in the foot. Her ladyship's whole family were great martyrs to gout, but she had been much less afflicted with gout than formerly, since she underwent the hypnotic treatment. Now, however, she had got a very smart attack in one foot, and what made her the more anxious about it was her past experience, for she told me that whenever she was attacked in the foot, she had *always* been laid up with it for at least six months, even under the superintendence of the most eminent medical assistance to be procured. Her stocking being removed, I found the great toe and dorsum of the foot very red, and exquisitely tender to the touch, and the whole foot so tender, that the patient durst not place the foot on the floor. I requested her ladyship to recline on the sofa, and submit to be hypnotised, whilst I should make passes over the foot. In the course of twenty minutes I aroused my patient, who had **never lost consciousness all the while**; when both the patient and her lady's maid expressed themselves greatly surprised to find the *redness* had entirely disappeared, and that the pain was so much mitigated that she could permit me to touch it freely, and was even able to rest her foot on the floor. As her ladyship lived thirty miles off, I did not wish to trust entirely on the power of hypnotism, when it could be so seldom applied; and I therefore prescribed my usual medicinal remedies for gout, and at my next visit, two days after, I hypnotised her again, and on the third day of the attack I had the agreeable intelligence communicated to me that my patient had been able to walk from one room into another on the same landing; and after another dose of hypnotism, in a day or two more she was able to be downstairs, instead of being confined for six months, as she always had been before when the gout attacked her in the foot. I by no means wish to attribute this cure entirely to hypnotism, but I am satisfied that a large share of the happy result was justly attributable to it.

[Rheumatic Pain]
The following is also one of my latest cases, and is quite in point. A few months ago, I was called to a gentleman who was suffering severely from rheumatism of the lower extremities. He had been confined to the house the previous year, with a similar attack, for fourteen weeks, in defiance of the best attention and care of two most respectable and experienced medical gentlemen. On this occasion he had again been under similar treatment without relief, which induced him to request me to treat him hypnotically. Both his feet were very painful, so that he could not stand on them without great suffering, and he had considerable pain in the knees also. **I explained to him that he might not lose consciousness during the process and yet be benefited.** I put him through the process, extending the limbs after his eyelids closed. On arousing him in ten minutes, which I did by a clap of my hands near to one of his ears, **he protested that no effect whatever had been produced upon him. I told him I perfectly well knew that he had been conscious all the while, but that still I expected that a very decided effect had been produced upon the sensation and circulation of his lower extremities by my process. He protested that he could not believe this. I then requested him to try how he could stand now, when he candidly admitted that he felt much less pain in the feet and legs, but still he persisted that it was impossible the improvement could have resulted from what I had done. Two days thereafter I called again, and found the feet much relieved, but both knees were extremely painful. I hypnotised him once more, extending his extremities. It was with great difficulty he held them up at first from the acute pain in the knees, but by degrees they got easier, and became slightly cataleptic. On again arousing him, he contended he had not been affected at all, but, to his great astonishment, he found his knees so much better that he could walk across the floor. The next operation, the day after, enabled him before I left the house to walk to the door, and, with all his scepticism, he had the satisfaction of getting quite well by these three simple processes, and he has continued well ever since, and very grateful for what hypnotism achieved for him.**

About nine years ago, I was consulted in the case of a young gentleman who had been given up as a hopeless cripple, resulting from an attack of rheumatic fever. He had been attended from the first seizure by an eminent physician, and also by an eminent and experienced surgeon. After exhausting all their resources, he was sent to the sea-side, where he had the benefit of being attended by one of the most respectable and intelligent and experienced surgeons in the kingdom. The whole ordinary resources of medical and surgical science consequently had been brought to bear on this case; and the patient was then abandoned as totally incurable, his legs being fixed nearly at right angles with the thighs, and incapable of extension even when subjected to strong pressure from straps surrounding them when laid upon a board, whilst they were surrounded by warm vapour. He had been for a length of time crawling about the room on his knees and elbows, each of which was provided with a patent leather shield, and such was expected to be his fate for life, when he came under the hypnotic treatment. Notwithstanding the extreme rigidity of the flexors of the legs, during the first hypnotic operation I was enabled to extend them considerably, and still more so at the second, as also to infuse strength into other muscles which seemed to have been almost entirely paralysed previously, so that after the second operation he manifested a degree of power which surprised myself as well as his friends. I went on daily with my hypnotic operations, without any other means being tried, and he gradually gained more and more power. I always made him exert his volition to the utmost when he was asleep, and *every decided advance he made was FIRST manifested during the hypnotic state*, and then in a lesser degree the improvement was manifested after he was aroused from it. Without entering into tedious details, suffice it to say that at length he acquired the power of walking with the aid of crutches, and then without them, and now he can walk at the rate of three and a half miles an hour, with only a slight degree of lameness, and without even the aid of a stick. When I saw him a few days ago, he was walking at this rate; and, when I asked him how far he could walk in a day, he said he did not know, but that he occasionally walked *six miles before breakfast.*

[Waking Suggestion & Induced Nausea]
Moreover, **there are many important cures effected by manipulating patients during the *waking* condition, so as to change physical action, by the *mental* direction of the *mind* of the *patient*; and even without manipulation or any process whatever of a second party, beyond desiring the subjects to sit still and concentrate their minds on the ideas which we wish to be realised;** examples of which I have already referred to in reference to my experiments with the coloured water made to act as an emetic, and the anti-emetic phial, when determining the probable nature of the effects of medicines said to produce their effects through glass, and on the alleged "Od" force of Baron von Reichenbach.

I have frequently produced full vomiting in hypnotised patients, simply by giving them a mouthful of water to drink, and then suggesting to them in audible language that they had taken an emetic; or simply by moving my own lips and jaws, which they heard and imitated; and on my suggesting that they had taken an emetic, the idea alone was quite adequate to produce vomiting. [Cf. the subsequent use of nausea in hypnotic "aversion" therapy.] I have never, however, seen hypnotised, Mesmerised, or magnetised water produce specific effects, without some mode of suggesting the idea to the mind of the patient, by words spoken or movements made, or by the peculiar manner of the operator or someone present, as has been alleged by the Mesmerists to take place with some of their patients.

[Bitter Laxative Effect]
With many hypnotised patients I have also produced action on the bowels *in a few minutes* by similar suggestions, or by audible suggestions, accompanied by drawing the tips of the fingers gently along the course of the colon, so as to excite its peristaltic motion. The following is a remarkable instance of this, and how an idea suggested during the sleep may manifest its powers for a length of time after the patient awakes. I had hypnotised a gentleman for some time, with considerable benefit, for epilepsy of long standing, and which had resisted all ordinary treatment prescribed by first-rate medical men. On one occasion I moved my lips, and imitated the act of swallowing, which acts he heard and immediately imitated. I then suggested that he had taken some [bitter] *aloes* [i.e., a strong laxative], the mere idea of which made him assume all the physical expression of disgust (and also to utter words through that effect) at the well-known bitterness of the drug. I then said it would soon give him still greater cause of uneasiness by its action on his bowels, and very soon he began to writhe his body as if he were labouring under the griping influence of an active cathartic. I said nothing further, but, in four or five minutes he arose from his seat and walked up stairs to the water-closet, and came down again, still asleep, after having left unmistakeable proof in the pan of the water-closet of the success of my experiment. On being aroused from the sleep, this patient had no idea of what had happened, but he complained of a very bitter taste in his mouth. When this gentleman called upon me next afternoon, he told me that the bitter taste which he complained of when he awoke out of his sleep the previous day, had been so disagreeable, that when he got home he tried to wash it out of his mouth, but could not do so. Every morsel of food or mouthful of drink was disgustingly bitter, both at tea and supper, notwithstanding he had tried to get rid of it by repeatedly washing his mouth. On awaking in the morning the bitter taste remained the same, his breakfast being as bitter and unpalatable as his tea and supper had been. He again tried to wash it away by assiduous gargling, but without effect, and the bitter taste never ceased to haunt him until some time about noon, when, his attention had become withdrawn from it through some cause of excitement which he met with in town.

[Overcoming Hallucinatory Odour]
I shall now give a case in which a disgusting odour had made a painful and lasting impression on a person in

the waking condition, and which was speedily removed by hypnotism, after all other means resorted to had failed. Mrs ——, the mother of a large family, and at the time in question in perfect health, in July 1849 had gone to the house of a deceased friend when the body was in a state of advanced decomposition. She felt distressingly affected by the disgusting odour, and for several days thereafter she never could enjoy a moment's pleasure for this disgusting odour, which haunted her night and day when awake, notwithstanding she had tried all sorts of fragrant scents, salvolatile [ammonia solution used in smelling salts], snuff, *etc.*, and had even burnt Lucifer matches [strong-smelling Victorian matches] and tobacco under her nostrils, but still the disgusting odour was as potent and persistent as ever. I hypnotised this patient, and, **by audible and muscular suggestion**, I led her mind to dwell on the idea of inhaling fragrant scents, and in five minutes I aroused her with this impression on her mind, when she expressed her delight with the fragrance with which she was now surrounded and feasted. She had no return of the disgusting odour, not even when on several occasions she tried, by an effort of attention, to recall it. Fourteen months after, however, I hypnotised this patient in the presence of several scientific friends, whom I had previously told that I should endeavour to recall this idea and impression in the sleep, and carry it into the waking condition. The patient had no idea of my intentions, but after she had been in the sleep a short time, by applying one finger to her nose and sniffing, whilst with the other hand I corrugated her brows, drawing them downwards over the root of the nose, the patient began to sniff, and speedily expressed her disgust with the smell of putrid meat – "that old smell come back again". On arousing her with this mental impression, and asking her how she felt, she replied, "That old smell has come back again." Having then had the full manifestation I wished to exhibit, for she explicitly described the peculiar smell she meant, I immediately hypnotised her again, and excited the opposite ideas in her mind, and awoke her feasting on more than all the fragrance of Arabia.

[Lactation, Breast Enlargement, Bowel Movement, & Menstruation]
Having told a gentleman that the expectant idea in the mind of a patient was quite adequate to produce a corresponding change in the physical function of any organ or part of the body to which it was directed, he expressed his incredulity. I asked him if his wife was not then nursing, to which he replied she was; and I therefore offered to prove my position, if he chose, by **causing an increased flow of milk to come into ONE of her breasts**, by directing her attention particularly to *that* breast during the sleep. This gentleman's wife had been a patient of mine some eight months previously, and was then cured of violent headaches by hypnotism; and I knew she was one of those subjects who pass into **the second-conscious or full state**, and upon whom the power of suggestion manifests its greatest influence. The lady was sent for, and asked if she had any objections to being hypnotised, for her husband to have an opportunity of seeing her in that state. She readily gave her assent, and whilst standing on her feet, I held my lancet case over her head, in my usual way, and requested her to gaze upon it, and speedily her eyelids closed, with the twitter peculiar to the hypnotic sleep. After she had remained in this state a little while, I gently drew the tips of my fingers two or three times over the left mamma, when the patient slowly raised her left arm towards her breast. I then inquired "What is it?" To which she replied "Baby." "What about baby?" To which she answered, "Oh this is so tight," pointing to her left breast. In this state I allowed her to remain for a few minutes, her mind riveted to the idea of her baby, and the fullness of her breast. With a clap of my hands I now aroused the patient, **who had no recollection whatever of anything said or done when she was asleep.** [Spontaneous amnesia being a characteristic of the "double consciousness" stage.] I asked if any part of her body felt different from its usual condition. To which she replied, pointing to the left breast, "This breast feels very tight." I asked her what had made it so. To this she replied, she could not tell, but that it felt so. Her husband now remarked, "That is what Mr. Braid said he would do – he said he would bring a rush of milk into it." To this the lady replied, "That will be no easy matter, for my baby is fourteen months old, and I have scarcely any milk." I requested her to bring baby and try, as I felt assured that *now* there would be no lack of milk in that breast. The baby was applied to that breast, and, notwithstanding he was fourteen months old, the flow of milk was so copious that it nearly choked him.

A few days thereafter **this lady complained that I had disfigured her, as I had made her over-protuberant on the left side**. I said I can soon settle that matter, for, by putting you to sleep again, I can take it down as readily as it was increased in size during former sleep. She most willingly assented to this, but when she was asleep, **instead of taking it down (which a suggested idea to that effect would have done), I acted on the other breast in precisely the same manner as on the left breast, and with precisely similar results**. The most important point, however, still remains to be told – *viz.*, that although her child was fourteen months old, and before being hypnotised she complained of having had very little milk, these hypnotic processes had given such a stimulus to the mamma, that **this lady was enabled to continue to suckle her child from an overflowing breast for *six months longer*.** [Braid appears to have enlarged both breasts by inducing lactation, and the child was breast-fed until it was a year and eight months old.]

Another important fact I have to communicate connected with this case. This patient was one of those ladies who menstruate during lactation, and, previous to my hypnotising her the first day, she had gone two weeks beyond the usual period for the appearance of the catamenia. The stimulus to the mamma, however, through sympathy, had brought on that discharge also within half an hour after she was hypnotised. The consequence of this was, that the lady wished to know whether the like process could be made available in the case of her niece, who was a well-developed young lady, sixteen years of age, but never had had the slightest indication of the catamenia. I told her my opinion and experience were favourable to a trial of hypnotism in such a case. The young lady was hypnotised accordingly, and during the sleep I made non contact passes over the mamma, and slight contact passes over the ovaria, with the view of producing excitement of sensation and circulation in these organs. She was not in the condition more than ten minutes, and was standing on her feet all the while. Next day the aunt told me that it had not produced any effect in the way intended, but that another remarkable result had taken place, namely, that her bowels had moved shortly after I hypnotised her, without her having taken medicine for that purpose – a circumstance which was most extraordinary, as the whole of her family were liable to obstinate constipation of the bowels, always requiring the use of aperients medicine, and that this young lady never had more than *one stool in SIX DAYS even with the aid of powerful medicines* – such as six grains of calomel and half a dram of jalap, followed by three or four ounces of black draught. I told the aunt that I had no doubt but I could hypnotise the young lady, and thereby excite her bowels to act again *before I left the house*. With all she had seen and felt, the lady could not imagine this possible, but she had no objections to my trying to experiment. I acted accordingly, drawing the tips of my fingers gently along the course of the colon, from the *caput coecum* to the *sigmoid flexure*, with the view of exciting the peristaltic action of the bowels, **at the same time suggesting, in audible language, frequently repeated – "This will soon make the bowels act."** In the course of six or eight minutes it was obvious, from her manner, that the patient was suffering from all the tormina [acute abdominal pains] of a violent cathartic, under which feeling I awoke her; and, at my request, in order to guard against all possibility of mistake as to the result, her aunt caused her to use a close stool, and thus I had ocular demonstration of the efficiency of my process before I left the house: and, moreover, the same afternoon and evening she had two more copious and violently purged stools. From that period I never saw this young lady for eight months; but I had the gratification to learn that my operation had effected a complete change on her constitution, as far as regarded the state of her bowels, as from that period she had required no more purgative medicines, as her bowels had acted DAILY *of their own accord*, and the young lady had been enjoying excellent health ever since, only she had not yet menstruated.

During this period the patient had left the aunt at whose house I hypnotised her, and the other friends, under whose care she was then placed, were afraid to have any farther trials of what appeared to them so mysterious, both in its nature and effects, as to appear more like magic or witchcraft than legitimate treatment. When this patient again returned to the aunt at whose house she was hypnotised, it was determined on, both by the patient and her aunt, that she should be hypnotised daily, with the object in view of exciting the catamenial flow, and they had no cause to regret their decision, for within eight days after I began to hypnotise her with this view, this important function was established, without the slightest inconvenience to the patient. All went on well with this lady subsequently, and she has now been many years married, and is the mother of several healthy children.

In like manner, by hypnotising patients labouring under violent diarrhoea, and imprinting on their minds by audible suggestions during the sleep the certainty of the process arresting the diarrhoea, in several cases in which I tried it, the success was as complete as immediate, both pain and purging being entirely arrested within a few minutes, and not recurring again after arousing the patients.

[Epilepsy & Waking Suggestion for Menstruation]
I have had many other cases where the catamenia have been excited in a few minutes by the hypnotic processes; but I must make the following case suffice, **as it has clearly proved that the expectant dominant idea is adequate to produce such result, not only in the hypnotic state, but even in the waking condition**; and not only of exciting it when suspended or deficient, but also of arresting or suppressing it when in excess.

In July 1849, I was called to attend Mrs ——, thirty years of age, married, and the mother of three children. She had suffered severely from epilepsy for four years, for which she had been under the care of several medical men. The attacks became a little less frequent for some time, but again increased in frequency and severity, until, at the period when I was consulted, notwithstanding she was under the constant care of a physician, and was taking medicines prescribed by him repeatedly every day, still she was getting worse, so that at this period she had as many as twenty-eight fits daily, besides what occurred during the night, when her attendants were asleep. The day before I first operated on her, she had thirteen violent fits in the space of eight hours; and, when I first saw her, she was jaw-locked, as the sequel to one of her epileptic attacks. Her friends told me, that whenever this state of locked-jaw occurred, they were never able to open her mouth for many hours, however much force they might apply to effect it. They were, therefore, not a little surprised to observe that, by one of my usual processes for reducing the cataleptic state of muscles during hypnotism or Mesmerism, I was enabled, *in a few seconds*, to open her jaws, and open her mouth, without the slightest difficulty or force. This patient was speedily thrown into the hypnotic condition by my usual method, and the results of my first operation, which was not of more than a quarter of an hour's duration, was this – that the patient had only *four* fits in eight hours, instead of the thirteen fits which she had during the corresponding period on the day previous.

This patient was operated upon by me twice each day subsequently, and on the fourth day the catamenia, which had been suspended for several months, reappeared, and, in the course of a week, the fits were almost entirely arrested. Indeed, since that period she has only had four or five fits, and these were brought on by causes of greater mental excitement. The catamenia recurred regularly for the next six months, and the results realised from the use of hypnotism, when they again became suspended, beautifully and conclusively illustrate the value of this mode of treatment in such affections.

At six successive periods I had occasion to resort to hypnotism for this purpose, and in *every* instance with *entire success*, by *a single operation of from ten to eleven minutes each*. Moreover, I ascertained that this important result could be effected **without either touch or pass of a second party, but by mental concentration and direction of the *mind of the patient alone***, and the management of the circulation, without farther mental or physical aid on my part, beyond simply requesting her to put herself to sleep and elevate her limbs, her attention being at the same time directed to and concentrated upon the idea of the expected result. On several other occasions when I hypnotised this patient for neuralgic or rheumatic pain in a leg or arm, through the mode of managing and directing the attention and expectant idea, the pains were immediately removed, without exciting any visible manifestation on *any* special organ or function.

Subsequently to this report, which was published in 1850, on six other occasions I resorted to the same process as in this case, and with the like success on *every* occasion. It now occurred to me that, inasmuch as it was my opinion that the change in the physical action resulted *entirely* from the fixed mental attention of the patient, with a predominant idea and faith on her part in the power of these processes to produce such results, it would be highly interesting to ascertain whether such results might not be realised by mental concentration of the patient alone, **when she remained wide awake**. On the 4th of April 1851, I proposed to test this. The requisite means were had recourse to for determining, with the utmost accuracy, the actual physical condition of the patient *before* commencing the experiment. Four ladies and one gentleman, besides myself, were present. Having requested the gentleman to note the time accurately, the patient being seated in an easy chair, **I addressed her in the following words, which were heard by all present:– "Now, keep your mind firmly fixed on what you know ought to happen."** All remained silent; and, in order to withdraw my own mind as much as possible from the patient (and thereby to prevent all idea of my will or other mental powers having any share in effecting the results) I took up an interesting book, and engaged myself in reading it. **At the end of eleven minutes**, I asked the patient if the desired effect had been produced – to which she replied she did not know. However, on proper examination being made, I had incontestable proof of the success of my experiment. Next month she did not require a repetition of the process; but, on the 2nd of June, it was again tried, in the presence of two professional gentlemen, and with equal success as on the 4th of April. On the 28th of July, I again had occasion to resort to this process with this patient; and I was then particularly anxious that it should succeed, as a lady was present who required similar aid, and a good example in point was likely to assist me greatly in influencing her the more certainly. My mind, therefore, was unusually intent on the accomplishment of the desired result. At the expiration of eleven minutes, I inquired if it had taken effect, when she replied she could not tell. On examination, however, it was ascertained **it had been a failure on this occasion. The patient hereupon remarked that, before sitting down, she thought it would *not* succeed *to-night*. I inquired why? To which she replied, "Because I *could not fix my mind on it to-night*, from having been put out of my way just before I came here." To this I replied, "Well, if you cannot fix your mind on the idea when awake, I know that I can command the requisite attention when you are asleep, and therefore I will hypnotise you."** This I then did, at the same time exciting the circulation by elevating the limbs. It very soon **became apparent, from the expression of her features and the movements of her body, that the spell was in active operation; and, on arousing the patient in eleven minutes, there was positive proof adduced that the experiment had not been tried in vain; and all went on satisfactorily subsequently.**

It merits special attention, that notwithstanding *my* mind was particularly active in *willing* the desired effect when the patient was awake, no success followed, because the requisite *mental* condition of the *subject* was wanting. This failure, therefore, was as positive proof in support of my theory as the successful results. In fact it was even more so; for, on other occasions my mind had not been so intently desiring the immediate result, and yet the experiment succeeded, but now I was most active in willing success, and even with greater confidence in consequence of former successes; but now I was doomed to be disappointed, because the requisite *mental condition* of the PATIENT *was absent*.

Next month my assistance was not required, but on the 8th of October, in the presence of her mother, the waking experiment was again tried with complete success. On the 8th of November 1851, her mother, and my esteemed friend Dr. William Stevens, well-known as the author of the saline treatment of cholera and yellow fever, being present, I once more tried the waking experiment, with complete success, in eight minutes. From that period it had never required to be repeated, till July 1852. On the 19th of that month, as the patient had exceeded the proper period by two weeks, I once more requested her to sit down and fix her attention on the certainty of thereby producing the desired result. In the meantime I engaged myself by reading an interesting book, so that the patient was **kept at her fixed act of attention, with the expectant idea in her mind, for *thirteen* minutes**; at the expiration of which period it was ascertained that the catamenia were flowing copiously. **The result of this more prolonged act of fixed attention was an** unusually copious flow, which continued for three weeks uninterruptedly, and was exhausting the strength of the patient. To arrest this, I desired the patient to sit down and keep her mind steadily fixed on the confident assurance that the discharge would thereby be arrested. I kept her at this task for ten minutes, and within *one hour* the menstrual discharge had entirely ceased. In a week thereafter, it returned in moderate quantity for three days; and from that period it has recurred monthly, up to the end of March 1853. On the 15th of April 1853, as this patient had exceeded her menstrual period by three weeks, in the presence of my much esteemed friend Dr. W. B. Carpenter and another gentleman, I once more tried the waking experiment with entire success in eleven minutes; and the two succeeding months all has gone on satisfactorily.

[Hypnotic Childbirth]

The following is another highly interesting case of the influence of mental impression changing physical action. The patient was one of those subjects who pass into the **second-conscious state** of hypnotism, and had been cured by hypnotism of paralysis, both of sense and motion, of one side of the head and face. The following effect of the expectant idea, however, relates to what occurred when she was in the waking condition. This patient, Mrs ——, was the mother of three living children, the last of which was a cross birth, delivery being accomplished with great difficulty. The two subsequent births were of largely developed children, both still-born, both having been shoulder presentations, the labour far advanced, and the shoulder and arm advance within the pelvis before medical assistance arrived. Upon careful examination of the bones of the pelvis of this patient, it was clearly ascertained that there was such advancement forward, and depression of the promontory of the sacrum and lumbar vertebrae, as to preclude the hope of her ever giving birth to a full-sized living child; and, therefore, when she again became pregnant, I explained how matters stood to her husband, as well as to the patient, and recommended that premature labour should be induced, as affording the only chance of her bearing another living child, and as affording the greatest safety, moreover, for the mother. Both parties were perfectly satisfied to abide by my decision on this point, so that I was to consider myself at perfect liberty to act in the matter as I thought best, both as to the method to be adopted for accomplishing such purpose, and also in regard to the time when I was to induce premature labour. About two weeks beyond the seventh month was the period which I had fixed on for inducing labour. I had seen the patient a few days before this period, and found her in excellent health, experiencing no inconvenience of any sort. I told her that in three or four days I intended to do something for her to bring on labour as had previously been agreed upon should be done. She was quite agreeable to this proposal, and seemed to entertain no anxiety whatever on the subject. In two days thereafter, however, I was sent for to the patient, and ascertained that the mere mental impression had been sufficient to bring on labour, for the *os uteri* was not only fully dilated, but, as in the three former labours, the shoulder was presenting. In this case, from the small size of the infant, I was enabled with great ease to turn and deliver the mother of a living child.

[Critique of Homeopathy]

The last proof which I shall adduce in support of my position is the number of *recoveries* which take place *during* (*not* of *cures* effected *by*) the use of infinitesimally small doses of medicines, as in what is called homoeopathic practice. According to the principles which I have demonstrated, there are a number of individuals who may be benefited and cured by whatever means their minds can be confidently and persistently concentrated on and engrossed with, so as to excite a lively expectant idea as regards a particular result. Besides changing the physical action directly, it also does so indirectly, by changing the current of thought, and withdrawing it from the unhappy train in which it was wont to flow. This latter effect alone does much to benefit the patient, by leaving nature free and unfettered, to carry out the salutary purposes of the "*vis medicatrix naturae*". ["The healing power of nature", i.e., the body's ability to heal *itself*.] This, together with good nursing and suitable regimen, are adequate to effect many recoveries and cures without the aid of a single particle of medicine.

The infinitely small doses of medicine, therefore, may benefit the patient, not by their physical or chemical qualities, but as sensible signs involuntarily to change or fix the current of thought, and thus to modify physical action [i.e., as placebo pills]. But, that the billionth, quintillionth or decillionth of a grain, or drop of any substance in nature, could, on *physical or chemical principles only*, do either good or harm to any human being, is what I do not believe; and I only feel surprised that any rational person can believe what, to me, appears to be such a palpable absurdity. It is just like the Lama amongst the Tartars, who, when short of the required medicine, writes its name on a piece of paper, and rolls it up in small pills, and desires the patients to swallow them, under the conviction that to swallow the *name* has the same efficacy as to swallow the medicine itself. Dr. Simpson's calculations in his work, clearly prove the exiguity of homoeopathic doses, when he demonstrates, that for any person taking billionths of a grain *every second of time*, night and day, would require to go on at this rate, without intermission, for *thirty thousand years*, before he consumed *one* grain of a substance which might be taken by any adult man or woman, at least in a full grain dose, and some of them in fifty grain doses, with perfect impunity. But, if you go to quintillionths, it would require a mass of sugar equal to *sixty-one globes the size of the earth to compound a single grain of said drugs!*

I am aware that some of the practitioners of homoeopathy contend that *dose* is *nothing*, but the proper selection of the medicine *everything*. Now to this dogma I cannot assent for two reasons – first, it is at variance with reason and common sense; second, it is at variance with fact and experience, when I have brought it to the test of experiment and observation. [Braid means that homeopathy is subject to both *a priori* (logical) and *a posteriori* (experimental) criticism.] Thus, I have never seen indubitable effects produced from such medicines, when administered by some of its most noted professors, in infinitely small doses; nothing beyond what might be anticipated from the expectant idea, or an accidental coincidence [i.e., spontaneous remission] occasionally. Moreover, I have prescribed half-drop doses, every half hour, of the tincture of aconite [a herbal sedative used in orthodox Victorian medicine, but also used by homeopaths in minute doses] in delirium with cerebral congestion, with the most marked benefit, but, on diminishing the dose on the subsidence of the symptoms, the delirium returned, and was again relieved, and finally cured, by increasing the dose, and persisting with these *increased doses a little longer*. No sophistry can gainsay such an obvious fact as this displays, that *much* depends on the *amount of dose given*, as well as on the adaptation of the medicine to the case.

Here is another good illustration of the same fact. In the case of a child about two years and a half old, *after other means had failed*, I had *prescribed* arsenic, for a troublesome eruption over most of his body. I gave half a drop of Fowler's solution [an arsenic solution used for skin conditions] for a dose twice a day, and still very little amendment followed. Another member of the family having occasion to take a mixture with the same arsenical preparation, the little fellow got hold of that bottle by accident, and swallowed so much as must have contained at least four or five drops, in one day, not only without inconvenience, but with most decided advantage, for there was an immediate and marked improvement of the eruption on the child from that day forward.

[The "Placebo" Power of Dominant Ideas]

With such evidences as these cases afford of the power of a dominant expectant idea in changing or modifying physical action, either in the second-conscious [or "full"] hypnotic state, or in some subjects in the waking condition, there seems to be no reasonable ground to doubt the fact, and therefore it would only be a work of supererogation to occupy space with the record of additional cases, which I could easily cite from my own experience were it necessary. Nor do I consider it at all proper, considering the great length to which this essay has already extended, to quote cases already recorded by others, where grave diseases have suddenly cured by powerful mental impressions, or where grave diseases have been suddenly induced, or even death itself, by sudden and intense mental impressions, either of joy or sorrow. These all can read at their leisure. **I must not, however, omit to call attention to the cures effected by spells, charms, and amulets, sacred relics, and by various nostrums [quack remedies], as all these furnish powerful corroboration of the main position I am here contending for.** The cures effected at the grave of the Abbé Paris, at St Medard in Paris, in like manner afford clear proof of the influence of mental and moral causes in changing physical action according to the expectant idea in the mind of the patient at the time. Surely few will believe that these cures were effected by the transmission of the "exuberant life of the healthy, to repair and sustain the deficient vitality of the weak" (which would be the notion according to the Mesmeric theory of Mr. Newnham), for how could exuberant LIFE of the *healthy* have come out of the ashes of the dead saint, so as to have produced these cures? The moral influence of a lively faith, hope, and confidence, however, in the efficacy of a visit to the grave of this notable personage, were quite competent to produce such results, on the principles which I have endeavoured to expound.

[Physical Effects of Hypnosis Beyond Suggestion]

Whilst the expectant idea modifying or changing physical action is undoubtedly an important agent in most cases of hypnotic treatment, still it is not the *only* cause by which such cures are effected; as the altered condition of the circulation of the blood, and the quality of that fluid during the cataleptic or reverse condition of the body, as formerly explained, makes a powerful impression on the brain and spinal cord, and ganglionic system of nerves, as also on the heart's action, and must thus produce an alterative effect on the whole system, independently of any fixed idea or special train of thought in the patient's mind.

In proof of the above statement, I could readily adduce cases in which no benefit had accrued to the patients when hypnotised with the *one* state of the circulation, and yet so soon as I threw them into the sleep, and acted on them in all respects as previously, *excepting as regarded the condition of the circulation during the sleep*, they were not only speedily benefited, but entirely cured.

The nervous sleep seems to act powerfully on the nervous and capillary systems, and in an extraordinary degree as regards the function of the skin, **perspiration being generally excited**, even in a few minutes, in cases which had resisted every other mode of treatment resorted to for that purpose. **This was strikingly verified in my own case when, in September 1844, I threw myself into the condition for a severe rheumatic attack, which had resisted other means. I sat down, suffering the utmost anguish, being unable to move my head, to lift my arm, or to draw a full breath, from the stabbing** pain accompanying the slightest motion. In *nine minutes*, I was aroused *quite free from pain*, and *literally bathed in perspiration*. I could then move my head and arm in any direction, and draw a full breath without the slightest pain; I slept comfortably all the following night, and next morning I was a little stiff, but had no pain. A week thereafter I had a slight return, which was removed by another operation, and I have had no return of it since, now upwards of eight years. Three severe cases of scarlet fever treated in this manner also proved the wonderful power of hypnotism in producing perspiration, and diminishing the velocity of the circulation. In ten minutes, all three patients were bathed in perspiration, the frequency of the pulse was much diminished, their headaches were gone, and in fact a crisis had been induced, so as to have converted a violent disease into a mild and moderate affection.

For the mode of producing sleep at will, I must refer to my late work, entitled "Magic, Witchcraft, Animal Magnetism, Hypnotism, and Electro-Biology" [1852].

["Hydro-Hypnotism" for Inducing Sleep]

The following method of producing and prolonging *sleep at will* – which may be designated hydro-hypnotism – is adopted by the peasantry residing among the Himalaya Mountains. An aged female is generally appointed to watch a number of infants whilst their mothers are engaged out of doors in agricultural labours. The infants are wrapped up like little mummies, laid on their backs arranged in a semicircle, and from a number of small spouts, a little of water is made to fall upon and flow over the head of each infant. The natives believe that this process strengthens the children, and makes them hardy. However this may be, it appears to be a most effectual method of sending them into a state of sleep and quietude, for, at page 272 of *Lloyd and Gerard's Travels*, they state, as eye-witness of the fact, frequently seen by them, "The most refractory imp, when tied up, let it yell never so loud, will, when the stream has for a few seconds bathed its head, fall into a most noiseless slumber."

[Concluding Remarks]

The length to which this essay has already extended in developing my views as to *general principles*, precludes the opportunity of giving more cases in detail. Nor is this particularly called for, after the numerous cases already published by me of the success of this mode of treatment of a variety of diseases which resisted ordinary treatment.

It is but proper, however, that I should here explain, that although most of the cases which I have published in this article, and in my other publications, were purposely selected from those which were so *speedily* benefited under the *hypnotic* treatment, as to leave no room to doubt that the treatment and cure stood in the relation to each other of cause and effect, still there have been many other cases which required a *protracted* course of hypnotism, and were at last relieved or cured by it, notwithstanding they had been quite intractable to much longer courses of other and more usual modes of treatment.

In conclusion, I beg leave to remark, that I have advanced nothing as fact which has not been verified in my own practice, by experiments frequently repeated, and with the utmost care, so as to satisfy myself and many scientific friends of the reality of the effects and phenomena; and I feel assured that the same amount of evidence must carry conviction to the mind of every honest and candid enquirer, as to the reality of the phenomena, whatever mode of explanation he might prefer as to the cause of their production. Of the correctness of the main position of my theory I am satisfied, but I am too well aware of the intricacy of the inquiry, involving as it does **the philosophy of *mind as well as of matter*, and their reciprocal action upon each other**, to imagine that I have succeeded in disclosing *all* which can be learned of their capabilities and powers in relation to each other. I trust that I may be able to prosecute my own investigations with increasing effect and increasing knowledge; and my ardent desire is that other minds may be brought to co-operate with me in **a research which is full, indeed, of novelty in its details, but which deals with principles and powers in themselves long recognised; and which, I trust, I have here shown as acting according to known laws, even in the condition of *nervous sleep*.**

I beg farther to remark, if my theory and pretensions, as to the nature, cause, and extent of **the phenomena of nervous sleep, have none of the fascinations of the transcendental to captivate the lovers of the marvellous, the credulous and enthusiastic, which the pretensions and alleged occult agency of the Mesmerists have, still I hope my views will not be the less acceptable to honest and sober-minded men, because they are all level to our comprehension, and reconcilable with well-known physiological and psychological principles.**

What I wish is to court inquiry, and to offer every facility in my power to aid candid inquiry into a department of science which is interesting in *many* respects, and which, when properly conducted, I feel convinced may be rendered, in some forms of disease, one of the greatest boons to the cause of suffering humanity.

Burlington House,
Oxford Street,
Manchester.
June 1853.

Appendix

In the course of last spring [1852] I sent, by desire of the members, an elaborate "Essay on Hypnotic and Mesmeric Phenomena", to be read and discussed at the Edinburgh Royal Medical Society. In that Essay my views were set forth briefly, on *every* brand of the subject, including the *modus operandi* of hypnotism in the relief and cure of disease, illustrated by most of the cases published in this article. The Society devoted three nights to the reading and discussion of my Essay, when many of the extraordinary, as well as the ordinary, members attended, and took part in the debate. Immediately after the last night's discussion, Professor Gregory, who had attended and taken part in the debate on the two last evenings, was so kind as to write me a very long letter, from which I make the following extracts:–

> Your paper, which is an excellent one, was very well received. My colleagues, Drs. Balfour and Bennett, were also present last night. What struck me most in the whole matter was that these gentlemen, and most of those who spoke, not only admitted all your facts, but adopted your theoretical views; and, what is more, were anxious to show that they must necessarily embrace the whole subject of Mesmerism, which you know is not my opinion. Now, when I remember what was the state of the profession only three years ago, nay, what it still is in the majority, I cannot but perceive a most manifest and remarkable progress. Dr. Bennett candidly admitted that it was the Mesmerists (including you of course) who had forced these most important facts on the profession. Of course the facts I mean are, the production of the nervous sleep, or the state of somnambulism, by artificial means, which is still denied by many, and was, very lately, denied by all; and the extraordinary or incredible effects of suggestion on persons in that state, or indeed sometimes on such as are only half in it, and occasionally on persons in the ordinary state; in short, all the phenomena so absurdly called biological, as well as all the suggestive phenomena occurring in the Mesmeric or somnambulistic state or sleep. Now, I not only admit all the facts recorded in your Essay, but I have always done so.

My learned friend then goes into a long disquisition, to convince me that clairvoyance, and the other higher phenomena of the Mesmerists, are equally true as those which I believe in and assert are producible by my usual hypnotic processes. As I do not claim any such high pretensions as attributes of *hypnotism*, once for all I beg to state, that I leave the Mesmerists in undisputed sovereignty in this higher department of the science. At the conclusion of his very long and interesting letter, Professor Gregory winds up thus:-

> Although I cannot adopt all your views, yet I agree with all you have stated, both as the subjective action and suggestion, only bearing in mind that these do not exhaust the subject. I regard your Essay as a very valuable one, more especially in a practical point of view, and my chief objection is to the summary opinions expressed, without proof, on the disputed points.

In the Essay submitted to the Royal Medical Society, I entered very fully into the consideration of the influence of dominant ideas in the minds of parties in exciting or depressing function in accordance with the purport of these ideas, whether originating spontaneously, or from previous associations, or from the direct suggestions of a second party. This led me to advert to Dr. Carpenter's term, ideo-motor, used by him to signify unconscious muscular motion from an idea, in contradistinction to voluntary motion. I then said that term was admirably well chosen for characterising the single phenomenon which he was describing, but that, inasmuch as a dominant idea might *arrest* as well as *excite* muscular motion and other functions, it was highly desirable to adopt some terms which might characterise the *whole* range of phenomena which might arise from dominant ideas in the minds of individuals. I have now come to the conclusion that the following would be most appropriate for the purpose:–

> 1st To *ideize*, would be to induce the state of abstraction or mental concentration favourable for manifesting the power of suggestion, and of predominant ideas.[49]

> 2nd *Ideized* would indicate the state of condition of the person when so impressed.

> 3rd *Ideo-dynamic*, or ideational phenomena, would indicate the character and intensity of the phenomena to be anticipated, according to the all-absorbing idea with which the mind of the subject was occupied, coupled with the known temperament and susceptibility of the subject.

It must be obvious that these terms would comprehend every conceivable variety of phenomenon, according to the function of the part on which the dominant idea of the subject was concentrated, and the liveliness of his faith. Thus, let the mind of the person be engrossed with the notion, that he is to be irresistibly drawn, repelled, or paralysed, or catalepsed, and the ideo-dynamic or ideational condition of the muscles corresponding to this idea will take place, without any conscious volition of the subject to that effect. It is this

---

[49] Causing individuals to look for a considerable length of time, with fixed attention, at any unexciting inanimate object, is generally the most speedy and certain mode of inducing this condition.

very ideational or unconscious muscular action which is the cause of "table-moving", which has lately so much astonished and excited the public. The experimenters perceive the fact that the table moves; but not being conscious of putting out any voluntary effort, they imagine that the table is drawing them, whilst all the while their own muscles are imparting the requisite impulse to the table, although they are unconscious that they are doing so. This theory of "table-moving" I published anonymously on the 30th of April last, in the *Manchester Examiner and Times*, from which I make the following extract:–

> This unconscious muscular influence from dominant ideas in the minds of subjects, Dr. Carpenter, Sir Henry Holland, and Mr. Braid, all bring to bear upon and explain the phenomena of the gyrations of the *odometer* of Dr. Mayo, the *magnetometer* of Mr. Rutter, and the *divining rod*; and we know that Mr. Braid attributes the supposed levity [i.e. levitation] of a human body, in an experiment described by Sir David Brewster, *as well as these furniture movements, to the same cause, viz.*, the extraordinary influence of dominant ideas in the minds of some individuals, in producing muscular action in accordance with those ideas, without any conscious effort of volition on the part of said subjects. It therefore becomes a complete illusion as regards the parties so experimenting, as is seen in [electro-]*biologised* subjects; and others witnessing the experiments become so engrossed by watching and anticipating the movements, as to overlook their real exciting cause.

In this paragraph, I referred to Dr. Carpenter's lectures at the Manchester Royal Institution, so recently reported in the Manchester newspapers, where I said, "The key to the solution of this mystery may be found." By this mode of expression, I did not mean to intimate that Dr. Carpenter had made any special or direct reference to "table-moving", either in these lectures, or in that at the London Institution, which was reported in the *Athenaeum* for the 12th March 1852, for I well knew that his observations in *both* institutions had reference to the ideo-motor, or unconscious muscular action as the cause of certain *biological* phenomena, and of the movements of Dr. Mayo's odometer, of Mr. Rutter's magnetoscope, of the diving rod, and of rings and other objects suspended from the points of the fingers, which he very graphically designated "the swing-swangs", all of which results he (Dr. Carpenter) viewed as coming under the same category. Still, although Dr. Carpenter did not refer to "table-moving", that was so much akin to the others, and the Doctor's ideas and my own coincided so entirely on the nature and cause of ideo-motor or unconscious muscular action, and the influence of dominant or expectant ideas in modifying physical action, that I felt assured if ever he brought his acute mind to investigate the phenomena of "table-moving", he would be certain to arrive at the same conclusion as I had done and I know he has since done so. Indeed, it is now some five or six years since I published a letter in the *Manchester Courier*, making a *similar* application of this, to me, familiar physiological principle, to explain the feats of a French peasant girl, who was then astonishing the Parisians by her feats of table and chair moving, and by even moving a heavy trunk with a strong man seated on each side of her. This was alleged to be produced by some extraordinary development of electrical agency in the girl, but, after my unconscious muscular action theory, from some predominant idea or delusion in the girl's mind, was published, the affair was speedily seen in this light, and the girl's marvellous feats were no more heard of. If there is any little merit, therefore, attaching to priority in promulgating this unconscious muscular force theory of furniture moving, by persons in a physical contact with such objects, I would have an undoubted right to claim it as due to myself.

Since my paragraph of the 30th April last was published, I expressed the same opinions at a public conversazione on table-moving at the Manchester Athenaeum, on the 2nd of June last, which was extensively reported in the newspapers, and I have also published several letters since, supporting the same views, as also cautioning the public against the dangers of trying such experiments too frequently. In one of these letters I said:–

> In addition to what I advanced in the Athenaeum, I beg to state that, inasmuch as my experience of the influence of dominant ideas being sufficient to produce corresponding muscular action unconsciously, involuntarily, or in some cases even in *opposition* to the will of the subject (that is, according to the predominant idea in the patient's mind at the time); *a fortiori*, when the *will and lively faith go along with the dominant idea*, the effect should be still more potent and efficient for accomplishing the expected result. In short; the only difficulty is to believe that, under these circumstances, the motor muscular impulse is *entirely* involuntary, for to *will* the table to move from some impulse of a mysterious nature streaming from our finger-points, held in contact with the body to be moved, and to will the voluntary muscles, at the same time, to be still and inoperative, seems to be contradiction in terms. **I believe the more strictly accurate mode of expressing the matter will be this – and the whole of this paragraph was written ten days ago for a different purpose – that the ideo-motor principle *might* be adequate to effect the result *without* volition, or even in *opposition* to volition, provided the dominant idea was sufficiently vivid; but in these cases of table-moving, when honestly conducted, the ideational motor impulse is supplemented by *volition, so slightly exerted as to be unconscious to the persons so exercising it*; their attention and will being, as they suppose, entirely concentrated on the table, instead of on impinging the nervous force into the muscles, the action of which is required for producing the motion. The illusion, therefore, becomes complete, the force being partly ideational and partly voluntary, but partaking so slightly of the latter quality as not to be cognizant to the subjects engaged in the said experiments.** I have been led to this conclusion regarding the true cause of these phenomena, from observing that someone of the party always announced, in audible language, the direction in which they were to *will* the table to move, and in every case

which I observed closely, the tables took the direction indicated. As to the *tendencies* of such experiments, if frequently repeated, it is quite obvious to me that it is not so harmless an amusement as many may suppose. It has a direct tendency to destroy the mental power of discriminating between ideo-motor or unconscious movements and voluntary motion, and to weaken the controlling power of the brain and will over the reflex or automatic muscular apparatus, and thus will be engendered a tendency to spasmodic or convulsive diseases, such as St Vitus' dance, hysteria, epilepsy, and catalepsy.

I also directed attention to the mischievous influence of excited imagination, sympathy, and imitation, as manifested during the dancing mania of the middle ages, the *convulsionnaires* in France, and the violent spasmodic disease from religious excitement, which seized 4,000 people within a very short time in the south and west of England and Wales, and also in America; and **I would also beg to remind my readers, that, in America, nearly two hundred individuals have been sent to lunatic asylums, and a number of suicides have taken place, as the result of this spirit-rapping and table-turning mania.**

A valuable report from four most intelligent medical gentlemen, advocating the same views, appeared in *The Medical Times and Gazette* three weeks ago, and a letter from Professor [Michael] Faraday, on the same side of the question, appeared in last Thursday's London *Times*. I consider the report of these gentlemen, and Professor Faraday's experiments in particular, as most satisfactory and conclusive on the point which I have always contended for, namely, that the movements were entirely due to unconscious muscular force; and I doubt not this view of the subject will very soon be the generally accepted mode of accounting for these phenomena – although there may always be some who will cling to the mystical and transcendental view, as it is the natural tendency of a certain class of minds to feast on the marvellous and mysterious, and to reject all common sense views of most subjects.

I observe that *The Zoist* for this month contains three articles on the subject of "table-moving", and "spirit-rappers", one from the pen of the Rev. George Sandby, vicar of Fixton, Suffolk, another from the Rev. C. Hare Townshend, and the third, entitled "The Departed Spirits", by Dr. Elliotson – three gentlemen of very great talents and attainments, all thorough going Mesmerists, and, as a matter of course, decidedly opposed to my "unconscious muscular action theory". Notwithstanding such a powerful phalanx is opposed of candour, and with an honest desire to arrive at truth. As I have the greatest possible dislike to be misrepresented, or to misrepresent anyone, by garbled quotations, I shall cite a few passages from these gentlemen so fully as shall fairly exhibit their opinions in their own words. At page 178, Mr. Sandby says, "With pure and simple Mesmerism in its primary action, there can be no question that this discovery (table-moving) is closely allied, if it be not, as I believe, one and the same thing."

> I have always contended for and believed in that theory which Mesmer originally promulgated, *viz.*, that some external agent, analogous to a fluid, or perhaps to the sparks that proceed from an electrical machine, does proceed in the act of Mesmerising from one human being to another. This invisible, imponderable agent, I have seen many reasons to regard as being of a quasi electrical character, if I might not even call it an actual electrical manifestation under the modification of physiological action. Dr. Scoresby's scientific investigations on this point have added greatly to our arguments in favour of this view. Reichenbach's elaborate researches confirm the notion. [...] We Mesmerise water, metals, leather, and paper, as we learn from the effects produced upon our patients; and this action of the tables, induced by continued contact with a chain of human fingers, is nothing but simple Mesmerism developing itself in an unexpected phase. – P. 179.

> And the value of this discovery is considerable. We cannot, indeed, say whether it will lead to any ulterior facts, or be useful in promoting more extended information in science; but it adds an important, it might be said conclusive, amount of evidence towards the establishment of Mesmerism as a physical truth. The theory of imagination will not hold good with wooden matter. – P. 179.

Now, with all due respect for the Rev. Mr. Sandby's talents and worth, I am bound to say that all my experience, which has been considerable, and all my convictions, are opposed to what he has here advanced. I beg respectfully to remind the reverend gentleman that whilst *imagination* and other mental faculties could not be supposed to influence the "wooden matter", for Mr. Sandby has more good sense than to refer the movements to the operation of a *spirit* in the table, still, imagination and the expectant idea *might* influence, and I maintain that they *do* influence the blood, and nerves, and muscles, which compose the *other* part of the apparatus, for, let it be observed, it is a *compound* apparatus, consisting of *human bodies and "wooden matter" combined*. Until Mr. Sandby and other opponents of the "unconscious muscular action theory" of these movements, therefore, shall succeed in producing incontestable evidence that they can effect these movements of inanimate matter by the force of their *will alone*, when all possibility of muscular action, either conscious or unconscious, is entirely excluded, they have no satisfactory proof to adduce in opposition to the evidence which the experiments of myself and others has furnished, that it is quite possible that such movements may be effected through unconscious muscular action, when the hands of fingers of the experimenters are brought into contact with the inanimate matter to be set in motion. The onus of such proof, therefore, necessarily devolves upon these gentlemen.

At page 181, first paragraph, Mr. Sandby seems to have overlooked the almost incredible rapidity with which unconscious muscular contraction, and even catalepsy, may take place in some subjects, from very slight exciting causes. Again, in the next paragraph, Mr. S. alleges that it is impossible that the grave and scientific narrators of certain experiments could have been mistaken in what occurred when the table was in *rapid motion*; but I am quite of a different opinion, for I believe that this was the very time of all others when they were *most likely to be deceived*, and rendered incompetent to distinguish what amount of momentum had previously been imparted to it *unconsciously*, and which might then be enabling it to move on for some time by its acquired momentum.

Again, at page 183, the reverend gentleman says, "The efficient cause of these marvellous phenomena is *nothing but electricity*; and the rotator movements of the tables towards the north, and towards the south, are brought about in accordance with the well-known laws which [Hans] Oerstedt and Faraday have established." It is certainly most unfortunate for this theory, and most fortunate for mine, that Professor Faraday published a letter in the London *Times* on the very day before the publication of the last number of *The Zoist*, containing these views by Mr. Sandby, in which this profound and most acute philosopher (Faraday) repudiates *all* causes of "table-moving", *but* the *unconscious* muscular force one. Indeed Faraday not only repudiates *all other* causes, but he also clearly demonstrates the fact by a number of ingeniously contrived and conclusive experiments. He particularly repudiates the notion of *electricity* or *magnetism* having anything to do in the matter; and we have no higher authority than Faraday to refer to on these matters. Moreover, Faraday invented a simple apparatus, by which he had been enabled so thoroughly to convince the experimenters of the source of fallacy, in supposing it anything else than their own muscular force which moved the tables, that the effects ceased so soon as thy steadily directed their vision to his tell-tale index.

The Rev. Mr. Townshend does not attribute table-moving to *electricity*, but he attributes it rather to the "Mesmeric medium" and he believes that this can be accumulated in the "*wooden matter*", for he says, at page 189, "When *once* the table has been affected, it seems much more easy to do it again, and once more he says, "I do really infer the action of a fluid from all this, and a certain accumulation of fluid (or vibratory action of a fluid, or medium)." Again,

> We know that the muscles are only moved by the nerves, and by nerve-galvanism. Now this last power may possibly be continued on, out of the mere animal frame, so as to constitute in itself a motive agency. And this will not seem wonderful to a Mesmerist, who so often projects a force beyond his own body. Mind, I only say all this problematically, and as a seeker after truth.

Dr. Elliotson sends the rapping spirits to flight with hearty good will. He admits that many cases of "table-turning" may be the result of "unconscious muscular action" but he inclines to agree with the two reverend gentlemen, whose papers have been referred to as preceding his, in believing that there are other cases which are independent of muscular action. Thus, at page 193, Dr. Elliotson says, "But may not such movements frequently result from other causes – from an occult agency?" Again, "The table always slid away from their fingers and mine, so slightly did we all touch it. It moved faster than the fingers of any of us, and got in advance of us."

Here, then, we have got all these three distinguished gentlemen agreed that the tables *may* be moved *independently of the muscular force, either conscious* or *unconscious*, of *the "table-turners"* and they are all agreed, moreover, that it is their old friend the *magnetic* or *Mesmeric medium*, which is the efficient agent that sets the inanimate matter in motion, and keeps it in motion independently of the muscular action of the experimenters. Table-moving is, therefore, deemed a most satisfactory proof of the existence of a Mesmeric medium or independent imponderable physical force, which can be directed and controlled by the human *will*, so as to produce various effects, and amongst others, this movement of inanimate matter, irrespective of the physical agency of the human muscles. According to Mr. Sandby, it "adds an important, it might be said a conclusive, amount of evidence towards the establishment of Mesmerism as a physical truth".

Moreover, a small book on table-moving was lately published by a London "physician", in which he states that, according to his computation, the average physical force exerted on a table by each "table-mover" is *five ounces*. Well, according to physical laws, this force may be exerted as well and effectively in *lifting perpendicularly*, as in drawing or shoving inanimate matter. We are therefore now in the position to propose the *experimentum crucis* to these gentlemen. Let five, or ten, or twenty, ascertained efficient table-movers stand or sit round a table, and exert the force of their *will* to raise a *single ounce* of lead, copper, wood, or marble, from the centre of the table, and hold it suspended in the air for a single minute, say twelve inches above the table, when no human hand is in contact with it, and no trickery or mechanical contrivance has been applied to effect such result, and I will admit that my theory has failed, and that a greater marvel has been presented before me than turning a table on castors weighing a ton, *when a number of human hands are held in contact with said table*. This test I proposed in my first letter, bearing date 15th June last; and I find that Professor Faraday has since proposed the *lifting* experiment, but that he has met with no one who could succeed in doing so. Now, I beg leave to remind the Mesmerists that, according to their own belief, they *ought to be able to do so*, for they allege that they can *project* the Mesmeric medium from their bodies, and direct its impingement by the force of their *will*, so as to make it act at prodigious distances, producing immediate effects. Thus, Dr. Ashburner has stated, in his notes to Reichenbach's translation, that he can do so to the distance of *seventy miles*, producing immediate effects; and, that, in this manner, he can telegraph messages to the distance of two miles, without any conducting medium other than his Mesmeric or odylic medium, or influence, emanating from his brain and set in motion by the force of *his will*. At page 32, Dr. Ashburner says he has come to the conclusion that "a force which is a material agent, attended by or constituting a coloured light emanates from the brain of man when he thinks – that his will can direct its impingement – and that it is a motive power". Nay, more, this gentleman avers that he can make this force *visible* to the eyesight of some individuals, so that they shall perceive it as a rope passing from his eyes to their heads, and *irresistibly drawing them towards him*, when he is engaged in exerting his will to that effect. There ought, therefore, according to Mesmeric notions, to be no insuperable difficulty to parties, standing or sitting round a table, being able to project their Mesmeric force to the centre of the table, so as to *lift a single ounce* weight, and suspend it in the air as I have proposed; but, I will dare to predict that, whenever they venture on such an experiment, the full force of the will of a score of the most obstinate and energetic of them will be proved inadequate to lift *a single farthing*. Or they may try to lift a penny or a sovereign at the end of a stick, or of a wheel made of a light hoop, with cross bars, and a central shaft, at right angles, placed upright, the lower end of the shaft resting on the object to be lifted at the lower end of the shaft by the force of their will, exerted to lift it instead of to turn the wheel. Or let two people, instead of turning a hat, lay hold of a wooden pencil or pen-holder, and lift a shilling at the lower end of either of them whilst they are held perpendicularly, which will be equally satisfactory, if they succeed, in supporting their theory of a special occult influence or force, and opposed to my unconscious muscular force theory. But, if they still wish to cling to the horizontal motion, then they may try the following plan:– Let them sit or stand round a table, but a few inches distant from it, and let them be provided with a number of leather straps or cords, the one end of which shall extend from the opposite hands of each couple of experimenters, and be allowed to lie loosely on the top of the table. In such cases, there would be the same facility of conducting the alleged *Mesmeric medium* to the table from the persons operating, as when the hands are in contact with it; but all chance of fallacy, from unconscious muscular action, would be effectually removed, so that, if the table really moves, it cannot be by muscular force, when the bond of communication between the muscles of the experimenter and the table is merely lying loose upon the table. My experiment at the *Athenaeum* conversazione with the circle of brass wire, held by five ladies at a short distance from the table, with a prolongation of the wire extending from each hand of the ladies to the table, where a coil was made so that it might rest loosely on the table, fulfilled this indication, as well as proved to others what was evident to myself before I proposed it – the fallacy of supposing the movement dependent on an accumulation of electricity in the table, whilst it was in direct communication with the earth. The ladies continued their task for half-an-hour without any movement of the table, although I observed the right hand of one of them advance two or three times to the extent of six inches in the direction the table was willed to move. When the wire was removed, and the hands applied, so that unconscious muscular force could again come into play, the table very soon moved as briskly as at first trials.

These experiments, with a repetition of Faraday's most unexceptionable and conclusive physical tests, ought to be quite adequate to determine such a question as this, and I feel very confident that the result will be in support of my theory of the nature and cause of such phenomena, *viz*.,

> [...] the extraordinary influence of dominant expectant ideas in the minds of some individuals, in producing muscular action in accordance with those ideas, without any conscious effort of volition on the part of said subjects. It therefore becomes a complete illusion as regards the parties so experimenting, as is seen in *biologised* subjects; and others witnessing the experiments become so engrossed by watching and anticipating the movements, as to overlook their real exciting cause.

I beg leave, therefore, to remark, that inasmuch as my own experience, as well as that of others, has proved that such movements of inanimate matter may take place from the unconscious muscular action of parties laying their hands in contact with the objects moved, *without* their alleged new force, the onus necessarily lies with our opponents to prove that they can veritably produce such physical movements of inanimate matter by the force of their *will alone*, when all possibility of such unconscious muscular action, as we allege is the cause of the movements, has been entirely excluded. Let these gentlemen, therefore, prove the sincerity of their belief in the principles which they avow, by trying the crucial experiments which I have suggested, and let them publish the results in an early number of *The Zoist*. There can be no satisfactory mode of determining such controversy but by such a course as this, *viz*., by repeating experiments under the guidance of the corrective suggestions, which may be conveyed to us by comparing the different points of view in which phenomena present themselves to different minds.

As to table gesticulations, table-talking, or spirit-rapping, keep all hands off, and all mechanical contrivances for moving the table away from it; and then, when the table replies by lifting one leg and giving the required number of raps on the floor with said leg, the time may have arrived when it may be worth our while to speculate about the cause of such a mysterious phenomenon, but certainly not until then. There can be no reason to doubt that unconscious muscular action, according to dominant ideas in the minds of patients, may be adequate to effect some of these phenomena, as certainly as they produce rotator movements of such inanimate matter; for, considerable pressure on one side of a table, of suitable construction, would no doubt cause the table to incline in that direction, and thus to do its manners or to elevate one leg from the floor and bump upon it alternately, according to the ideas in the minds of the experimentalists; but to those who deny this, and will still insist, on touching the tables during such experiments, I think we might with some degree of propriety apply the remark, "the pleasure is as great in being cheated as to cheat" for assuredly I can only consider they are persisting in a course of experiments calculated to deceive themselves, as well as others who are not alive to the source of fallacy which I have pointed out.

The influence of expectant ideas in the mind of persons pointing to the letters of the alphabet, in varying the action when they arrive at the letter which they allege may be the one to be indicated, and the change on the expression of the features of unwary subjects when doing this, and in the tones of their voice when calling letters, may all very readily enable the "medium" to make happy guesses as Mr. Lewis has suggested – just as ordinary fortune tellers have long been well aware of, and profited by. Indeed this phenomenon of physical manifestations, in accordance with mental emotions and dominant ideas in the minds of subjects, is so familiar, and is acted on so largely every day by consul, judge, and jury, when sifting evidence in our courts of law, that the great marvel is, that so many respectable and intelligent people in all ordinary matters, should have suffered themselves to be so much duped by such a transparent trick as these spirit-rapping mediums have palmed upon them as supernatural gifts. But let a screen be interposed between the medium and tester, so as effectually to prevent the former from seeing the features of the latter, or his modes of pointing at the card, and let the letters be pointed at irregularly as regards their alphabetical arrangement; and if there is only one medium in the room, I suspect the fallacy of such pretensions will soon become apparent, provided the tester is careful neither to lead nor to mislead the "medium".

But there is still another important consideration and objection to be urged against these spirit-rapping experiments, *viz*., that they must necessarily have a direct tendency to engender in the minds of the experimenters the grossest superstition. To bring one's self to believe that a table, or any other piece of inanimate matter, is possessed by a spirit of divination, which can reveal secrets to the credulous inquirer or worshipper at said shrine, is quite as bad, in the midst of Christian and civilised society, as the ignorant and benighted idolaters of heathen lands, whose folly we deplore in cutting down a tree, one part of which they burn, and another of which they make a graven image, and fall down and worship as a god, possessed of the power not only of revealing all knowledge to them, but also of succouring and supporting them under every trial, difficulty, and danger. Is this what we are to come to in Great Britain, in this year of grace 1853? God forbid! But such, I apprehend, is the obvious tendency of such practices, if they are zealously persisted in.

James Braid.
Burlington House, Oxford Street.
Manchester, 2nd July 1853.

"Psycho-Physiology & the Ideo-Motor Reflex"
(1853)

Editor's Preface
Donald Robertson

Of the many eminent physicians and scientists who endorsed Braid's work, perhaps the most notable is the physiologist Prof. William Benjamin Carpenter (1813-1885) of University College London and the Royal Institution. Carpenter was a highly distinguished academic with a special interest in psychology and neurology. His work can be seen as prefiguring Pavlovian conditioning theory in certain respects, e.g., in the training of children and animals. Carpenter coined the term "ideo-motor response" (or "reflex") to describe the causal effect of ideas upon the musculature of the body, independent of direct volition, referred to as the "reflex actions of the Cerebrum". He was a staunch critic of pseudoscience and used the ideo-motor theory to debunk many examples of popular Victorian spiritualism, e.g., table-turning, levitation, Ouija boards, pendulum dowsing, etc. The observation of the same muscular phenomenon had been made several decades earlier by the French pharmacist, Michel Eugène Chevreul (1833), as Carpenter acknowledges.

> The continued concentration of Attention upon a certain idea gives it a *dominant* power, not only over the mind, but over the body; and the muscles become the involuntary instruments whereby it is carried into operation. [...] But it is the characteristic of the state of mind from which these Ideo-motor actions proceed, that the Volitional power is for the time in abeyance; the whole mental power being absorbed (as it were) in the high state of tension to which the Ideational consciousness has been wrought up. (Carpenter, 1874: 293)

In his book on *Mesmerism, etc.,* (1877) he praises Braid's work for recognising the reality of certain Mesmeric phenomena but adopting a new and more credible 'scientific *rationale*'. Elsewhere writes,

> In fact, the positions taken in regard to Mesmerism by my friend Dr. [Daniel] Noble, as far back as 1845, and more fully developed by myself a few years later on the basis of Mr. Braid's experiments and of my own Physiological and Psychological studies, have, not only in our own judgement, but by the general verdict of the Medical and Scientific world, been fully confirmed by the subsequent course of events [...] (1877: 28)

From at least 1847 onwards, Carpenter and Braid seem to have had sufficient personal contact to exchange ideas in detail, and it is clear that Carpenter had directly observed Braid's work on many occasions and had also experimented with hypnotism himself. In *The Critics Criticised* (1855) Braid is even forced to correct the misapprehension that he and Carpenter had co-authored an article together, that was in fact written solely by Carpenter. This otherwise trivial confusion serves to illustrate the degree to which Carpenter and Braid were perceived as scientific collaborators and allies. In the same booklet, Braid responds thus,

> I cannot feel it otherwise than a great compliment to find that a gentleman of Dr. Carpenter's mark, who had enjoyed many opportunities of investigating along with me my various opinions, and the practical illustrations as the reasons thereof, had so thoroughly set forth my views in the said article as to have led even the clairvoyant carping critics in *The Zoist* to suppose that certain portions of it must have been written by myself [...].

Braid thoroughly assimilated Carpenter's theory of ideo-motor reflex action into his later writings, theory, and terminology. Indeed, Braid's new term for hypnotism, "monoideism", is apparently meant as an extension of Carpenter's terminology. In *The Physiology of Fascination* (1855), Braid therefore states,

> In order that I may do full justice to two esteemed friends, I beg to state, in connection with this term *monoideo-dynamics,* that, several years ago, Dr. W. B. Carpenter introduced the term *ideo-motor* to characterise the reflex or automatic muscular motions which arise merely from ideas associated with motion existing in the mind, without any conscious effort of volition. In 1853, in referring to this term, Dr. [Daniel] Noble said, *"Ideo-dynamic* would probably constitute a phraseology more appropriate, as applicable to a wider range of phenomena." In this opinion I quite concurred, because I was well aware that an idea could *arrest* as well as *excite* motion automatically, not only in the muscles of voluntary motion, but also as regards the condition of *every other function of the body*. I have, therefore, adopted the term *monoideo-dynamics,* as still more comprehensive and characteristic as regards the true mental relations which subsist during all dynamic changes which take place, in every other function of the body, as well as in the muscles of voluntary motion.

To *monoideise* (Braid) is quite simply to enhance the *ideo-motor* response (Carpenter), or more generally the *ideo-dynamic* response (Noble), by focusing the mind unnaturally upon a single idea or train of thought, i.e., through *mono-ideo-dynamic* action as Braid calls it.

It should be noted that Carpenter based the ideo-motor reflex theory upon an everyday ("common sense") observation which 'like many other mental phenomena, has not attracted the notice it merits, simply because it *is* so familiar' (Carpenter, 1874:281). Hence, he illustrates it by reference to everyday examples, such as the fact that we do not think about the individual movements our mouth makes as we speak or the steps we take as we walk down a street, but merely allow ourselves to respond automatically to the intention to act. Our involuntary facial expressions are another familiar example of the power of an idea over the musculature of the body, to the extent, e.g., that we may grimace visibly without even *realising* that we do so, when contemplating the memory of a painful experience.

Analysis of Dr. Carpenter's Lectures on the Physiology of the Nervous System (1853)

> According to both Bramwell's and Kravis' bibliographies of his writings, this newspaper article, from The Medical Times, was *written* by Braid, although his name does not seem to have been attached to the original publication, and the text refers to him in the third person ('Mr. Braid'). The contents are of considerable interest, however, in illustrating the close connection between Braid's observations and Carpenter's theories.

[Introduction]

In our last Saturday's paper we gave a report of the sixth and last lecture of this course at the Royal Institution. However, from the high character of Dr. Carpenter in this walk of science, we have resolved to furnish our readers with a more interesting analysis of the general scope of the inquiry than detailed reports of each lecture separately were likely to convey.

Dr. Carpenter commenced by showing the importance of scientific knowledge of the physiology of the nervous system, in forming our judgment as to what to believe and what to disbelieve of those unusual phenomena to which public attention has of late been attracted, under the names of Mesmerism, hypnotism and electro-biology. He showed that without such knowledge the most extravagant notions might be formed and believed in by otherwise intelligent and trustworthy individuals. He then sketched the nervous system in its relation to the animal body; that its elementary structure consisted of ganglionic centres for generating nerve force, and nerve-trunks for conducting that force. Nerve force was different in kind from electricity and all other forces, although it resembled them (electricity and galvanism in particular) in some respects, and might be excited into activity by them. Its simplest form was that of a single ganglion with afferent and motor fibres – i.e. to carry impressions to the ganglion and motor impulses, from that to the motor apparatus or muscles, which reflex actions were called excito motor, and occurred independently of sensation. The first stage of complication consisted in a multiplication of similar ganglia, as in the higher radiated and lowest articulated animals. The second complication consisted in the addition of ganglionic centres of dissimilar function, as shown in the higher articulated and *molluscous* animals. In these cases distinct evidences of sensation were presented; so that sensory motor actions were super-added to excito-motor actions, and these together constituted all the varieties of instinctive action, so remarkable in the class of insects. The nervous system of *vertebrated* animals in its lowest grades, presents an essential conformity with the preceding; the spinal axis and sensory ganglia everywhere being its fundamental constituents; and evidence was adduced of their independent operation as excito-motor and sensori-motor action in various kinds of automatic (unconscious) movements, even to man.

Dr. Carpenter next proceeded to the consideration of the nervous system in its relation to mental action. The super-addition of a brain to the other ganglia constituted the communication between consciousness and the external world. The gradual augmentation of the brain in size and increase of its complexity in structure, exhibited in the ascending series of vertebrated animals, seemed to prove its probable instrumentality in the production of ideas, in the production of the emotional states connected with these, and in the performance of intellectual processes based upon them, seeing the hemispherical *ganglia*, as the brain had been called, bore a certain ratio of complexity of structure and increased size, in accordance with the intelligence of the creatures up to man, who stood at the top of the scale, both for development of the brain and intelligence. There was also a gradual subordination of instinct to intelligence, in a ratio corresponding to the higher development of the cerebrum (the brain).

The lecturer then explained the relation of the will to the nervous system; that many of the cerebral actions were of a reflex or automatic character, and that **the influence of suggestion** exercised a prodigious power over many individuals; that emotion and **ideo-motor movements** might take place, proceeding directly from mental states, without any agency of volition, the will being in abeyance at the time. The volitional power was exerted, not by acting directly on the particular muscles required to be called into action to produce specific movements, but through the automatic apparatus, the mind being entirely concentrated on the idea of the result, and the confident expectations of it being realised. The will had an equal controlling power in directing the automatic action of the mind, and in directing and controlling the current of thought, and the vast importance and influence which it thus obtains in the well-disciplined mind, were pointed out and illustrated by the unhappy consequence of deficiency of these qualities in the cases of Coleridge and Mozart. The whole of these states were illustrated by reference to various drawings and diagrams of a very instructive and suggestive character.

[On Sleep & Dreaming]

The state of sleep in a physiological point of view, was that of a period of temporary response to certain portions of the nervous system, during which reparative actions took place, to compensate for the too rapid waste which had taken place in them during the waking state of energy and activity. In perfect and profound sleep, contrary to the opinion of some, he believed that there was no dreaming, the activity of the whole cerebrum, as well as that of the sensory ganglia, being suspended. The activity of the spinal cord was still maintained, however, because without that the functions of respiration and circulation, necessary to the maintenance of life, could not be carried on. This activity through the spinal cord was also maintained during insensibility, such as apoplexy, which was distinguished from sleep by not being refreshing. In the insensibility arising from narcotic poisons, or apoplexy, we found that the torpor extended downwards; first the individual lost the use of his intellectual powers, then he ceased to feel, and finally, when the torpor reached the spinal cord, the vital functions of respiration and circulation were not performed, and he died. He (the lecturer) agreed with Sir Henry Holland in thinking that sleep was not a single state, but rather a series of ever varying conditions or states, from profound sleep to waking vigilance. In falling asleep the will is first lost, or the power of controlling the current of thought, and then by degrees he becomes unconscious. In awaking, the process is reversed, the person first becoming conscious of his existence, and then by degrees recovering the power of his will. Certain forms of somnambulism, more particularly that which had been called **electro-biology**, precisely corresponded with that stage of transition between sleeping and waking in which the power of the will was lost. Sleep may be induced by a variety of modes, and the most powerful influence for its production was that of **monotony, or the recurrence to a certain set of unexciting sensations or ideas in the mind.** These might be either sights or sounds, or the remembrance of past impressions.

Dreaming was a departure from the perfect inactivity of the cerebrum. It was a state characterised by activity of the cerebrum with complete suspension of the will, which was common to all the states he would have occasion to bring under their notice. In dreaming there was no creation, no production of ideas which had not previously been in the mind. Sometimes, though rarely, our trains of thought were coherent in dreams; and when such was the case, there had generally been some idea dominant in the mind before going to sleep. He was satisfied that in dreaming, a long train of thought passed through the mind in an instant, as well-known to have been the case with many people when in instant fear of death, as in drowning, when the whole events of their previous lives have been presented before them in an instant. **The duration of sleep, and the modes by which we may be aroused, may be determined, and in the case of many individuals are determined, entirely by previous and dominant ideas**. It was the habitual impression which determined the effect of any particular sound in producing a recall from sleep to the waking condition and many individuals had the power of determining, to a few minutes, the time at which they would awake. This power could only be accounted for by admitting that the strong impression with which the individual went to sleep determined the changes which took place in his brain during his sleep.

The connecting link between dreaming and insanity was exhibited in delirium, which seemed to depend rather upon the state of the blood, than of that of the brain. The effect of alcohol, opium and hashish, was to increase the activity of the automatic apparatus, and to weaken the controlling power of the will. This weakness of the will was also the condition induced by insanity, the first defect observed in the mind of any person being usually a want of power to control and direct his thoughts. **He then had a tendency to brood over some particular set of odd ideas, which gradually acquired dominion over him; and then a very extraordinary set of aversions often resulted.** The essential distinction between a sane and insane man was that the former had complete power of will, while the latter had no such power. There were many persons counted sane who really possessed little more control over themselves than others who were admitted to be insane. However strange might be a man's ideas, yet if he could compare these with others, so as to exercise a judgment upon them, he could not be accounted insane. Many individuals saw spectral illusions, but they knew they were illusions, and must therefore be accounted sane. But let them lose the power by which they judged them, they then began to believe in them, and must be regarded as no longer responsible or sane.

[On Braid & Hypnotism]
The lecturer now directed attention to the states of **reverie, abstraction, day dreaming, and absence of mind**, all of which he believed the expression of one and the same condition, a condition in which the mind was, in a great degree, **withdrawn from contemplation of external objects, and was attending chiefly and entirely to its own trains of thought, and in which the will did not exercise its power of controlling or directing those trains of thought**. In these states the inlets of sensation were not entirely closed against impressions from external objects, but the mind was very little, or not at all influenced by such impressions. In all these states strange misapprehensions often occurred. Persons made the most singular mistakes and sometimes even forgot their own names, or believed themselves to be different persons. What had been termed electro-biology was, in his opinion, simply a state of **induced reverie or induced abstraction**, and **all its phenomena were, several years before it was brought before the public, shown to him by Mr. Braid**, in the person of a gentleman well-known in this town, and utterly incapable of deception. This gentleman possessed in a marked degree the power of spontaneous abstraction, and when his attention was for a few seconds fixed on any subject so he completely lost the power of voluntary control, that he did anything he was told to do, and his whole mind was for a time possessed with whatever ideas might be communicated to him by another. This was the essential character of this condition, the power of

the will over the current of thought entirely suspended, the sensorium more open to external impressions than it was to ordinary reverie, but otherwise the condition essentially the same, and the mind so **completely possessed by the idea with which it was occupied, that no other could come into collision with it.** The power of the will being entirely suspended, there was nothing whatever to connect the state of consciousness with the ordinary experience, and therefore when the state was complete, the individual was surprised at nothing, his **whole consciousness was entirely given up to the suggestions of another party. A great deal had been said about the will of the subject being completely brought under the domination of the will of the operator. It would be more correct to say that the will of the subject was for the time paralysed. It was not everyone whom in this state could be induced. Experience showed that somewhere in between one in ten and one in twenty [5-10%] could be brought into this condition.** [Braid elsewhere states that 10% of his clients entered the state of double consciousness, accompanied by amnesia, which is presumably the state referred to here.]

When the state had been induced, the subject was told by the operator, in an authoritative tone, that he could not open his eyes, or perform certain muscular movements, and when he endeavoured to do so he found he could not. Now, he believed that the real explanation of this was not that it was an expression of will on the part of the operator which influenced the subject, but that the operator possessed the mind of the subject with the idea that he could not open his eyes, or perform other movements, and that, the will being suspended, the subject was obliged to act in accordance with this idea. The operator frequently went through a variety of other processes which seemed very marvellous but all of which might, he thought, be explained in the same manner. **Sometimes when the state was not completely induced, there was a struggle between the idea suggested to the individual and his sensation. Generally speaking those were most susceptible of this state whom were most prone to involuntary abstraction or reverie, and who had imagination sufficient to place themselves in the position of others. Those who might be induced to believe they were persons whom they really were not were generally those who had most imagination. By the power of imagination our best actors and actresses were enabled to identify themselves with the characters which they represented; and the assumption of character in the electro-biological states was only a similar condition.**

In all respects electro-biology confirmed the conclusions which Mr. Braid arrived at some years ago [*On the Power of the Mind*, 1846], with regard to a curious class of phenomena to which attention had been directed by the researches of Baron Reichenbach who stated that susceptible persons could see flames proceeding from magnets and some other bodies. The fact was, that he (Baron Reichenbach) had fallen in with a number of persons whose minds readily received ideas suggested to them, and by this suggestion he had induced them to believe that they had seen these flames. Mr. Braid soon induced persons to see flames where there was no magnet, but where they believed that there was one. There were individuals upon whom, even in the ordinary waking state, a strong mental impression would produce the same effect as if a real sensation from without had been impressed upon them. **This fact had been previously known, but no one had experimented with so much success and accuracy for determining this as Mr. Braid, as he had clearly proved that excited or arrested motion and power might be regulated and controlled by suggestions, and dominant expectant ideas, both in the waking and somnambulic state; and that the circulation and secretions, as well as sensations, might be changed by these means in many subjects.** Patients frequently applied to him, believing he possessed particular powers in this respect, which he frankly disavowed; but still, through their conviction on this point he (Mr. Braid) was enabled to produce effects which others could not.

Mr. Braid had also clearly proved the sense of smell that came so quickened in some subjects through somnambulism, as enabled them to perform, by its aid, feats which by the Mesmerists were attributed to some more mysterious power, such as detecting individuals known to them by smell only, as also the owners of gloves and other articles. **He (the lecturer) had on one occasion, by way of experiment, picked out one subject from a number of somnambules remarkable for the poverty of his muscular development, and who, on being assured by Mr. Braid that a twenty eight pound weight might be lifted by him with ease, seized it with his little finger, and swung it round his head with perfect ease, whereas, after being awoke, he durst not attempt to lift it with his whole hand for fear of straining himself.** In this state they are entirely controlled by the dominant idea in their minds at the moment. An instance of this was found in the case of a butcher, in Edinburgh, who, while hanging up a piece of meat, having fallen so the hook had caught his coat sleeve, experienced sensations similar to those which would have been produced had his arm been caught by the hook; not only so, his pulse became feeble and he burst into a cold sweat.

[On the Ideo-Motor Reflex]

Analogous to the phenomena which he had mentioned were those in which involuntary movements, such as the will attempted to control, were produced entirely under the influence of ideas. Doctor [Herbert] Mayo had stated that if a button, or ring, or other light body, were suspended from the finger [i.e., by a thread, making a simple pendulum] it would vibrate in a certain direction; but that if a person of the opposite sex took the hand of the person to whose finger the button was suspended it would move in a different direction. **Now it had**

been found that this certainty of motion and the change were entirely the result of the slight motion in the finger of the individual which was caused against his will, by his expecting that the change would take place. Similar results, obtained by Mr. Rutter of Brighton, from an instrument which he called the magnetometer, depended upon the same cause. The phenomena of the [dowsers'] divining rod might be explained in the same manner. The motion of the rod was occasioned by an involuntary motion of the part of the individual holding it, which arose from his thinking that below the particular place over which it was held there was a lode of metal or a stream of water.

If the account given in the preceding lectures of the condition of the mind and of the mode of its operations on the body, in the states of natural and artificial reverie and abstraction, be correct, all the actions being performed in these states must be regarded as essentially automatic, in their nature, and the course of thought being entirely determined by the associations previously formed and all the bodily movements being the direct manifestations of the ideas which possess the mind at the time, just as the ordinary movements of 'expression' are of its emotions. And it is, therefore, in these remarkable phases of psychical existence that we have the clearest manifestations of the power of which cerebral changes possess to produce muscular movement independently either of volition or emotion; an action which may be distinguished as *ideo-motor*, **since it only takes place when these changes are of a kind to awaken the ideational consciousness, and which is true 'reflex' action of the cerebrum.**

The same designation ["ideo-motor"] may be fairly applied also to all those actions performed by us in our ordinary waking condition, which are rather the automatic expressions of the ideas which dominate in our minds at the time, than prompted by distinct volitional effort. It is the dominant idea, then, which determines the movement, the will simply permitting it; and the more completely the volitional power is directed to other objects, the more completely automatic are the actions of this class. They may, indeed, come to be performed even without consciousness, or at least without the remembered consciousness, of the agent. All that is here stated is in perfect accordance with the general principle laid down, that in proportion as the higher channels of activity are obstructed will the excitation of nerve force manifest itself through the lower. For, whilst the ordinary sequence is for external impressions to excite sensations, for sensations to excite ideas, and for ideas (after becoming the subject of reasoning processes of greater of less complexity) to issue in volitional determinations, the direct action of ideational changes in the cerebrum or the motor system, when either the will is in abeyance or is entirely directed to mental operations, seems quite as natural as the immediate reaction of the sensational changes through the sensory ganglia, or of impressional changes through the spinal cord.

[On Hypnotic Somnambulism]

The phenomena of somnambulism are no less important in a scientific point of view, when they are regarded under the same aspect. They differ from those already described, in that they occur in a state of consciousness so far distinct from the ordinary waking condition as not to be connected with it by the ordinary link of memory; and although the course of thought in somnambulism usually manifests the directing influence of previous habits, and the knowledge of persons and things possessed during the waking state may be readily brought before the mind, yet nothing which occurs during the state of intense somnambulism is ever retraced spontaneously, or can be brought back by an act of recollection during the waking condition. Impressions upon the nervous system, however, are sometimes left by strong emotional excitement, which give rise to subsequent feelings of discomfort, of whose origin the individual is entirely unconscious.

The phenomena of somnambulism are so various, that it is difficult to give any definition that shall include the whole; but it is a condition which is common to all forms of this state, that the controlling power of the will over the current thought is entirely suspended, and that all the actions are directly prompted by the ideas which possess the mind; and the differences chiefly arise out of the mode in which the succession of ideas is directed, this being in some cases a coherent sequence through the whole of which some one dominant impression may be traced, whilst in other instances it is more or less completely determinable by external suggestions.

The first of these phases, which is nearly akin to the state of abstraction, is frequently seen in natural somnambulism; in which a train of reasoning is often carried out with remarkable clearness and correctness, and its results expressed in appropriate language, or otherwise acted on. Thus, a mathematician may work out a difficult problem, an orator make a speech appropriate to the occasion on which he supposes himself to be called up or an author may compose and commit to writing poetry or prose, upon the subject which occupies his thoughts. But it is a frequent defect of the intellectual operations carried on in this condition, that, through the complete absorption of the attention by one set of the considerations, no account is taken of others which ought to modify the conclusion; and this, although it may be palpably inconsistent with the teachings of ordinary experience, is not felt to be so, unless the latter should happen to present themselves unbidden to the thoughts.

The second of the phases which is especially seen in the artificial somnambulism, induced by the so-called Mesmeric process, or by the fixed gaze at a near object, as practised by Mr. Braid,

under the name hypnotism, is essentially the same as that of the "biological" condition, save in the different relations which they respectively bear to the waking condition; for there is the same readiness to receive new impressions through the senses (the visual sense, however, being generally in abeyance), and the same want of persistence in any one train of ideas, the direction of the thoughts being entirely determined by the suggestions which are introduced from without. In either of these extreme forms of somnambulism, and in the numerous intermediate phases which connect the two, the consciousness seems entirely given up to the one impression which is operating upon it at the time; so that whilst the attention is exclusively directed upon any object, whether actually perceived through the senses, or brought suggestively before the mind by previous ideas nothing else is felt. Thus there may be complete insensibility to bodily pain, the somnambulist's whole attention being given to what is passing in his mind; yet in an instant, by directing the attention to the organs of sense, the anaesthesia may be replaced by ordinary sensibility; or, by the fixation of the attention on any one class of sensations, these shall be perceived with most extraordinary acuteness, whilst there may be a state of complete insensibility as regards to the rest. So, again, when the attention of the somnambulist is fixed upon a certain train of thought, whatever maybe spoken in harmony with this is heard and appreciated, but what has no relation to it or is in discordance with it, is entirely disregarded.

[Muscular Suggestion]
It is amongst the most curious of the numerous facts which Mr. Braid's investigations upon artificial somnambulism have brought to light, that the suggestions derived from the "muscular sense", have a peculiar potency in determining the current of thought. For if the face, body, or limbs, be brought into an attitude that is expressive of any particular emotion, or that corresponds with that in which it would be placed for the performance of voluntary action, the corresponding mental state – that is, either an emotional condition affecting the general direction of the thoughts, or the idea of a particular action – is called up in respondence to it. Thus, if the hand be placed upon the vertex [the crown of the head], the somnambulist will frequently, of his own accord, draw his body up to its fullest height, and throw his head slightly back; his countenance then assumes an expression of the most lofty pride, and the whole train of thought is obviously under the domination of this feeling, as is manifested by the replies which the individual makes to interrogatories, and by the tone of voice and manner in which they are delivered; where the first action does not of itself call forth the rest, it is sufficient to straighten the legs and spine, and to throw the head somewhat back, to arouse the emotion, with its corresponding manifestation, to its full intensity.

If, during the most complete domination of this emotion, the head be bent forwards, and the body and limbs be gently flexed, the most profound humility then takes its place. So, again, if the angles of the mouth be gently separated from one another, as in laughter, a hilarious disposition is immediately generated; and this may be made to give place to moroseness, by drawing the eyebrows towards each other downwards upon the nose, as in frowning. The lecturer had not only repeatedly witnessed all these effects, as produced by Mr. Braid upon hypnotised subjects, of whom several had never been previously in that condition, and had no idea whatever of what was expected from them; but he had been assured by a most intelligent medical friend, who had paid special attention to the psychological part of the inquiry, that having subjected himself to Mr. Braid's practice, and having been only partially thrown into the "hypnotic" state, he distinctly remembers everything that was done, and could retrace the uncontrollable effect upon his emotional state which was produced by this management of his muscular apparatus.

So, again, if the hand be raised above the head, and the fingers be flexed upon the palm [in a gripping motion], the idea of climbing, swinging or pulling at a rope, is called up in such as have been used to this kind of exertion. If, on the other hand, the fingers be flexed when the arm is hanging down at the side, the idea suggested is that of lifting weight. And if the same flexure [making a fist] be made when the arm is advanced forwards in the position of striking a blow, the idea of fighting is at once aroused, and the somnambulist is very apt to put it into immediate execution. On one occasion in which the lecturer witnessed this result, a violent blow was struck, which chanced to alight upon a second somnambulist within reach; his combativeness being thereby excited, the two closed, and began to belabour one another with such energy, that they were with difficulty separated by Mr. Braid and another gentleman. Although their passions were at the moment so strongly excited, that, even when separated, they continued to utter furious denunciations against each other, yet a little discreet manipulation of their muscles soon calmed them and restored them to perfect good humour.

[Concluding Remarks on Hypnotism]
The lecturer also read the following beautiful description of hypnotism (Mr. Braid's system of Mesmerism) from Mr. Wilkinson's book, entitled "The Human Body":–

> The preliminary state is that of abstraction, and this abstraction is the logical premise of what follows. Abstraction tends to become more and more abstract, narrower and narrower, it tends to unity, and afterwards nullity. There, then, the patient is, at the summit of attention, with no object left – a mere statue of attention – a listening, expectant life – a perfectly undistracted faculty, dreaming of a lessening and lessening mathematical point, the end of his mind sharpened away to nothing. What happens? Any sensation that appeals is met by

this brilliant attention, and receives its diamond glare, being perceived by force of leisure, of which our distracted life only affords the rudiments. External influences are sensated, sympathised with, to an extraordinary degree; harmonious music sways the body into graces the most affecting; discords jar it as though they would tear it limb from limb; cold and heat are perceived with equal exaltations, so smells and touches. In short, the whole man appears to be given to each perception; the body trembles like down with wafts of the atmosphere; the world plays upon it as upon a spiritual instrument finely attuned. This is the natural hypnotic state, but it may be modified artificially. The power of suggestions over the patient is excessive. If you say, 'What animal is it?' the patient will tell you it is a lamb, a rabbit, or any other. 'Does he see it?' 'Yes.' 'What animal is it *now*?' putting depth and gloom into the tone of *now*, and thereby suggesting a difference. 'Oh,' with a shudder, 'it is a wolf.' 'What colour is it?' still glooming the phrase. 'Black.' 'What colour is it now?' giving the now a cheerful air. 'Oh, a beautiful blue,' spoken with utmost delight. And so you lead the subject through any dreams you please, by variation of questions, and of inflections of voice; and he sees and feels all as real. Another curious study is the influence of the patient's postures on his mind in this state. Double his fist, and put up his arm, if you dare, for you will have the strength of your ribs rudely tested. Put him on his knees, and clasp his hands, and the saints and devotees of the artists will pale before the trueness of his devout actings. Raise his head while in prayer, and his lips pour forth exulting glorifications, as he sees heaven opened, and the majesty of God raising him to his place; then, in a moment, depress the head, and he is dust and ashes, an unworthy sinner, with the pit of hell yawning at his feet; or compress the forehead so as to wrinkle it vertically, and this little attitude of gloom glooms the whole mind, and thorny-toothed clouds contract in from the very horizon; and what is remarkable, the smallest pinch and wrinkle, such as will lie between your nipping nails, is sufficient nucleus to crystallise the man into that shape, and to make him all foreboding; as again the smallest expansion, in a moment, brings the opposite state, with a full breathing of delight. [...] In this state, whatever posture of any passion is induced, the passion comes into it at once, and dramatises the body accordingly. Moreover, the patient's mind directed to his own body does physical marvels. He can do in a manner what he thinks he can. Tell him that a tumour on his body is about to disappear, and his mind will often realise your prophecy. [...] A patient in the full state obeys all motives in the most natural direction. If the arm is placed up, there it will stay; but a waft of air will cause it to fall. Why? Because it is already up, and the new motive changes the direction. If the arm be down, another waft will raise it. If down, and prevented from moving up, the impression will send it sideways. When the frame is erect, a touch behind the bend of the knees will send it into genuflexion, which will at once suggest prayer, as noticed before. [Wilkinson, *The Human Body*, 1851]

The lecturer considered the attentive and scientific study of the phenomena of the hypnotism of our [Manchester] townsman, Mr. Braid, and of electro-biology, would tend to eliminate the true from the false in Mesmerism, more effectually than any other method of procedure.

Much had been done by the inquiries of Mr. Braid, who discovered the hypnotic mode of inducing artificial somnambulism, and who has carefully studied the phenomena of the hypnotic state, and he felt it due to that gentleman farther to mention, that very soon after the publication of the first edition of Baron Reichenbach's researches on odyle, Mr. Braid discovered their true explanation, and exhibited to him (the lecturer) many of the odylic phenomena, **as the result of *suggestion*** in certain individuals, whom he had discovered to have the power of voluntarily inducing a state of abstraction or artificial reverie, closely corresponding to what is now termed the electro-biological condition. He (the lecturer) had no doubt of the genuineness of the Mesmeric sleep in various degrees in certain individuals, to the extent he had explained, as conformable to the physiology of the nervous system, and as witnessed by *him* in cases of natural somnambulism and hypnotism, which he had scrutinised with the utmost care and attention; but he had seen no satisfactory evidence of the special objective influence which the Mesmerists contended for as the *cause* of the phenomena or for the reality of *clairvoyance* and the higher phenomena, alleged by the Mesmerists as manifested by some of their patients. He thought these were legitimate point for farther inquiry, but *clairvoyance* and the higher phenomena seemed to him to admit of no necessary relation with the nervous system, as at present known (nor is *clairvoyance,* and these alleged higher phenomena, ever manifested in any of Mr. Braid's hypnotised subjects). The phenomena of somnambulism and hypnotism threw important light on the nature of various forms of insanity, and on the general study of psychology, on which grounds they merited a greater degree of consideration, and more extensive study, than had hitherto been accorded to them.

We must now, in order to avoid repetition, refer our readers to what was published in our paper of Saturday the 23rd for some additional remarks on a few other points, and with these we feel that they will be put in possession of all the most important bearings of this interesting and instructive course of lectures.

Braid, J., "Analysis of Dr. Carpenter's Lectures on the Physiology of the Nervous System." *Manchester Examiner and Times,* (Part I) Saturday 30th & (Part II) Wednesday 3rd April 1853.

Appendix: "The Psycho-Physiology of Suggestion" (Carpenter, 1874)

The Ideo-Motor Reflex

But further, even the Cerebrum responds automatically to impressions fitted to excite it to reflex action, when from any cause the Will is in abeyance, so that its power cannot be exerted either over the muscular system or over the direction of the thoughts and feelings. Thus in the states of Reverie, Dreaming, Somnambulism, etc., whether spontaneous or artificially induced, *ideas* which take full possession of the mind, and from which it cannot free itself, may excite respondent *ideo-motor* actions; as happens also when the force of the Idea is morbidly exaggerated, and the Will is not suspended, but merely weakened, as in many forms of Insanity.

The general views here put forth in regard to the independent and connected actions of the several primary divisions of the *Cerebro-spinal* apparatus, may perhaps be rendered more intelligible by the following Table; which is intended to represent (1) the ordinary course of operation, when the whole is in a state of complete functional activity, and (2) the character of the Reflex actions to which each part is subservient, when it is the highest centre that the impression can reach. [Carpenter, *The Principles of Mental Physiology*, etc., 1874: 125.]

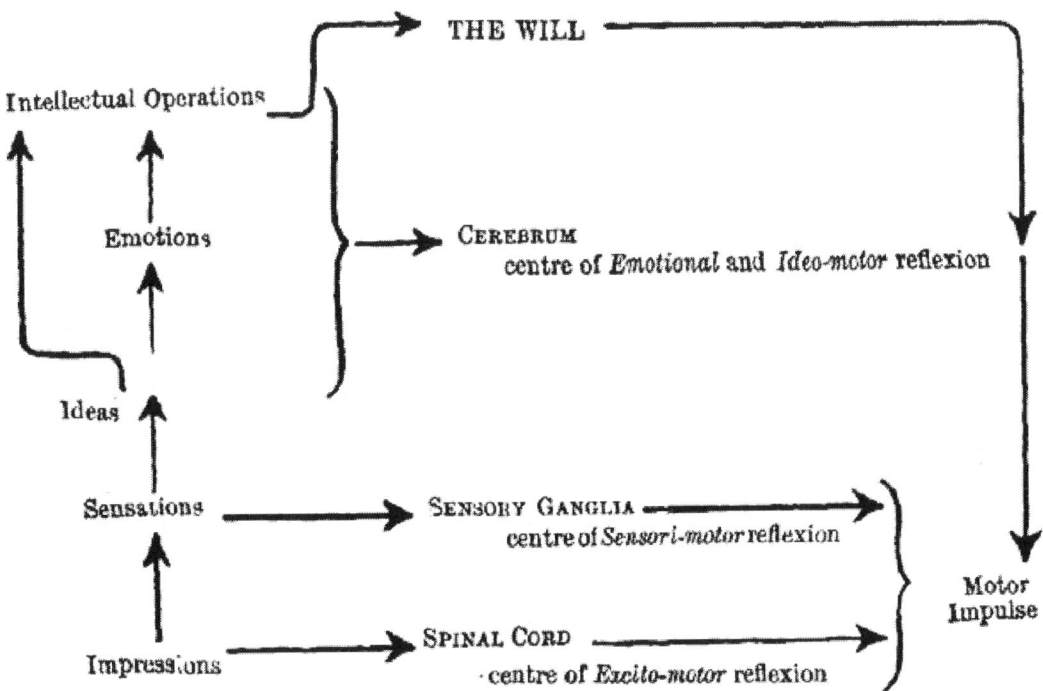

Monoideism

In the course of that important series of researches, carried on about thirty years ago by **the late Mr. Braid of Manchester, by which, in the Writer's opinion, more light has been thrown upon the reflex actions of the Cerebrum than by any other investigations**, Mr. B. discovered that there are many persons in whom a state may be artificially induced, resembling profound *reverie*; save that the subjects of it are yet more amenable than the subjects of natural reverie, to external suggestions conveyed to their minds through their Senses; whilst, in the absence of such suggestions, the Mind (having in itself no power of altering the current of its Ideas) remains as completely "possessed" by its own internal train of thought as it is in profound *abstraction*. This state may be superinduced in certain susceptible or "sensitive" individuals, upon the ordinary waking state, without a previous passage through the stage of insensibility; it being often sufficient for its induction, that the attention should be *fixed* for a few minutes, or even for a few seconds, upon any object whatever. By "leading" or suggestive questions addressed to his "sensitives", Mr. B. could not only bring them to feel any kind of sensation (pricking, burning, streaming, creeping and the like) which he chose that they should describe, when magnets were drawn along their limbs, or elicit descriptions of small volcanoes of flame seen by them to issue from the poles of the magnet; but he could cause their hands to be powerfully attracted towards magnets or crystals, or to be repelled by them in short, he could repeat all the phenomena adduced by Baron von Reichenbach as proofs of "odylic force", and this *as well without magnets as with them*, provided only that the "subjects" believed that some operation was being performed, and were led to expect some result

The Writer himself witnessed a most remarkable series of such experiments, about the year 1847, upon a gentleman of high literary and scientific attainments, who possessed in an unusual degree the power of self-concentration. It was sufficient for him to place his hand upon the table, and to fix his attention upon it for half a minute, to be entirely unable to withdraw it, if assured in a determined tone that he *could not possibly* do so. When his gaze had been steadily kept for a short time upon the poles of a Magnet, he could be brought to see flames issuing from them, of any form or colour that one chose to name. And when he had been desired, to place his hand upon one of the poles, and to fix his attention for a brief period upon it, the peremptory assurance that he could not detach it was sufficient to hold it there with such tenacity, that Mr. Braid positively dragged him round the room, in a manner that most amusingly realised the German fairy story of the Golden Goose. Some may, perhaps, think the Writer rather credulous in at once yielding his assent to the genuineness of such a strange performance. But the character and position of the "subject" of it were such as to place him beyond the suspicion of intentional deceit; and the Writer's previous inquiries had prepared him to find nothing too strange for his belief, that could be referred to the one simple and intelligible principle of "possession" by a "dominant idea" excited through *suggestion*.

Notwithstanding that Mr. Braid's investigations were thus carried on for several years, with every disposition on his part to enable the public to judge of their nature and results, they did not attract by any means the amount of general attention that might have been anticipated for them. But about the year 1850, "the world was turned upside down" by a couple of itinerant Americans, who styled themselves "professors" of a new art which they termed *Electro-Biology*; asserting that, by an influence of which the secret was known only to themselves, but which was partly derived from a little disc of zinc and copper held in the hand of the "subject" and steadily gazed on by him (whence the designation which they adopted), they could subjugate the most determined will, paralyse the strongest muscles, pervert the evidence of the senses, destroy the memory of even the most familiar things or of the most recent occurrences, induce obedience to any command, or make the individual believe himself transformed into anyone else – all this, and much more, being done while he was still wide awake. They soon attracted large assemblages to witness their performances; and there was an appearance of good faith about them which made a favourable impression, as they showed themselves ready to operate upon any who might offer, and seldom failed to elicit some of the most remarkable phenomena from individuals whose honesty could not be called in question, and who had previously been entire strangers to them. Ever on the watch, however, for any novelties in his favourite study, Mr. Braid set himself to inquire into the real nature of the so-called "electro-biological" process: and he soon proved that the little disc of copper and zinc may be replaced by any object which furnishes a *point d'appui* [supporting point] for the fixed gaze ; the whole secret consisting in the induction – through the steady direction of the eyes to one point, at the ordinary reading distance, for a period usually varying from about five to twenty minutes – of a state of reverie, in every respect similar to that which had previously fallen under his notice. Thus, in place of a few peculiarly susceptible "subjects" difficult to be met with, and open to suspicion on various grounds, every member of the public came to be furnished with a ready means of experimenting for himself upon his own family and friends, the student upon his fellow-students, the officer on the members of his mess; everybody, in fact, upon somebody else on whom he felt that he could place reliance. "Electro-biology", or "Biology" (as it came to be very commonly designated), was not merely introduced at scientific *réunions*, but became a fashionable amusement, in some circles, at ordinary evening parties. And thus it happened that a very large proportion of the public became familiarised with its phenomena; though still labouring under the perplexing difficulty of not knowing what to believe as to their genuineness, or to what scientific principles to refer them if their genuineness were admitted.

Considered in their relation to other states in which the Mind is "possessed" by "dominant ideas", and acts in accordance with them, the Biological phenomena are so far from being absurd or incredible, that they are simply manifestations of a condition to which we may frequently detect very close approximations within our ordinary experience; the most special peculiarity which attends them, consisting in the *method* by which the peculiar condition in question may be *artificially induced* – in such individuals, at least, as are constitutionally susceptible of its influence. In some "subjects", five, ten, or twenty minutes may be necessary to produce the effect; in others, a single minute, or even half a minute, is sufficient. It may be regarded as certain that the "biological" state may be thus induced in individuals who were previously quite incredulous in regard to its reality; so that it does not require any mental preparation on the part of the "subject". But it seems no less certain that the anticipation of the result tends to produce it in a shorter time than would otherwise be necessary; and it is for the most part among individuals who have repeatedly subjected themselves to the operation, that the greatest facility presents itself. The longer the steady gaze is sustained, the more is the Will of the individual withdrawn from the direction of his *thoughts*, and concentrated upon that of his *eyes*, so that at last it seems to become entirely transferred to the latter; and, in the mean time, the continued *monotony* is tending, as in the induction of Sleep or of Reverie, to produce a corresponding state of mind, which, like the body of a cataleptic subject, can be moulded into any position, and remains in that position until subjected to pressure from without. [Carpenter, *The Principles of Mental Physiology*, etc., 1874: 548-552.]

Magic, Witchcraft, Animal Magnetism, etc. (1852)

Braid's Critique of Victorian Energy Therapies

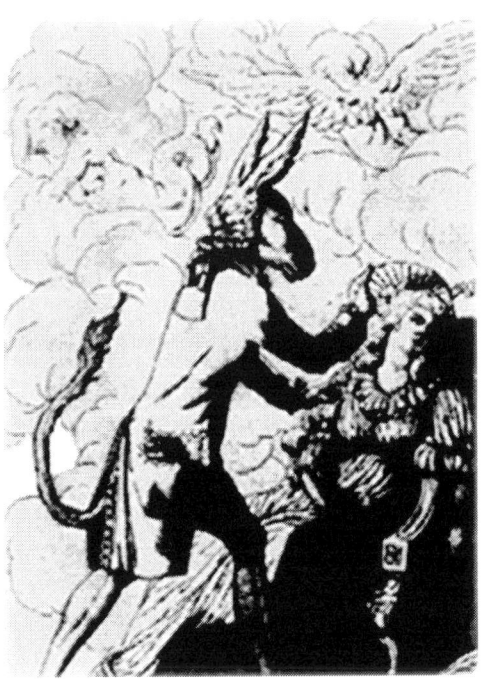

Republished in its entirety, James Braid's original work formerly entitled,

Magic, witchcraft, animal magnetism, hypnotism, and electro-biology; being a digest of the latest views of the author on these subjects.

Editor's Preface
D. Robertson

This short book was originally published by Braid specifically as a defence of his views in response to a set of erudite volumes on the history of occult practices by the Mesmerist, and former Scottish MP, John Campbell Colquhoun, entitled *An History of Magic, Witchcraft, & Animal Magnetism* (1851).

In the *Preface* to his work, Colquhoun had openly criticised Braid in a somewhat personal manner. Braid states that these comments forced him to rush into print with a rebuttal. In the process of answering Colquhoun's criticisms, though, Braid elaborates on the specific differences between his psycho-physiological theory of *hypnotism* and rival theories which tended to explain similar phenomena by reference to various hypothetical forms of *energy*, i.e., magnetism, electricity, vital power, or yet more supernatural and ethereal forces. Braid's supporters specifically label these theories as "pseudo-scientific" and he repeatedly provided evidence suggesting their effects were due to (what we now call) the "placebo effect".

Placebo Effects & Pseudoscientific Theories

Braid's main target was the "animal magnetism" theory of Franz Anton Mesmer and his followers. One of the basic principles of scientific method, the principle of parsimony or Occam's Razor, requires that new forces are only postulated if existing concepts are proven insufficient to explain the observations in question. Braid famously contended that all of the phenomena attributed by the Mesmerists to the effects of animal magnetism were in fact due to a variety of *well-established* psychological and physiological factors, primarily,

1. Verbal suggestion ("audible suggestion").
2. Role-modelling ("sympathy and imitation").
3. Autosuggestion ("predominant ideas").
4. Prolonged or focused attention ("monoideism").
5. Nervous arousal ("excitation") or fatigue ("nervous sleep").
6. Mental conditioning ("association" and "habit").

As Braid himself realised, these factors constitute what we now call the "placebo effect" – a term not commonly used until the 20th century. Indeed, Braid refers throughout his works to the use of saline injections, "bread pills" and other *inert* substances prescribed by Victorian physicians as deliberate placebo remedies. Ironically, the concept of the medical placebo forms, to a large extent, *positive evidence* used to support Braid's concept of hypnotism. Whereas other forms of complementary therapy have traditionally been susceptible to accusations that their perceived effects are due to the "placebo" response, hypnotism has largely *disarmed* this criticism by deliberately basing itself upon the same psychological and physiological mechanisms assumed to *explain* the placebo effect itself.

Braid introduced the concept of hypnotism specifically to offer a credible scientific explanation, "in accordance with generally admitted physiological and psychological principles", as he puts it, for the effects widely *misattributed* to animal magnetism and other hypothetical energies. Throughout his career, he undertook many experiments to debunk the claims of Mesmerists and others, and to demonstrate the explanatory value of the factors constituting hypnotism, i.e., attention, imagination, suggestion, etc. In doing so, it is fair to say that Braid made a reputation for himself, not only as the *discoverer* of hypnotism, but *also* as one of the most rigorous and influential 19th century critics of pseudoscience in medicine. His ideas attracted the explicit support of a pantheon of highly-distinguished Victorian scientists and academics, many of whom he mentions or cites in this work. These men seem frequently to have observed Braid's experiments themselves, either in private or at public lectures, or even to have been personally hypnotised by him.

Braid's Reaction to the Charge of Materialism

> [...] the nature of the charge in which I was implicated – unintentionally or inadvertently, probably, on his [Colquhoun's] part – was of such a grave character, that justice to myself, to my family, and friends, compelled me to endeavour to refute it as publicly as it had been diffused [...] (*footnote*)

Braid is likely to seem, to a modern reader, to have *over*-reacted to Colquhoun's comments. There are a number of reasons, however, for believing that Braid's response was necessary given the context and circumstances.

First and foremost, it should be noted that the apparent charge of "materialism", insinuated by Colquhoun, was synonymous with *atheism* in 1850s England. The orthodox Christian God is decidedly *immaterial* and therefore simply does not *exist*, if viewed from the perspective of most materialist philosophies. Moreover, in Victorian England, the word "materialist" undoubtedly carried the popular *connotation* that one was an atheist, and was widely used by contemporary Christians as an accusation of heresy.

As a Christian himself, Braid took offence at this accusation, and it should be remembered by modern readers that the insinuations made by Colquhoun could have had very serious professional implications for him. Perhaps it will suffice to note that Charles Darwin's *On the Origin of the Species* was published *seven years later* in 1859 and met with a well-documented storm of controversy from the clergy because of its apparent "materialism". Braid therefore felt compelled to publish a detailed refutation of Colquhoun's views on *magnetism* and, simultaneously, a defence of the empirical "psycho-physiological" stance adopted by *hypnotism*.

Magic, Witchcraft, Animal Magnetism, Hypnotism, & Electro-Biology; Being a Digest of the Latest Views of the Author on these Subjects

BY

JAMES BRAID, M.R.C.S. EDIN., C.M.W.S. etc.

Third Edition, Greatly Enlarged,
Embracing Observations On
J. Colquhoun's "History of Magic," *etc.*

"Amicus Plato, amicus Socrates, sed magis amica veritas."
["I love Plato as a friend, I love Socrates, but greater love have I for truth itself." – attrib. Aristotle]

LONDON:
John Churchill, Princes Street, Soho.
Adam and Charles Black, Edinburgh.
1852.

"No men of independent habits of thought can be driven
into belief: their reason must be appealed to,
and their objections calmly met."
– *British and Foreign Medical-Chirurgical Review.*

Preface

In the first edition of these "Observations", [*Observations on J.C. Colquhoun's History of Magic, etc.*, was the original title] I merely intended to shield myself against the more important points upon which I considered Mr. Colquhoun had misrepresented me. In the second edition I went more into detail, and quoted additional authorities in support of my theory of the nature, cause, and extent of hypnotic or Mesmeric phenomena. In the third edition I have gone so much more into detail, as to furnish a periscope [overview] or vidimus [an inspection and formal authentication] of my views on all the more important points of the hypnotic and Mesmeric speculations.

By this means, after perusal of a Mesmeric manual, any intelligent person can easily compare the two systems, and determine for himself which he most approves of; and by this means, moreover, I am making up, in some measure, for the delay in the publication of another edition of my work on *hypnotism*, which has long been out of print, and so frequently called for. That call I hope shortly to be able to respond to, with fullness of detail as the importance of the subject merits; more particularly as regards its practical application to the relief and cure of *some* forms of disease, of which numerous interesting examples will be adduced.

Burlington House, Oxford Street, Manchester.
20th February 1852.

Observations on
J.C. Colquhoun's History of Magic, etc.

[Preliminary Comments]
A work in two volumes has just issued from the press, entitled "An History of Magic, Witchcraft, and Animal Magnetism, by J.C. Colquhoun, Esq., author of 'Isis Revelata', etc." The author has brought a flood of light to bear upon his subject, and has produced a book which will amply repay anyone for its perusal, being agreeably and ably written, and embodying much matter which is both entertaining and instructive. Still there are some parts of the book which I must dissent from, both as to the matter and manner in which the learned and ingenious author has drawn from certain premises.

There is one topic, in particular, which Mr. Colquhoun has undertaken to discuss, which, in my humble opinion, had better have been left in a profound magnetic slumber – and that is his attempt to prove that there is no reality in the belief in the *mythos* of the Devil – that there is no such personage as his Satanic Majesty – and that his existence is a mere allegory of Pagan or Zoroastric origin, borrowed by the Jews from that source, and introduced by them into the sacred scriptures. At pp. 258-9, vol. I., Mr. C. says:–

> We formerly observed that the actual existence of such a personage as the Devil was not originally a Jewish, but a Zoroastric notion – a Chaldean or Babylonish hallucination – which had been borrowed by that people (the Jews) and transferred into their religious code at or after their captivity and exile. Even the doctrine of good and bad angels, and their continual interference in the affairs of this sublunary sphere, appears to have been derived from the same source. Ideas of this nature, however, besides being unwarranted, are calculated to pervert religion, and to embarrass and distort the minds of mankind. [...] The metaphorical notion of the Devil himself, in the conceptions of mankind, is generally admitted, by all cultivated minds, to represent the evil and perverse dispositions which deform the nature of man, or the diseases, moral or physical, by which human beings may be afflicted.

For my own part, I cannot see how these views can be entertained, without rejecting the obvious interpretation of various important parts of scripture. Nor can I approve of his contrasting cures by prophets and apostles with Mesmeric processes and cures. Mr. [Henry George] Atkinson [a Mesmerist] and Miss [Harriet] Martineau [an early feminist and political philosopher] lately attempted to persuade mankind that their Mesmeric researches had enabled them to come to the conclusion that there was no God, that man had no immortal soul, and that there was no future state of existence after death [in their controversial book *Letters on the Laws of Man's Nature and Development*, 1851]. For this, Mr. Colquhoun rated them right well, and most deservedly, as I thought. Now, however, he himself, although a religious and Christian man, puts forth the above opinions, which will be startling to many, and may raise an unmerited prejudice in the minds of some against the whole inquiry, as leading to unchristian, unscriptural principles; and will, no doubt, ensure for the learned gentleman and his science, *the benefit of clergy* [the right under English law for ministers of the Church to be treated more leniently].

The great object of Mr. Colquhoun's investigations has been to prove, by drawing from the history of all people, and of all times, that phenomena, similar to those which have been recognised in later times as producible at will in certain individuals, by what have been termed the processes of animal magnetism, have existed and been recognised from the earliest ages, in every clime, and amongst every people, under various designations; occurring spontaneously, or from unknown causes occasionally; at other times brought into play from religious or political excitement, and then diffused extensively through the power of sympathy and imitation; on other occasions and places, as the result of mystical processes, as in the temples, for the purposes of divination, soothsaying, or the cure of diseases, *etc. etc.* Having proved the existence of such conditions for so long a period, and occurring under such divers circumstances, and so universally diffused, the learned author contends that they ought the more readily to be admitted in our own time, when so much better understood, and more readily produced by known processes. Mr. C.'s examples, instead of opposing, actually furnish strong support to my subjective or personal theory. In the case of the Convulsionaries of St. Medard, in particular, I would beg leave to ask how a *nervous* or *vital* force could have passed from the *ashes* of the *buried* saint, and produced the effects realised at the grave of the Abbé Pâris? Mental emotion, imitation, and faith or confidence, however, were quite adequate to account for all which was there manifested.[50]

In a little *brochure* which I published in 1850, entitled "Observations on Trance, or Human Hybernation," the following remarks occurred:– "I believe that the great cause of the opposition which has been offered to the acceptance of the truth of the genuine phenomena of *hypnotism* and *Mesmerism*, has arisen from the extravagance of the Mesmerists, who have contended for the reality of *clairvoyance* in some of their patients – such as seeing through opaque bodies, and investing them with the gifts and graces of

---

[50] [See appendix (originally a lengthy footnote) 'On Newnham's *Human Magnetism*.']

omniscience, Mesmeric intuition, and universal knowledge – pretensions alike a mockery of the human understanding, as they are opposed to all the known laws of physical science."

[Braid Defends Himself Against the Charge of Materialism]
It appears that these remarks have excited the bile of my ingenious, learned, and esteemed friend Mr. Colquhoun, to such an extent as induced him to give vent to such "sensitive ebullitions" as compel me, in self-defence, to offer a few observations on his slashing lucubrations. Had the strictures referred to been of the ordinary character of legitimate criticism, or even had they exceeded these bounds to any reasonable extent, the great respect which I entertain for the author, as a scholar and a gentleman, and as one with whom I have personally, and more particularly by letter, had much agreeable intercourse, I should most willingly have allowed his remarks to pass without note or comment. These very circumstances, however, which would have induced me to be silent under an ordinary, a severe, or merited castigation from the pen of this gentleman, render it the more imperative a duty for me to repel the aggression, and endeavour to set myself right with the public, when he has gone so far as even to merge me with the materialists – namely, with those who maintain that the mental functions are a mere secretion of the brain, as the bile is of the liver. Now, that any man should attribute such opinions or sentiments to me – and more particularly a friend like Mr. Colquhoun – passes my comprehension, because, in *all* my writings – and Mr. C. has had presentation copies from me of the *whole* of them, I believe – I have ever stoutly contended for the *very opposite sentiments*.

In proof of this I beg leave to refer to pages 81, 87, 88, 89, and 91 of my work on "Hypnotism", [*Neurypnology*] published in 1843, where I entered into a rather elaborate *refutation* of the *doctrine* of *materialism*; adducing various arguments as the basis on which my dissent from that doctrine was founded. I also quoted the opinions of Drs. [Thomas] Brown and [John] Abercrombie, Dugald Stewart [three philosophers of the Scottish school of "Common Sense" academic philosophy] and Plato, in support of my *opposition* to the doctrine of materialism.

Now, in the face of all this, was it not an unwarrantable, inconsiderate imputation in Mr. Colquhoun to represent me as a materialist? And what else but this could he hope to convey by the innuendo contained in the following sentence:– "Does Dr. Braid, then, acknowledge no science but the merely *physical*?" After having promulgated in my writings such sentiments as those referred to, I am sorry to say that I cannot see how Mr. Colquhoun, or anyone else, should endeavour to rank me amongst the materialists, unless from a reckless perversion of legitimate inference, or a determination to misrepresent and injure me, because I would not accept their transcendental notions about the *higher* phenomena, as they style them, of Mesmerism or animal magnetism.

In July last I published a pamphlet, entitled, "Electro-Biological Phenomena considered Physiologically and Psychologically", [1851] a copy of which was sent by me to Mr. Colquhoun several months before the publication of his book containing the strictures of which I complain. The object of that publication was to prove the subjectivity of the hypnotic, Mesmeric, and the so-called "electro-biological" condition, in opposition to the theory of the Mesmerists and electro-biologists; the former of whom contended for an occult or special influence, or the "od force" of Reichenbach as the *cause*; whilst the latter attributed it to an electrical influence, excited and directed by the will and manoeuvres of a second party. My theory was this – **that the phenomena resulted from the concentrated mental attention of the patient acting on his own physical organism, and the changed condition of the physical action thus induced reacting on the mind of the patient. I contended, and endeavoured to prove that, by the patient concentrating his attention on any part of his body, the function of the part would, to a certain extent, be altered or modified, according to the predominant idea and faith which existed in his (the patient's) mind during the continuance of such fixed attention. I proved – and I had done so, indeed, more than five years previously [in his *The Power of the Mind Over the Body*, 1846] – that these ideas might arise in the minds of patients, and become operative on them, through their own unaided acts, or from the mere remembrance of past feelings, without any co-operation or act of a second party; and that, in certain subjects, they might also be excited by audible, visible, or tangible suggestions from another person, to any extent whatever – even before they passed into the state of sleep**. My object, then, was to prove, by these results, the wonderful "power of the *mind*" of the *patient* over *his* OWN body. Did this look as if I recognised "*no* science but the *merely PHYSICAL?*"

But, farther, had I not devoted three pages and a half of the appendix to the above-named pamphlet ['Electro-Biological Phenomena,' etc., 1851] (an 8vo., small type, closely set) to expose the folly and impiety of the infidel, atheistical principles set forth by Mr. Atkinson and Miss Harriet Martineau, in their late publication "On the Laws of Man's Nature and Development", [1851] in which, as the enlightenment which they had drawn from their Mesmeric clairvoyants, they denied their belief "in a God or the future", and declared that "philosophy finds no God in nature – nor sees the want of any"; in short, that they acknowledged "no science but the merely *physical*"? Was this of itself not enough to have convinced Mr. Colquhoun (whose daily avocation, as a Barrister and Sheriff of a county, is to sift evidence) or any other candid and rational man, that my sentiments were the very reverse of those of the materialists? It is therefore matter of astonishment to me, that a learned and ingenious man like Mr. Colquhoun – professing himself to be my friend too – should have been so excited by my remarks regarding the transcendental Mesmerists, as induced him to publish such an unjust and injurious attack upon me, merely because my theoretical views, and limited extent of my confession of faith, as to the higher phenomena of Mesmerism, were at variance with theirs, and I had presumed to say so. And, be it observed, my remarks were made with reference to the transcendental Mesmerists as *a class*, whilst Mr. Colquhoun's attack is made against me as *an individual*, which, of course, greatly aggravates the injury, both as regards the apparent intention and the fact.[51]

[Colquhoun's Other Criticisms]
Had I not been compelled to defend myself against the charge of being a *materialist*, I should not have deemed the other charges of my learned friend of sufficient importance to demand a formal reply. However, having been forced to enter the lists, it may be as well to take a brief glance at the *other* charges this gentleman has brought against me. He charges me with having been "uncandid, uncourteous, and unjust towards my fellow-labourers in the magnetic mine". To the first count in this indictment I plead *not guilty*, and for this reason, that it cannot be "*uncandid*" to declare what one honestly believes to be the truth; and such, assuredly, was the case with me in all which I said on that occasion. To the second count, "uncourteous", I must plead guilty, but with justification of the offence, in consequence of certain circumstances connected with my observations. I am aware that it may be considered "uncourteous", on some occasions, to speak the truth; still, circumstances may arise to render it requisite that the truth should be spoken, and such I considered was the case in that instance. To the third count, "unjust", I plead *not guilty*, because that the views which I have taken, in opposition to those of the animal magnetists, I believe to be much nearer the truth than theirs. I might, with much more propriety, apply the term "unjust" to the conduct of Mr. Colquhoun, in reference to myself, not merely on the point already discussed, but also when he says, "Is he (Mr. Braid) acquainted with *all* the laws even of physical science, with all their various modifications under peculiar circumstances?" Mr. C. had no right, by such an innuendo, to impute to me any such arrogant pretensions, seeing that, in the very words he had quoted from my work, only two sentences before this charge, I expressed myself thus:– "Pretensions alike a mockery of the human understanding, as they are opposed to all the KNOWN laws of physical science." I spoke only of "all the *known* laws", therefore it was both uncandid and unjust in the learned gentleman to impute to me any greater pretensions than I had actually alleged myself possessed of.

Mr. Colquhoun says he has not had the good fortune to meet with any scientific Mesmerist who invested his patients "with the gifts and graces of omniscience". But what else, let me ask, is investing them with the clairvoyance which the Mesmerists contend for (which Mr. C. declares, at page 47, he conceives "equally capable of being demonstrated as any other portions of the science,") but investing them "with the gifts and graces of omniscience"? The grand scope of Mr. C.'s book is to prove, by drawing from the records of all people and of all times, that the phenomena of catalepsy, trance, somnambulism, extase, the gift of prophecy, magic, witchcraft, the second sight, divination, universal knowledge by intuition or inspiration, thought-reading; the power of *seeing* from the pit of the stomach, or any other part of the body, without the use of the eyes; of seeing through opaque bodies; of tasting and feeling through the physical organs of others instead of their own; of enabling them to see and describe what may be transacted at any moment of time, past, present, or future by any party, at any part of the habitable globe, or even throughout any part of creation; to invest parties uneducated in medical science with the faculty or power to discover the nature, cause, and cure of any disease, even without seeing or touching the patient, but merely by sending the clairvoyant a lock of the absent patient's hair or his hand-writing – such as the address of a letter written by him – to the entranced Sibyl; all these marvels, and much more, Mr. Colquhoun endeavours to prove have existed in all ages and in all countries, arising spontaneously occasionally, or from unknown causes; and he contends that a similar condition may be produced, in certain subjects, at any time by the Mesmeric processes. Now, if this really is a *fact*, that the mere exercise of the silent will of the Mesmerist, or the wafting of his hand through the air, so as to make a few Mesmeric passes, can impart to his patients all these alleged wonderful powers, is it not very like investing their subjects "with the gifts and graces of omniscience"? And, be it remarked, Mr. Colquhoun repudiates the notion that any of these wonderful feats are accomplished by a process of reasoning from known facts to probable results, but seems to suppose that they acquire "universal lucidity" ("Clairvoyance", page 108) as an instinct, or "immediate intuition of the soul, without any assistance from the reasoning faculties". – p. 51.

[Braid's Critique of Mesmerism]
I cannot better express my views regarding the presumed Mesmeric-clairvoyance than by the following quotation from my recently published pamphlet. At page 27, I said:–

> Professor Gregory thinks that I have gone too far in denying the existence of clairvoyance and what are called

---

[51] That the sole cause of this attack was merely a splenetic ebullition as I have alleged, excited by the perusal of the observations above quoted from my work on "Trance", will be obvious to anyone who shall take the trouble of comparing the style in which the author referred to me and my writings, at vol. I. page 112, and vol. II. page 118, which had been written *before* reading said remarks, with what he wrote in the preface *after* their perusal.

the higher phenomena. It is quite possible that it may be my misfortune to have such a constitution of mind as requires too great an amount of evidence before I can be convinced that certain phenomena are facts; still, when I state *this* fact, that I have had many opportunities of investigating the pretensions of alleged clairvoyants of the first water, and, from knowing and attending to the sources of fallacy requiring to be guarded against, that I found *every individual clairvoyant wanting*, even including trials by myself and others, on several occasions, with a subject who has been adduced by the Professor, in his recent work, as *one of the most lucid examples on record*; under such circumstances, I think few can feel surprised that I should still be somewhat sceptical as to the *bona fides* of these transcendental phenomena, which are said only to manifest themselves *occasionally*; and that, again, only *in a few individuals*; and, moreover, before those only whose foregone conclusions incline them, unwittingly, to overlook sources of fallacy of vital importance in such an investigation, and to accept vague generalities as clear and satisfactory replies, on points which ought to be determined with the utmost rigour and unmistakeable accuracy. To say that ninety-nine negatives will not gainsay or disprove *one* positive fact, as many argue, I readily admit; but I admit it only on the following *conditions* – provided always that the assumed *positive fact* can be clearly and satisfactorily proved to be a *fact*. In such a case as that, however, I would look very charily at the solitary alleged fact, from a fear that, after all, it might not be a *real*, but only a *spurious* result – a mere illusion – arising out of the numerous chances of error, having deceived me, in some way, in this solitary successful case. From all which I have seen, read, and heard, on the subject, I think I am fully entitled to say that, if we are not warranted to pronounce the things supposed to be performed by clairvoyants *impossible* – feats which never *can* be proved by any possible amount of evidence – still I consider myself justified in saying, that it is highly improbable that such a power or faculty will ever be realised so as to be satisfactorily proved to the conviction of mankind at large. [*Electro-Biological Phenomena, etc.*, 1851]

It has always appeared to me as a strong argument against such a power being delegated to man, that it would upset the whole fabric of society, in the present state of its existence – in which so much depends on each individual being able to confine a knowledge of the state of his affairs and intentions to himself and his friends only, and give his chief attention to his own concerns.

However, I most cordially agree with the judicious remarks of the reviewer of Mr. Colquhoun's book in the "Critic", of the 15th January, page 32, where he says – "Obviously, science is a question of *fact*. It is useless to assail asserted facts by *reasons* for their non-existence. There is but one way of disproving them, and that is by trying the experiment. [...] Verbal controversy is a most wasteful method of trying physical truths. It takes so much more time. The *experiment* may, probably, be tried in a few hours; an *argument* at probabilities and possibilities may extend over years." In reference to the veritable clairvoyance of the Mesmerists, according to the above canon of the reviewer, I am entitled to offer an opinion, because "I *have* tried, and found them to *fail*. I *have* put the asserted experiment to the proof, and it has *not* yielded the result". And, moreover, I have made these experiments honestly and fairly, and frequently, with *my own patients and friends*, as well as with some of the most noted clairvoyants of others; still nothing satisfactory was realised by such investigations.

The following was the result of a trial with a noted clairvoyant – so noted, that her fee, when in London, was *five guineas for a single consultation* when she called on the patient, or three guineas when consulted at her own residence. In order to prove to my satisfaction, and induce me to give a certificate of her wonderful powers at detecting and prescribing for diseases by Mesmeric-clairvoyance, her husband offered to put her to sleep; and, when in this state, she voluntarily offered to prove her clairvoyant powers, by describing and prescribing for *my own complaints*. As she had never seen me before, I considered this was an unexceptionable offer. She then made the examination by applying the tips of her fingers to various parts of her own person, raising them again and again before her face, as if reading the required information from the points of the fingers. I determined to watch carefully all that was said and done, and say nothing which could either *lead* or *mis*lead the clairvoyant sibyl. She detected and described minutely, and prescribed for, *three grave complaints*, which she discovered me labouring under; but, more satisfactorily for myself than the clairvoyant and her husband, I was bound in candour, at last to declare, that neither then, nor at any period of my life, had I suffered from any one of the three grave diseases she alleged I was afflicted with.

But what, after all, let me ask, would be the value of the clairvoyance contended for by the Mesmerists, in a *practical* point of view, even if they could satisfactorily prove its existence in certain cases? For, according to their own showing, the capriciousness and uncertainty of this alleged faculty would render it worthless, because of the difficulty of determining when the enunciations of clairvoyants were true, and when they were erroneous. Even Mr. Colquhoun admits this at page 216 of volume II., where he says – "We cannot always depend upon the same accuracy of instinct; for there are many confused magnetic states in which truth may be mingled with error; and such annunciations, therefore, may mislead the bystander; and, for this reason, they ought always to be received with great caution!" And, again, at pages 218-19, he says – "The conclusion, therefore, to which, we are disposed to come, in regard to this matter of instinct of remedies, is this – that, in many cases, this instinctive feeling is natural and just, and may be depended upon; but that, in other cases, it may be impure and merely fanciful; and that it requires a great deal of tact and experience on the part of the observer, in order to enable him to distinguish the true from the false."

This is also fairly admitted by Dr. Haddock, regarding his subject Emma, who is held up for admiration by Professor Gregory and others, as being one of the most remarkable clairvoyant subjects who has been met with; and the reports of her alleged visits to Sir John Franklin at the North Pole, of course, invested her with no ordinary degree of notoriety. At page 114 of the second edition of his work, entitled "Somnolism and Psycheism", the author says – "I would by no means wish the reader to suppose that Emma was always successful. In some cases there have been no means of proving or disproving her statements; in others, she has apparently mixed up the *past with the present*, and thus presented a confused and erroneous picture." Then, after enumerating other sources of error in her revelations, the doctor adds:– "The reader will thus see the difficulties attending these inquiries, and observe the many sources of error. Clairvoyance has its *uses*; and, unfortunately, from the enthusiasm of some parties, and knavery of others, its *abuses*. But it ought, by no means, to be considered as equalling, much less of superseding, the investigations and conclusions of the normal, rational faculty."

Such an admission as the one contained in the last sentence of the above quotation, coming as it does from a gentleman who makes constant professional use of said clairvoyant, for the purposes of diagnosis, prognosis, and the treatment of diseases, is highly significant, and fully justifies the humble estimate which I made of its *practical* value at the beginning of the paragraph, page 17. It is, obviously, merely a dream spoken and acted out, directed and modified by suggestions of those present, and partakes of the peculiar character of dreaming, which is to accept every idea arising in the mind, or suggested to it through impressions on the senses, as present realities, with a tendency, as in insanity, to reason correctly, occasionally, from the erroneous premises which had been assumed as true. Like dreaming and fortune-telling, moreover, the answers, like those of all oracular predictions, are given in very vague phraseology; so that they may admit of any variety of interpretation which may best suit the fancy of the parties interested in the issue of the inquiry."[52]

[Braid's "Discovery" of Hypnotism; its Ancient Precursors]

The observations contained in the paragraphs pages 36-7 of Mr. Colquhoun's "Preface", are calculated to convey most erroneous notions regarding me. **They implicate me in making undue attempts to claim for myself the credit of being an "original discoverer", and endeavouring to supplant Mesmerism by its younger brother, *hypnotism*.** Mr. Colquhoun was as well aware as myself that the method devised by me for demonstrating the fallacy of the Mesmeric theory, about a magnetic fluid or force being the *cause* of the phenomena educed by these various processes, *in as far as I was aware at that time*, was entirely new – or, if he prefer that term, **it was a *discovery*; for, I was not then aware of it having been resorted to by anyone else.** However, having undertaken the investigation of the habits of the Hindoos and Magi of Persia, in 1844-5, I was enabled to publish a series of papers in The Medical Times, on "Magic, Mesmerism, Hypnotism, *etc.*, Historically and Physiologically Considered". In these papers I stated that I had found in the writings referred to, "many statements corroborative of the fact, that the **eastern saints are all self-hypnotisers – adopting means essentially (but *not identically*, I wish it specially to be observed) the same as those which I had recommended for similar purposes"**. I added, that it was "a curious and important fact, clearly demonstrated by my investigation, that what observation and experience had led me to adopt and recommend as the most speedy and effectual mode of inducing the nervous sleep and its subsequent phenomena, had been practised by the *Magi of Persia* for ages before the Christian era – most probably from the earliest times; was known to Zoroaster, who followed in their steps, 550 years before Christ; and from this found its way into India in those days, where it has been employed by the Hindoo saints and religious mendicants, Jogees [i.e., yogis], Fakirs, and others". **I farther added:– "Whilst there is this remarkable coincidence, however, between my own views and theirs, as to the mode of *inducing* the *sleep* and *some of the phenomena*, in the sequel it will be found that our theoretical views as to the nature and cause of the *subsequent and ulterior* phenomena, 'are wide as the poles asunder'."** Now, these are the very papers which Mr. Colquhoun has referred to in such flattering terms at page 112, vol. I.; and can he really think, under such circumstances, that he was warranted in making such remarks as those contained in his "Preface", imputing to me a desire to conceal what I knew had been long ago done by others, in order that I may appropriate to myself what belongs to them?

Strictly speaking, perhaps there is really nothing new under the sun – that is to say, there may be no idea of the present day which may not, in some shape or other, be alleged to have occurred to the mind of

---

[52] Another point in which it seems to resemble dreaming is this, that through the multiplicity of ideas rushing through the mind in a confused manner, it is easy for the person who remembers his dreams on awaking to allege that such and such occurrences are foreshadowed or revealed to him in this manner, or to imagine to himself, after their actual occurrence, that such and such things really had been prefigured to him. Moreover, there are not wanting occasional instances of individuals having in their sleep exercised a process of reasoning, so as to solve difficult problems, or complete and perfect literary compositions, with which they had been puzzled and perplexed and were unable to accomplish during their waking moments. This actually occurred with myself, when I was a school-boy; and it has also occurred to several of my friends, and to others of whom I have read accounts, some of whom had recorded in their sleep, or spontaneous somnambulism, the result of their labours, unknown to themselves on awaking, whilst others remembered all which had occurred during their sleep. Still, these are such rare exceptions to the general stuff of which dreams are made up, that I believe few individuals would be rash enough to hazard important enterprises by a minute and strict adherence to the revelations communicated to them in dreams. Just as there are always some who attach great importance to ordinary dreams, through the occasional coincidences and alleged successes which occur, so will the like occasional coincidences and apparent successes always secure a certain class as believers in the importance and truth of clairvoyant revelations. Even Mesmeric clairvoyants, however, with all the aids which they enjoy over the natural dreamer, by suggestions caught from the leading questions, observations, looks, and gestures of those around them (for many of them are seeing through their *partially closed eyelids*, and scrutinising all which is going on, by the aid of the ordinary organ of vision, and other organs of sense, whilst the bystander is not at all aware of this important fact) – I say, even with all these aids, one of the most noticeable things about the *instinct* of Mesmeric clairvoyants, compared with that of animals, is this – that the *instinct* of animals is *generally right*, whereas the instinct of Mesmeric clairvoyants is *generally wrong*.

some other human being, long deceased or still alive. But it is not the vague, and confused, and dreamy idea which is of importance and of real practical value. **It is only when an individual has been enabled, in some measure, to explain the nature and cause of certain phenomena, or at least to devise means for gaining such certainty and precision to processes and their sequences and relations, as shall give a definite form and practical bearing to the ideas, that they really come to merit the appellation of *a discovery*. Now, all which I have ever laid claim to, was simply the discovery of more certain and speedy modes of producing the hypnotic state, and of applying it with the more advantage for the relief and cure of disease, than by "the old-established modes of Mesmerising"; and also that my method has enabled me to demonstrate that the influence is subjective, or personal, and *not objective*, or the result of the transmission of an occult, magnetic, or odylic, or vital, or nervous influence or fluid, passing from the operator to the patient.** In respect to the attempts of Mesmerists to give the merit due to me in this matter, and to this extent, to any dead or living man, rather than to the author of *hypnotism*, I may be consoled, perhaps, by reflecting on the following shrewd remark:– "In the progress of improvements, it is always a good sign of their appreciation when attempts are made to rob the authors of the merit due to them."

Throughout the whole of my inquiries my chief desire has been to arrive at what could be rendered most practically useful for the relief and cure of disease; and I hesitate not to say, that, in the hands of a skilful medical man, who thoroughly understands the peculiar modes which I have devised for varying the effects in a manner applicable to different cases, *hypnotism*, besides being the speediest method for inducing the condition, is, moreover, capable of achieving *all* the *good* to be attained by the *ordinary Mesmerising processes*, and MUCH MORE.

[Conditioning to the Hypnotic Induction]

However, after the susceptibility has been fairly stamped upon patients who are naturally highly impressionable, I adopt either my own usual process or the common Mesmerising modes indifferently, because either will so speedily induce the state favourable for varying the mental and physical conditions, according to the indications in each particular case. After the susceptibility has been engendered, the modes of working out the subsequent results, so as to produce the specific effects required in each case, I consider the most important part of the whole affair. **There is obviously one remarkable result of a fixed act of attention, and which I insist on, if it does not arise spontaneously, from the simple act of gazing steadily at some unexciting and empty thing, and that is the suppression of the respiration which accompanies such act.** The influence of suppressed respiration on the state of the oxygenation of the blood, and in preventing the elimination of carbonic acid, I doubt not, plays an important part in making the slight organic changes on which the hypnotic and Mesmeric condition is at *first* engendered. **Subsequently, however, habit and expectation play the most important part for inducing the sleep.**

[Hypnotism More Credible & Scientific than Mesmerism]

Of course there is one point which renders *hypnotism* less an object of approbation with a certain class of society – *viz*., that I lay no claim for it to produce the marvellous or transcendental phenomena [such as telepathy, levitation, clairvoyance, etc.]; nor do I allege that the phenomena manifested have any relation to a magnetic temperament [a supposedly innate gift of those practising Mesmerism] or some peculiar or occult power possessed in an extraordinary degree by the operator. These are all circumstances which appeal powerfully to the feelings of the lovers of the marvellous, and therefore tell in favour of Mesmerism; and, moreover, seeing that, for conducting the hypnotic processes with any degree of certainty and success, I contend that, in many cases, a knowledge of anatomy, physiology, pathology, and therapeutics are all requisite, it is obvious that such requirements must be less calculated to secure the approbation of *non-professional* Mesmerists and amateurs, whose magnetic creed taught them to believe that the mere possession by them of the magnetic temperament – of a surcharge by nature, within their own bodies, of a magnetic fluid, or odyle – is quite sufficient to enable them to treat any case as efficiently as the most skilful medical man in the universe, simply by walking up to the patient with the *will* and *good intention* of doing him service, or by adding thereto, occasionally, the efficacy of Mesmeric touches, passes, or manipulations.

All I claim for hypnotism is now willingly admitted by the great majority of scientific men, who have investigated the subject without previous prejudice in favour of Mesmerism; and even Mr. C. himself admits, at page 188, vol. II, that, in the course of my researches in hypnotism, I have brought forward "many curious facts and illustrations which well deserve the attention of all who take an interest in the investigation of the subject".

[Hypnotism Developed to Oppose Mesmerism]

But further, in reply to Mr. Colquhoun's remarks at pages 36-7 ("Preface"), I beg leave to state, that the sole object which I had in view, in undertaking the experimental investigation of animal magnetism, was to devise **a simple and satisfactory mode of demonstrating that the real cause of the phenomena manifested was subjective [i.e., psychological] or personal, and not objective, or the result of any magnetic fluid or force passing from the operator to the patient; and, as I succeeded by this attempt in producing all** the *ordinary* and *useful* phenomena, (useful in a curative point of view, I mean) more speedily and certainly than by the ordinary Mesmerising methods, whilst I never succeeded in producing clairvoyance and the higher phenomena, I thought it better to discuss the phenomena producible by my method under a new name, and adopted the term hypnotism, or nervous sleep.[53] By this means I hoped that hypnotism might be prosecuted quite independently of any bias or prejudice, either for or against the subject as connected with Mesmerism, and only by the facts which could be adduced. Like the originators of all new views, however, hypnotism has subjected me to much contention; for the sceptics, from not perceiving the difference between my method and that of the Mesmerists, and the limited extent of my pretentions, were equally hostile to hypnotism as they had been to Mesmerism; and the Mesmerists, thinking their craft was in danger – that their mystical idol was threatened to be shorn of some of its glory by the advent of a new rival – buckled on their armour, and soon proved that the *odium Mesmericum* ["hatred of the Mesmerists"] was as inveterate as the *odium theologicum* [the notorious (and ironic) hatred of rival theologians for one another]; for they seemed even more exasperated against me for my slight divergence from their dogmas, than would have been the case had I continued an entire sceptic, denying the whole as a mere juggle or imposture.[54]

[Review of Learned Journals' Reports on Hypnotism]

Notwithstanding all the opposition which I have had to contend against, however, I have persevered in my course, with firm determination to hold to that which I believed best and nearest the truth; and I shall now adduce a few quotations from our leading reviews and other sources, which will show the relative position in which the two theories or systems now stand, in the estimation of men in all respects well qualified to be arbiters in this scientific strife.

In a review of my work "On Trance", which appeared in the October number of *The Edinburgh Medical and Surgical Journal*, 1850, they say:–

> Some four years ago, Mr. Braid published a very ingenious treatise on what he denominates hypnotism; that is, a state of induced sleep, different from natural sleep. Mr. Braid rejects altogether the doctrine of what is called animal magnetism and Mesmerism, but he admits the facts such as they are observed to take place, and these he refers to the state to which he gives the name of hypnotism, or nervous sleep, by which he understands a peculiar condition of the nervous system, into which it may be thrown by artificial contrivance, and which differs, in several respects, from common sleep, or the waking condition.
>
>> Since the publication of that essay, Mr. Braid has been considering all those facts, and classes of facts, which might illustrate the doctrines therein proposed. – Page 421.
>
> Mr. Braid has also evinced great ingenuity in referring the alleged facts to a general principle. [...] His book deserves attentive perusal, both for the statements which it contains, and for the reasonings with which the author has connected them. – Page 443.

Then in *The British and Foreign Medico-Chirurgical Review* for October, 1851, which gives an elaborate and able article, embracing the whole speculations of animal magnetism, Mesmerism, hypnotism, the "od" force of Baron Reichenbach, and electro-biology, etc., the following passages occur in support of my views:–

> Although many of the phenomena are real, the 'od' force is imaginary, and the scientific basis altogether unsound. Animal magnetism presents to the medical practitioner a new means of investigating the functions of the brain and nervous system, and of elucidating their physiology, pathology, and therapeutics; and, therefore, the phenomena and alleged phenomena are most deserving the notice of the profession. [...]
>
>> We cannot omit this opportunity of congratulating Messrs. Braid, Bennett, and Wood upon their efforts to place Mesmerism and Mesmeric doings in their true position, in a way calculated to reach and enlighten the popular mind. – Page 383.
>
> It cannot be doubted that 'electro-biology' (that is, the power of suggestion, and expectation, and belief) is not only amply sufficient to show that *all* the phenomena described by Baron von Reichenbach as objective phenomena are really subjective, but that all the phenomena of animal magnetism belong to the same category. – Page 406.

---

[53] The original term which I had adopted was "Neuro-Hypnotism", but, for the sake of brevity, I proposed to omit the prefix "Neuro". My adopting the term 'hypnotism', therefore, could be no intended plagiarism.

[54] I could furnish ample proofs of the persecution and misrepresentation to which I have been subjected by the Mesmerists, but the following example shall suffice. In consequence of my *hypnotic heresy* and my honest endeavours to protect myself and hypnotism against the most unfair and wilful misrepresentation by a chief in the Mesmeric school [probably John Elliotson, editor of *The Zoist*], this gentleman, who, as well as his friends, had raised a mighty outcry against the cruelty and injustice, illiberality and persecution which the medical profession had manifested towards him, in consequence of his having adopted the Mesmeric notions and practice in some cases, carried his spleen and persecuting spirit against me to such a pitch, that he raised such determined opposition at head quarters as deprived me of an official appointment, which had been most kindly and voluntarily offered to be secured for me by the chairman of a public board; and which election, I have good reason to believe, would have been decided in my favour, but for the implacable opposition to me, for the above-named cause, of this illiberal vindictive, and persecuting Mesmeric Autocrat.

We ask Dr. Gregory [the English translator of Reichenbach and an advocate of magnetic theories], with ample reason for the inquiry, *why HE has not pointed out the striking similarity between 'electro-biological' and 'odylic' methods and phenomena*?

Yet a greater fault remains to be noticed. Mr. Braid had already, in 1846, demonstrated, in his essay, entitled 'The Power of the Mind over the Body', that the phenomena of the 'od' force, as described by von Reichenbach, *could be produced to any extent by suggestion alone*. Now, Dr. Gregory not only has omitted to notice the analogies referred to, and neglected to analyse and investigate those phenomena by the light which the experiments of Dr. Darling [a leading British electro-biologist] and others have thrown upon them, but has made no reference whatever to these conclusive experiments of Mr. Braid. In the 'Edinburgh Monthly Medical Journal' for June, 1851, Mr. Braid has published a very interesting paper on this subject, recalling attention to his researches, and restating the results of his experiments. We subjoin one or two illustrations; and first as to the 'od' power of magnets:–

> With nearly all the patients I have tried, many of whom had never been hypnotised or Mesmerised, when drawing the magnet or other objects slowly from the wrist to the points of the fingers, various effects were realised, such as a change of temperature, tingling, creeping, pricking, spasmodic twitching of muscles, catalepsy of the fingers or arms, or both; and reversing the motion was generally followed by a change of symptoms, from the altered current of ideas thereby suggested. Moreover, if any idea of what might be expected existed in the mind previously, or was suggested orally during the process, it was generally very speedily realised. The above patients being now requested to look aside, or a screen having been interposed, so as to prevent their seeing what was being done, and they were requested to describe their sensations during the repetition of the processes, similar phenomena were stated to be realised, even when there was nothing whatever done, beyond watching them and noting their responses.

Then as regards the odylic light and the aurora borealis [the "Northern Lights", a genuine optical illusion appearing in northerly skies, but falsely supposed to be the emanation of magnetic energy]:–

> A lady upwards of fifty-six years of age, in youth a somnambulist, but now in perfect health, and wide awake, having been taken into a dark closet, and desired to look at the poles of the powerful horse shoe magnet of nine elements, and describe what she saw, declared, after looking a considerable time, that she saw nothing. However, after I told her to look attentively, and she would see fire come out of it, she speedily saw sparks, and presently it seemed to her to burst forth, as she had witnessed an artificial representation of the volcano of Mount Vesuvius, at some public gardens. Without her knowledge, I closed down the lid of the trunk which contained the magnet, but still the same appearances were described as visible. By putting leading questions, and asking her to describe what she saw from *another* part of the closet (where there was nothing but bare walls), she went on describing various shades of most brilliant corruscations and flame, according to the leading questions I had put for the purpose of changing the fundamental ideas. On repeating the experiments, similar results were repeatedly realised by this patient. On taking this lady into the same closet after the magnet had been removed to another part of the house, she still perceived the same visible appearances of light and flame, when there was nothing but the bare walls to produce them; and two weeks after the magnet was removed, when she went into the closet by herself, the *mere association of ideas was sufficient* to cause her to realise a visible representation of the same light and flame. – Page 410-11

Mr. Braid details, in his essay just mentioned, a number of experiments like those made on persons in the waking state, to the complete overthrow of all the more important experiments and observations of von Reichenbach, and the extinction of the whole odylic philosophy based thereon, yet Dr. Gregory takes no notice whatever of them, so that he has neither experimented crucially himself nor noticed the crucial experiments of others. – Page 411.

It now only remains for us to draw the general conclusion, that the phenomena described by von Reichenbach and Dr. Gregory *afford no proof whatsoever of the existence of the new force*, and that, consequently, all the theories and hypotheses founded upon the assumed demonstration of its existence are altogether baseless. The phenomena themselves have long been recognised, more or less, by those physiologists and pathologists who have specially directed their researches to the nervous system; and although curious and interesting, they have never been thought inexplicable, provided *all the conditions* under which they occur be stated. Mr. Braid, Professor Simpson, Dr. Bennett, Dr. Wood, and others, who have carefully investigated the matter, all agree in this. Mr. Braid very justly observes […]

[Braid Cited as Critic of Pseudoscience in Medicine]

Here a quotation is given from my essay, **limiting the extent of phenomena which I have met with to those "in accordance with generally admitted physiological and psychological principles"**. The reviewer then adds:–

> Dr. Gregory, indeed, allows this, as it respects the greater proportion of the phenomena (as we have already seen), but, at the same time, he maintains that in those of clairvoyance there are a number of residual phenomena, to the explanation and classification of which modern neurology is unequal. Now, this conclusion

we not only altogether deny, but we assert that it is reached by the same unsatisfactory method by which Dr. Gregory has attained to other conclusions, palpably erroneous. – Page 412

The slightest consideration of this matter will excite the deep conviction that a duty has devolved on the medical profession which has hitherto been foreign to it. The medical practitioner must now be so fully acquainted with the physiology and pathology of the nervous system as not only to treat its diseases, but to demonstrate the origin of the popular delusions, which those diseases (when artificially excited) will (with the general circulation of the works before us) inevitably cause, even in the minds of otherwise highly-educated persons. He must be able to demonstrate the scientific and pseudo-scientific fallacies, and to assign good and sufficient reason for a large number of phenomena, that to the non-professional person appear nothing less than supernatural; he must be equally able to say when the practices by which those phenomena are produced are dangerous to the healthy action or the cerebrum; when beneficial to the cerebrum, if functionally or structurally diseased; when applicable to the alleviation of pain. The three essays last on our list (Wood's, Bennett's, and Braid's) have each their respective value for these ends, and will be useful to the practitioner. We here propose to add something to the views their writers have advanced, and to criticise others.

Mr. Braid has given the most useful index to the causation of these phenomena by his special inquiry into the physiology and pathology of *attention*. In looking at the methods by which that morbid condition of the cerebrum is produced, which Mr. Braid designates *hypnotism* (a term we propose to use generally, in place of the words Mesmerism, animal-magnetism, etc.), it is obvious that they all, without exception, are calculated to *excite the attention*. This point Mr. Braid has seized, and has expanded and elucidated views respecting the physiology of attention, and its influence on the cerebrum and system generally, which had been already advanced by several writers, but especially by Dr. Holland. The examination of the matter is, however, only cursory and superficial. Dr. Alexander Wood notes another point in the methods by which hypnotic phenomena are excited, namely, that the *volition* or will, of the individual is particularly brought into action; omitting, however, to consider the concurrent influence of attention. Dr. Bennett considers the influence of both the attention and the will but very generally. Dr. Mayo, we ought to add, now and then gets a glimpse of the true state of things, although, unfortunately, he quickly runs off after some will-o'-the-wisp of an 'od' force or Mesmeric influence. He can see the nature of the relations which attention bears to ordinary sleep; but when we hope he will carry out the analogy so as to illustrate the trance-sleep, he stops. The following passage regarding sleep is interesting – Page 416:

The attention alone slumbers; or, through some slight organic change, it is unlinked from the other faculties, and they are put out of gear. This is the basis of sleep. The faculties are all in their places; but the attention is off duty – itself asleep, or indolently keeping watch of time alone.

Each nerve having special endowments, and each portion of the encephalon its appropriate powers, the phenomena will vary according to the nerve upon which attention is concentrated, or the class of ideas which are suggested or attempted to be realised. – Page 424.

The group of diseases induced by hypnotism (for diseases they are in the same sense as any alteration of the normal action by medicine may be called so), is constituted of a well-marked class of cerebral affections, long known to pathologists. The novelty regarding the majority is, that they can be artificially produced; and regarding several, that they can be excited temporarily and evanescently by operating on the brain by means of the attention. This is a real and solid addition to the physiology and pathology of the nervous system. – Page 425.

As my article on "Electro-Biology" [1851] was written as the basis of a *conversazione* at the Manchester Royal Institution, I was compelled to compress my observations so that the whole could be read in little more than an hour, which will account for the subject of *attention* having been treated by me much more cursorily than its importance merited.[55] I have, therefore, great pleasure in referring the reader to the above very able article, from which I have made so many extracts, where he will find the author has gone into a minute analysis of the hypnotic phenomena, as well as of the normal phenomena of *attention*; and this he has done with so much ability, as will amply repay anyone for a careful perusal of what he has written on this curious and important subject.

The North British Review for May, 1851, contained a very able article on animal magnetism, in which the writer supported my views in the warmest manner, in preference to those of the Mesmerists; and he narrated the results of experiments, made by himself, which completely disposed of the self-deceiving "Odometer" of Dr. Mayo.

[Mesmerism Struggles to Exclude the Influence of Psychology]
In fact, in the whole of their experiments, the Mesmerists are never in a position to be able to prove that the expectant idea, or influence of habit, in the patient, may not be the *real* producing cause of the phenomena realised; because the crucial experiments of myself and others have satisfactorily demonstrated, that these subjective influences *alone* are quite adequate for their production, without any influence whatever passing to the subject from another person; whereas the Mesmerists *cannot* prove that these subjective influences are *not* in operation *during* the exercise of their Mesmeric processes.

---

[55] See appendix (originally a lengthy footnote) 'Experiments on Mesmerism at Aberdeen University'.

The *Critic* for the 1st November, 1850, in reviewing my work on "Trance", [*Observations on Trance*, 1850] says:–

> As Mr. Braid is rather opposed to the Mesmerists, whom he accuses of going too far, and asserting too much, our readers will feel the more confidence in the following statement of his experiences of the condition of patients in the Mesmeric sleep.

After a long quotation, describing the extraordinary exaltation of the senses of smell, touch, hearing, and the muscular sense, and the gift of phonic imitation, which enabled an uneducated girl to imitate [the world-renowned soprano] Jenny Lind in singing songs in Swiss, German, and Italian, catching the sound of both words and music, and imitating them so quickly, that it was scarcely possible to detect that both were singing, so perfectly did they accord in giving both words and music simultaneously as if each had previously been equally familiar with the songs, the reviewer adds:–

> Such statements are the more valuable, as coming from such a quarter. It is the testimony of one who has at least looked into the subject with an impartial eye. Some other cases collected in this volume are extremely interesting and curious, and will reward perusal by all who desire to unravel the mysteries of existence. – Page 526.

In like manner I could refer to many of the most scientific and able writers of the day, in support of my views. Amongst these, I have much gratification to know that Professors [William Pulteney] Alison [a highly distinguished professor of medicine and social reformer] and John Hughes Bennett [the father of medical physiology], men of world-wide reputation, are to be ranked. The latter gentleman has said in his published lectures, *vide* page 175:–

> In all these and various other cases which might be cited, it must be evident that the effect is produced by operating on the mind of the individual, and through that on his bodily powers. In short, predominant ideas, whether originating spontaneously, or suggested by the words and actions of others, seem to be the exciting cause in individuals affected with a peculiar condition of the cerebral functions. As regards the nature of this condition, it seems analogous to that of sleep or dreaming, in which certain faculties of the mind are active, and may be stimulated into excessive action, whilst others are suspended. Hence, it has been very appropriately called hypnotism by Mr. Braid. [...]
> The labours of Dr. Esdaile in India, and of Mr. Braid, of Manchester, exhibit a worthy commencement in the rational treatment of disorders by the means now alluded to; and there can be little doubt that in no long time its influence, when further studied, will be acknowledged.[56] – Page 178.

[Effect of Medicine Irreducible to Suggestion or Mesmerism Alone]

Having been constantly engaged in the study and practice of the medical profession for nearly forty years, I presume I ought to be as competent to express an opinion upon the matter referred to in the note below, as Mr. Colquhoun, whose chief study has been law, literature, and science. Under the terms "literature and science", I ought to include an intimate knowledge of the anatomy and physiology of the nervous system, which I understand Mr. Colquhoun has studied with great care and attention, and, consequently, must be intimately acquainted with. Moreover, having devoted a considerable share of his time and attention, for many years past, to the study of Mesmerism, with the aid of his splendid collection of books on that subject, he may safely be pronounced one of the best informed, as far as regards the literature of that science, of any magnetist in Europe. I am not aware, however, that Mr. Colquhoun has devoted so much attention as myself to the study of the therapeutic effects of medicines, therefore, I venture to say, whilst I most readily admit that the efficacy of medical treatment may be greatly aided by the peculiar manners, looks, and language of the person who prescribes the medicines, and the confidence engendered by these means in favour of his prescriptions, still, I feel assured that there is *a positive and obvious effect to be expected from some medicines, altogether irrespective of the physical or mental qualities and manners of the individual who prescribes them.*

Were I not thoroughly convinced of this, as a matter of course, I should consider it quite unnecessary for *me* to prescribe active medicines in *any* case; since it is alleged by the Mesmerists themselves that, by nature, I possess an unusually powerful *magnetic temperament*, and that it is through the influence of *this peculiar temperament* that I have been so successful in producing the hypnotic or Mesmeric state with my

---

[56] Whilst I have had the most satisfactory proof of the value of the hypnotic mode of treating some forms of disease, when it is judiciously applied, I repudiate the notion of holding it up as a panacea or universal remedy; or believing that the efficacy of medicines mainly depends upon "the peculiar idiosyncrasy, or magnetic temperament", of the prescriber, as alleged by Mr. Colquhoun, in the following extraordinary paragraph:– "For our own part, we are disposed to be of opinion that, in many cases of disease, much less of the ultimate effect depends upon the character of the medicines prescribed than upon the peculiar idiosyncrasy of the physician, who prescribes them. The magnetic temperament is of more efficacy in the cure of diseases than all the drugs enumerated and classified in our pharmacopoeias; and the magnetic method of cure is of far more general use in practice, in as much as it may be employed in, almost, all the diseases to which the animal frame is subject." – vol. II, page 226.

patients.[57] According to this theory (to which, however, I by no means subscribe) and Mr. Colquhoun's expressed opinion in the note above quoted, and the theory of other Mesmerists referred to by him at pages 292-3 of vol. I, the whole efficacy of the means used is attributable to the *magnetic temperament and the energetic Will and good intentions of the Mesmeriser or medical prescriber.* Mr. C. writes this at page 292-3, vol. I:–

> The magnetists hold it as a fundamental principle, that the intention of doing good is the very soul of their art. The verbal formulas (and passes and manipulations also, of course) are merely the accessories which ignorance, quackery, and superstition have elevated into real causes.

I say then, according to these theories of the Mesmerists, all which I ought to have occasion to do in any given case, in order to insure the recovery of my patient, would be merely to approach him and exercise my *will and good intentions in his behalf.* This assuredly would be making short work of it, and would save me a vast deal of mental labour, as well as pecuniary outlay, in devising, as well as procuring, the requisite medicines for my patients. It is well-known, however, that I use *hypnotism* ALONE *in a certain class of cases* ONLY, to which I consider it adapted; and that, in some other cases I use it in conjunction with medical treatment; but that *in the great majority of cases, I do not use hypnotism at all,* but depend entirely upon the efficacy of active medicines, which I prescribe in such doses as are calculated to produce sensible effects. I can honestly say that, whichever of these modes I am adopting in any given case, it is always done, not merely with the *will,* but also with the *earnest intention and desire,* for the speedy relief or recovery of my patient; still, notwithstanding all this, I am bound to admit that, with *neither* method, nor even with *all* these means combined, can I always succeed in curing some of my patients. Like other medical men, I have found that death will come at last, in defiance of all human efforts to oppose it; for it is the law of nature – man is born to die.

> "Nascentes morimur, finisque ab origine pendet."
> ["From the day of our birth we are dying, the end of life is appended to its beginning."
> – From Manilius' *Astronomica*]

[The "Placebo" Effect in Medicine]
Nevertheless, I feel convinced that with implicit faith, hope, and confidence on the part of the patient, many disorders may be recovered from, even whilst the patients are merely taking a drop of plain water occasionally, or a particle of bread, or *any other harmless substances,* which shall suffice as visible and tangible agents, to keep their minds involuntarily fixed on the idea that the innocent ingredients used are agents fraught with great virtues for effecting certain purposes. The stronger the intellect, the more certain are the results to be realised, provided the imagination is sufficiently brilliant, and the faith proportionately fervent, to fix the mind steadily on the confident and pleasing contemplation of the certainty of the cure. **Every strong mental impression produces a concussion [i.e., a powerful impact] on the centres of the nervous and circulating systems, and by thus changing physical action, in many instances, acts as an alterative [i.e., a medical drug]; but, whether for good or for evil to the individual, depends very much upon the character and persistency of the predominant idea. I believe that this is the real philosophical explanation of the temporary success of certain medicines and fanciful modes of treating some disorders – they rapidly rise in the estimation of a certain class of society, whilst novelty and ardent faith inspire their votaries; but, at length, having attained to the culminating point of their fame and favour, as they have no root in them, they speedily wane, to give place to some fresh novelty or nostrum [quack remedy].**

Still, all patients are not susceptible of being so influenced [Beecher (1955) famously calculated that 35% of subjects in placebo control groups respond on average], and hence the inefficient visible appliances, which, through fixed mental impression [i.e., suggestion], and giving time for nature to manifest her powers of conservation [i.e., "spontaneous remission"], prove successful with the former, would utterly fail with the latter and *larger* class. Nor is it wise in the former exceptional class to hazard their safety, in important cases, in such a frail bark, when they might, in addition to the influence of the mind and fixed attention, hope, and confidence, add thereto the certain aid of active medicines. Those who act in this manner are still more indiscreet than the other class, who content themselves with simply prescribing drugs, without paying the slightest attention to the management of the minds of their patients. **For my own part, it is always my endeavour to combine *both* agencies, so far as is consistent with truth and honour, and a sincere desire to benefit my patients.** I am aware that, in some cases, it might be possible to enhance the

---

[57] In proof of this, I may mention the following anecdote:– On calling, for the first time, on a chief in the Mesmeric ranks – one who applauds the speculations of Baron von Reichenbach to the echo, urging every Mesmerist to procure and read his work and who was willing to stand sponsor for it, having distinctly recorded that he felt that every word said by the Baron must be true, and that every one of the phenomena had been confirmed by his own experience years before, this gentleman told me he had read accounts of my doings and remarkable success in hypnotising patients. He then added, moreover, that, on reading the results of my experiments, he had attributed my success to the possession by me of an unusually powerful magnetic temperament; and that he had expressed himself sure that I had a large brain, a large, capacious chest, and great mental energy, i.e., that I possessed a determined *will.* He farther added, as a proof of his sagacity:– "And now that I see you, you are just the person I supposed, for you have them all." *I* attributed my success, however, to a very different, and less mystical or special cause.

effect and apparent importance of hypnotic processes, by involving them in mystery, and alleging that I could bring some occult or special influence into play, and thereby produce extraordinary effects; but, inasmuch as I entertain no belief in the existence and transmission from the operator to the patient of such an agency, I could not honestly do so; and I therefore prefer trusting to the simple explanation and modes of changing physical action already advanced by me, which are so much more susceptible of definite control, and are level to the comprehension of most men, and consequently are the more likely to secure the approbation of those who are not hopelessly enamoured by the love of the marvellous and transcendental. The advantages of combining moral [i.e., psychological] and medical means have been well expressed in the following remarks – the first paragraph by Professor Alison, the present eminent Professor of the Practice of Physic in the University of Edinburgh:–

> However minutely the physician may have examined the anatomy of the brain and nerves, and however accurately he may have noted the effects of injuries, these parts in experiments on animals and in observations on disease, still, unless *he has carefully considered and generalised the* MENTAL PART OF THE PROCESSES, *of which the brain, and nerves are the instruments,* HE HAS DONE BUT HALF HIS WORK. [...]
> The generality of medical men attach too exclusive an importance to the mere drug. They deal with people as if there were nothing psychical in them. If their diagnosis be correct, they write their prescriptions, and there is a stop to their operations. If part of the frame be diseased, there is no reason why the whole should not combine against the enemy. Faith saves physically as well as morally; and to lull the trembling mind to ease is to stay the heart's rapid pulsations, to allay the blood's fever, and to stop life in its quickening flight, with strengthened wings from the human tenement. – *Medical Times.*

[Imagination & Suggestion in Hypnotism & Mesmerism]
Many sceptics have endeavoured to throw discredit on the importance of hypnotic processes as a means of cure, by attributing the whole results to the power of *imagination*. They are willing to admit that certain effects are produced, and are content if they can only damage the importance of the facts, by associating them with what *they* consider a *bad name*. Their admission of the *facts*, however, is something; and we shall now devote a few moments to the consideration of the power of imagination over the physical organism of man. Those who suppose that the power of imagination is merely a mental emotion [i.e., purely subjective], which may vary to any extent without corresponding changes in the physical functions, labour under a mighty mistake. It is notorious to those who have carefully studied this curious subject, that imagination can either kill or cure; that many tricks have been played upon healthy persons, by several friends conspiring, in succession, to express themselves as surprised, or sorry, or shocked to see them looking so ill; and that very soon a visible change has come over the patients, and they have actually gone home and been confined there for days from bodily illness thus induced. Not only so, but there are even cases recorded, in which we have the best authority for the fact, where patients who were previously in perfect health, have actually died from the power of imagination, excited entirely through the suggestions of others. Nor are the suggestions by others of ideas of health, vigour, hope, and improved looks less influential with many people for restoring health and energy both of mind and body. Having such a mighty power to work with, then, the great desideratum [the primary goal] has been to devise the best means for regulating and controlling it, so as to render it subservient to our will for relieving and curing diseases. The modes devised, both by Mesmerists and hypnotists, for these ends, I consider to be a real, solid, and important addition to practical therapeutics; and not the less curious and important that it is done simply through appeals to the *immortal soul*, to assert and demonstrate its superiority and control over the *mortal body*.

The following remarks upon this subject, from the pen of that eminent philosopher, Dugald Stewart [a distinguished academic philosopher of the "Scottish School of Common Sense"], are interesting and important:–

> It appears to me, that the general conclusions established by Mesmer's practice, with respect to the physical effects of the principle of imagination (more particularly in cases where they co-operated together), are incomparably more curious than if he had actually demonstrated the existence of his boasted science: nor can I see any good reason why a physician, who admits the efficacy of the *moral* agents employed by Mesmer, should, in the exercise of his profession, scruple to copy whatever processes are necessary for subjecting them to his command, any more than that he should hesitate about employing a new physical agent, such as electricity or galvanism. – *Elements of the Philosophy of the Human Mind.*

[Hypnotic Treatment of Monomania]
The experiments in what has been so absurdly styled "electro-biology", lately exhibited publicly, fully demonstrated that, with some individuals, predominant ideas and fixed attention, whether arising spontaneously or from the suggestions of others, are sufficient, of themselves alone, even in the waking condition, to change physical action, and produce the expected results; whilst they also demonstrate the important fact, that, **through the influence of suggestion, existing predominant ideas may be removed, and *any other ideas whatever produced in their stead*, which the operator chooses to indicate by word, look, or gesture.** This at once points to an important practical fact, as regards the most

rational, simple, and successful mode of treating *monomania* – *viz.*, by engaging the mind of the patient so strongly on some *new* idea, as shall, as much as possible, withdraw it from the previously existing morbid delusion. By the temporary suspension of the morbid delusion thus effected, its activity and power become less and less enthralling, and the mind more and more capacitated for entertaining new and healthy trains of thought. In this manner, I have succeeded very speedily in curing several cases of monomania [a form of paranoid psychosis characterised by obsession] and delirium tremens [acute delirium due to withdrawal from alcohol or other drugs]. Of course, there are some cases which will not yield to this method; but, I believe that, in almost all cases of monomania in patients who pass into the second conscious state of hypnotism [characterised by spontaneous amnesia, also known as "artificial somnambulism"], a far more speedy cure may be calculated on by this mode of treatment than by any other.

[Intelligence & Concentration Required]
It is a curious fact, and tells strongly in support of my subjective [i.e., psychological] or personal mental theory, that, whilst many insane patients, particularly cases of monomania, may be readily enough hypnotised, I have never yet been able to affect an *idiot*. Where there was no mind capable of being aroused to an act of sustained, fixed attention, I have never succeeded in hypnotising the patient, although I have made many persevering attempts to do so. The following is also an important fact, bearing on the same point:– In the case of a patient, who was highly susceptible, and had been frequently hypnotised with decided benefit, on one occasion, when she was delirious from fever, and had not slept for several nights and days, as it was highly desirable to procure sleep for her without the administration of opiates, I made a persevering attempt, with the strongest desire on my own mind to put her to sleep; but it was all in vain – the mental chord of the patient was unstrung, and hence there was not the wonted harmonious response, even to *my most anxious and strenuous efforts*. Could a better proof than this be adduced, that success depended neither upon *my will* and *intentions, nor physical efforts*, but on the influence which could be produced by the *mind* of the patient over her *own* body?

The truth of all the above statements was demonstrated by my experiments, published in 1845, and still more extensively in 1846.[58]

In the *Psychological Journal* for July last, in a most able and acute article on "The Progress of Thought, or Electro-Biology", the following quotations from my writings with comments by the reviewer occur, in refutation of the doctrines of von Reichenbach:–

> "It is an undoubted fact," observes Mr. Braid, and *the profession will agree* with him, "that with many individuals, especially with the highly nervous, imaginative, and abstractive, a strong direction of inward consciousness to any part of the body – especially if attended with the expectation or belief of something being about to happen – is quite sufficient to change," or rather, we should say, to *modify* the physical action of that part, and produce such impressions from this cause alone as Baron Reichenbach attributes to the new force. – Page 357.

Then regarding the alleged odylic lights, and their different sizes and colours, as seen by different patients, the author comes to the same conclusions as myself, *viz.*:–

> That there would clearly not have been this discrepancy had there been a physical reality in the alleged flames and colour.

He then adds:

> All doubt on the subject is, however, set at rest by the fact, that, in several of Mr. Braid's experiments, when he deceived the patients by pretending to use a magnet, all the abnormal sensations were produced by the mere imagination of the patient; as in Dr. [John] Haygarth's case [who exposed Perkins' tractors as a placebo] – the key of his portmanteau [a doctor's holdall] – when the patient imagined it to be a magnet, produced effects as singular as if it had been endowed with the new imponderable magnetic force discovered by the Baron's patients.

---

[58] After the amount of evidence which has been furnished, both through the press and by public exhibitions, for anyone to deny the power of audible suggestion, sympathy, and imitation to affect *some* individuals irresistibly, according to the import of the words they have heard spoken, or the physical acts they have witnessed exhibited before them, no man with a candid and competent mind could deny the fact *after fair investigation*. The power of influencing patients at a distance, however, where they can neither see nor hear, in the common acceptation of these terms, the suggestions intended to be conveyed to them, is entirely a different affair, and it would require much clearer and more unexceptionable evidence to establish the existence of such a faculty than has yet come under my notice, either by reading or personal observation. The report of the Aberdeen committee, referred to [in the appendix], is a good illustration as to what value is to be attached to the *alleged facts* of less cautious and searching inquirers. I by no means wish to deny that the Almighty may cause an influx of ideas into the minds of men through spiritual agency; or that, on special occasions, and for important purposes, he may exhibit remarkable manifestations of a sort of inspiration – far exceeding the ordinary current of events – but, for my own part, I cannot, without indubitable evidence to the contrary, bring myself to believe that the Almighty Creator of the universe would condescend to confer such gifts, as alleged, upon a few individuals, for such paltry purposes as those for which they are generally represented as called into requisition.

[Braid's Stage Demonstration with Fourteen Subjects]
In like manner, my *mental* theory of explaining the cause of hypnotic phenomena has the unqualified support of this able writer, in preference to the special-influence theory; and he gives, as an example, the experiment tried by me before 800 people, when I invited strangers to come forward who had never submitted themselves to any Mesmerising process, of whom ten out of fourteen male adults were reduced to a state of sleep more or less profound – some even remembering nothing of what had happened during their sleep; and all this was accomplished simply by their gazing at inanimate objects, and the subjects fixing their attention as much as possible upon the simple act of looking attentively at the end of corks tied on their own heads, so as to project horn-ways from the middle of the forehead of each; and some others of the patients were desired to fix their gaze and attention on points of the gas apparatus, or other parts of the room by which means, all commencing the operation at the same time, ten of the fourteen [i.e., 71%] went to sleep, although I never touched any one of them until their eyelids had closed involuntarily. None of them seemed able to open their eyes; some became cataleptic, others were insensible of pain from the prick of a pin, and one or two [*c.* 10%] forgot all that had occurred. [Likewise, Braid states in *The Physiology of Fascination* (1855) that only 10% of his patients entered the double consciousness, or "somnambulistic", state characterised by full spontaneous amnesia.] Moreover, during these proceedings, three more of the audience threw themselves, of their own accord, and without my knowledge, into a state of profound sleep, by fixing their gaze and thoughts in the same way, upon other single points in the room. The reviewer, then, very justly remarks:–

> But supposing, instead of the piece of cork [used by Braid], a disc of zinc [used in electro-biology], or a common brass button were substituted, and the same attention to it enjoined, would it be at all wonderful if the same effect were produced? Certainly not. Nay, we can easily understand that, when the vision becomes confused and the mental faculties bewildered, erroneous impressions and illusions, ocular and aural, (and tactual, motorial, olfactive, and gustative, he might have added,) may easily be suggested.

In the numbers of *Fraser's Magazine* for June, 1844, and July, 1845, two very able articles appeared on the subject of "Animal Magnetism and Neuro-Hypnotism", from which essays I might make many quotations furnishing most important support to my views. I prefer, however, referring the reader to a careful perusal of the *entire articles*, where much will be found both to amuse and instruct him regarding the subjects brought under consideration. In my book on "Trance", at pages 38-9, I cited from these dissertations some remarks which, to me, appeared lucidly expressed, and were in exact accordance with my own convictions, as to the mode of explaining, upon natural or generally recognised principles, many results which, by the magnetists, are alleged as clairvoyant feats, or direct "intuitions of the soul", instead of being the results of a process of reasoning, regarding the natural relations of things, presented before the mind during their entranced state. Mr. Colquhoun took occasion, in his *Preface*, to animadvert upon the quotation referred to with far greater severity than, in my opinion, legitimate criticism warranted, on a careful consideration of the real import and obvious meaning of that part of the said articles which I thought so appropriately illustrated my views. Inasmuch as Mr. Sowler, barrister-at-law, is known to the public as the real author of these papers in *Fraser*, and many remarks have been made to the prejudice of that gentleman, in reference to the sharp castigation which Mr. Colquhoun had dealt out to the alleged *anonymous* author from whom I had quoted – I should be wanting in the duty which I owe to Mr. Sowler, as a scholar and a gentleman, and one who is well versed in the science of *hypnology*, and who had been drawn into the affray by my having quoted and announced him as the author of said articles in *Fraser* – he being, moreover, as well as Mr. Colquhoun, a personal friend of mine, of many years standing – were I not to afford him an opportunity of saying a word or two in vindication of himself (as I have done in my own behalf), by publishing the subjoined letter which he has addressed to me on the subject:

Clarkshill, Stand,
February 2nd, 1852.

My dear Braid,

I am very much obliged to you for affording me an opportunity of perusing Mr. Colquhoun's brace of volumes on "Magic, Witchcraft, and Animal Magnetism". I have read them with pleasure and profit as I always read everything from the pen of Mr. Colquhoun. He appears to me to have produced, out of his large and varied experience, in this particular branch of physiological and psychological investigation, a very valuable "History", that must be read with intense interest. The only part of the book to which I object is the *Preface*. You did me the honour, in the course of your very admirable "Observations on Trance", (a *big* book in a small compass), to refer to certain observations which I made in *Fraser's Magazine*, in June, 1844, and July, 1845, and to mention me by name as the author of those articles. This was a compliment to be appreciated, coming, as it did, from a "master" in the empire of psychological science, whose theories have been most triumphantly sustained in practice. You made some extracts from the articles in question, and proclaimed your assent to the principle and the reasoning therein contained. This appears to have given Mr. Colquhoun great offence. He thinks that I have not shown sufficient gallantry towards the *Pythoness* [the famed oracle of Apollo at ancient Delphi], and that I have treated her rather peculiar blandishments with undue contempt. I can only very deeply regret that her ladyship does not live in the days of Alexis [a young clairvoyant tested in The Medical Times] and Mr. Colquhoun; for I imagine, that, if she had been bodily amongst us, you and I *might* have been able to detect and rout her sorceries even if Mr. Colquhoun had been her first lieutenant. I regret deeply that Mr. Colquhoun has not given me an opportunity of replying to his attack upon me under my own name and by my own authority, for he has carefully avoided any mention of me by name – although you, in your book, had given my name, as the author of the obnoxious articles – and although he had written to me a very handsome letter on the subject of the first article, and inscribed to me a copy of his book, "*Isis Revelata*". I cannot imagine that "professional courtesy" has deterred our Edinburgh friend from addressing his strictures directly to me, because I do not see in what respect the subject he has taken so ably in hand is related either to the law or to private intercourse. Surely I may attack Mr. Colquhoun, or he may attack me, on an abstruse subject of curious investigation, without violating the rules of the one or the courtesies of the other! and my deliberate opinion is, that he has not treated either of us with that fairness and candour which his high character, as a scholar and a gentleman, entitled us to expect. However, I am glad to hear that *you* intend to answer him. I should have done so too if he had attacked me by name. I am prepared to do so whenever he shall think fit to transfer his strictures and his sneers from the shoulders of an *incognito* in *Fraser's* (not an *incognito* to *him*!) to the shoulders of the real "Simon Pure". Even a giant in this particular department is not entitled to play such tricks as he has played in his *Preface*; and that he is a giant I most loyally confess – reminding us of Homer's and Virgil's monster –

"Ουρανω εστηριξε χαρε, και επι Χθονι βαινει."
[The goddess Strife... raises her head to the Heaven while her feet tread upon the Earth.]

Iliad, iv, 443

"*Mox sese attollit in auras,*
"*Ingrediturque solo, et capit inter nubila condit.*"
[Rumour... soon she lifts into the air, on the ground she goes, and hides her head among the clouds."]

Aeneid, iv., 177.

I give you leave to make what use of this note you may think fit. I hope to receive an early copy of your reply to "Magic, Witchcraft, and Animal Magnetism".

    Believe me, my dear Braid,
        Ever yours faithfully,

    ROBERT S. SOWLER.

To James Braid, Esq., *etc., etc.*,
    Burlington House.

["Divination" by Intensified Perception & Reasoning]

No man knows better than Mr. Colquhoun that the ancients believed in *two* modes of divination – one "by means of the intellect, the other by inspiration"; for, in vol. I., page 50, he has referred to Plato, and Cicero, and the Stoics, in proof of this, as the following quotation will show:–

> Plato, in his *Phaedrus*, as is well-known, distinguishes two modes of divination – the one by means of the intellect, the other by inspiration. Cicero mentions that the Stoics also assume two modes of the exercise of this faculty: *unum (genus) quod particeps erat artis, alterum quod arte careret* [one kind requires skill, and the other lacks art] the former derived from observation of the present, and a conjecture founded upon this observation, in regard to the future; the latter being produced solely by a peculiar exaltation of the mind, or spiritual faculties, to a *presentiment* of futurity: i.e., either a conclusion drawn from given premises, or an immediate intuition of the soul, without any assistance from the reasoning faculties. The latter – the immediate intuition of the future – was the most highly appreciated by the ancients, as the most pure and infallible – the more immediate and more precious gift of the gods. *Carent autem arte ii*, says Cicero, *qui non ratione aut conjectura, observatis ac notatis signis, sed concitatione quadam animi, aut soluto liberoque motu futura praesentiunt.* ['Those diviners employ art, who, having learned the known by observation, seek the unknown by deduction. On the other hand those do without art who, unaided by reason or deduction or by signs which have been observed and recorded, forecast the future while under the influence of mental excitement, or of some free and unrestrained emotion.' Cicero, *On Divination*, Book One, §18]

Now Mr. Sowler was cited by me, because he had so well expressed opinions which I had long avowed, and *still believe to be true* – *viz*., that the *whole* of the really striking achievements of Mesmeric clairvoyants –

which were not simply occasional coincidences and shrewd guesses – were merely results of concentrated attention, quickened memory, exaltation of the natural organs of special sense, with self-confidence, and accurate deductions as to what might be calculated upon regarding the future, from contemplation of the circumstances in the existing case, compared with what was known from past experience. *We* believe that the whole is derived from observation of the past and present, and that all regarding the future – and what of the present is not cognisant to the quickened organs of special sense – is mere conjecture, founded upon these observations, from a process of reasoning – in fine, that they are conclusions drawn from given premises, when contemplated with a quickness of perception, conception, and memory, and with a force of reason, unknown to us during the ordinary diffused, and distracted, or ever varying state of our attention during the ordinary waking condition. Mr. Colquhoun, however, and the magnetists generally, who contend for clairvoyance and the higher phenomena of Mesmerism, seem to wish us to infer that these achievements are accomplished by a sort of inspiration – or through "an immediate intuition of the soul, without any assistance from the reasoning faculties". Having thus endeavoured to set both views fairly before the public – for I wish, as far as possible, to do full justice to Mr. Colquhoun and all who coincide with him – I leave it to my readers to decide which theory is more likely to be true.

[Dr. J.J.G. Wilkinson's Account of Braid's Work]
That eminent philosopher, Sir David Brewster [a distinguished Scottish scientist], has expressed his *entire* concurrence with the explanation given by me of the phenomena of "electro-biology". Sir David also informed me, in confirmation of the correctness of my views, that he had lately had occasion to talk over the subject with Sir Benjamin Brodie and an eminent London physician, both of whom most willingly admitted the wonderful power of fixed mental attention in changing physical action in some abnormal conditions of the nervous system. This is entirely in accordance with my views, as stated at page 10. Mr. James John Garth Wilkinson [a doctor and popular writer who had been hypnotised by Braid], in his interesting book, "The Human Body", after giving certain details, adds:–

> We presume it is evident to the reader what a power Mr. Braid has methodised and called into play for the treatment of disease. As a curative agent, hypnotism contains two elements, each valuable in its kind:– 1. Where it produces trance, it has the benefits of the Mesmeric sleep, or furnishes so strong a dose of rest, that many cases are cured by that alone. But 2. The suggestion of ideas of health, tone, duty, hope, which produce dreams influential upon the organisation, enables the operator by this means to fulfil the indication of directly ministering to that mind diseased, which always accompanies and aggravates physical disorders. We have a direct proof of the continuation of the mind through the body, in the way in which suggestions, directed to the mind, respecting the organs, operate upon the latter. In the hypnotic state, the operator can play upon the emotions by a variety of suggestive means, and in this way give power to impotent parts, and hand them over to the will. Mr. Braid's devices for these ends stamp him as a man of inventive genius; and we are surprised that such a piece of combined intellectual and scientific sagacity as hypnotism has not placed him, long ago, in the first rank of metropolitan physicians. The virtue of hypnotism, where it succeeds, is just this, that for the moment it unweeds the human soil so completely, that whatever faith is impressed can work and grow. We regard hypnotism as the most intellectual phenomenon which has yet been produced by the *phrenopathists* [Wilkinson's term for mind-body therapists in general]. – Pages 476-80.

Without at all wishing to arrogate to myself that I deserve the amount of approbation and praise Mr. Wilkinson has here accorded to me, still, I have quoted these remarks with those of others, as a set off against the observations respecting the prospects of hypnotism which Mr. Colquhoun had presented to my consideration, in the passages of his *Preface*, pages 36-7, above referred to.[59] Regarding Mr. Wilkinson, however, I may observe that he possesses a mind of the *very highest order*, and was, therefore, peculiarly fitted for dealing successfully with the *psychological* part of the question. Another circumstance which gives so much greater value to his opinions is his *practical* experience of *hypnotism* in his *own person as well as in others*. Mr. W. not only carefully watched many cases when operated upon by me, and has continued ever since to practise the art when suitable, but he also submitted himself to me several times to be hypnotised; and, as he is one of those who remember when awake all which occurs during the condition, he was enabled to describe, with the greater accuracy, not only what he *saw* but also what he *felt*.

[Prof. William Carpenter's Account of Braid's Work]
Mr. Wilkinson is the gentleman [Braid's hypnotic subject] to whom reference is made in the following remarks

---

[59] I cannot deny myself the pleasure, and Mr. Colquhoun the justice, of publicly acknowledging that gentleman's great liberality and kindness to me on all former occasions, and of thanking him for the respectful terms in which he alluded to my labours in what he terms "the magnetic mine", both in his works and his private correspondence – which latter has been most interesting to me. I have also to thank him for presentation copies of all his valuable and highly interesting works, including his lately published "History of Magic, Witchcraft, and Animal Magnetism", which was heralded by a very kind letter from the author, received some time before the arrival of the book, in which he intimated to me that, in his Preface, he had made some strictures on my "Observations", which he hoped I would take *good-naturedly*. There are few men to whom I should be disposed, *good-naturedly*, to submit so much as to Mr. Colquhoun, for reasons already stated at page 8; still, the nature of the charge in which I was implicated – unintentionally or inadvertently, probably, on his part – was of such a grave character, that justice to myself, to my family, and friends, compelled me to endeavour to refute it as publicly as it had been diffused by its publication in the work of a gentleman of the high position, and great talents and attainments, of the ingenious and learned author of "*Isis Revelata*".

by Dr. Carpenter, the eminent physiologist (Examiner in Physiology and Professor of Medical Jurisprudence, in University College, London), in his article on sleep, in the "Encyclopaedia of Anatomy and Physiology". After describing my experiments and confirming my views on *various* points, Dr. Carpenter adds:–

> It is one of the most curious and important of Mr. Braid's discoveries, that the suggestions conveyed through the muscular sense are among the most potent of any in determining the current of thought. Not only have we witnessed all these effects repeatedly produced upon numerous 'hypnotised' subjects, but we have been assured by an intelligent friend, who has paid special attention to the psychological part of this inquiry, that having subjected himself to Mr. Braid's manipulations, and being only partially thrown into the 'hypnotic' state, he distinctly remembers everything that was done, and can retrace the uncontrollable effect upon his state of mind, which was produced by this management of his muscular apparatus.

Dr. Carpenter gives his testimony still farther in favour of hypnotism thus:–

> We consider that the experimental researches of Mr. Braid throw more light than has been derived from any other source upon the phenomena of *Mesmerism*. That there is much of reality mixed up with much imposture in these phenomena is a conclusion to which most candid persons have arrived who have given their attention to them; and we have little doubt that a searching investigation, carried on under the guidance of his results, would lead to something like a correct discrimination between the two.

[Braid Defines Hypnotism]

With such testimony in support of my views, I feel no great anxiety for the fate of *Hypnotism*, provided it only has "a fair field and no favour". I am content to bide my time, in the firm conviction that truth, for which alone I most earnestly strive, with the discovery of the safest, and surest, and speediest modes of relieving human suffering, will ultimately triumph over error.

I feel pretty confident that whoever will undertake the investigation of hypnotic phenomena with a candid mind, and untrammelled by any previous prejudices in favour of the mystical and transcendental, may very soon satisfy himself that **the real origin and essence of the hypnotic condition, is the induction of a habit of abstraction or mental concentration, in which, as in reverie or spontaneous abstraction, the powers of the mind are so much engrossed with a single idea or train of thought, as, for the nonce, to render the individual unconscious of, or indifferently conscious to, all other ideas, impressions, or trains of thought. The** *hypnotic* **sleep, therefore, is the very antithesis or opposite mental and physical condition to that which precedes and accompanies** *common sleep***; for the latter arises from a diffusive state of mind, or complete loss of power of fixing the attention, with suspension of voluntary power.**

> The attention alone slumbers; or, through some slight organic change, it is unlinked from the other faculties, and they are put out of gear. This is the basis of sleep. The faculties are all in their places; but the attention is off duty – itself asleep, or indolently keeping watch of time alone. – Dr. Mayo.

The following remarks, from the pen of Mr. J. J. G. Wilkinson, are interesting, as well as elegantly and lucidly expressed:–

> The atom of sleep is diffusion; the mind and body are dissolved in unconsciousness; they go off into nothing, through the fine powder of infinite variety, and die of no attention; common sleep is impersonal. The unit of hypnotism is intense attention, abstraction – the personal *ego* pushed to nonentity. The unit of Mesmerism is the common state of the patient, caught as he stands, and subjected to the radiant ideas of another person; it is mediate – or both personal and impersonal. Patients can produce the hypnotic state upon themselves, without a second party; although a second will often strengthen the result by his acts or presence, just as one who stood by and told you that you were to succeed in a certain work would nerve your arm with fresh confidence.

The state of mental concentration, however, which is the basis of the hypnotic sleep, enables the subject to exhibit various passive or active manifestations, such as insensibility or exalted sensibility, rigidity or agility, and entire prostration or inordinate energy of physical power, according to the trains of ideas and motives which may arise spontaneously in his mind, or be addressed to it by others, through impressions on his physical organs.

> The preliminary state (of hypnotism) is that of abstraction, and this abstraction is the logical premise of what follows. Abstraction tends to become more and more abstract, narrower and narrower; it tends to unity, and afterwards to nullity. There, then, the patient is, at the summit of attention, with no object left – a mere statue of attention – a listening, expectant life – a perfectly undistracted faculty, dreaming of a lessening and lessening mathematical point, the end of his mind sharpened away to nothing. What happens? Any sensation that appeals is met by this brilliant attention, and receives its diamond glare, being perceived with a force of leisure of which our distracted life affords only the rudiments. External influences are sensated, sympathized with, to an extraordinary degree, harmonious music sways the body into graces the most affecting; discords jar it as though they would tear it limb from limb; cold and heat are perceived with equal exultation, so also smells and

touches. In short, the whole man appears to be given to each perception, the body trembles like down with the wafts of the atmosphere, the world plays upon it as upon a spiritual instrument finely attuned. – Wilkinson.

[Different Stages of Hypnosis]
The above is a beautiful description painted in elegant and most felicitous language, of the phenomena manifested by a *certain class of patients*, and *at a certain stage of the sleep*; but **at another stage the very opposite state manifests itself: for the abstraction may be so intense as to render the patient unconscious even of inflictions the most severe; and the muscles may be locked in immovable, cataleptic rigidity, or dissolved in the most entire passive flaccidity according to predominant ideas or impressions on the senses, which immediately preceded the full intensity of the all-absorbing abstraction.**

As is the case in reverie or abstraction, so also is it in the hypnotic state – there are *different degrees* of mental concentration; so that from some of them, the patient may be aroused by the slightest impression – whilst in other stages, he can only be influenced by very powerful impressions on the organs of sense. Moreover, in the hypnotic condition, as in the state of reverie or abstraction, the subject may be so partially engrossed in his train of thought as to be susceptible of receiving suggestions from others – through words spoken or movements made in his presence – which shall involuntarily or unconsciously change his current of thought and action, without entirely dissipating his condition of mental abstraction.

[Braid's Hypnotic Induction Technique]
My usual mode of inducing the sleep is to hold any small bright object about ten or twelve inches above the middle of the forehead, so as to require a slight exertion of the attention to enable the patient to maintain a steady, fixed gaze on the object; the subject being either comfortably seated or standing, stillness being enjoined, and the patient requested to engage his attention, as much as possible, on the simple act of looking at the object, and yield to the tendency to sleep which will steal over him during this apparently simple process. I generally use my lancet case, held between the thumb and first two fingers of the left hand; but any other small bright object will answer the purpose. In the course of about three or four minutes, if the eyelids do not close of themselves, the first two fingers of the right hand, extended and a little separated, may be quickly, or with a tremulous motion, carried towards the eyes, so as to cause the patient involuntarily to close the eyelids, which, if he is highly susceptible, will either remain rigidly closed [a phenomenon now termed "eyelid catalepsy"], or assume a vibratory motion – the eyes being turned up, with, in the latter case, a little of the white of the eyes visible through the partially closed lids. If the patient is not highly susceptible, he will open his eyes, in which case request him to gaze at the object, *etc.*, as at first; and, if they do not remain closed after a second trial, desire him to allow them to remain shut after you have closed them, and then endeavour to fix his attention on muscular effort, by elevating the arms if standing, or both arms and legs if seated, which must be done quietly, as if you wished to suggest the idea of muscular action without breaking the abstraction, or concentrative state of mind, the induction of which is the real origin and essence of all which follows.[60]

[Effect of Imagination, Belief, & Habit]
There is great difference in the susceptibility to the hypnotic impression, some becoming rapidly and intensely affected, others slowly and feebly so. Moreover, those who are naturally highly susceptible, at length become so much so as to be liable to be affected entirely through the power of imagination, belief, and habit, *i.e.*, the expectant idea will produce it in such subjects when no process whatever, either near or distant, is going forward; whereas if they are made to believe the contrary, through the requisite attention and expectation being otherwise engaged they may not become affected by processes which would naturally throw them into the sleep.

[Suggestive Effect of Sympathy & Imitation]
Whatever mode is adopted for producing sleep at first trials, whether my usual mode just described, which is the most speedy and most generally successful method, or that of causing the patients to look steadily and attentively at fixed points, or the ordinary Mesmerising processes may have been resorted to, **there can be no doubt of the fact that they will be rendered much more efficient by previously affording the patients an opportunity of watching others when submitted to the processes.** The influence of

---

[60] My first experiments were devised for the purpose of proving the fallacy of the magnetic theory – of the phenomena of the sleep depending upon the transmission from the operator to the patient of some peculiar influence during his processes of thumbing and staring, pointing with his fingers at the eyes of the patient, or making passes near to his person. By causing patients to produce the sleep on themselves, by maintaining a steady, fixed gaze at any inanimate object, it appeared to me that this was clearly demonstrated; for not only were single individuals thus thrown into the sleep, at first trials, but, on one occasion, before eight hundred people, out of fourteen male adults, ten were so affected – all commencing at the same time to fix their thoughts and sight, some upon corks, bound so as to project from their own foreheads, others by looking at fixed points in the room. Within ten minutes, the eyelids of ten of these subjects became involuntarily closed; some remained conscious, some were cataleptic, others insensible to pain from the prick of a pin, and some forgot all which had occurred during their sleep. Three more of the audience sent themselves to sleep, unknown to me, by the same process of fixed gazing at points in the room. – *Vide* Pages 10 and 45.

sympathy and imitation are thus brought into play, and increase the susceptibility in a marked degree. Of this fact I have had many striking proofs. Where patients exhibit considerable resistance, therefore, it is always desirable to bring the power of sympathy and imitation to bear upon them, as well as the influence of direct auricular suggestion and expectation, excited by the confident tone and deportment in the operator so as to inspire them, as far as possible, with the conviction that the influence cannot be resisted.

I am satisfied that all the Mesmerising processes produce their effects from what is essentially the same exciting cause as that which induces hypnotic phenomena, *viz.*, by producing a state of mental concentration, through the attention becoming so exercised by watching the manoeuvres or suggestions of the operator, as, for the nonce, to render the subject dead or indifferent to all other sensible impressions or trains of thought.[61]

[Suggestive Effect of Voice Tonality]

In this condition the whole attention of the subject is given to every existing or suggested idea; and thus it works wonders in changing or modifying the existing condition of the physical frame. Moreover, suggestions may be given either through words spoken or sensible impressions made on any of the organs of special sense – for the mind is naturally drawn to the part signified or impressed, and thus ideas are excited, connected with, or corresponding to, the function of that organ or part; and the appeal being made to the mind at the very summit of its abstraction, every sensation is met by **the "diamond glare" of this "brilliant attention"**; and consequently is "perceived with a force of leisure of which our distracted life affords only the rudiments. External influences are sensated, sympathised with to an extraordinary degree". In this stage of the sleep the power of suggestion on the patient is excessive. **Whatever idea is suggested to his mind, whether by the natural import of the words spoken, or modified by the tone of voice in which they are uttered, is instantly seized upon by the subject and interpreted in a manner to surprise many, and lead them to believe it has been accomplished by a sort of intuition or inspiration. In this way you may vary or modify the ideas suggested in the most remarkable manner, and the patient sees, and feels, and speaks of all as real, without the slightest desire to impose upon others.** Thus, if you say,–

> "What animal is it?" The patient will tell you it is a lamb, or a rabbit, or any other animal or thing. Does he see it? "Yes." What animal is it *now?*' – putting depth and gloom into the tone *now*, and thereby suggesting a difference. "Oh!" with a shudder, "it is a wolf." "What colour is it?" – still glooming the phrase. "Black." "What colour is it *now?*" – giving the *now* a cheerful air. "Oh! A beautiful blue," spoken with the utmost delight. And so you lead the subject through any dreams you please, by variation of questions and of inflections of voice, and he sees and feels all as real.
>
> Another curious study is the influence of the patient's postures on his mind in this state. Whatever posture of any passion is induced, the passion comes into it at once, as well as into the mind, and dramatises the whole body.
>
> Moreover, the patient's mind, directed to his own body, does physical marvels: he can do, in a manner, what he thinks he can. Place a handkerchief on a table, and beg him to try to lift it – observing, however, that you know it to be impossible – and he will groan and sweat over the cambric as though it were the anchor of a man-of-war. On the other hand, tell him that a fifty-six-pound weight is a light cork, to be held out at arm's length on his little finger, and he will hold it out with ease. Tell him that a tumour on his body is about to disappear, and his mind will often realise your prophecy.
>
> A patient in the full state obeys all motives in the most natural direction. If the arm is placed up, there it will stay; but a waft of air will cause it to fall down. Why? Because it is already up, but the new motive changes the direction. If the arm be down, another waft or touch will raise it. If down, and prevented from moving up, the impression will send it sideways. When the frame is erect, a touch behind the bend of the knees will send it into genuflexion, which will at once suggest prayer, as noticed before, etc. [Wilkinson, *The Human Body*]

The last four paragraphs are all but verbatim quotations from Mr. J. J. G. Wilkinson's interesting book, "The Human Body", as descriptive of what he saw manifested in some of my hypnotised patients, as illustrations

---

[61] The ordinary magnetising processes are very numerous. Those most commonly resorted to are – laying hold of the patient's hand after he has been comfortably seated in an easy-chair, or of the two hands, or the thumbs – the operator and patient maintaining a steady, fixed gaze into the eyes of each other until the eyes of the patient become dim, the sight confused, and the eyelids drooping. When this period arrives the two first fingers of the right hand, extended and held a little apart, are darted towards the eyes; and, when they have closed, the operator commences making passes – that is, he draws one or both hands slowly, and with a tremulous motion, over the head, face, chest, or upper extremities, or even over the legs also. They may be near to, but not touching the body; or they may be gently pressed on the body; in which latter case they are called contact passes. Or the patient and operator may simply stare into each other's eyes until the tendency to close the eyes supervenes; or he may desire the patient to look steadily at the operator's fingers; pointed at his eyes; or he may simply make passes with the fingers drawn slowly from the head down before the face, or behind his back; or this may be done whilst the left hand is held on the patient's head. The patient is to be a consenting party, or, as much as possible, to remain passive, which greatly aids the result – the operator concentrating his energies and will, apparently with great determination to produce the effects. So soon as sleep manifests itself, the passes are resorted to; and when the passes are made, whilst the patient remains awake, they are still considered, by the magnetists, to be influential on the patient by the transmission to him, from the body of the operator of the exuberant life, nervous or odylic influence, so as to modify and sustain the deficient vitality or morbid condition of the patient. My mode of explaining the influence of passes is set forth at pages 10 and 61-2; to which I beg to refer my readers. By calling muscles into play by elevating the limbs, or touching, or tickling, or making sensible impressions upon the integuments over them, by passes or otherwise, they become rigid or cataleptic – then the circulation becomes quickened in a ratio corresponding to the class and number of muscles so affected; and the intensity of the rigidity or the cataleptic condition can generally be more readily produced, at first trials, when the hypnotising methods are adopted than when they are acted on in the less active state of mental concentration which results from the ordinary Mesmerising processes.

of what I had told him could be exhibited according to the theoretical views which I had propounded to him.

[Suggestive Effect of Mesmeric Hand Passes]
From all this it may readily be perceived that the efficacy or influence of Mesmeric passes and touches – of the *tractim tangere* of the Romans [healers employed to stroke the body from head to foot with their hands] – does not arise from any special influence or virtue passing from one human being to another; but that they act merely as sensible impressions, assisting the patient in concentrating or drawing the mental attention vividly *to* parts, and thus increasing their action beyond the natural activity of their functions, or diffusing or withdrawing it *from* certain parts, and thus diminishing the natural activity of function of such organs or parts from which the attention has been withdrawn. Curiously enough however, these results, which should naturally be calculated on to arise according as I have here stated, may each and all of them be modified or subverted by a spontaneous or suggested *predominant idea*; so that the result shall be in accordance therewith, rather than with what otherwise would be the natural or spontaneous result. **The instinctive feeling which everyone has to rub any part which has sustained a blow or other injury and by which the pain is moderated, does not produce its soothing or salutary influence from any special virtue imparted to the injured parts from the hand, either of the patient or other party who rubs it, but from making a sensible impression on an *extended* surface, and thus *diffusing or withdrawing the attention FROM the injured point*. Such is my mode of explaining the efficacy of the *tractim tangere*, or gentle rubbing, or touching with the human hand.** To quote from a former publication of my own on this subject:–

> That there is nothing occult or specific in the pass with the hand, is manifest from this, that a similar agitation of the air by the blast from a pair of bellows will produce precisely similar results as the like current of air from the wafting of the human hand, as I have proved to the satisfaction of hundreds of intelligent individuals.
>
> A pass, therefore, as a visible or sensible impression, aids the patient in concentrating his mental attention to a given organ or part, and thus influences the function, through giving a special direction to a power residing within the patient's own frame, but it no more imparts a virtue of an occult nature from the operator to the patient, than the lens produces the light and heat which it makes visible and perceptible to the senses, through concentrating the luminous and calorific rays of the sun, and drawing them to a focus. Both the pass and the lens aid in concentrating and manifesting the respective influences; but neither the operator nor the lens is the source or origin of the power or influence so manifested.

[Positive & Negative Effects of Suggestion]
It is quite possible, however, to subvert the whole of these *natural* suggestions, by a system of training such as by speaking aloud in the hearing of the patients, and in a language known to them, the idea you wish to make predominant in their minds, by suggestions associated with certain sensible impressions. The associations once formed will always thereafter come up and be predominant, whenever the like sensible impressions are made. Whatever faith is imprinted, at the proper stage of the sleep, will work and grow, either for good or for evil to the subject, and will be recalled to mind, in the most susceptible, as mere acts of memory (according to the law of double consciousness), when in that stage of the sleep subsequently. **And in this way, also, some patients having predicted that certain effects will be manifested in their persons, at a certain time specified, the predominant idea will often realise the prophecy. [Braid here, as elsewhere, recognises the possible role of *negative autosuggestion* in causing problems such as neurosis or psychosomatic illness.]**

[Tranquilising versus Stimulating Forms of Hypnotism]
If tranquilising is the object in view, let the patient remain in a recumbent and easy posture, with all the muscles relaxed to the utmost, and let the mind he sustained by encouraging expressions, and such as shall withdraw attention *from* the part most requiring to be tranquilised. If stimulation is required, then the limbs must be extended, and they will speedily pass into a rigid state, during which the circulation and respiration become much quickened, and by directing the patient's attention and expectation to any organ of sense, its function will naturally be quickened; and so of the function of any other organ or part of the body. Still, even in the state of excitement of the circulation and respiration, a suggested idea may be made so completely to engross the patient's attention, as to subvert results which ought to have followed, and would have followed, but for this all-absorbing suggested idea.[62] The first point to be determined, therefore, in this hypnotic mode of treating suitable cases, is the same as is required in any other mode of treatment – *viz*., to endeavour, by careful examination, to ascertain what is the real nature and cause of the existing symptoms, and whether they require stimulating or depressing [i.e., tranquilising] measures to be adopted, locally or generally; and to what extent, in either direction, the excitement or depression ought to be carried. It is also requisite

---

[62] [Here, as elsewhere, Braid describes the induction, for different therapeutic purposes, of two opposing hypnotic states: stimulating and tranquilising, or cataleptic and somnambulistic.]

in order to determine this to make out whether the disease is of an acute or chronic character; for, in such cases, not only have we *similar* symptoms arising from *different* causes, but they can only be successfully treated by the very opposite modes of acting. It must, therefore, be obvious, to any sensible person, that the superintendence and direction of medical men are as requisite for conducting the hypnotic mode of treating disease, with anything like precision and general success, and adapting it in the best manner to each individual case, as for treating them by ordinary medical means. Not but that those ignorant of medical science could be made to stimulate or depress locally or generally, according to the methods which I have devised for that purpose, when they had been instructed *how* and to *what* extent they were to conduct the processes *in each individual case*, under the superintendence and direction of some skilful medical man, who understands the hypnotic system, the pathology of the disease, and the therapeutic indications to be fulfilled. Until a number of assistants have been provided, who could be employed by medical men to act under them in this manner, I have no hope of the hypnotic mode of treatment having a fair trial; because it takes up *too much time* for medical men in general to adopt it, even in suitable cases, when they must operate personally; and, for those ignorant of medical science to do so, without professional superintendence is a mere haphazard mode of procedure, which never can be expected to become so successful as it might be, when conducted on scientific principles. This is one of the very reasons why I have ventured to say that when skilfully conducted, hypnotism is capable of producing *all* the *good* to be effected by the *ordinary Mesmerising processes*, and *much more*; and the other is that they have so much reliance upon the efficacy of their alleged magnetic or odylic influence, that they overlook the important effects, and the certainty of their production, which are attainable by **regulating the state of the circulation in the various modes which I have methodised, through the influence of the muscular system and management of the minds of the patients, effected by sensible impressions and auricular suggestions.**

[The Waking, Partial & Full Hypnotic States]

These various modes of suggestion are most successful when resorted to with patients who pass into the full or double conscious stage of the sleep; but they influence all, to a greater or lesser extent, who submit themselves honestly and fairly to the processes for **inducing a state of mental concentration, whether they remain with their eyes wide open, or have their eyes involuntarily closed, but retain their consciousness, and remember, on awaking, all that was said or done; or pass into the double conscious stage of the sleep.** By the latter term, I should observe, is meant, a condition in which they, forget, on awaking all which was done or said during the sleep, but which they will have a perfect recollection of when they pass into the sleep again. I have had striking instances of this in most respectable and intelligent patients, who have a minute recollection of what took place during the sleep six years ago, and have remembered and described the same facts many times since, when hypnotised, but who have never had the slightest recollection of the subject, when awake, during these six years.

The most curious and important fact of all, however, is this – that by engendering a state of mental concentration, by a simple act of sustained attention, fixed upon some unexciting and empty thing – "for poverty of object engenders abstraction" – the faculties of the minds of some patients are thereby thrown out of gear, (*i.e.*, their ordinary relations are changed) so that the higher faculties – reason, comparison, and will, become dethroned from their supremacy, and give place and power to imagination (which now careers in unbridled liberty), easy credulity, and docility or passive obedience; so that, **even whilst apparently wide awake, and conscious of all around**, they become susceptible of being influenced and controlled entirely by the suggestions of others, upon whom their attention is fixed. In fact, such subjects are in a **sub-hypnotic condition** – in that intermediate state between sleeping and waking, when the mind becomes wavering, the attention off duty, or engrossed with a predominant idea, so that, in reality, the subjects are only half conscious of what is passing around; and their minds, therefore, become **easily imposed upon by any suggestion, audibly expressed or visibly exhibited before them.** Thus they may be made to perceive and mistake for realities, whatever mental illusions or ideas are suggested to them. In common parlance they *see* and *feel* AS REAL, and they consider themselves *irresistibly* or *involuntarily fixed, or spell-bound, or impelled to perform whatever may be said or signified by the other party upon whom their attention has become involuntarily and vividly riveted* until a new idea has been suggested, by which the spell is broken, and the subject is left in a condition again to be subjugated and controlled by other suggestions of his temporary fascination. **This is just similar to what we see occurs to anyone spontaneously engaged in deep abstraction, who is instantaneously aroused to consciousness of all around by a tap on the shoulder, or by a word sharply addressed to him.**

[Effect of "Commanding & Confident" Tone of Voice]

It requires considerable tact to manage this, adroitly and successfully, with *some* patients; for the will and belief of certain subjects can only be successfully subjugated and controlled by **an earnest and energetic, and confident and authoritative manner, on the part of the operator; such as by his *insisting* that *such* and *such* MUST be the case, according to his audible suggestions, or visible manoeuvres for influencing the subjects through the power of sympathy and imitation.** I have had ample evidence to convince me of the fact, that, in cases where these waking illusions and delusions could not be excited by giving the suggestions in an apparently doubting tone of voice, or with a hesitating manner, they became quite efficient for the purpose, the instant I assumed a commanding and confident tone of voice and deportment. By these means the *Reason* and *Will* become temporarily paralysed; they lose their freedom of action, through the mind being so much engrossed by the suggested thought, as to allow every idea which has been vividly and energetically addressed to such individual, to assume all the force of present reality – just as we know occurs, spontaneously, in cases of *monomania* and *delirium tremens*.

[The Subject Rejects Objectionable Suggestions]
Such are the effects realised in this **sub-hypnotic or partial state of the nervous sleep**; but with all who – pass into the **full or second-conscious stage**, the power of suggestion is still more prompt and almost unlimited. Curiously enough, however, (and, as it appears so ordained by a special providence,) **any suggestion involving a grave assault upon a moral principle, in persons with well constituted minds, will instantly arouse consciousness and self-control, and induce and enable the subject to protect himself against the real or imaginary moral assault or suggestion.**

[Suggestion & the Art of Rhetoric]
Nor, after all, is this power of suggestion, or persuasion, or concealed fascination, so remarkable or unaccountable as at first sight it appears to be. The secret of success with all sophistical [i.e., rhetorical] writers and orators is of a similar nature. They make repeated appeals to the feelings, as well as to the reason, until the minds of their readers or hearers get bewildered and withdrawn from the true bearings of the main points of the case; and the assumed, and apparent sincerity and energy, of the writer, and still more so of the orator, who, to his other aids of words and arguments, adds that of his physical manifestations, to captivate and carry his entranced hearers along with him, through the power of sympathy and imitation, and fixed attention, at last irresistibly moulds them to his will. In support of this I might appeal to the personal feelings and experience of most people who have watched the effect upon a jury of a powerful and eloquent special pleader; or observed the effect of an accomplished actor or actress on the stage, over an audience excited and entranced by the felicitous impersonation of fictitious dangers and difficulties, pains and perils, joy or sorrow, fear or courage, compassion, hatred, or revenge. The historical fact, however, recorded of the powerful effect of eloquence upon the whole House of Commons, by the brilliant speech of Sheridan, in the trial of Warren Hastings [Governor-General of British India, impeached in 1787 for corruption], is more than sufficient for my purpose; for it is recorded that, in that instance, it was deemed requisite to suspend the sitting of the house, and postpone it till another day, as it was felt that no one could be expected sooner to have the power of emancipating himself from the spell thrown over the senators by such a flood of eloquence, and prepare himself for exercising sober judgment, in voting upon that important case.

All who have duly considered the workings of the human mind must have observed that, for forming a correct judgment upon an important matter, it is requisite that an individual should be able so to control his attention, that it can be constrainedly fixed on any one point, and from that directed to any other, and *every point in succession*; bearing upon the issue of the inquiry, as he may consider requisite for forming a correct appreciation of the bearings of the whole. The intense abstraction of hypnotism, therefore, which, at one stage, rivets the attention to a *single idea or train of thought*, without the power of voluntarily directing it to the various points in succession, is obviously as inimical to correct reasoning and the exercise of sound judgment, as the discursive state of mind, which renders it impossible for the person to fix his attention sufficiently on any given point of the subject, but permits it to roam hurriedly and vaguely, or inattentively from one idea to another.

[Revivification of Memory, Confidence, & Performance]
When in that stage of the sleep, however, which gives a more healthy tone to the power of fixing attention than obtains in the waking condition, or in **that which gives a degree of brilliancy to the imagination, and more rapid flow of ideas, with a revivification of memory**, **which thereby recalls thoughts and actions long forgotten** – all these circumstances, combined with the self-confidence in their own powers, which such patients generally possess may prove mighty aids in **enabling them intellectually to trace out the relation of things and circumstances with so much greater facility and felicity than in the waking condition, as to lead many to imagine such feats are achieved through intuition or direct inspiration.** So is it as regards their powers of writing correctly without the use of their eyes, entirely through the quickened muscular sense, and their attention firmly fixed on the one subject in hand. So also the power of phonic imitation; by which one of my subjects who, when awake, was even ignorant of the grammar of her own language, and had very little knowledge of music, but naturally possessed of a good voice, was enabled, when in the hypnotic sleep, to imitate Jenny Lind [a world-renowned soprano known as "The Swedish Nightingale"] so accurately, in songs sung by that lady in different languages, never before heard by the somnambulist, that she caught the sound so promptly as enabled her to give both words and music so correctly and simultaneously, that several parties present could not discriminate whether there were only one or two voices, so entirely did they accord, both in tune and vocal enunciation of the foreign languages. This

patient has frequently done so with equal success before others, and I have had other patients who could do the same; *but not one of them comprehended the meaning of the words which they uttered so correctly in the foreign language.* Such is my experience on these points.

[Categories of Suggestion versus Animal Magnetism]
I am well aware that all subjects are not susceptible or being affected in this manner, either in the partial or complete hypnotic state; for some are speedily and intensely affected – others slowly and feebly so. Moreover, **compliance with certain conditions is generally required at first trials**. Enough, however, has been ascertained, incontestably to prove, that **there is a considerable number of individuals, in every community, who may be thus *completely* subjugated and controlled; whilst there are many more who may be influenced in a slighter degree.** I wish, however, particularly to record, as my own present conviction, that these means can only prove efficient for producing such results when,

> [1. Auditory Suggestion[63]:] the patients *hear the ideas suggested when uttered in a language known to them*; or
> [2. Written Suggestion:] when they see them written (which is sufficient to affect many); or
> [3. Sympathy:] when they can see, by ordinary vision, the movements made in their presence which it is intended they should be forced to imitate, through the power of sympathy and imitation; or
> [4. Association:] when they feel sensible impressions [i.e., physical sensations], associated with certain ideas or previous feelings; or
> [5. Muscular Suggestion:] which call subjacent muscles into action [i.e., when the body posture or facial expression is manipulated so as to evoke the corresponding state of mind]; or
> [6. Focused Attention:] direct attention to the special organs of sense, which excites ideas corresponding with the functions of these different organs, or arouses former ideas arbitrarily or accidentally associated with such and such sensible impressions. [As in the experiments on attention, debunking the Reichenbach phenomena, which show that prolonged or focused attention *alone* can create spontaneous hallucinatory sensations.]

Of the power of influencing patients at a distance, however, through *silent willing* [i.e., Mesmer's theory of animal magnetism], I have had no satisfactory proof in my own patients; nor, from all which I have seen read, and heard on the subject, do I believe such a power is possessed by others. I am familiar with so many sources of fallacy, requiring to be guarded against in such inquiries, from the power of imagination, habit, and the expectant idea over certain susceptible subjects, that, without the least desire to impugn the testimony either of patients or operators who have alleged that such influences have been manifested in their cases, I beg respectfully to say, that I consider it far more probable that they have been deceived, in some of the ways which I have pointed out, than that the phenomena manifested were *bona fide* the product of the *silent will* and gesticulations of the operators, on patients at considerable distances from them.

The following is the *resumé* of the result of my experience on these points, which was quoted with approbation in the article in the *British and Foreign Medico-Chirurgical Review*, page 412, from my essay on "Electro-Biology", after the remark, "Mr. Braid very justly observes":–

> I have never yet seen any phenomena during either the hypnotic or Mesmeric sleep, or during the state for manifesting vigilant phenomena, which were not in accordance with generally admitted physiological and psychological principles. The senses and mental powers may be torpified [i.e., dulled] or quickened to an extraordinary degree; but I have never seen anything to warrant a belief that individuals could thereby become gifted with the power of reading through opaque bodies, [...] and other transcendental phenomena, called by the Mesmerists the *higher phenomena*. The power of a strongly fixed attention, vivid imagination, and self-confidence, however, enables them to perform some extraordinary feats of phonic imitation, and writing and drawing by touch, without the use of their eyes; discovering parties who own certain articles worn by them, through the quickened sense of smell; overhearing conversation in a distant apartment, which they could not do in a waking condition; of recalling to mind things long forgotten when awake; and also of deducing conclusions, manifesting uncommon shrewdness, from premises suggested to them, or arising in their minds spontaneously from recollection of past events, to which they have directed their concentrated attention.

[De-hypnotising Patients]
Having described the modes of inducing the full condition of sleep and the sub or partial condition for manifesting the **waking phenomena**, I must now state the modes of *arousing patients from these states*. If I wish any predominant idea, or *physical* change which has been induced, to be carried strongly into the waking condition, I arouse the patient abruptly, by a clap of my hands near his ear, when at the full height of the desired condition; if tranquillising is intended, then he had better be aroused slowly and softly – such as by gently wafting with the hand, or a fan, or open handkerchief, over the face, or by placing the thumbs gently on the eyes of the patient, or on his eyebrows, and carrying them laterally a few times, so as to

---

[63] [I have taken the liberty of reformatting and numbering Braid's classification of different forms of suggestion in order to highlight the scope of his distinctions.]

produce gentle friction, to which may be added gentle fanning when required. If the patient is in the sub or half-waking condition, a word spoken or a visible movement of any sort made, so as to break his abstraction, excited temporarily by previous suggestion, will suffice.

The Mesmerists divide passes into Mesmerising and deMesmerising passes – those made longitudinally, from the head or face downwards, over the body and extremities, being called *Mesmerising passes*, those made crossways, *deMesmerising passes*. The first are considered to induce certain effects; the others to remove them when existing. I have reason to believe that the patient may be aroused as readily by one sort of pass as by another, unless when he has got a mental impression somehow excited, that there is a speciality in each. In that case the result will be according to the faith [i.e., the expectation] of the individual.

[Alleged Difficulty Arousing from State]
One decided advantage in favour of hypnotism is this – that I have **never experienced the slightest difficulty in arousing any of my patients even from the most profound stage of the sleep which they may pass into**; nor do they experience any annoyance from other persons than the operator approaching to, or touching them, during the sleep – both of which inconveniences frequently manifest themselves, in a marked degree, in the ordinary Mesmeric state, for some Mesmerised subjects will be thrown into the most violent agitation, with intense catalepsy or convulsions, merely by another person touching them – which is called cross-Mesmerism – or they may remain for many hours, and sometimes even for *days* in the sleep without being able to be aroused. I consider this merely arises from a predominant idea or conceit in the mind of the patient, and the operator, not knowing the key to the puzzle, presents the great difficulty of unlocking him from the condition.

I was once called upon to arouse a Mesmeric lecturer from the sleep induced in him by a friend, who became alarmed when he could not arouse him after he had been twenty-four hours in the condition. After some trouble, I succeeded in arousing him, for twenty minutes, from his maniacal excitement; but he spontaneously passed into it again, and remained so, with only one or two short snatches of consciousness, for nearly two days more. No such distressing event ever occurred to any of **my hypnotised patients; they have always been capable of being aroused almost instantly.**

[Common Sources of Fallacy in Mesmerism]
I am not ignorant that there are many men with great abilities, distinguished alike for their high rank and superior attainments in literature and general science, as for their moral worth, who avow their belief in magnetic or Mesmeric clairvoyance. But inasmuch as the feats alleged by them as facts are of such an extraordinary nature, so much opposed to the generally recognised laws of mind and physical organisation, I consider it is the imperative duty of every man to investigate such a subject with great care and caution, before accepting as facts, what, from the difficulty of the inquiry, and the numerous sources of error with which it is surrounded, are very likely to be fallacies or illusions. Such has been the case with myself; for, knowing as I do, so many of the fallacies requiring to be guarded against, I have soon been enabled to prove the alleged clairvoyant powers of some of the most noted of the class were mere illusions, shrewd guesses, or ingenious frauds on the part of the entranced subjects, contrived by them from a passion for notoriety and a desire to excel and astonish others by their apparently wonderful powers. Moreover, some of them may actually resort to these artifices, during the sleep, without any recollection on their awaking of such tricks having been perpetrated by them during their entranced condition. Amongst the marvels alleged by the Hindoos, as resulting from this condition, was the power of walking on the water; and Professor Gregory has recorded his belief that Mr. Lewis could suspend a man in the air, through his magnetic powers merely by holding his hand above the patient's head; and Dr. Ashburner has declared, in print, that the material force emanating from his brain by the power of his *will*, is such as to enable him to compel the precious metal, gold, to ignore the vulgar law of gravity, and actually advance towards him when, in the form of a ring, it has been suspended by a thread from a glass rod, securely attached across the top of two upright glass rods fixed in a table. These experiments admit of easy proof, if rightly set about; and combining the two first would be the most clear mode of determining whether any man could suspend another in the air, through the mere force of magnetic attraction; for there could be no doubt of the fact, if he could so elevate and hold him suspended above a good sized eight-feet-deep water-cistern.

The remarkable discrepancies in the Mesmeric camp, however, and that even amongst some of the chief officers, on points of vital importance as regards the first principles of their science, certainly do not inspire one with the notion of their infallibility. Thus Baron Reichenbach lays it down as one of the remarkable properties of odyle [Reichenbach's supposed energy, similar to animal magnetism], that it is so subtle as to pass through every form of matter, including *glass*, in which particular it differs from *electricity*. To all this Professor Gregory, the translator and sponsor of Reichenbach's work, gives in his adherence; whilst Dr. Ashburner, the other translator (?) and expounder of the Baron's views, declares that he can, by the mere power of his silent *will*, extrude odyle from the points of his fingers, or send it direct, by the force of his *will* "into a wide-mouthed phial of a pint capacity", in which he can carry it into another room, and pour the fluid or substance upon the body of a patient and thereby produce its specific effects. It is certainly ludicrous to hear this gentleman gravely telling us that he can *will* this fluid into a vessel, and carry it into another room, in what, according to Reichenbach and Gregory must have been a *bottomless vessel – a mere sieve –* since they declare that unlike electricity, it passes *through* GLASS and *every other substance!*[64]

[Post-Hypnotic Suggestion]

An unsuspected but fertile source or fallacy is this, that we all receive suggestions, both when asleep and when awake, from impressions in the waking state so slight as never to have aroused consciousness; or from suggestions of others, or ideas arising spontaneously during sleep, which have long lain dormant, but become active when certain exciting causes or correspondences come into play to arouse the silent chord to harmony. This will frequently resemble prevision or intuition. It is certain that **suggestions may be given during the hypnotic or Mesmeric sleep, of which the subject shall have no remembrance on awaking; but, through the influence of which, nevertheless, when the time fixed on for the manifestation arrives, he will feel a sort of desire or instinctive impulse to act according to previous suggestion. Nor is this more wonderful than the fact that some individuals can go to bed and sleep soundly, and awake at the exact moment which they had determined upon the previous evening.**

[Intelligence is Associated with Hypnotisability]

There may, no doubt, be some self-sufficient, dogmatic sceptics who, glorying in their shame – for they avowedly speak and write authoritatively, without having practically investigated the subject regarding which they set themselves up as censors or judges – who will be ready to poo pooh all this alleged power of producing either the *major* or the *minor* phenomena, especially the waking phenomena, unless upon credulous, ignorant, and weak-minded men, and *hysterical* women. I take the liberty to tell such individuals that their *merely theoretical* notions are not worth a rush, when brought to oppose the stern facts of cautious experimentalists. I have myself hypnotised a noble lord, who, for intellectual attainments and moral worth, is one of the most distinguished and influential of the British Aristocracy; and I have both succeeded in producing **the full or double-conscious condition**, and the sub or waking state, for eliciting the vigilant or waking phenomena, in some of the most intellectual and strong-minded men and women in the kingdom; whereas, **I never yet could hypnotise an *idiot*! The boasted power of resisting such influence, therefore, may be of a very *equivocal character*, and the very opposite of what such individuals wish should be inferred, from their vain-glorying about *their* non-susceptibility.**

[Critique of Dr. James Esdaile's Mesmerism]

As a proof of the unmitigated folly, and presumption, and thoughtless inhumanity of those self-conceited obstructers of human progress in the relief and cure of their suffering fellow creatures, I shall adduce a single example, about which there can be no reasonable ground of cavil [i.e., quibbling], as the whole proceedings to which I allude took place in a public hospital, where there was free access to all honest inquirers; and the operations and experiments were not performed upon paid servants, or those known to the intrepid and excellent man who so gallantly fought and so nobly triumphed over every obstacle which prejudice, cabal, and combination had raised against him and his humane efforts. The most important surgical operations were performed on utter strangers, and that even from distant provinces throughout a great part of British India. Dr. [James] Esdaile is the gentleman to whom I refer – a man who, by his intrepid and indomitable courage and success, in introducing painless surgery into India, on a large scale, by operating upon patients reduced to the state of Mesmeric unconsciousness, has raised for himself "a monument more enduring than brass". In a most interesting and friendly letter which I received from Dr. Esdaile last October, he kindly furnished me with a *resumé* of his Mesmeric experience in India, with permission to make any use of it which I chose. I therefore gladly avail myself of this privilege on the present occasion; and as that gentleman's theoretical notions, and the extent of his confession of faith in the *higher phenomena*, are more in favour of Mesmerism than of hypnotism, (although he admits the influence of hypnotism too, but has not tried it extensively), the reader will thereby perceive that the principle by which I am swayed in conducting scientific inquiries is – "Nought conceal, nor set down aught in malice."

After acknowledging the receipt of some of my publications on hypnotic phenomena, and thanking me for them, Dr. Esdaile says:–

> I shall find much in the books to interest and instruct me, as I did in your first work on Hypnotism; but I shall not wait to read them before replying to your communication.
>
> I have not seen any of the papers you allude to in the journals; but am glad to hear that the doctors are, at last, condescending to turn their attention to one of the most interesting and important subjects ever submitted to the consideration of the physiologist, the metaphysician, and natural philosopher. [...] Regarding the reality and cause of the Mesmeric phenomena, if I venture to differ from you even, who are so much better prepared to investigate the subject (than certain individuals to whom the Doctor had referred), it is for reasons which I hope you will consider worthy of your attention. I am fully aware that there are various modes of

---

[64] [Braid could have also observed that these pseudo-energy theorists assume that the odyle or animal magnetism is stored in their *own* bodies, yet is also capable at will of passing through the skin and into the bodies of others and being stored *there*. Is human flesh naturally a *barrier* to it or not; why at some times but not others?]

inducing the Mesmeric symptoms, to a certain extent, without the probability, or even possibility, of any vital force proceeding from the operator being concerned in the matter. But I have never (except for experiment) produced the Mesmeric state of the system by the exhaustion of any organ, such as the eye, (here the Doctor has overlooked the important part which the mental act of *fixed attention* plays in this matter, *vide* page 53-7) or by acting strongly on the imagination, or by any means that could favour self-Mesmerisation, as you will perceive from the following *resumé* of my practice:–

During the last six years I have performed upwards of 300 capital operations of every description, and many of them of the most terrible nature, without inflicting pain on the patients; and, *in every instance*, the insensibility was produced in this fashion.

All knowledge of our intentions was, if possible, concealed from the patients, and if they had never heard of Mesmerism and painless operations, so much the better. They were taken into a darkened room, and desired to lie down and *shut their eyes*. A young Hindoo or Musulman [i.e., Hindu or Muslim] then seated himself at the head of the bed, and made passes, without contact, from the head to the epigastrium [around the navel area], breathing on the head and eyes all the time, and occasionally resting his hands for a minute on the pit of the stomach. This often induced the coma deep enough for the severest surgical operation in a few minutes; but the routine was for me to examine the patient at the end of an hour, and if he was not ready, the process was repeated daily. Taking the average, the operation, of whatever description, was usually performed on the fourth or fifth day.

Probably as many more cases were subjected to the trance for medical purposes, and were usually treated in the same way, for its convenience to both parties.

The enclosed remarkable case of clairvoyance, with transference of the senses to the epigastrium [i.e., the Mesmerised subject "seeing with" their own belly], will show that the Mesmeric control of the system may be obtained, when the patient is not only asleep, but in a state of intense natural coma.

I have also entranced a blind man, and made him so sensitive, that I could entrance him *however employed*, (eating his dinner, for instance,) by merely making him the object of my attention for ten minutes. He would gradually cease to eat, remain stationary a few moments, and then plunge, head foremost, among his rice and curry.

Numbers of madmen have been entranced in the lunatic asylum of Calcutta, and I performed a Mesmeric operation on one man who had cut his throat.

I frequently desired the visitors of my hospitals to pretend to take the portraits of patients, and to engage their attention as much as possible, by conversing with them. I then retired to another room, and reduced them to statues, without the possibility of their suspecting my intentions.

How such phenomena can be accounted for, without presuming the existence of a physical power transmitted from the operator to the subject, passes my comprehension, that the Mesmeric virtue can be communicated to inanimate matter, is a physical fact, of which I am as well convinced as of my own existence. It was my common hospital practice to entrance patients *for the purpose of having their sores burned with Nitric Acid*, by giving them Mesmerised water to drink.

Community of taste, and thought-reading, are among the most common of the higher Mesmeric phenomena, and how they are to be explained, except by the transmission of the operator's sensations, through his *thought-stamped*, nervous fluid, sent to the brain of the subject, I cannot conjecture.

"Important, if true," you will probably say. I can only say that healthy senses, a natural power of seeing things as they really are, and an earnest desire to know the truth, whatever it may be, are perfectly useless for the acquisition of knowledge, if all I have related is not perfectly true.

Till such facts are known to medical men and natural philosophers, it is surely premature to dogmatise about the *only* source of the Mesmeric phenomena.

It happened curiously enough, that the sleeping Fakir of Lahore had attracted my attention about the very time your interesting account of him appeared, and I had actually written to Sir Henry Lawrence [an influential British statesman and soldier in India], begging him to procure us information on the subject; but my departure from India, shortly after, prevented my prosecution of the subject.

Such was the experience of Dr. Esdaile, whose firmness of nerve, and dexterity of hand, and scientific skill, in every way stamped him as a man eminently qualified for being a leader in his profession. Most sincerely do I wish that the like processes could be rendered equally available in this country as they were in India, for annulling the pain incident to surgical operations. I am well aware, from my own experience, as also from what I have read as the results with others, that Mesmerism, or hypnotism, may be successful for this end with *some* patients; but, I fear it will not become so generally successful in this country as in India, or as chloroform has been proved to be in Europe. Mesmeric anaesthesia, however, has this great superiority when it succeeds – that no injury has ever resulted to the patient from its use; for the recoveries under Mesmeric surgical operations in Dr. Esdaile's hospital were far beyond the average success. Why, therefore, should it not be fairly tried in this country as well as in India, when no danger to the patients can result from such trials? My own convictions, from trials of both methods, are in favour of chloroform, as being *more speedy and certain in its effects with patients in this country*, and I know that, with due care and caution, it may generally be used with safety in surgical operations, as well as in midwifery; but I should think it interesting, in every point of view, that the Mesmeric or hypnotic modes should be fairly tested, so that we may know how far Dr. Esdaile's method, described above, can be made available in this country, with British subjects on British soil, for suspending the anguish of mind and body, during surgical operations, by such a safe and simple process. [In fact, Braid seems to have been right to express the need for Esdaile's claims to be tested, possibly a sign of slight reservation on his part. Esdaile, who had recently returned to Scotland, in

June 1851, subsequently *refused* to demonstrate his Mesmeric technique of surgical anaesthesia with British subjects, complaining that he found them too difficult to entrance (*q.v.* Forrest, *Hypnotism: A History*, 1999: 187), and serious doubts were cast on the accuracy of his claims regarding painless operations by at least one of the doctors who had originally reported positively on his work in India (*Ibid*.: 185-186). Braid now proceeds also to question Esdaile's conclusion that paranormal powers were exhibited by his Mesmerised subjects.]

Agreeing, as I so cordially do with Dr. Esdaile, as regards the great value of the practical application of Mesmerism, I am sure he will forgive me if I venture to differ somewhat from him, theoretically, in the conclusions which I have come to regarding some of the results which he has particularised, as proofs of "the existence of a physical power transmitted from the operator to the subject"; because it is only by examining and comparing with each other, the different modes of explaining phenomena, which occur to different minds, that we can hope to arrive at a true solution of such difficult problems.

In the case of the blind man, I am so well aware of the remarkable quickness of hearing which many acquire from *loss of sight*, and being compelled to rely upon that, and the sense of touch and smell, that I can easily imagine that he might perceive the doctor's presence, and fixed position, and suppressed respiration, concomitant upon a fixed act of attention, and thus catch the idea of his intention and then the power of imagination and habit would produce the result named. Then, in respect to entrancing the patient from another room, many such patients become so quick in catching the requisite ideas from the slightest peculiarity in the looks and tone of voice and manners of those around them, that the individual referred to might readily have caught the idea of something being intended, from the manners and looks of the *pretended artists*, and then the usual result would naturally follow. The efficacy of Mesmerised water admits, if possible, of still easier explanation; for there is an aroma peculiar to every individual, both as regards the exhalation from the lungs and skin; hence the dog can trace his master through a crowd, by smell, or anyone else he has been set on the trail of. Either breathing on water, or wafting over it with the fingers, therefore, might readily impart a physical quality to suggest, by means of smell, ideas connected with some individuals, such as the doctor's Mesmerisers, and the ideas thus excited, through the laws of association, would produce the wonted results. Nay, even the very *mode of presenting* it might be sufficient, of itself alone, to produce the sleep in highly susceptible subjects, after having been impressed. Hearing, and sight, and smell, would require to be annulled, before I could readily believe in community of taste and feeling, which all will easily comprehend who have closely observed the powers of suggestion, in giving such vividness to ideas as shall delude the patients, even in the wide-waking state, and make them mistake mere ideas for realities.

The above are merely *my opinions* on these points; but I shall now state what I know to have been a positive fact. I had heard much of an interesting case of a highly susceptible lady – so susceptible to ordinary Mesmeric processes, that she might be sent off into the sleep by the most simple attempt to produce it – and so sensitive of the influence of magnets, that she was quite uncomfortable if a magnet were near her, in any room; and in the dark she could point out any part of the room where a magnet of very moderate power was placed, from her *seeing* the light it produced, streaming all around it. I was kindly invited to spend an evening at this lady's house, to afford me an opportunity of seeing and hearing more particulars of these wonders. I had the pleasure of sitting very near the lady, and of enjoying a long and interesting conversation with her and her husband, who was a most respectable and intelligent gentleman, and no manifestation whatever took place during the whole time, until after I had explained my views regarding the power of an *act* of *fixed attention*, directed to any part, in modifying the natural condition of the part so regarded. She was requested to direct her fixed attention to her hand, and watch the result, without anything being done, either by her husband or anyone else. She did so, and very quickly fell asleep, and the arm to which she had directed her attention became rigidly cataleptic. Sometime after being aroused, and when the shades of deep twilight had set in, the most interesting experiment was proposed, which was this, that she should walk round the room and find a magnet, which had been hidden behind some pictures when she was out of the room, in order to prove to me her power of *seeing* its light, and thus detecting it. She walked cautiously round the room (wide awake, for she did not require to be asleep to manifest this faculty), her husband repeatedly urging her to seek about and persevere until she should find it. I feel satisfied that *he* had no intention of aiding her; but, from his long silence when she approached the place where the magnet was hid, *I* should myself have caught the suggestion that I was *near to it*, or, in nursery phraseology, that it was then getting *very hot*. After she had passed it a little she sat down on a chair, but said she could not *see* it tonight, and then came up to where we were, shortly after which we sat down to supper. The lady showed no symptom of being uncomfortable from the proximity of a magnet, until requested to look at, and fix her attention upon, her hand; and, after being aroused, all seemed right again, until she was told that the *dreaded magnet was hidden somewhere in the room*, and she was requested to go round in the dark and endeavour to find it. The husband thought her sitting down in the chair proved that she *felt* the influence of the magnet, although she could not *see* the *light* from it; but, what seemed conclusive evidence to *my* mind that it was the *mere idea*, and *not* any *physical* influence in the magnet, which affected the lady, was this – that all the time I had been sitting so close to her, conversing with her and her husband, I had had a *fourteen-pound lifting magnet*, with the armature unattached, *in my side pocket next to the lady* – and that was a magnet, of *more than double the power of her husband's*; and yet *no visible* effect was produced by *my powerful*, but *unsuspected* magnet.

[Sympathy & Imitation in Hysterical Dancing Epidemics]

As regards sympathy and imitation, every medical man is well aware of their wonderful power, especially on certain temperaments. From the wag who sets a whole company a yawning, against which the very dog below his master's table cannot protect himself, to the recent public exhibitors of experiments in "electro-biology" we have abundant proofs of their power, as well as of the **influence of audible suggestions**. In particular, we have the history of its extensive prevalence in the middle ages, in the dancing mania, the St. Vitus' and St. John's dancers. Again, the dancers who had the disease, induced by the alleged poisonous bite of the tarantula, or venomous spider, likewise spread extensively in Italy, "where, during some centuries, it prevailed as a great epidemic".

> From the middle of the fourteenth century, the furies of the Dance brandished their scourge over afflicted mortals, and music, for which the inhabitants of Italy now, probably for the first time, manifested susceptibility and talent, became capable of exciting ecstatic attacks in those affected, and then furnished the magical means of exorcising their melancholy. – *Hecker's Epidemics.*

I have already referred to the convulsionnaires in Paris.[65] Even in recent times, however, and in our own country too, the power of sympathy and imitation was vividly portrayed in the south and west of England, where, from this influence, within a short period, about 4,000 people became affected by a violent convulsive malady. It is recorded of this epidemic that "hundreds of people who had come thither, either attracted by curiosity, or a desire, from other motives, to see the sufferers, fell into the same state". The like condition was also manifested very lately in the Shetland Isles; and the power of suspending moral and physical maladies of the sort, by *moral* means, is beautifully illustrated by the following anecdote:–

> An intelligent and pious minister of Shetland informed the physician (the late Dr. Samuel Hibbert Ware), who gives an account of this disorder as an eye-witness – that, being considerably annoyed, on his first introduction into the country, by those paroxysms, whereby the devotions of the church were much impeded, he obviated their repetition by assuring his parishioners that no treatment was more effectual than immersion in cold water; and as his kirk was fortunately contiguous to a fresh water lake, he gave notice that attendants should be at hand, during Divine service, to ensure the proper means of cure. The sequel need scarcely be told. The fear of being carried out of church and into the water acted like a charm. Not a single naiad was made. [None of the parishioners were dunked in the water, that is.] – *Hecker's Epidemics.*

Let those who deride the notion of *their* being susceptible of such impressions, from *such* causes, have a care that they do not trifle too confidently at the attempt to prove how far *they* can surrender their self-control, for a time, for the purpose of imitating others. They may very probably, in the end, find to their cost and sorrow, that their *will* having been for a time surrendered into another's keeping, may not return at their bidding and that what they believed to be a mere delusion or fraud in others, has proved to be a grave reality with themselves. They ought to remember the fate of the distinguished prelate, Jo. Baptist Quinzato, Bishop of Foligno, who "having allowed himself, by way of a joke, to be bitten by a tarantula, could obtain a cure in no other way than by being through the influence of the tarantella, compelled to dance". Now, it is fully ascertained that the bite of the tarantula is not at all poisonous, and the bishop was fully persuaded of this when he perpetrated the joke; still, the idea having at length taken possession of his mind, that it possibly might be poisonous after all, he became a victim to this imaginary poison. From the state of public opinion in that age, it has, moreover, been recorded, "that even the most decided sceptics, incapable of guarding themselves against the recollection of what had been presented to the eye, were subdued by a poison, the powers of which had been ridiculed, and which was IN ITSELF INERT in its effects". – *Hecker's Epidemics.*[66] Even at the end of the seventeenth century, Tarantism,

> [...] showed such extraordinary symptoms, that Baglivi, one of the best physicians of the time, thought he did a service to science by making them the subject of a dissertation. He repeats all the observations of Ferdinando, and supports his own assertions by the experience of his father; a physician at Lecee, whose testimony, as an eye-witness, may be admitted as unexceptionable. – *Hecker's Epidemics.*

> Against the effect produced by the tarantula's bite, or by the sight of the sufferers, neither youth nor age afforded any protection, so that even old men of ninety threw aside their crutches at the sound of the tarantella (the name given to the music played to those seized with the dancing mania, excited through the bite of the tarantula) and as if some magic potion, restorative of youth and vigour, were flowing through their veins, joined the most extravagant dancers. Ferdinando saw a boy of five years old seized with the dancing mania, in

---

[65] For an interesting account of the convulsionaires, and cammisards and nuns of Loudun, *vide* Mr. Colquhoun's "History"; also, Hecker.

[66] [The dancing epidemic of Tarantism was blamed upon a species of wolf spider misleadingly called a "tarantula", common in the region surrounding the town of Taranto in Italy, whose bite is utterly harmless to humans, but which legend claimed to be deadly unless cured by frenetic dancing, from which the Italian tarantella dance reputedly derives.]

consequence of the bite of the tarantula; and, what is almost past belief, were it not supported by the testimony of so credible an eye-witness, even deaf people were not exempt from this disorder – so potent in its effect was the very sight of those affected, even without the exhilaration caused by music. – *Ibid.*

The powers of sympathy were also strikingly manifested, in 1787, at Hodden Bridge, in Lancashire, where a girl put a mouse into the bosom of another girl, who had a great dread of mice. The girl was instantly thrown into a fit and continued in it with the most violent convulsions for twenty-four hours. On the following day three more girls were seized in the same manner; and on the second day there were six more attacked. The alarm was now so great that the whole works – where from 200 to 300 hands were employed – were totally stopped, and the idea prevailed that the plague had been introduced among them from opening a bag of cotton. On the two following days fourteen more were seized making, in all, twenty-four victims to this excitement of terror in sport. Of this number twenty-one were young women, two girls under ten years of age and one man who had been much fatigued by holding the girls. The symptoms were so violent as to require four or five persons to hold the patients, so as to prevent them from tearing out their hair and dashing their heads against the floor or walls. So soon as the public became assured that the complaint was merely a nervous disorder, easily cured, and not introduced by any poison from the cotton bale, no other person was affected although previously several persons had become affected when at several miles distance from the centre of excitement, merely from hearing reports of the symptoms manifested in others.

To dissipate their apprehensions still further the best effects were obtained by causing them to take a cheerful glass and join in a dance. On Tuesday the 20th, five days after the first case occurred, they danced, and the next day they were all at work, except two or three, who were much weakened by their fits. – *Hecker's Epidemics.*

The **beneficial effects of dancing**, for dissipating the baneful influence of fixed morbid impressions and associations, is proved by the experience which has been had on this point, since this mode of amusement and exercise has been introduced into some of our public lunatic asylums.[67]

The effects of sympathy and imitation and excessive excitement, manifested amongst certain religious sects at their camp meetings in North America, in recent times, prove that, with all our boasted advancement in civilization, beyond those who inhabited Europe during the middle ages, the human mind is still susceptible of these strange mental delusions and physical manifestations, excited entirely through the power of sympathy and imitation in those who place themselves in circumstances favourable for their development.

The following curious and exciting scene occurred, a few years ago, in a maritime town well-known to me:– Two captains of merchant vessels arrived in port at the same time, and both went to take up their quarters in their usual lodgings. They were informed by the landlady of the house, however, that she was very sorry that she could not accommodate them on that occasion, as the only bed-room which she could have appropriated for their use was occupied by the corpse of a gentleman just deceased. Being most anxious to remain in their accustomed lodgings, almost on any terms, rather than go elsewhere, they offered to sleep in the room wherein the dead body was laid out. To this the landlady readily gave her assent, considering it better, so far as she was concerned, to have three such customers in her room than only one, and he a dead one. Having repaired to bed, one of the gentlemen, who was a very great wag, began a conversation with the other by asking him whether he had ever before slept in a room with a corpse in it, to which he replied, "No." "Then," said the other, "are you aware of the remarkable circumstance, that always, in such cases, after midnight, the room gets filled with canaries, which fly about and sing in the most beautiful manner?" His companion expressed his surprise at this. But no sooner said than realised; for, the candle having been put out, presently there was a burst of music, as if the room really was full of canaries, which were not only heard, but at length the horrified novice in the chamber of death avowed that he both *saw* and *felt* the birds flying in all directions, and plunging against him. In a short time he became so excited that, without taking time to do his toilet, he rushed down stairs in his night-dress, assuring the astonished household of the fact, and insisting that the room really was *quite full of birds*, as he could testify from the evidence of his senses, for he had not only heard them, but also seen and *felt them, flapping their wings against him*.

The origin of this extraordinary and exciting scene was simply this: his companion had provided himself with a straw or small reed, cut so as to imitate the notes of the canary, when blown through, the end of it being dipped in a glass of water. Here, then, the ear alone was impressed, but the mind superadded thereto illusions of *two other senses* – sight and touch – and that in the case of a brave sea captain too.

The powers of sympathy, imitation, and suggestion were remarkably evinced in the extraordinary delusion which occurred to a multitude of people, on the banks of the Clyde, below Lanark, Scotland, in 1686, when,

---

[67] [It might be noted in this connection that laboratory evidence suggests muscular movement is capable of reducing anxiety even in animals, whereas restriction of movement is well-known to increase anxiety in behavioural experiments, as even Pavlov observed.]

Many people were gathered together, for several afternoons, where there were showers of bonnets, hats, guns, and swords, which covered the trees and ground; companies of men marched in order on the water side – companies meeting companies, going all through each other, and then falling to the ground and disappearing; other companies immediately reappeared, marching the same way.

Now it is recorded that *two-thirds of those who went to witness these strange sights bore testimony to their reality*, not merely by their words, but also by their physical manifestations of fright and trembling, which were visible to those who could see nothing of such apparitions and martial array themselves. No doubt all this apparent marvellous appearance resulted from excited imagination, and the confusion of vision consequent on overstraining the eyes, by constant and persevering efforts, to see the invisible phantasms. Had there been any *reality* in the objects of observation, they ought to have been obvious to the *whole* spectators. The concluding remark in Walker's history of the transaction merits particular attention: "Those who *did* see them *there*, whenever they went abroad, saw a bonnet or a sword drop in the way."

[Braid's Special Hypnotic Technique for Insomnia]
I shall now advert to one of the most important points connected with my hypnotic investigations, and that is, to record the result of my experience, corroborated as it is by the experience of others who have fairly tried my method, as regards the most simple speedy and certain, and safe mode for inducing *sleep at will*, without the use of opiates. It is well-known that there are many who dare not use opiates in any form, from their baneful influence, in some way or other, on their constitutions, their damage, in other respects being greater than can be compensated for by the disturbed sleep induced by their aid. As I have already said, I consider the hypnotic mode of treating certain disorders is a most important ascertained fact, and a real solid addition to practical therapeutics, for there is a variety of cases in which it is really most successful, and to which it is most particularly adapted; and those are the very cases in which ordinary medical means are least successful, or altogether unavailing. Still I repudiate the notion of holding up hypnotism as a panacea or universal remedy. As formerly remarked, I use *hypnotism* ALONE *only in a certain class of cases*, to which I consider it peculiarly adapted – and I use it *in conjunction with medical treatment, in some other cases*; but *in the great majority of cases, I do not use hypnotism at all*, but depend entirely upon the efficacy of medical, moral, dietetic, and hygienic treatment, prescribing active medicines in such doses as are calculated to produce obvious effects. **A method of producing *sleep at will*, however, *without the use of opiates*, may be most advantageously resorted to, on certain occasions, by *most people*; and I shall, therefore, briefly describe the method devised by me for that purpose.**

In [*Neurypnology*] my work on hypnotism, published in 1843, I explained how "tired nature's sweet restorer, balmy sleep", might be procured, in many instances, through a most simple device by the patient himself. All that is required for this is simply to place himself in a comfortable posture in bed, and then to close the eyelids, and turn up the eyeballs gently, as if looking at a distant object, such as an imaginary star, situated somewhat above and behind the forehead, giving the whole concentrated attention of the mind to the idea of maintaining a steady view of the star, and breathing softly, as if in profound attention, the mind at the same time yielding to the idea that sleep will ensue, and to the tendency to somnolence which will creep upon him whilst engaged in this act of fixed attention. Or it may be done with still more success, in certain individuals, by their placing some small, bright object in a similar aspect with a distant light falling thereon, the party looking at the object with open eyes, fixed attention, and suppressed [i.e., relaxed] respiration. Other modes of producing a state of mental concentration directed to some unexciting and empty thing, and thus shutting out the influence of other sensible impressions, may also prove successful for inducing calm sleep, by monotonising the mind – just as we see effected in the case of children, who are sent to sleep by rocking, patting, or gentle rubbing, or monotonous, unexciting lullabies – but none are so speedy and certain in their effects, with patients generally, as the modes which I have briefly explained. Mr. Walker's method of procuring "sleep at will", by desiring the patient to maintain a fixed act of attention, by imagining himself watching his breath issuing slowly from his nostrils, after having placed his body in a comfortable position in bed – and which was first published to the world by Dr. Binns, a few years ago – is essentially the same as my own method, which I had promulgated some time prior to the publication of the *first* edition of Dr. Binns's work on sleep.

In reference to my hypnotic devices, Professor Gregory makes the following gratifying observations, at page 200 of his "Letters to a Candid Inquirer":–

> Let us now attend for a moment to the hypnotism of Mr. Braid. I have had the pleasure of seeing that gentleman operate, and I most willingly bear testimony to the accuracy of his description, and to the very striking results which he produces.

After describing my usual process for hypnotising, the Professor adds:–

> In a short but variable time, a large proportion of the persons tried are not only affected, but put to sleep. Nay,

> there is, as I have proved on my own person, no plan so effectual in producing sleep, when we find ourselves disposed, in spite of our wish to sleep, to remain awake in bed.

After describing the induction of sleep effected by reading a class of books of a dry, unexciting character, he adds:–

> But let these persons try the experiment of placing a small, bright object, seen by the reflection of a safe and distant light, in such a position that the eyes are strained a little upwards or backwards, and at such a distance as to give a tendency to squinting, and they will probably never again have recourse to the venerable authors above alluded to. A sweet and refreshing slumber steals over the senses; indeed, the sensation of falling asleep under these circumstances, as I have often experienced, is quite delightful, and the sleep is calm and undisturbed, though often accompanied with dreams of an agreeable kind. Sir David Brewster, who, with more than youthful ardour, never fails to investigate any curious fact connected with the eye, has not only seen Mr. Braid operate, but has also himself often adopted this method of inducing sleep, and compares it to the feeling we have when, after severe and long continued bodily exertion, we sit or lie down and fall asleep, being overcome, in a most agreeable manner, by the solicitations of Morpheus [god of dreams], to which, at such times, we have a positive pleasure in yielding, however inappropriate the scene of our slumbers.

Such testimony, from two such philosophers, regarding the efficacy of my method of inducing *sleep at will*, in their own persons, by such a simple process, I consider a boon to the public, as well as gratifying to myself to have had it recorded by Professor Gregory, and thus diffused so much more widely than when confined to my own publications alone.

[Group Experiment on Attention & Spontaneous Sensations]
Before concluding these "Observations", I shall briefly record the results of two classes of experiments, which must convince any unprejudiced person that the changed or modified action which takes place during hypnotic processes, is due entirely to the influence of the mental concentration of the *patient over his own physical functions*. At the same time, however, **I fully admit that another person being present may modify the results produced by audible, visible, or tangible suggestions**, in the manner explained at pages 61-2.

I requested four gentlemen, all in perfect health, and varying from 40 to 56 years of age, to sit down, and lay their arms on a table, with the palms of their hands upwards, and each to look at the palm of his own hand for a few minutes with fixed attention, and watch the result, entire silence being enjoined. In about five minutes, the first, one of the present members of the Royal Academy, stated that he felt a sensation of great cold in the hand; another, who is a very talented author, said that, for some time, he thought nothing was going to happen, but at last a darting, prickling sensation took place from the palm of the hand, as if electric sparks were being drawn from it; the third gentleman, lately mayor of a large borough, said that he felt a very uncomfortable sensation of heat come over his hand; and the fourth, secretary to an important association, had become rigidly cataleptic – his arm being firmly fixed to the table. Now, here all commenced the operation at the same time, and all were sitting round the same table, and **not a word was spoken**, not a movement made by anyone, to aid or influence the results which followed. In this instance, therefore, of the four senses in the hand, *viz*., common feeling, heat and cold, and the muscular sense, the one which was naturally most active manifested itself in each case; but, had I suggested what should be expected in each case, the probability is that, in some of them, the *suggested* idea might have been realised instead of the natural one. It is obvious that my will could not have produced four such different results at the same instant of time, and at first trial too.

[Experiment on Waking Autosuggestion & Menstruation]
At page 58 of my book on "Trance" [*Observations on Trance or Human Hybernation*, 1850] I recorded the case of Mrs. ——, 30 years of age, married, and the mother of three children, whom I had speedily cured, by hypnotism, of epilepsy of a most formidable character, and of four years standing. All ordinary treatment had previously utterly failed. I stated the fact that, within four days of my first hypnotising her, one of the most important of the female functions [i.e., menstruation], which had been suspended for many months, reappeared, and recurred regularly every month subsequently for the next six months; and when it again became suspended, the value of hypnotism was beautifully illustrated, as the following quotation will show:–

> At six successive periods I had occasion to resort to hypnotism, for this purpose, and in *every* instance with *entire* success, by *a single operation of from ten to eleven minutes each*. Moreover, I ascertained that this important result could be effected without either touch or pass, but by mental concentration and direction of the *mind of the patient*, and the management of the circulation alone, without farther mental or physical aid on my part, beyond simply requesting her to put herself to sleep, and elevate her limbs – her attention being directed to the expected result [i.e., restoration of the menstrual cycle]. On two or three other occasions, when I hypnotised this patient for neuralgic or rheumatic pain in a leg or arm, through the mode of managing and directing the attention and expectant idea, the pains were immediately removed, without exciting any visible manifestation on any special organ or function.

Subsequently to the publication of that report, on six other occasions I resorted to the same process as in this case, and with the like success on *every* occasion. **It now occurred to me that, inasmuch as it was my opinion, that the change in the physical action resulted entirely from the fixed mental attention of the patient, with a predominant idea and her faith in the power of the processes, it would be interesting to ascertain whether the result might not be realised by mental concentration alone, when she remained wide awake.** On the 4th of April, 1851, I proposed to test this. The requisite means were had recourse to for determining, with the utmost accuracy, the actual physical condition of the patient *before* commencing the experiment. Four ladies and one gentleman were present. Having requested the gentleman to note the time accurately, the patient being seated in an easy-chair, I addressed her in the following words, which were heard by all present:– "Now, keep your mind firmly fixed on what you know should happen." All remained silent; and, in order to withdraw my own mind as much as possible from the patient, I took up a volume of "Southey's Life", [a biography of Lord Nelson] and engaged myself in reading it. At the end of eleven minutes I asked her if the desired effect had been produced – to which she replied she did not know; but, upon proper examination, I had incontestable proof of the success of my experiment. Next month she did not require a repetition of the process; but, on the 2nd of June, it was again tried, in the presence of two professional gentlemen, and with equal success as on the 4th of April. On the 28th of July, I again had occasion to resort to the process with this patient; and I was then *particularly* anxious that it should succeed, as a lady was present who required similar aid, and a good example in point was likely to assist me considerably in influencing her the more certainly. My mind, therefore, was unusually intent on the accomplishment of the desired result. At the expiration of eleven minutes I inquired if it had taken effect, when she replied she could not tell. **On examination, however, it was ascertained that it had been a failure on this occasion. The patient hereupon remarked that, before sitting down, she thought it would *not* ensue *that night.* I enquired, "Why?" to which she replied, "Because I could not *fix my mind* on it *to-night*, from having been put out of my way just before I came here." To this I replied, "Well, if you cannot fix your mind on the idea when awake, I know that I can command the requisite attention when you are asleep, and therefore I will hypnotise you. This I did at the same time exciting the circulation. It very soon became apparent, from the expression of her features and the movements of her body, that the spell was in active operation; and on arousing her in eleven minutes, there was positive proof adduced that the experiment had not been tried in vain; and all went on satisfactorily subsequently.**

It merits special attention that, notwithstanding my mind was particularly active in *willing* the desired effect when the patient was awake, no success followed, because the requisite *mental* condition of the *subject* was wanting. This failure, therefore, was as positive proof in support of my theory as the successful results; in fact, it was even more so. For, on other occasions my mind had not been so intently desiring the immediate result, and now I was most actively engaged in willing it, and even with greater confidence, because of former successes; but I was doomed to be disappointed, because the requisite *mental condition* of the PATIENT *was absent*.

Next month my assistance was not required, but on the 8th of October, in the presence of her mother, the waking experiment was again tried with complete success. On the 8th of November, 1851, her mother, and my esteemed friend Dr. William Stevens, well-known as the author of the "Saline Treatment of Cholera and Yellow Fever", being present, I once more tried the experiment, with most complete success, in eight minutes. From that period it has never required to be repeated, as all has gone on in the natural course.[68]

It appears to me that nothing could be more conclusive and interesting for determining the correctness of my subjective or personal, psychical [i.e., psychological] or mental theory, than the evidence furnished by these cases; nor more important than the last for proving the value of hypnotism for curative purposes. I may also add that, on the 2nd of June, after exciting the [menstrual] function by mental concentration, whilst the patient was simply reposing in an easy-chair, by causing her to try it for two minutes more with the legs and arms extended, so as to quicken the circulation, a greatly increased effect was produced; **proving the importance of regulating the circulation, for modifying the subsequent results.**

[Group Experiment on Self-Hypnosis]
Another point worthy of remark, in support of my subjective or mental theory, is this – that not only may the requisite mental concentration be induced by the personal acts of the patients alone [i.e., autosuggestion or self-hypnosis], as already explained – such as by keeping their minds engaged in the continuous act of contemplating some part of their own bodies, or some ideal [i.e., imaginary] or inanimate objects, or the mere remembrance and expectation of the recurrence of past sensation, – but I have caused patients to hypnotise themselves, or each other, at the same instant of time,

---

[68] [Note that Braid appears to be demonstrating both i) that the intention ("silent will" supposed by the Mesmerists to telepathically influence the client) of the hypnotist is not necessary, ii) that concentration on an idea enhances the effect of waking suggestion, but that when such concentration is disrupted the induction of hypnotic "sleep" may be indicated in order to restore it.]

simply by staring at each other, or joining hands, etc., after the fashion of the ordinary Mesmerising processes. On one occasion I requested twenty-two patients to lay hold of each other's hands whilst standing in a semi-circle, and watch the result, and the whole twenty-two subjects speedily passed into the sleep, which is decidedly subversive of the *polar* theory of the magnetists; for, according to that theory, those only should have passed into the condition who had become surcharged with their alleged occult force passing from one set of patients into the others; and, consequently, those who supplied this Mesmeric, magnetic, odylic, nervous, or vital charge to the others, having thereby sustained a *diminution*, and thus being *under* par, ought to have remained awake. It is obvious that the same effect of sleep ensuing in every case, at the same time, could not have flowed from two such *opposite* PHYSICAL causes.

[Critique of Baron von Reichenbach's "Odylic Force"]
Another proposition of Baron von Reichenbach is this – that sensitive patients sleep better when in bed, and feel more comfortable in other places, when nestled in bed with their heads towards the north, or when seated elsewhere, such as in church, in a similar aspect. In my work on "The Power of the Mind over the Body", [1846] I stated that I had tried this experiment with a highly sensitive patient – and I know of others who have been so tested – without any such result following as the Baron had indicated. At the same time, I directed attention to the strange anomaly which this would present in the constitution of man, if proved to be true; because his most agreeable posture would be in direct opposition to what it ought to be, according to the physical constitution of his nature. For, according to Faraday, the very highest authority we have upon such speculations, the body of man is *dia*-magnetic, so that, were it hung up by the middle, it would naturally point east and west, instead of north and south, like the mineral magnet. A predominant idea or conceit, however, in the patient's mind may, no doubt, cause some individuals to realise such results as the Baron supposed; but were it a physical and physiological fact, as he alleged, what an amount of misery must people have entailed upon themselves, especially in large towns, where they nestle themselves in bed in all points of the compass! Is it conceivable that experience would not have taught them better, in the course of six thousand years? Moreover, would it not seem strange that the clergy, with all their learning and natural sagacity, should have built their churches in the very opposite direction to which they ought to have placed them in for comfort and attraction, according to the Baron's views, and that public halls and private dwellings should have been built without due regard to the Baron's alleged natural laws?

Baron Reichenbach has given the result of two experiments with the daguerreotype [an early photographic method], by Carl Schuh, as a physical proof of the optical nature of the odylic flames, threads, and smokes, described as seen, by sensitives, issuing from the poles of magnets. Regarding these experiments, the reviewer in the *North British* says they are:–

> Utterly unsatisfactory. Certainly these two poor experiments prove nothing. The experiment with two plates lasts a few hours; the experiment with only one, and therefore without a check, lasts sixty-four, the check in the former was rendered null by want of care about the box and the drawer, and there was no check provided in the latter. The experiments of Mr. Braid are much better.
>
> They were made with nine plates, prepared by Mr. Akers, of the Manchester Photographic Gallery – a man professionally engaged in daguerreotype experiments, and therefore quite as likely to be an adept as Herr Schuh. Three of the plates were exposed to the action of a powerful horse shoe (originally able to lift eighty pounds, but somewhat reduced by use) in seclusion from light. Another three were treated precisely in the same manner – only two sheets of black paper were placed between the magnets and the plates, so as to intercept the real or supposed radiance of its poles. A seventh was confined in a box at a distance from the magnet. They were all kept in these several circumstances from sixty-six to seventy-four hours; but in no instance was there any appearance of the photographic action of light – the only changes being such chemical modifications of the surfaces "as generally arise from keeping prepared plates for some time before exposing them to mercury".
>
> The other plates were enclosed in a camera, and exposed at such distance as must have given a picture of the poles of the magnet, and flames issuing from them, according to the Baron's statement regarding the focal distance of odyle. One was left sixty-six, the other thirty-five and a half hours so exposed; but no photographical indications were manifested.
>
> "Now it is to be noticed that these are three (four) positive results. Those of Schuh, such as they were, were at the best only negative ones. In his two experiments, it is not the least impossible but that common light reached the plates; and it does not appear that he was on his guard against those chemical changes which, generally arise from keeping prepared plates for some time." But in the experiments of Braid and Akers, metallic sensitives were positively and indubitably submitted to the prolonged action of a powerful magnetic force, but no photographic effects ensued. This is the positive observation not that; although, at first sight, it seems to be the reverse. In every point of view, in fact, the experiments of the Manchester surgeon are greatly superior to those of the Viennese authority on meteoric stones; and they settle this part of the question in the meantime. – Pages 145-146.

Regarding the experiments with the lens, the reviewer raises a very reasonable objection to them, as embracing such vagueness of testings as are "far below the mark of scientific accuracy, as it is practised and demanded in these days". And he then adds:–

> But here appears the avenging Nemesis of Reichenbach's contempt for the older Mesmerists. If he had studied their works, he could neither have made nor published this set of his experiments. Braid, the hypnotist, would more especially have furnished him with both facts and thoughts for his guidance. Dr. Holland, who is neither hypnotist nor Mesmerist, would have put him on his guard against the effects of expectant attention on certain exceptional nervous systems. In fine, our otherwise accomplished investigator would have been all the better for a little more knowledge of the physiology and pathology of the cerebro-spinal axis, considered as the instrument of the mind, and a little less knowledge of meteors. At all events, these experiments with the lenses will carry conviction into the judgment of neither physicist nor physiologist, especially if he is cognizant of the phenomena to be evoked in the Mesmerised nervous system by a word, by a sign, by absolutely next to nothing; and still more especially if he has seen how perfectly self-conscious the possessor of such a nervous system may appear to be, even when seeing water become white, a handkerchief turning into paper, and so forth. – Page 147.

According to Baron Reichenbach's own admission, a magnet suspended from one end of a beam, and balanced by weights at the other end, never moved when a cataleptic hand was advancing towards it with much force, even when allowed to approach close to it, and was hindered from touching and clinging to it only by the stronger arm of the operator or others holding the patient. It must be obvious that, were the attraction mutual, the magnet would advance towards the hand when the latter was restrained, after being near it. I, therefore, quite concur with the reviewer, when he says:–

> It is astonishing that, knowing, as he does, that there is no mutual attraction between the magnet and the cataleptic limb, he should not have defined it as an irresistible following of the removed magnet on the part of the limb. This phenomenon, in fact, considered as a phenomenon of motion, is altogether subjective in the patient. The magnet does not draw the hand, but the hand seeks towards the magnet; and an experimenter's fist, or a large crystal, is as good as a magnet.

[Critique of Dr. John Elliotson's Mesmerism]

I have hitherto omitted to advert to the alleged Mesmeric influence of certain metals and the non-Mesmerising quality of others. Dr. Elliotson had set forth that nickel was powerfully magnetic, so that drawing it along the palm of the hand would send a patient to sleep, and produce catalepsy; whilst, lead had no such quality – in short, that one class of metals enumerated would produce specific effects, whilst the others would reduce them, or prove neutral. He offered to prove this to the satisfaction of T. Wakley, Esq. M.P. [founder of *The Lancet* medical journal, and England's leading critic of Mesmerism], by giving him the respective metals into his own hands to operate with. According to this gentleman's statement, when he operated "with the lead, the patient believing it to be nickel, the effect of nickel came; and when he used the nickel, the patient supposing it to be lead, no effect followed. The effects were thus active or passive, according to the expectation or belief of the patient; and this exactly coincides with my own experience on this point – either that there are no such opposite effects in the different metals, or that the difference is so insignificant that it may be entirely superseded by the power of suggestion, or by a predominant idea. By this means I could, with most patients, invest metals, or any other substance, with whatever qualities I might imagine and audibly suggest to them. These experiments of Mr. Wakley [conduced in 1838] have always appeared to me as well devised and adroitly managed, for determining the physical fact, as to whether or not Dr. Elliotson was correct in maintaining that nickel was powerfully Mesmeric, whilst lead was wholly inert; and they clearly proved that Dr. Elliotson's hypothesis was erroneous in this respect. It was an unwarrantable, hasty conclusion, however, for Mr. Wakley to assume that the patients gave the manifestations realised from sheer deception, and, consequently, that the whole of what has been designated the Mesmeric state and Mesmeric phenomena was a tissue of unmitigated imposture. Even supposing the Okeys [two young sisters favoured by Elliotson as demonstration subjects] had been impostors in what resulted in these trials, (which I believe was not the case, but that the manifestations resulted from the powers of belief, habit, imagination, and the influence of predominant ideas over them, as explained elsewhere), surely it would have been a most unwarrantable deduction that there could not be an honest person in the world, merely because Mr. Wakley had met with two rogues? It was perfectly natural, however, for a person of enthusiastic mind, to impugn the honesty of the patients, and draw inferences unfavourable to the *bona fides* of the whole phenomena, when the results were so subversive of Dr. Elliotson's theory or explanation, and where the real state of the matter was then so imperfectly understood. Now, however, that we have so much clearer a comprehension of the real nature and cause of these phenomena, it behoves every candid minded man, and honest inquirer after truth, to modify his hostility and opposition accordingly.

[Mesmerism Refuted by Suggestion Experiments]

My investigations, supported as they are by the researches of many men of the highest rank and intelligence, fully prove that the solution of the problem is this – that many patients, who are naturally highly susceptible of such influence, become, at length, liable to be affected entirely through the force of imagination, belief, and habit, and that they do not exhibit these manifestations from any desire to deceive others, but because they are self-deceived through their implicit credulity, belief, and fixity of their attention on the ideas suggested in their hearing, or in any way associated in their minds with certain processes and combinations of circumstances. The late public experiments, on a large scale, in what has been called "electro-biology", and of which I gave examples, as well as my *rationale* in 1846, in my work on "The Power of the Mind over the Body". [a detailed critique of Reichenbach] fully demonstrated this influence over many patients, even in the waking condition; and my own experiments on a Mesmerised patient, recorded in that work, in which every variety of result which I audibly suggested was manifested on the said patient, merely by touching her with my portmanteau key, or placing it in her hand, or suspending it from her fingers, all proved the same fact. In Mr. Wakley's experiments in 1838, he used *different* substances, and the results changed according to his suggestions or the expectation of the patient; in Dr. [John] Haygarth's experiments with the wooden tractors in 1799, results were realised similar to those when Mr. Perkins' metallic tractors [metal pins drawn across the surface of the skin] were used, whatever variety of wood was tried, painted so as to represent the metallic tractors; but, in my experiments with my portmanteau key, in 1846, many different results flowed from using the *same article*, and these effects were always in exact accordance with my audible suggestions. All these three classes of experiments, therefore, although tending to prove the same ultimate fact, *viz.*, the power of expectation, belief, and a predominant idea, over certain patients, were, in themselves, essentially different from each other.

[Conclusion]

In conclusion, I beg leave to remark that, from ample experience, I feel pretty confident that all the phenomena alleged by me as producible in the above-named manner are veritable *facts* – that they are NOT *fallacies*. I believe, moreover, that the explanation which I have endeavoured to propound is quite adequate to account for all which I represent as true, **without violating any of the recognised laws of physiology and psychology**. From a consideration of the whole, therefore, I am led to infer that my subjective [i.e., psychological] or personal theory is, at all events, a step in the right direction, and somewhat nearer the truth than the theories of the Mesmerists and electro-biologists. Even the Mesmerists themselves are willing to admit that, in the production of the phenomena of "electro-biology", there is no more *electricity* than there is in all the operations of nature; and that there is nothing of a special influence, a magnetic fluid, an "od" force, or transmission of a nervous or vital force from one human being to another, as the *efficient* CAUSE, either of the phenomena of "electro-biology" or the ordinary phenomena of Mesmerism. I consider the experiments and observations which I have published during the last ten years, together with the experience and opinions of others quoted in this little treatise, should be sufficient to demonstrate, to the conviction of all whose minds are not sealed by dogmatic scepticism, or [electro-]*biologised* by some previous predominant idea about the existence of an "od" force or Mesmeric influence. For my own part, however, I am quite open to receive instruction and guidance in my search after truth, from whatever quarter it may be presented for my consideration; because I believe that, as yet, we are only on the threshold of this curious, interesting, and most important inquiry.

> It is the great rule of the inductive hypothesis, that the investigator invent nothing new if possible; it is the second, that he adduce the minimum of causation for the maximum of effect; and it is the third, that he proceed from the known to the unknown. It is humbly submitted that the doctrine now explained fulfils these conditions.
> – *North British Review*.

Appendices
1. Letter of Apology from J.C. Colquhoun (February 1852)

It has been remarked by someone, and frequently repeated by others, that the most important part of a lady's letter is generally to be found in the postscript. Whether or not such may be the fact in respect to the letters of the fair sex, I pretend not to decide; but I have no hesitation in saying, that the most pleasing part of the duty which has devolved upon me connected with the subject of this discussion, will be found in my concluding remarks, which are written for the purpose of fully and freely exonerating Mr. Colquhoun from the imputation of having published the remarks which I have criticised, with any *desire* or *intention* whatever, on his part, to injure me. In the note at [the beginning of this book], I had alleged it as probable that the charges of which I complained might have been written by him "unintentionally or inadvertently", merely from a little momentary irritation, arising out of my remarks against what appeared to me to be extreme views of the Mesmerists, of whom he was one of the most distinguished, and which had roused his enthusiasm, and excited him to take up the gauntlet and fight in support of a theory which he had long espoused, and ably and warmly supported. Now, I have that gentleman's earnest and candid declaration to that effect, which was so promptly given (for he wrote the moment he heard I considered that he had misrepresented me), and so frankly expressed by him in the subjoined letter, as to require neither note nor comment from me to bespeak for it a favourable reception and due appreciation, by every honourable-minded man, as it does equal credit to the heart as to the head of the *ingenuous* [i.e., sincere], as well as ingenious and learned writer:–

> Edinburgh, 14th February, 1852.
>
> My Dear Sir,
>
> Our friend, Mr. S——, has just mentioned to me that you are displeased with what I have said of you in my last work. I regret this very much, if it be so. But you must recollect that you had, upon different occasions, made certain pretty severe remarks upon the magnetists for believing in the higher phenomena of their science; and I thought it fair to defend myself, and those who entertain the same views. Nothing could be farther from my intention than to give you serious cause of offence; for, besides the friendly terms which have always subsisted between us, I have ever been disposed to look upon your labours as valuable, and always expected that you would ultimately arrive at the same results as the Mesmerists. Mr. S—— mentioned that you seemed to think that I had charged you with being a materialist. I am not aware of this, and certainly had no such intention. You had said, when speaking of the pretensions of the Mesmerists, that they were "alike a mockery of the human understanding, as they are opposed to all the known laws of physical science". I then asked, "Does Mr. Braid, then, acknowledge no science but the merely physical?" I never thought of such a thing as charging you with being a materialist. I merely wished to remind you that there are moral as well as physical laws; and, it appears to me, that both are co-operative in producing the higher phenomena of animal magnetism. I trust, therefore, that you will take no offence at these expressions. They are surely less severe and objectionable than those you have used in speaking of the Mesmerists, of whom I am one. Let there be no quarrel, then, between you and me. I should sincerely regret such a thing.
>
> You are probably aware that the higher phenomena of clairvoyance have recently been most clearly and beautifully developed in this city. My friend, Mr. Napier – whose first case I printed, at his request, in the appendix to my late book – has since, in association with Professor Gregory, brought out similar, and even more striking phenomena: in other cases, of which, perhaps, you may be aware.
>
> From a conversation I lately had with Dr. Esdaile, of Indian celebrity, I find that he is perfectly convinced of the reality of clairvoyance – has himself produced the phenomena in many instances – and laughs at those who deny them. I think it likely that he will publish something upon this subject before long. I repeat, then, let there be no dryness or coolness between you and me. Let each prosecute his own researches, and I have no doubt that the truth will ultimately emerge out of free and open discussion; and I sincerely trust, without any breach of friendship. I should be exceedingly sorry to have any quarrel with you upon this or any other subject.
>
> I am, my dear Sir,
>   Very sincerely yours,
>
>   J. C. Colquhoun.

Most heartily do I reciprocate the kindly feeling and desire expressed by Mr. Colquhoun, that there should be no coldness or diminution of friendly feeling between us arising out of our doing battle for the support of our respective theories, or modes of explaining the nature, cause, and extent of magnetic or hypnotic phenomena. Notwithstanding Mr. C. had no unfriendly intention against me in publishing his remarks – particularly the unfortunate query which, by innuendo, implicated me in the charge of being a materialist – still, that would not have been enough to shield me against the evil effects which might result therefrom, in the minds of those who perused what he had published. It would, therefore, have been requisite for me to have replied, in self-vindication of the erroneous impressions regarding me, which might have originated with those who perused Mr. Colquhoun's interesting and learned book, (the great merits of which will insure for it an extensive circulation and eager perusal) even had I privately received that gentleman's letter before I had gone to press. Had I received that letter sooner, I certainly should have modified some expressions made use of by me when criticising Mr. Colquhoun's remarks regarding myself and hypnotism; but it is particularly gratifying that the said letter came to hand before the present edition was completed, and although it was not written with the intention of being published, that I was able to obtain Mr. C.'s permission to publish it as an appendix to my "Observations" on his History; because it exonerates *both* parties from any desire, wantonly and intentionally, to misrepresent or injure each other personally, whilst entering into free and open discussion upon scientific subjects. For my own part, I believe that truth, in such inquiries, can only be arrived at through the collision of intellect, and the different points of view from which the subjects are contemplated by different minds.

2. Self-Hypnosis & Hindu Yoga Meditation

I shall now cite from a paper published by me in The Medical Times for December 28th 1844, a few of the wonders recorded in Ward's "History of the Hindoos", which they represent as facts and as special gifts imparted to them in token of the great superiority of their religious system, of inducing a state of **self-hypnotism**, or ecstatic trance. They produce this condition by certain postures or modes of sitting – the minds of the devotees being engaged in acts of fixed attention, by looking at some parts of their own bodies, or at inanimate or ideal [i.e., imaginary] objects; at the same time holding their breath, i.e., suppressing their respiration. My modes of explaining these alleged marvels are given within parentheses. I may premise, however, that whatever idea occupies the mind of the subject before he passes into the condition, or whatever may have occurred to it accidentally or through the suggestion of others subsequently, will ever after be realised, under similar combination of circumstances, in consequence of the power of suggestion and double-conscious [dissociated] memory, as manifested in some patients even in the sub-hypnotic or waking condition, when what have been called the vigilant or waking phenomena are producible; and still more certainly during the full, active, double-conscious condition. These principles alone, and the vivid state of the imagination, explain most of the marvels; but, with the parenthetic explanations, I trust to make them sufficiently obvious to any candid and intelligent person.

> The Yogee [i.e., master of yogic meditation] who has perfected himself in the three parts of sungyamu [yogic "self-mastery"] obtains a knowledge of the past and of the future (quickened memory and excited imagination); if he apply sungyamu to sounds, to their meaning and to the consequent results, he will possess, from mere sound, universal knowledge (hypnotic patients imitate, with the utmost precision and with the greatest facility, the vocal enunciation of any language, but do not understand the meaning of the words which they utter). He who applies sungyamu to discover the *thoughts* of others will know the thoughts of all. (He will believe and talk as if he did so.) He who does the same to his own form, and to the sight of those whose eyes are fixed upon him, will be able to render his body invisible, and to dim the sight of the observers. (Through the force of imagination, or fixed attention, or suggestion.) He who, according to these rules, meditates on his own actions, in order that he may discover how he may most speedily reap the fruits of them, will become acquainted with the time, cause, and place of his own death. He who, according to these rules, meditates on the strength of the powerful, so as to identify his strength with theirs, will acquire the same. (Through concentrated attention and conviction of their physical energy, there is a most amazing manifestation of increased muscular power.) He who meditates, in the same manner, on the sun as perfect light, will become acquainted with the state of things in every place. (He will believe and speak as if he really did.) By similar application of sungyamu to the cup at the bottom of the throat, he will overcome hunger and thirst; by meditation on the basilar suture, he will be capacitated to see and converse with deified persons, who range through the aerial regions; by meditation on extraordinary presence of mind, he will obtain a knowledge of all visible objects; by meditating on the seat of the mind, or on the faculty of reason, he will become acquainted with his own thoughts and those of others, past, present, and future; by meditation on the state of the Yogee who has nearly lost all consciousness of separate existence, he will recognise spirit as unassociated and perfect existence. (Belief and vivid imagination.) After this he will hear celestial sounds – the songs and conversations of the celestial choirs; he will have the perception of their touch in their passage through the air, his taste will become refined, and he will enjoy the constant fragrance of sweet scents. (All this I can easily cause hypnotic patients to realise, through suggestion and their fervid imagination.) When the Yogee, by the power of Samadhi [meditation], has destroyed the power of those works which retained the spirit in captivity, he becomes possessed of certain and unhesitating knowledge; he is enabled to trace the progress of intellect through the senses, and the path of the animal spirit through the nerves. After this he is able to enter into any dead or living body, by the path of the senses – all the senses accompanying him, as the swarm of bees follows the queen bee; and, in this body, to act as though it were his own. (Now, all this extravagance I can easily make hypnotic patients imagine themselves accomplishing – but, of course, it is *only imaginary*, just as such feats are accomplished in dreams.)
>
> The collected power of all the senses is called the animal soul, which is distinguished by five operations connected with the vital air, or air collected in the body. The body of the Yogee who, according to the rules of Dharanu, Dhyanu, and Sumadhee [concentration, meditation, and mystic union], meditates on the air proceeding from (...) to the head, *will become light as wood*, and will be able to *walk on the fluid element*. He who, in the same manner, meditates on the ear and its vacuum, will hear the softest and most distant sounds, *as well* as those uttered in the celestial regions, etc. (This accords with my proposition, that calling attention to any organ or function will exalt the activity of the function positively, as well as excite ideas connected with such organ or function.) He who meditates on vacuum will be able to ascend in the air. (Imaginary ascent.) He who meditates, by the rules of sungyamu, and in a perfect manner, on the subtle elements, will overcome and be transformed into those elements; he will be capacitated to become as rarefied and atomic as he may wish, and proceed to the greatest distance; in short, he will be enabled to realise in himself the power of Deity, to subdue all his passions, to render his body invulnerable, to prevent the possibility of his abstraction being destroyed, so as to subject himself again to the effects of actions.
>
> "By applying sungyamu to the division of the four last minutes of time, he who perfects himself in this will obtain complete knowledge of the separate elements, atoms, etc., which admit not of division of species, appearance, and place. This knowledge brings before the Yogee all visible objects at once, so that he does not

> wait for the tedious process of the senses. (Imagination, lively faith, and fixed attention, until ideas became too vivid to be corrected by an appeal to the senses and sober reason.)

The following paragraph is from the "Dabistan" [*Dabistān-i Mazāhib*, a 17th century Persian religious text of a syncretistic nature]:–

> The Sipasian [an ancient Zoroastrian sect] and the historians relate that, whoever carries this process to perfection rises above death; as long as he remains in the body, he can put it off and be again reunited to it; he never suffers from sickness, and is fit for all business.

So much for the lively fancy and fervid faith of these religious enthusiasts, during their dreams, in the state of self-induced hypnotism, through fixing their thoughts or sight upon some part of their own bodies, or on some ideal [i.e., imaginary] or inanimate objects, and holding their breath, or suppressing their respiration. By an appeal, therefore, to the feats of the Hindoos, I might claim for hypnotism, or **self-induced trance**, quite as high pretensions for its capability of inducing clairvoyant marvels as anything adduced by the animal magnetists or Mesmerists, with all the exoteric or alleged aid which they profess to communicate or impart to their subjects, by whatever name they may call it – whether magnetic, Mesmeric, odylic, nervous, or vital force transferred from the operators into the bodies of their subjects.

3. Braid Exposes a Bogus Clairvoyant

"A chiel's amang you takin' notes,
And faith he'll prent them." [– Robert Burns]

I append the following narrative, believing that it may be interesting to some of my readers, especially as it has a direct bearing on the question regarding the truth or error of what has been asserted as the special gifts of Mesmeric clairvoyants. It may also aid them in conducting similar investigations in future, so as to guard against some of the many sources of fallacy with which such an inquiry is necessarily surrounded.

Whilst the last sheet of this little book was passing through the press, M. Lassaigne and Mdlle. Prudence Bernard, of Hungerford Hall notoriety, made their appearance in Manchester, to astonish us by their wonderful Mesmeric, clairvoyant, and supersentient feats. In their circulars, Monsieur Lassaigne was heralded as "The First Magnetiser in Europe", and Mdlle. Prudence as "the best Clairvoyante known"; and, in support of these high pretensions, thirty-two paragraphs were appended from the London Newspaper Press.

Under these circumstances, and having been urged by an Edinburgh friend to test this lady's wonderful pretensions, I did not see how I could refuse to go and witness at least *one* of their public exhibitions, without subjecting myself to the charge of acting like the philosophers in the days of Galileo, who refused to look through his telescope, from a dread that they might thereby be compelled to admit the alleged fact, which they had so strenuously denied. I, therefore, went to the *séance* announced for Friday, the 27th of February, 1852, and secured one of the best seats on the platform, so that I might have an opportunity of observing, with the greater accuracy, all which might be said or done by M. L. and his Mesmeric clairvoyante.

I was perfectly well aware that many of the feats announced in the programme were capable of being accomplished by a system of collusion, so devised that it might be difficult to detect the sources of fallacy, particularly on a public platform; but there were others, and those the more important pretensions, which I knew that I could test in such a simple and satisfactory manner as must convince everyone in the room, either that she possessed the supersentient gifts [in other words, "ESP"] asserted, or that she possessed them not; and I, therefore, went prepared to test this fairly, should a favourable opportunity offer.

The first point which arrested my attention, after the lady was announced as being in the Mesmeric state, was this – that she was one of those subjects who, during the Mesmeric condition, have the use of their eyes, i.e., seeing through, or rather from under, their partially closed eyelids. I am quite aware that many of the Mesmeric phenomena may be feigned, as, indeed, every other condition may be, and daily is, on the stage; and it is, therefore, quite *possible* that Mdlle. Prudence Bernard was not in the Mesmeric state at all, which some seemed to suppose was the case. For my own part, however, I think it much more *probable* that she was in the so-called Mesmeric state, and for this reason, that during the state of mental concentration peculiar to that condition, all the organs of sense which are called into action become prodigiously quickened, so that they can hear at much greater distances than when awake; and some have the sense of smell so exalted that they can readily detect the owner of a glove in a room full of company, by *smell* – for, if their nostrils are stopped, they cannot do so. (The blind boy, Mitchell, recognised people by smell in his ordinary state; and he formed a favourable or an unfavourable opinion of them when first introduced to him, according to the peculiar odour from their persons.) The sense of touch and resistance, and of heat and cold, and no doubt taste also are in like manner greatly quickened.

Many of the first experiments of the evening were, in my opinion, quite vitiated, from the request to do such and such feats having been given to M. Lassaigne, or the interpreter in a whisper, which, I well knew, any attentive Mesmerised subject might overhear, from their quickened sense of hearing I called attention to this source of fallacy, and suggested that all future requests should be conveyed to M. Lassaigne in writing. This proposal was at once most readily acceded to; and she still continued to give proofs of her power of understanding M. Lassaigne – although both myself, and others near me, observed, in certain instances, that suggestions were now given which were "not in the bond" – such as, "You are near him," audibly expressed, before she gave the flower to the reporter – which was the order proposed on this occasion, and was to have been conveyed to the clairvoyante silently, and by the mere force of M. Lassaigne's will. At first she passed by the reporter, and went up to several other persons seated behind him, and fenced about as if she expected it should be some of them; but, at length, judging from their looks and manners that she was off the proper scent, she drew back and stood still for a little, as if quite at a loss what to do next; but the instant the words "You are near him," were audibly uttered, she turned round and gave the flower to the reporter, who was the person nearest to her at that moment. It was, therefore, easy for her to fix upon the reporter, seated at a table by himself, and near to where she was standing, when the audible suggestion was given regarding their proximity. A similar hesitation took place before giving a book to the proper person; so that, instead of what I saw, being *clear* seeing, I considered it *dim* seeing and artful dodging. Moreover, M. L.'s mode of walking behind his clairvoyante when he wished her to advance, and standing still when she had gone to the extent desired, was a mode of suggestion which did not escape observation. When to all this is added the mode of giving suggestions through watching the eye of another, and signals communicated through slight movements felt and heard by the patient, though unobserved by the audience, there is no difficulty in comprehending how M. L. succeeded with almost all the experiments tried by him and his clairvoyante whilst I was in the room, without the possession by her of any supersentient gift of the nature which he alleged. Even. M. Robin's experiments with the bell, with his blindfolded clairvoyante, were still more remarkable; and yet he avowed that they were done *entirely by collusion*, and by means so simple, too, that he could scarcely restrain himself from laughing outright when thinking of the ease with which the audience could be deceived by those experiments.

But now arrived the experiment which I considered by far the most interesting of all on the programme, *viz.*, playing at cards and reading, when her eyes were to be so securely blindfolded that not a ray of light could reach them, in the common acceptation of the term. To effect this, folds of cotton wadding were placed across the forehead, eyes, and nose, and over the face as far as the point of the nose, and then a white handkerchief folded several times, so as to be about 2½ inches wide, was bound round the head and eyes, so as to maintain the cotton in its place. This done, M. Lassaigne triumphantly asked anyone to examine his subject, and say whether it was *possible* for her to see through all this apparatus. Someone having exclaimed "no," the lady sat down at a table to challenge anyone present to play a game of cards with her. Whilst they were making arrangements for the game, even without being Mesmerised, I was sufficiently clairvoyant to observe the lady pensively lay her face upon her hands, so as to enable her very conveniently, and *by mere accident no doubt*, to give the proper twist and finish to the apparatus for *excluding* light from her eyes. I observed this manoeuvre by the lady *twice*, and called the attention of some friends to it, who can also testify to the fact. The clairvoyante now became very lively; described the personal appearance of her opponent, played dexterously, and beat him. She also did the same by another gentleman who tried a round with her; and with a third gentleman, a friend of my own, who, by my suggestion, had taken a new pack of cards with him, she proved her power of describing his personal appearance correctly, and playing well, but she lost on this occasion from having bad cards.

As the lady was now considered to have proved her clairvoyant powers to the satisfaction of all present, I stepped forward and announced my desire to have the privilege of applying a test which would be far more satisfactory to *my* mind, because I had no confidence in the supposed efficacy of the blindfolding then in use, for effectually accomplishing what it professed to do. I told the audience that I felt convinced that the patient was seeing through interstices between the cotton and the face, near the side of the nose. My proposal for guarding against such a source of fallacy as this was simply to place a thin sheet of brown card board under her chin and round her neck, so as to guard against the possibility of the deception which I suspected. This I intended to have accomplished by tying the sheet of pasteboard around her neck, proceeding from the bottom of the throat upwards in a conical form, after the fashion of the Elizabethan frill, extending considerably higher than the head, so as to prevent the possibility of her raising her hands or lowering her head sufficiently for seeing over it, without exciting the attention of the audience. Indeed, whoever had had the opportunity of observing the clairvoyante, as I did, during this card scene, must have felt that he would be permitting an insult to be perpetrated upon himself and upon the whole audience, were he not to endeavour to expose what appeared to me to be such an absurd farce. I was aware that my test would be objected to, on the ground that she did not profess to read *through card board* (although I must confess my surprise that a person who can see and read through stone or brick walls, should not be competent to penetrate through thin card board), so I, therefore, offered to remove that objection, by cutting out a piece of the card board, and covering the hole with the cotton wadding and folded handkerchief, which *she actually professed to see through* but, although the audience were almost unanimous in their opinion that my proposed test was a fair one, and such as they wished to see tried, M. Lassaigne well knew that it was too certain and obvious a mode of testing to answer his purpose, and, therefore, under various pretexts, and in a most rude manner, he obstinately refused to try it. I therefore withdrew from the platform and left the room, feeling the force of the remark – "*Ex uno; disce omnes.*" ["From one (such example), learn about them all."]

Had M. Lassaigne, like M. Robin, admitted that his feats were done by ingeniously contrived collusion, I should have considered it perfectly fair for him to refuse submitting to any mode of testing which might destroy the interest of his *future* public exhibitions. Here, however, we had a different sort of pretensions to deal with, for M. Lassaigne represented that there was no collusion in the matter, but that all was accomplished by supersentient gifts imparted to his patient by his Mesmerising processes. According to this notion, that the mind of the subject could hold intercourse with the outer world without the aid of the physical organs required for such purposes during the waking condition, I consider the audience not only had a right to expect, but to *demand*, that they should have satisfactory proof adduced, that all chance of the subject deceiving us by using her natural physical organs of sight, hearing, feeling, and smell, when we thought these excluded, should be clearly demonstrated to be impossible, under existing circumstances. Such was the sole purport of my test, which was perfectly fair, and would not have been refused had she really possessed the power alleged; for, be it observed, I was willing to cut a hole in the pasteboard, and cover it merely with the wadding and handkerchief which she really *professed to see through*; that is, to take them *off* the *eyes* and cover the aperture in the mask with the *same materials*. Inasmuch, then, as the objects to be seen and described and the light were still to remain in the same relative position to the eyes, wherein existed a difference between the mode she professed and the one I suggested – unless in the facility for deceiving us by the *former* mode, and the impossibility of doing so by the latter?

At their first *séance* at Manchester, on the 24th of February, 1852, a gentleman went prepared to test the lady's power of reading without seeing through interspaces. He had written a short sentence from a French book, in a plain hand, and folded and enclosed it in a common letter envelope, so that, including the envelope, four folds of paper would have required to be read through. The gentleman has written to me, and enclosed the test unopened. After detailing various alleged clairvoyant feats done by the lady, such as playing at cards, and reading written words with the eyes covered with cotton and a handkerchief, he adds,

> When these experiments were concluded, I rose and said – "Now that the balls of cotton and the cloth are removed from the lady's eyes, will she read a few words, plainly written, on a slip of paper, and enclosed in a common envelope?" "No," replied the interpreter, "that is a very difficult experiment." "But some of Dr. ——'s patients have done it." "It cannot be done, except light falls in some way on the words to be read." "Oh!" said a gentleman in another part of the hall, "that throws *light* on the proceedings." I was of the same opinion, and did not again interfere.

This gentleman's test was really not a very severe one, had she possessed any remarkable quickness of vision, for I find that, with the aid of *transmitted* light, I can myself see to read the writing through *two* folds of the paper, and surely *four* folds ought not to be impossible for a clairvoyante who pretends to see through stone or brick walls innumerable, or even through mountains, and to the other side of the globe, or, what is being transacted by living men or their departed spirits, throughout any part of illimitable space. Mdlle. Prudence Bernard, moreover, had the double chance of reading the silent *thoughts* of the *writer*, which was one of her *professed feats*.[69]

As my object in attending M. L.'s *séance* was neither simply to be amused, nor to be deceived by mere illusions, but to investigate what was proposed for our consideration with some degree of philosophical accuracy – although a public platform is by no means a favourable place for doing so – when I found the latter was to be peremptorily denied us, I could not condescend to remain and countenance a mere *sham* investigation, which might be set forth to the world, hereafter, as having been exhibited before me and not demurred to. Had fair and full investigation been permitted, there were several other experiments in the programme which I wished to have tested, with as much accuracy as a public platform would have permitted; but I must have a fair field and no favour when testing, or totally decline being a party to any proposed scientific, but merely *sham*, investigation. I understand, moreover, that, after I had left the room, it was represented to the audience that M. Lassaigne had been so polite as to invite me to his *séance*, and that, in return for that kindness, I had rudely come and interrupted the harmony of the meeting. The audience must, naturally, have inferred from this, that M. Lassaigne had presented me with a free ticket of admission, but such was not the case. The only civility of the sort which I am aware of was this – that one of his circulars was left at my house, as they were at other houses in Manchester, in order to tempt me to go and pay the usual admission fee, which I did pay, and therefore was under no such obligation to M. Lassaigne as he wished the audience to believe.

From my anxious desire to guard against every chance of misrepresenting, in any respect whatever, what really occurred at said *séance* of M. Lassaigne, before going to press, I submitted a proof of the above narrative to the inspection of three of the most intelligent gentlemen who engaged in testing Mdlle. Prudence Bernard, that evening, who are ready to vouch for its accuracy on *every point*.

[Conclusion]

In conclusion, I would beg leave only farther to observe, that the advanced state of physical and chemical science has now enabled us to explain, on scientific principles, many phenomena which, in former days, were looked upon as the results of Magic and Witchcraft. When to these are added the peculiar manifestations of nervous diseases, and **the power of imagination, sympathy, imitation, predominant ideas, easy credulity, fixed attention, habit, and suggestion in all its various forms, in changing or modifying mental and physical phenomena in many individuals, even in the waking condition, and**

---

[69] Many years ago reports were published of a remarkably clairvoyant boy, in ——— who could see through a mask of nine folds of silk stuffed with cotton wadding. Through all this his optics were said to enable him to penetrate when Mesmerised; so that he could play cards and read any book, or print new from the press, more fluently and elegantly than when awake. I wrote to the gentleman whose book this account appeared in, told him what I suspected, and how he was deceived. He could not believe it possible to trick him, and the hundreds of respectable people who had seen the boy, in the manner I supposed; but offered me an opportunity of testing him, by a friend who was visiting that city. The boy having played cards dexterously, as usual, with his mask on, my friend took him in hand according to the plan suggested by me, which was to guard against interspaces near the nose. The boy read the superscription of my letter to him, then, opened it and read on with fluency; but the moment my friend placed his card over the writing, or below the nose, the clairvoyance was gone but returned when he withdrew it, the same with a sheet of paper interposed; and, finally, by carrying his hand, holding the letter, sufficiently high to prevent any ray of light getting to the eye by the side of his nose, it was a dead pause, without covering the writing with any substance. This opened the eyes and understanding of all present to the source of fallacy through which they had been deceived; and they wrote and begged I would not publish the case; because the boy's father was such a respectable man, being one of the town council. I consider that Mademoiselle Prudence Bernard was clairvoyant on the evening when I saw her through the same means and the object of my test was simply to prove this to be a fact.

their almost unlimited control over those who pass into the second conscious stage of hypnotism – as explained in the foregoing pages – the whole of the well-ascertained apparent marvels of Magic, Witchcraft, Animal Magnetism, Hypnotism, Electro-Biology, Crystal-seeing, *etc.*, become level to our apprehension, and admit of explanation without violating any of the recognised laws of physiology and psychology.

An accidental circumstance having caused delay in printing off the last sheet of this little book enables me to add the following valuable testimony in support of my views, which I extract from the newly published volume entitled, "Chapters on Mental Physiology, by Henry Holland, M.D., F.R.S., *etc. etc.*, Fellow of the Royal College of Physicians, Physician Extraordinary to the Queen, *etc.*" That gentleman has long been well-known as one of the most ingenious, scientific, and learned writers, as well as accomplished practical physicians, in Europe; and his recent work fully maintains his high reputation, being one of the most valuable and masterly productions which has issued from the press for a long period, both as regards the important topics discussed by the author, the facts adduced, and the ingenious reasonings and philosophical deductions with which he has connected them. At page 30, the learned author acutely and justly observes:–

> Are these phenomena – admitted by all to be singular and striking – derived from a peculiar agent or influence, transmitted from one human body to another by certain modes of communication? Or are they the effects of various external excitements on the sensorium [i.e., the senses] and nervous system of persons of a peculiar temperament, analogous in nature and origin to phenomena with which we are more familiar in sleep, trance, hysteria, and other forms of cerebral or nervous disorder?
>
> These questions, involving the very reality of the Mesmeric theory, must ever be kept before us in all observation or reasoning on the subject. It is singularly important that this should be done wherever experiment is concerned; inasmuch as they suggest those particular tests which are essential to complete evidence, but which have been, for the most part, unaccountably neglected. In putting these questions, moreover, we indicate the absolute need of familiarity with the natural phenomena of health and disease just adverted to for the right prosecution of this inquiry. Without this knowledge, and without the just perception of what constitutes scientific evidence, we might as well be gazing at the feats of a conjurer at a public exhibition, as on those of animal magnetism in similar assemblies.
>
> Another point in this question, not sufficiently kept in mind, is the vast distinction between the two classes of Mesmeric phenomena – sleep, reverie, trance, and certain acts arising from them – and the miraculous assumption of clairvoyance, prophecy, and other powers, superseding all the physical laws of time and space of which we have any knowledge. These things are presented to us as parts of the same phenomenon, and produced by the same manipulations or personal contact. But they are in truth of very different nature, and totally incommensurate with each other. There is less distinction between the intellect of an infant and that of Bacon, Newton, or Laplace, than between the conditions thus brought into pretended connection. If the miraculous powers in question, for they admit no other name, be proffered to our belief, it must be upon evidence far more searching and stringent than is needed to verify those other conditions, which are so closely allied to the ordinary changes in health and disease. It is unnecessary to dilate on the importance of a distinction which every man of understanding will admit and appreciate.

And, at page 34:–

> Applying these facts to the more mysterious exhibitions of this influence, they cogently suggest the question, how it can happen that such manifestations of new and exalted power – the knowledge of events far distant in space and time – the instant recognition, without inquiry, of the seat and nature of internal disease and of the befitting treatment – vision, or that perception which is equivalent to it, through other organs than the eyes, etc. – how it happens, I say, that faculties so marvellous should be given to those of feeble, vague, or distempered mind, and wholly denied to men of the highest mental energy and intellectual powers – given, moreover, by persons who themselves possess none of the faculties which they thus miraculously bestow? This question, though stated merely as such, is in effect pregnant with argument; and deserved to be well weighed by all who incline to this separate and more mysterious part of Mesmeric belief.

At pages 9, 10, 24-35, 83-94, 123-128, 155, 160, 169, 172, 173, 223, and 280, Dr. Holland has given many admirable observations bearing on this subject, to which I beg to refer, in addition to the following quotations:–

> The observations of Mr. Braid, more especially, have done much to establish this fact of the altered character of sleep in effect of the manner in which it is brought on; and this may be regarded as a valuable part of his researches. – Page 89.

> We must not quit this topic without noticing the striking results of what has been termed *Hypnotism* – the sleep or trance produced, not by Mesmeric means, but by the act of the individual himself, made to concentrate his vision fixedly for a certain time upon some one object. It apparently facilitates the effect if this object be of small size; and Mr. Braid's interesting experiments would seem to show what may well be understood, that the posture of the head further favours the results. The simple fact, that the various physical character of the object gazed upon does in no way alter the effect will readily be received as sufficient proof that the trance induced arises from causes *within*, and not from influences *without*, the body of the person thus affected.

The evidence, indeed, furnished by these experiments in relation to Mesmeric sleep, is simple and convincing as respects the main assumption, that this state is brought on by the influence of one human body on another. The effects are less in degree, inasmuch as the means employed less powerfully excite the imagination. But they are expressly the same in kind; and justify the conclusion, that all these states depend on affections of the nervous system, in persons of a certain temperament, and under certain modes of excitement.

These researches of Mr. Braid on Hypnotism well deserve careful examination; as do also his valuable experiments connected with Electro-Biology; each inquiry illustrating the other by analogous facts and inferences. – Page 92

Additional Appendices
1. Experiments on Mesmerism at Aberdeen University

Whilst this little tract was going through the press, an interesting report of an "Examination of Mr. Lewis's Experiments on Mesmerism, at the Medical School of the University and King's College, Aberdeen" has come under my notice in the "Monthly Journal of Medical Science". The committee consisted of three professors, two medical men, and a clergyman, who undertook the investigation at the earnest solicitation of the pupils at the medical school, for whose benefit the inquiry was instituted. The experiments seem to have been conducted in a fair and liberal spirit, due care being taken to guard against all obvious sources of fallacy, but with every desire to give ample justice to the experimentalist. Three of the committee remained in the class-room where the patient was seated, whose duty was to consist in recording the time and the character of the movements performed by the patient, whilst the other three were in an adjoining room with Mr. Lewis, to suggest the various movements they wished him to excite by his silent will and physical gestures at different times, which were also correctly recorded. When the round of experiments was finished, these three gentlemen and Mr. Lewis returned into the room where the patient and audience were, and then both reports were read aloud and compared. The results I give in the words subscribed by the whole committee:–

> There was a total want of correspondence in point of time and character between the volitions and acts of the operator and of his subject, when in different rooms, which shows at once that Mr. Lewis exercised no influence whatever over the person whom he had deliberately chosen for that purpose, after he had tested his susceptibility. It is only necessary to point to Mr. Lewis's attempt to overcome the influence of gravitation, in his effort to make Mr. M. stand on one leg, with the same side of his body and his foot pressed close to the wall, to prove that in this case, at least, not the slightest influence of the kind was exerted. These experiments, therefore, afford no ground whatever for the opinion, that either Mr. L. or any other person can influence another at a distance from him, or in the least degree counteract the influence of physical laws.

These results and inferences are in entire accordance with my own experience and deductions on this branch of the inquiry, as may be seen recorded in various parts of my published observations. Regarding the pretensions of Mr. Lewis to *overcome gravity*, so as to enable him to raise a man from the ground, and hold him suspended in the air for a short time, simply by holding his hand above the man's head, and willing such a result, in my publication of July last (page 27), I distinctly stated that, for the reasons there adduced, such pretensions involved "*a physical impossibility*", and that such attempts would fail, whenever the experiment should be "fairly tested, before *sceptics as well as converts to this odylic faith*". To the Aberdeen committee's report I am now enabled to refer for a complete confirmation of this prediction. Moreover, according to Mr. Lewis's own admission to the committee, as recorded by them at page 172, the indications which he and others had mistaken for his power of overcoming the laws of gravitation, so as to enable him to suspend a man in the air by his odylic power, simply by elevating his hand over him, turns out to be precisely as I had alleged at page 27 of my last publication, *viz.*, "purely subjective or personal acts". In proof of this, I may remark that, after failing in his trials in the above experiment, Mr. L. admitted [according to the committee] "that he had no such power, and that he could only influence a person lying on the ground so as to make him start up, though others were endeavouring to hold him down." The inference, therefore, is obvious.

In reference to the *first* experiment, I may remark that only *one act* was proposed by the committee, namely, that Mr. Lewis should "make Mr. M. lie on the floor, with his face on the floor". Instead of exhibiting this characteristic act, however, which was proposed exactly at three o'clock, before any other manifestation was proposed by the committee, Mr. M. had made *fourteen* movements, not one of which corresponded, either in time or character, with that desired, as will be seen by the following extract from the report:–

Hour	Minute	
3pm	1½	– Raised himself up in the chair, and shook himself.
3	2	– Slipped down a little – got up and sat down – changed his seat.
3	2½	– Rubbed his hand (on his thigh), and his left arm with the right hand.
3	3¼	– Stamped on the floor and moved his feet sideways – then got up and changed his seat again.
3	3⅔	– Folded arms – put left hand behind.
3	4½	– Rocked his body from side to side.

At five minutes past three, and at nine minutes past three, other suggestions were proposed by the committee, with like results – fully warranting the inferences above quoted from the report of the committee, that "there was a total want of correspondence, in point of time and character, between the volitions and acts of the operator and of the subject, when in different rooms," etc. It is worthy of remark, moreover, that when

Mr. Lewis left the class-room, the audience was desired to remain quiet for a little, as another experiment was about to be tried. Hereupon most of the company directed their attention to Mr. M. and Mr. H., who having been previously acted upon, it was therefore conjectured that they would be the parties acted on in that instance. At twelve minutes past four, being seven minutes after the time Mr. L. was to Mesmerise Mr. M. from a distance, Mr. M. went down to the chair on which he had previously been seated, and having gone through certain manoeuvres, he rushed out of the room and went to Mr. L.'s apartments, impelled, as he believed, by the irresistible and silent *will* of Mr. L. to draw the patient to him, from such a distance as he could neither be seen nor heard through the physical organs. It was proved, however, that the intended experiment was quite different from what Mr. M. manifested. Mr. H. also became affected in a peculiar manner, and could not be induced to go home without paying a visit to Mr. L.'s lodgings, feeling himself irresistibly drawn thither by the *silent will* of Mr. L. It was ascertained, however, that *all this occurred without Mr. L. having directed his mind to this patient at all!* It was known to many present, as well as to Mr. H., that Mr. Lewis had, on former occasions, presumed that certain individuals had been drawn to him, at his lodgings, *by the power of his silent will*; and hence the origin of the idea in the mind of the patient, as also of many of those present on this occasion. The result, however, proved how readily some enthusiastic parties may be deceived, through overlooking very obvious sources of fallacy. These are certainly remarkable *proofs* of Mr. L.'s alleged power of influencing patients at a distance, simply by the power of his *silent will* and physical gesticulations.

2. On Newnham's 'Human Magnetism'

Allusion to this extraordinary epidemic has recalled to my mind certain reflections which occurred to me on reading Mr. Newnham's well-written work on "Human Magnetism", which was published in 1845. Whilst I willingly admit that Mr. Newnham's work was agreeably and pleasantly – indeed, *elegantly* – written, and that he made the most of the materials at his disposal for the support of the *magnetic* theory, still, I suspect that he was then more of a theoretical than a practical magnetist. He had, that is, read much on the subject, and taken for granted, as true, the *objective* theory of the Mesmerists, and contented himself with merely substituting the phraseology, "communication of the *exuberant life* of the healthy, to repair and sustain the deficient vitality of the sick", for the old term, "the transmission of a magnetic or Mesmeric fluid from the body of the operator to that of the patient". Thus, at page 17, Mr. Newnham says:– "Magnetism may be said to be the medicine of nature – to consist in the communication of the exuberant life of the healthy, to repair and sustain the deficient vitality of the sick. (…) This is a most important principle, Mr. N. adds, and in various ways will come before us, in several stages of our future remarks; but as it is the key-stone of the arch upon which rests the security of all future reasoning, it is now especially mentioned, that at every subsequent page it may be carried with us as our guide through doubtful or intricate passages." Mr. Newnham was well aware of the scenes enacted at the grave of the Abbé Pâris, at St. Medard. He knew that it was notorious that numerous important cures occurred there to patients whose cases had resisted all ordinary treatment, and even after the cemetery was shut up, that cures occurred to patients at their own homes, simply by addressing fervent prayers to the saint, in firm faith and confidence in his power and will to cure them, that in other cases the cures were effected by adding to the prayers the efficacy of some visible and tangible agency, such as a sacred relic, or a particle of earth said to have been taken from his grave, or by drinking a little water said to have been brought from a well near the resting place of the mortal remains of the Holy Deacon. Now, with a perfect knowledge of all this, did it never occur to Mr. Newnham to ask himself the question – How could there have been, in these recorded cures, a "communication of the *exuberant* LIFE of the *healthy*", passing from the ashes of the DEAD *saint*, "to repair and sustain the *deficient vitality* of the *sick*"? If the "key-stone of the arch upon which rests the security of all the future reasonings" of Mr. Newnham be what he has stated in these words – the communication of the *exuberant* LIFE of the *healthy*, to repair and sustain the *deficient vitality* of the *sick*", then, most assuredly, the above-recorded cures by the *ashes* of a DEAD *saint* prove that the reasonings and super-structure must be frail indeed, which are reared upon *such* a fragile "arch", as one provided with such a "KEY-STONE."

But not only were many important *cures* effected, as above narrated, on individuals visiting the tomb of the Holy Deacon, but the very *opposite* effects were also manifested to a much greater extent; for it is recorded that immense numbers of individuals who went to the cemetery of St. Medard, merely as spectators of the marvellous scenes being there enacted, although previously apparently in good health, became affected with the most violent convulsions. It is, therefore, obviously absurd to suppose that both a sanative and pestiferous influence of this sort could have flowed from the same cause – *viz.*, from the ashes of the dead saint. The power of mental emotion, however, a lively faith, hope, and confidence were sufficient to account for the cures in the one class; whilst fear, terror, sympathy, and imitation were quite adequate to account for the convulsions in the other class. On this subject the learned Hecker observes – "Every species of enthusiasm, every strong affection, every violent passion, may lead to convulsions – to mental disorders – to a concussion of the nerves, from the sensorium to the very finest extremities of the spinal cord. The whole world is full of examples of this afflicting state of turmoil, which, when the mind is carried away by the force of a sensual impression that destroys its freedom, is irresistibly propagated by imitation," *Hecker's Epidemics of the Middle Ages.* – Page 142.

If Mr. Newnham would only condescend to consider **the simple subjective theory which I have ventured to propound**, I think he might readily comprehend how **the new modes of excitement, or depression, or peculiar distribution of the nervous or vital influence *within the patient's own body,* might arise through the influence of *his own mind acting on his own physical organism*, and might thus account for all which is realised without the transmission of any occult influence from one human being to another. I readily grant, however, that the looks, words, and actions of a second party may furnish suggestions influential upon others – just as a word of encouragement, spoken or written by a friend, may nerve our arm with greater power, and inspire our tongue with greater eloquence – and that a lively companion, or encouraging expression may excite us; whilst a grave companion, or doubtful expression, would chill and depress – and that hope and confidence, or the contrary in the means used, may modify, to a remarkable extent, the results under *any* mode of treatment. Still, I believe that there is no positive interchange or transference of nervous or vital force from the operator to the patient as the *actual cause* of these results, as has been alleged by the Mesmerists.** I do *not* believe that, in such instances, A loses an amount of power equivalent to what B gains. I do *not* believe that a preacher, an orator, or an author loses an amount of vital force in exact ratio to the numbers influenced by his spoken printed ideas, sentiments, and illustrations – which would necessarily be the case were the magnetic theory true. On the contrary, I *do believe* that the perusal of a posthumous work may be equally influential as if the book had been printed when the author was alive – and that **the simple suggestion of new ideas to the mind of the reader, through the printed symbols of thought, is the *real* efficient cause of the future results. Such is the "keystone of the arch upon which rests the security of all my reasonings" regarding *hypnotism*.**

Lecture on Electro-Biology
(1851)

The Edinburgh Medical & Surgical Journal. Volume 76. 1851.

'Abstract of a Lecture on Electro-Biology,'
Delivered at the Royal Institution, Manchester, on the 26th March 1851.
By James Braid M.R.C.S., Edinburgh, C.M.W.S., etc. etc.

On Wednesday evening the last of the *conversazioni* for this session took place at the Royal Institution, Mr. Alderman Watkins in the chair, when Mr. Braid read a paper on "Electro-biological phenomena, physiologically and psychologically considered". [This seems to have been the article published in the *Monthly Journal for Medical Science*, June 1851] The audience was large and respectable.

Mr. Braid commenced by stating that his essay comprised the results of his own experience in the investigation of the reciprocal action upon each other of mind and matter. His chief object was to give an explanation of the phenomena lately exhibited in Manchester, Liverpool, and surrounding towns, in London, by Mr. Stone; and in Edinburgh and Glasgow, and other towns in Scotland, by Dr. Darling, on what was termed "electro-biology". These exhibitions had excited much interest.

After reading extracts from an article entitled "Experiments in Electro-biology", in *Chambers' Journal* of February 8th 1851, describing some successful experiments of Dr. Darling on a previous sceptic on the subject, Mr. Braid proceeded to notice his own experience. **Nine years ago [1842] he entered on the investigation of Mesmerism, believing it wholly a system of collusion or illusion; but he anon discovered a reality in some of the phenomena, though he differed from the Mesmerists as to their causes.** His experiments proved that similar phenomena of abnormal sleep, and peculiar condition of mind and body, might be self-induced by fixed gaze on any inanimate object, the mental attention being concentrated on the act. This proved the subjective or personal nature of the influence, and that it did not arise from any magnetic influence passing from the operator into the patient, as alleged by the Mesmerists.

Mr. Braid appealed to the result of his experience nine years ago, in sending numbers of subjects into a state of sleep, by causing them to gaze continuously at inanimate objects. **Thus the potency of his method he had demonstrated on the 8th December, 1841, before a Manchester audience of eight hundred individuals, when fourteen male adults came forward, all strangers to him, who had never been so tested before. Some were desired to keep a steady fixed gaze upon the end of a cork bound upon their heads, so as to project from the middle of the forehead, each to look at the cork bound upon his own forehead, and to fix his undivided attention on the act. Some were desired to fix their sight and thoughts on points of the gas apparatus in the room. All commenced the process at the same time, and ten of the fourteen [71%] went into the sleep, whilst he had never touched any one of them until after their eyelids closed involuntarily. None of them were able to open their eyes, some became cataleptic, others were insensible to the prick of a pin, and one or two forgot all which had occurred. During these proceedings, three more of the audience sent themselves into the condition, by fixing their gaze and thoughts upon points of the room, according to what he had indicated during his lecture, as sufficient to produce the sleep.** Mr. Braid knew nothing of their acts or intentions until called upon by their friends to unlock them from their profound sleep, from which they could not succeed in arousing them.

He was also equally successful in operating upon a number of strangers together, at a private *conversazione* given to the profession in London, in March 1842, sixteen out of eighteen [89%] having passed into the sleep, simply by maintaining a steady fixed gaze, and fixed act of attention, whilst gazing at the root of a chandelier. Mr. Herbert Mayo [a distinguished physiologist] tested them, and ran a needle from the back to the palm of the hand of one patient without the patient evincing the slightest consciousness of pain or remembrance of it after awaking. Mr. Braid appealed to these facts, and many of a similar character, and to the feats of the Fakirs of India in this respect for the last 2,400 years, and then added, "Inasmuch as similar results arise from all these personal acts, there can be no reason to doubt that the influence is essentially subjective or personal, and not the transmission of any magnetic or occult influence passing from the operator into the patient, which the Mesmerists contend for – and that the subsequent results are merely modified or intensified by others, by suggestions or impressions conveyed to the subjects through words spoken within their hearing, and other physical impressions acting on their organs of special sense. **The condition (he further added) is essentially one of mental abstraction or concentration of attention, in which the powers of the mind are engrossed, if not entirely absorbed, with a single idea or train of thought, and concurrently rendered unconscious of, or indifferently conscious to, all other ideas or impressions."**

In the condition of mental abstraction, or concentration of attention, thus produced, the imagination becomes so vivid as to invest with present reality whatever idea arises spontaneously to the mind, or is suggested to it by some person on whom the subject's attention has been specially fixed. The oftener these phenomena are excited the more easily may they be reproduced, through the laws of association and habit; and some patients may at length become so impressible as to be liable to lapse into the condition entirely through the force of imagination and fixed belief that some process is throwing them into the state, though no such be in operation. This he regarded as a great source of fallacy with those who assert that they possess the power of influencing patients at a distance through mere volition or secret passes.

Mr. Braid observed, "It is an undoubted fact, that there is great difference in the susceptibility to the Mesmeric impression, some becoming rapidly and intensely acted, others slowly and feebly so. This want of uniformity in the results has been seized upon by sceptics, as a warranty for their suspecting the whole phenomena manifested to be a tissue of collusion or illusion; whereas, when viewed in the light in which I advocate the science, as the result of a subjective or personal influence, we ought naturally to expect as great difference in the results as there are differences in the mental and physical constitutions of the patients subjected to the processes. Upon this principle, therefore, I contend that the variety manifested by different individuals is the strongest proof of the genuineness of the phenomena."

Mr. Braid then explained, that in some patients who went into a deep state of the sleep, "the imagination seems to assume a supremacy over the reason, will, and natural functions of the organs of special sense, and the concentrated state of mind enables them readily to be imposed upon, and induced to act out their dreams excited by suggestions, precisely in the manner referred to by Dr. Abercrombie, in the case of the officer, who could be made to talk in his sleep, and be convinced of anything by his fellow officers, or even led to act out the most foolish suggestions of his companions. The sense in action may, through suggestion, be rendered inordinately active, or its natural function may be temporarily suspended by mental impressions strongly imprinted on the minds of the subjects by repeated and appropriate suggestions, in short, in this condition, the mind seems already to accept as truth, the first suggestion, and, from its distractive tendency, becomes so absorbed with that, as to be dead, or comparatively indifferent to all else, during the dominance of that idea or train of thought – **a state similar to what is witnessed in individuals noted for absence of mind**." He then went on to explain that some individuals manifest this condition of mind, even before they close their eyelids or fall into the state of sleep, and that these subjects had long been known in this country to exhibit the "vigilant or waking phenomena" now brought forward by Mr. Stone and Dr. Darling as something new under the name of "electro-biology".

Mr. Stone caused his patients to gaze continuously **on a zinc disc, with a spot of copper in the centre**, held in the hand for ten or fifteen minutes, silence being enjoined, and the patients to keep their mind fixed on the act during that period. Those who showed no symptoms of being affected at the expiration of that period were desired to retire, as not being suitable subjects for manifesting the phenomena. The mode of operating with susceptible subjects was this – the lecturer desired the subject to close his eyes, and then said aloud to him, **"Now you cannot open your eyes," or desired him to sit down, and then predicted he would not be able to rise from his chair; or to stand up, and then audibly predicted that he would be unable to sit down; or gave him a glass of water, and then suggested aloud that it was wine, beer, spirits, vinegar, milk, coffee, tea, and so on in succession, when the patient would become influenced and deluded, according to the suggestions of the operator, until some audible, or visible, or tangible signal from the fascinator broke the spell.** Mr. Braid said that startling as these alleged pretensions might seem, nevertheless he knew, from ample experience that these and many other equally extraordinary phenomena could be produced in some individuals, without the slightest collusion or intended fraud on the part of such subjects; but he contended that they were to be accounted for, not as the result of any electric influence, but as examples of the power of imagination, easy credulity, and fixed mental attention, over a certain class of subjects. Mr. Braid proved, by quotations from his work, on "The Power of the Mind over the Body", published in 1846, that he had fully investigated this subject at that period, and proved the existence of this law of the reciprocal action and reaction of the mind and body upon each other, to his entire satisfaction; and his experiments had moreover proved, that wherever the mind is strongly and continuously directed, it changes the sensation and circulation in the part so regarded, and the more so according to the faith of the patient and vividness of his imagination, and belief in what is to happen. This he considered was the grand source of fallacy regarding Baron Reichenbach's alleged "new imponderable", or odyle force. The only test of this alleged force was admitted to be the human nerve, but, inasmuch as the mind of the patient must always constitute an element in the test of the results realised, he (Mr. Braid) could not consider it a satisfactory test, because the influence of the mind alone was sufficient, in such patients, to produce the results attributed to this alleged new force.

Mr. Braid then called attention to the fact that the process of these Americans [Stone and Darling] is merely a variety of his old process for inducing what he called the hypnotic or Mesmeric state; he remarked that the copper and zinc were **"merely visible and tangible objects for aiding the patients in fixing their attention, and inducing that state of mental abstraction which is the real origin and essence of all that follows"**. **"I know from experience,"** he added, **"that any other object would be equally efficient, provided the patients were impressed with that conviction. The auricular or audible suggestion and other impressions resorted to by these experimentalists (for they speak aloud within the hearing of the patient, the idea or act which they wish and intend to be manifested, or give some visible signal or tangible impression to excite ideas and actions in their subjects), are merely modes of influencing the minds of their patients, and of reflecting the habit of concentrated attention, superinduced by the first process, from one idea or purpose, and fixing it on another; and the expression, by the experimentalist, of 'all right' or a nod of his head, or other manoeuvre, for dissipating the existing delusion, are merely different modes of breaking down the previously existing ideas – just as a tap upon the shoulder will restore the individual, who was so rapt in mental contemplation as to have passed his friend without recognition, or been insensible to what was being said or done in his presence previously, to consciousness of all around.** Now, the repetition of these audible, visible, and tangible suggestions being requisite to insure the results, is a clear proof that the influence is psychical or mental in its nature, and that it is not a physical or electric influence, as the electro-biologists allege. For, if electric, there ought to be no more need for their auricular suggestions and manoeuvres to produce the results on the patients, than there would be for such to insure the one side of a Leyden jar [a primitive electrical capacitor] being charged negatively with electricity when the other is being charged positively, or for the attendant to speak aloud to the electric telegraph the message which he wishes it to convey. The few occasional examples adduced by them, in which they allege that they can convey their behests to subjects silently and unseen, through pure sympathy, and the power of their will, I consider inadequate to sustain their hypothesis. At best they are but exceptional cases; and when I have had opportunities of testing such patients I have soon been able to demonstrate the source of fallacy which had misled the operators."

Mr. Braid further added, "It is a well-established physiological fact, that the moment the trunk of a nerve is divided, all sense and voluntary motion is abolished in parts supplied by such nerve beyond the point of section. Now, are we to believe that it could be possible that such a degree of sympathy could exist between different individuals as to enable one, by the exercise of his volition, or other silent and unseen manoeuvres, to force his own nervo-vital influence beyond his own organism, so as to control the acts of the other at a distance, even when miles apart, when he could not propel it a fraction of a line beyond the section of the nerve in his own limb (the divided ends of the nerve being in close apposition), so as to produce a voluntary movement of his own member?"

After quoting at length a series of experiments given in his work on "The Power of the Mind over the Body", published by Mr. B. in 1846, experiments, in every respect similar to those of the electro-biologists, and performed on individuals whose character placed the facts above suspicion of complicity or trick in the manifestations referred to, Mr. Braid made the following quotations from the above work.

> Not only may patients in the waking state be made to believe that they see various forms and colours, and perceive variable sensible impressions, and irresistible powers, drawing, repelling, or paralysing them, from a strong mental impression, changing the physical action of the organ or part usually engaged in the normal manifestation of such functions, but I have, moreover, ascertained that the same influence may be realised in respect to sound, smell, taste, heat, and cold, in some excitable subjects when wide awake, without any actual objects; and merely by asking what tune, odour, animal, or substance the subject *now* perceived, the ideas thus suggested were frequently totally different from those in my own mind at the time.

And again:–

> The true cause of these phenomena is not a physical influence from without, but a mental delusion from within, which paralyses their reason and independent volition, so that, for the time being they are mere puppets in the hands of another person, by whom they are irresistibly controlled, so that they can only see or hear, or taste or feel, or act in accordance with his will and direction. They have their whole attention fixed upon what may be said or signified by this alleged superior power, and consequently perceive impressions through the excited state of the organs of sense, called into operation, which they could not perceive in their ordinary condition. It may have been interesting enough to have demonstrated that the human mind could be so subjugated and controlled, but I do not consider that the continual repetition of such experiments, in the waking condition, is at all proper, or free from the danger of throwing the faculties of the minds of such patients into a morbid condition.

Mr. Braid added,

> The processes, however, when prudently and skilfully conducted, are **perfectly harmless**, and are moreover, capable of being turned to the happiest results in the relief and cure of several affections, which are most intractable or altogether incurable by the ordinary modes of treatment, by the exhibition of medicines. By the former mode, we can excite or depress the state of sensation and circulation, locally or generally, and consequently the functions of any organ or part in a most remarkable degree, according to the mode of procedure, and the mental suggestion resorted to in each individual case, so that **in this way morbid delusions may not only be excised but cured in many instances, not only as regards the faculties of the mind, but also as regards the functions of the body. Whatever function can be paralysed or perverted by a given mode of procedure, and suggestion, and manipulation may be invigorated and corrected by an opposite mode of management.** This may be still more remarkably verified in patients who pass into the sleep.

It was for the public to judge whose theory of the phenomena was correct, his own mental and suggestive theory, or their electric theory. The repetition of audible, visible, and tangible impressions being requisite to insure the results were a clear proof that the influence was psychical or mental in its nature. Mr. Braid then made the following remarks:–

> I am as well aware as any sceptic can be that many of the phenomena manifested by such subjects, both when asleep and in the waking condition, are capable of being feigned. Indeed, I set about the experimental investigation of the subject with the full conviction that there was imposture, and with the determination,

moreover, if possible, to discover and expose the trick. With such evidence as presented itself before me, however, of the genuineness of the phenomena, as exhibited in parties known to me to be possessed of the strictest probity, honour, and Christian principle, it became impossible for me, with a proper regard for candour and honour, to persist longer in a course of dogmatic scepticism. I therefore confessed that my former notion had been erroneous, and set about the further investigation of the subject, with the honest desire to arrive at truth. It is important to remark, however, that these waking phenomena prove that a strongly fixed idea of determined scepticism may so possess the mind of an inquirer, as to render him a totally unfit person to be a valid witness in what are matters of plain fact and observation to those who are not so enslaved by prejudice. His imagination and fixed conceit may be so powerful and engrossing that, unconsciously, he is forced to interpret the ideas of his own mind as the facts, instead of what is actually presented before him. This view of the subject throws an important light upon the nature and value of evidence, in cases where parties point blank contradict each other, when describing occurrences of which they have both been eye-witnesses. A strong mental impression or prejudice may have deceived one or more witnesses, without the slightest intention to misrepresent facts.

The writer of an article in *Chambers' Edinburgh Journal* for the 8th of last month, Mr. Braid allowed, to a certain extent, had hit upon a true solution of the cause of the waking phenomena, *viz.*, that it was a play upon the will of the patient, and the influence of sympathy and imitation upon certain individuals. "This theory," he said, "readily accounts for all the phenomena in which muscular motion is concerned, but it does not at all account for a much larger and more surprising class of phenomena, *viz.*, suspending, increasing, or perverting impressions addressed to any or all of the organs of special sense. These results are to be accounted for only by an appeal to the power of an over-excited and vivid imagination and fixed idea changing physical action. **Those who suppose that the power of the imagination, and sustained mental attention, directed to any part of the body, is a mere mental condition, without being accompanied by any change in the physical organism, labour under a grave mistake. Sustained mental attention, directed to any part, changes both the sensation and circulation of the part so regarded; and in a more marked degree, according to the imagination and belief of the patient. From this cause the most grave and fatal diseases may be engendered; and by withdrawing the attention and fixing the train of thought on some *new* object or pursuit, relief and cure may be effected in cases which would utterly fail without such management of the mind.**" The lecturer then gave the following explanation:–

> Voluntary motion arises from mandate of the *will* giving a special direction to the nervo-vital influence, so as to excite into action the class of muscles which naturally produce such motion, whilst their antagonists remain passive. In these electro-biological experiments, however, the suggestion of the operator excites a greater flow of nervous force into the class of muscles which produce the action *suggested,* than the patient is able to throw into the opposite class. Both classes of muscles, therefore, are called strongly into action. But the suggested idea being the stronger, there is no efficient voluntary motion, notwithstanding a great amount of nervous influence may be expended by the patient, as evinced by his rapid exhaustion. Thus, he lately led a patient to suppose that a walking stick was so heavy that he could not support its weight; and, after struggling some time with misdirected muscular efforts, he fell on the floor, quite exhausted by his effort to support the imaginary load. Most people must have experienced a similar feeling and result from an attack of nightmare during common sleep. The struggle and exhaustion in both cases are analogous. On the other hand, if the suggested idea and strongly fixed belief go along with the will of the patient, his volition may thereby be so much intensified as to enable him to lift a weight which he would be quite incapable of doing in his ordinary state. The history of cases of panic in the army from slight causes, and deeds of daring, and achievements almost superhuman during fits of enthusiasm, are examples in paint, on a large scale. Neither a play upon the will, nor sympathy, nor imitation, can account for patients feeling insufferable heat or cold, or for having the organs of sense paralysed or perverted by an audible suggestion; but a strongly-fixed idea and vivid imagination are quite adequate to produce such results as witnessed in monomania, delirium tremens, intoxication, narcotism from opium, the hashish or bangue [i.e., cannabis sativa] of the East, and of other drugs, as well as in various morbid conditions.

He added,

> In all these states it is a well ascertained fact, that ideas may become so vivid as to assume all the force of reality and that whilst the individual so affected retains a certain amount of consciousness of all around, still he cannot emancipate himself from the erroneous impression, or that he may be so engrossed with the one idea as to be dead or indifferent for the nonce to all other impressions.

Mr. Braid then gave his views of the so-called Mesmeric passes, whether by contact or non-contact. The Mesmerists allege that the effects arise from some occult or magnetic influence – the odyle force of Baron Reichenbach – affecting the part in a particular manner. He attributed it to the mental power in the patient to change the physical action of the part to which his mind is continuously directed by a sensible impression or audible suggestion from another person, or by an effort of the patient's will, especially if done in the belief of some change being about to happen. One of the most puzzling classes of phenomena was that, exhibiting reverse results, apparently arising from the same sensible impressions – as the Mesmerising and deMesmerising passes. But he found that, on first going into the sleep, patients had sufficient mobility to be affected by certain impressions, and would approach to or recede from them, according as they were agreeable or the reverse in quality or intensity. Thus by titillating the skin, or agitating the air over it, the adjacent muscles are called into play, so as to bend the hand and raise the arm; and by similarly stimulating the opposite class of muscle, the hand and fingers become extended, and the arm falls. He subsequently ascertained that a class of muscles thus called into action and allowed to remain a short time in one position, a repetition of the impression on the same point which had produced the action, would now reduce it. At length he discovered the solution of the apparent mystery. The movements being instinctive or automatic, the impression merely gives a tendency to indication; the direction and character of the motion being the most natural motion under the circumstance. Thus, if a muscle is passive, it will become active, and *vice versa,* from the same exciting cause. If an impression be made on the hand or arm, on the patient's lap, as it cannot descend it will rise and become rigid: but, after remaining awhile in that condition, a like impression will induce the most natural motion – in this instance to descend. If an obstacle be interposed to prevent its rising or descending, and the impression be repeated, it will move laterally. **This mode of exciting action by sensible impressions may be confined to individual muscles or classes of muscle, and thus the muscles of expression may be so acted upon as to waken any passion or emotion in the mind – a mere inversion of the sequence which ordinarily obtains between mental emotion and the physical manifestations of such emotion.**

> That there is nothing occult or specific in the pass with the hand is manifest from this; that a similar agitation of the air by the blast from a pair of bellows will produce precisely similar results as the like current of air from the wafting of the human hand, I have proved to the entire satisfaction of hundreds of intelligent individuals.

But if with each touch, or agitation of the air, the operator aloud declares what should happen, this suggestion may be so strong as to cause the predicted manifestation to be realised, instead of the natural result. Thus we may have manifested an artificial as well as a natural set of phenomena, according to the mode and intention of the operator. Then some subjects, during the sleep, see through their partially closed eyelids, and thus catch the suggestion of even a fixed gaze by the operator on a leg or arm; and, imagining a movement of such limb is desired, their docility will obey the suggestion. In like manner, the remarkable tendency to sympathy and imitation in such patients, will induce them to observe and imitate every physical act of the operator. If a screen be interposed between them, the patients will rely on hearing instead of sight, and be only occasionally correct in their imitation of physical acts. All these phenomena may be realised without the patient intending deception on others or having any remembrance of the acts, on coming out of the sleep.

Mr. Braid then remarked that he had "never seen any phenomena, during either the hypnotic or Mesmeric sleep, or during the state for manifesting the vigilant phenomena, which were not in accordance with generally-admitted physiological and psychological principles". The senses and mental powers may be torpified or quickened in a remarkable degree, but he had never seen the clairvoyance which would enable patients to read through decidedly opaque bodies, and some other of what have been called by Mesmerists the higher phenomena. He, however, referred to apparently very astonishing feats which had occurred in some of his patients in imitating words and music of which they were previously quite ignorant, also of the exalted power of smell, and of the muscular sense which enables them to write and draw with some neatness without the use of their eyes; quickened hearing and exaltation of some of the mental powers, as was manifested by second-sight men in the Highlands of Scotland, and then added:–

> Several important inferences may be drawn from what has been adduced regarding the power of the imagination, belief and fixed act of attention in changing and controlling physical action, and of the state of the body thus superinduced reacting on the mind. It not only enables us **to comprehend, upon scientific principles, the cause and cure of many diseases**, where there has been no specific and adequate external physical agency to account for the results, but it also explains many phenomena which used to be attributed to demonology, witchcraft, ghost-seeing, being spell-bound, the power of the *obi* women who could cause their credulous victims to wither and die under their assumed malign power and malediction, the power of charms, spells, and amulets, of Perkins' metallic tractors, the efficacy of galvanic rings [popular, but fake, magnetised rings], **bread pills** [i.e., placebo pills], and such-like. It also explains the alleged clairvoyance of the Egyptian boys, after looking steadfastly at an inky globule held in the hands, narratives of which have been published by Lord Prudhoe and Mr. Lane; the revelations of [Edward] Kelly, recorded daily for Dr. [John] Dee, who was warden of Manchester during the reign of Queen Elizabeth, and which were alleged to be revealed to him by a spirit whilst gazing into Dr. Dee's celebrated show-stone; the fortune-tellers, who exercise a similar mode of looking into futurity by gazing into an unground glass egg, and the late revelations of the same sort published by Zadkiel in his almanac for this year, as the revelations of the angel in Lady Blessington's magic crystal, all come under the same category – merely the figments of fancy, excited by questions or otherwise, set down as visions seen and answers audibly uttered, or written in visible characters before them, by the said alleged spirits. We also thus acquire this salutary lesson, that in order to have a healthy state of mind and body, it is requisite that *all* our faculties should be duly cultivated, and that the attention should not be devoted too long and exclusively to any one object or pursuit, as the latter course has a tendency to engender a morbid state of mind as well as of body. Hence the advantage of relaxation and amusements of various kinds, so long as they are pursued in

reason and with moderation. We are also taught this important fact, that dogmatic scepticism, or prejudice, not only beclouds the reason, but also destroys or perverts the perceptive faculties. This truth seems to have been clearly perceived by Dugald Stewart when he penned the following notable paragraph:– "Unlimited scepticism is equally the child of imbecility as implicit credulity."

Mr. Braid concluded:–

My experiments have proved that the ordinary phenomena of Mesmerism may be realised through the subjective or personal mental and physical acts of the patient alone, whereas the proximity, acts, or influence of a second party would be indispensably requisite for their production, if the theory of the Mesmerists were true; moreover, my experiments have proved that audible, visible, or tangible suggestions of another person whom the subject believes to possess such power over him, is requisite for the production of the waking phenomena, whereas no audible, visible, or tangible suggestions from a second party ought to be required to produce these phenomena, if the theory of the electro-biologists were true. There is, therefore, both positive and negative proof in favour of **my mental suggestive theory**, and in opposition to the magnetic, occult, or electric theories of the Mesmerists and electro-biologists. My theory, moreover, has this additional recommendation, that it is level to our comprehension, and adequate to account for all which is demonstrably true, without offering any violence to reason and common sense, or being at variance with generally admitted physiological and psychological principles. Under these circumstances, therefore, I trust that you will consider me entitled to your verdict in favour of my mental theory.

[Discussion]

Mr. Caplin opened the conversation by speaking of what he conceived Mr. Alfred Smee had proved in his work on electro-biology, and detailing some experiments he had himself made on a little boy, who was then in the room, with their results. The boy had been afflicted with paralysis of one limb since he was sixteen months old; he (Mr. Caplin) had brought him completely under his control as a subject of electro-biology, and with the happiest results; he was fast acquiring strength, and the paralysis was giving way. He did not believe that the effect produced by the placing of coins in the hand was at all galvanic, but that the heating of the coin produced an electrical disturbance, indicated by certain palpitations of the muscle, as the disturbance went on from the head to the extremities. He offered that the boy should be operated upon in the presence of the audience, but it was against the rules of the institution. Mr. Braid, in reply, said that Mr. Smee's theory was so fanciful, and subjected him to such severe criticism, that he sought to shelter himself by taking legal proceedings against those who analysed his views. He conceived that there was no need of any outward manipulation, or means of fixation; for people could throw themselves into a condition of mental concentration; and as to the movement of the hand, it was merely the effect of concentrated mental attention directed to any part of the body. He had proved this by experiments on four gentlemen **(two of whom were then in the room)**, when experimenting on Baron Reichenbach's "new imponderable". **They were seated, each with his arm on the table, and they were requested to maintain a steady fixed gaze each on his own hand and watch the result. He knew that of the four senses of the hand – heat, cold, common sensation, and muscular sense – that most prominent in the individual would be brought out, provided he had no consciousness of what was to be expected.**

After a time one felt a cold sensation stealing over his hand, another felt a pricking sensation, as if sustaining galvanic shocks, the hand of another was hot, and the fourth became cataleptic, and the hand and arm were fixed to the table. Now, this was the power of the mind in the individual directed in each case. He did not doubt the value of the concentration of mental power as a remedial agent in the case of paralysis, if there was not organic disease. A woman that very day, labouring under paralysis, he had relieved in the course of ten minutes, and enabled her to raise an arm which she could not previously move. **As we can suspend the power of muscle, so can we increase or intensify it, by a suggestion.** There were instances of parties having wrenched iron bars from windows under great mental excitement; and during the fire in Market Street, a friend of his rushed into his room, tore out an iron safe containing his books, and dragged it out of the office, a task which it would have been impossible for him to effect, except under intense mental concentration and excitement. As to the agency of electricity, there was no thought without a change of the cerebral matter, and no change in that without a certain disturbance of the electrical influence; but in that case the thought was the cause of the disturbance, and not the electricity the cause of the thought.

Mr. Catlow said they had omitted to propose a vote of thanks to Mr. Braid for his paper, and perhaps such a motion would come well from himself. **He congratulated Mr. Braid on having come round to a common sense view, well adapted to a popular audience. Mr. Braid started originally with the theory that fixed gazing at some object, until the muscles of the eye were strained, was an absolute necessity in the production of these phenomena, and said nothing about the mind.**

Dr. Hodgson thought Mr. Braid was not to be disparaged for having **changed his views after nine years of study,** he was rather to be praised for his candour. He conceived that Mr. Braid's explanation of electro-biological phenomena was satisfactory. Mr. Stone might have the power of producing certain phenomena by silent volitions of will, but he did not do so in public, nor, indeed, could he well do so. He (Dr.

Hodgson) could not, however, go so far as Mr. Braid in respect to Mesmerism. His theory would not account for many apparently well-authenticated phenomena.

Mr. Prentice said a few words respecting an exhibition he saw at Mr. Braid's house, at which a factory girl very closely imitated a lady [Jenny Lind] who sang difficult music in several languages, so closely that the tone of voice of the two could scarcely be distinguished. He believed the clairvoyant cases were wonderful guesses arising out of suggestions. The Chairman confirmed Mr. Prentice's remarks, from what he had personally witnessed at Mr. Braid's, by the above patient imitating accurately words and music unknown to her.

Dr. Shelton Mackenzie also said a few words as to his personal experience in this matter, confirmatory of Mr. Braid's power of suggestion, as witnessed by him in the case of a boy, and also on his own person. – The vote of thanks was passed and the meeting broke up.

Electro-Biological Phenomena
Considered Physiologically & Psychologically
(1851)

Electro-Biological Phenomena
Considered Physiologically & Psychologically

(Lecture delivered at the Royal Institution, Manchester, March 26th, 1851.)

[Introduction]

In the following essay, I shall endeavour to submit to your consideration, in the most simple and comprehensible manner, the results of my experience, whilst investigating one of the most recondite and interesting departments of philosophy and science – namely, the reciprocal actions upon each other of mind and matter.

Most of you have no doubt seen or heard of the experiments in what has been designated "Electro-Biology, or the Electrical Science of Life", which were lately exhibited in Manchester, Liverpool, and the surrounding towns, and which are now being exhibited in London, by an American gentleman named Mr. Stone. The following announcement is contained in one of his hand-bills, of the 12th inst. [i.e., 12th March 1851], as to what he professes to exhibit in London, at the Marylebone Literary and Scientific Institution:–

> Persons in a perfectly wakeful state, of well-known character and standing in society, who come forward voluntarily from among the audience, will be experimented upon. They will be deprived of the power of speech, hearing, sight. Their voluntary motions will be completely controlled, so that, they can neither rise up nor sit down, except at the will of the operator; their memory will be taken away, so that they will forget their own name and that of their most intimate friends; they will be made to stammer, and to feel pain in any part of their body at the option of the operator – a walking stick will be made to appear a snake, the taste of water will be changed to vinegar, honey, coffee, milk, brandy, wormwood, lemonade, *etc., etc., etc.* These extraordinary experiments are really and truly performed without the aid of trick, collusion, or deception, in the slightest possible degree.[70]

These may no doubt be considered as startling announcements; nevertheless, I know as a fact, that such phenomena, and the very reverse effects, may be realised in certain individuals; but I account for them in a very different manner from the so-styled Electro-Biologists.

A similar class of phenomena has also lately been exhibited in Edinburgh, Glasgow, and various parts of Scotland, by another American named Dr. Darling. These exhibitions have excited great interest at Edinburgh and Glasgow, and have enlisted in the discussion the pens of Sir David Brewster, Professor Gregory, Professor J. Hughes Bennett, Mr. Robert Chambers, and other gentlemen of the highest character and scientific attainments. Amongst the contributions which have been published on the subject, I have been quite charmed by an article which appeared in the Number of *Chambers' Edinburgh Journal* for the 8th of last month, entitled "Experiments on Electro-Biology". The analysis therein given of the nature, causes, and tendencies of scepticism in mankind generally, and in certain coteries in particular, in reference to probationary sciences, is an admirable picture by a first-rate artist, which merits the candid study of the whole human family. The writer of the article alluded to had been a decided sceptic, and had accompanied a gentleman of his acquaintance, who was equally sceptical as himself, to a *séance* in a private family, where most of the company assembled consisted of persons in the upper ranks of society. The said friend offered to submit to the trial on himself, for the purpose of proving the fallacy of such pretensions; however, the result was very different from his anticipations, for the proud sceptic and derider was converted into a complete victim. Two ladies of the party, also well-known to the writer of the article, were likewise proved to be equally susceptible. Collusion and fraud being out of the question in all these cases, the writer was constrained, through the force of such unexceptionable evidence, to renounce his scepticism. From what has been stated by Professor J. Hughes Bennett, it appears that several members of the Medical Society of Edinburgh, who were most sturdy sceptics, were also victimised upon submitting to such trials. In short, there is now abundance of evidence of the fact that such phenomena may be produced in perfectly good faith in some subjects, in the waking condition, and consequently the chief point remaining to be determined is the *cause* of these remarkable phenomena.

The ingenuous and manly confession of the learned author regarding the scepticism of himself and his friend, and the interesting narrative of the immediate cause of their conviction as to the reality of certain phenomena manifested, at the *séance* depicted, by him, is just a transcript of my own feelings and experience in this department of science. I beg, therefore, to submit the following remarks, for your consideration, with the hope that they may tend to the elucidation of truth, and the overthrow of that unreasoning, uninquiring, dogmatic scepticism which *Chambers'* correspondent has so ably combated.

---

[70] [These performances clearly resemble modern comedy "stage hypnosis" shows, although they did not claim to be using hypnotism. Similar public performances were also given by Mesmerists many decades before hypnotism was introduced.]

[Braid's Public Demonstrations of Hypnosis]

Nine years ago I entered upon the experimental investigation of Mesmerism, believing, from what I had read and heard of it, that the whole was a system of collusion or illusion. I very soon discovered, however, that there was a reality in some of the phenomena, notwithstanding I had reason to differ from the Mesmerists regarding the cause. My experiments proved that similar phenomena of abnormal sleep and peculiar condition of mind and body, might be self-induced, by the patient's maintaining a steady fixed gaze at any inanimate object, the mental attention being concentrated on the act. This at once proved the *subjective* or *personal* nature of the influence, and that it did not arise from the transmission of any magnetic or occult influence passing from the operator into the patient, which the Mesmerists contended for. The potency of this method was proved by me at a public lecture in Manchester, before an audience of about eight hundred individuals. After explaining my views or theory, and exhibiting the phenomena on patients who had previously been subjected to such operations, I requested strangers who had never been operated upon, to come forward and try the effect of my process. Fourteen male adults came forward, all of whom were entirely strangers to me. Some of them were desired to keep a steady fixed gaze upon the end of a cork, bound on the head, so as to project from the middle of the forehead, each to look at the cork bound upon his own head, and to fix his undivided attention on the act. Some of the others were desired to fix their sight and thoughts upon a part of the gas apparatus in the room. All commenced the process at the same time, and ten of the fourteen [71%] went into the sleep, and that whilst I never touched any one of them, until, after their eyelids closed involuntarily. None of them seemed able to open their eyes, although they remained conscious; some became cataleptic; others were insensible to the prick of a pin, and one or two forgot all which had occurred. One, who remembered nothing of what had happened during his sleep, was a powerful mechanic, who was sent down, bribed by a medical man, to resist me, and this he tried by not complying with my conditions; but, nevertheless, when I at length signified that I observed he was acting falsely, he set about it with a look of grim defiance, when he was speedily caught, and became one of the best examples of the power of my process that evening. Another, a most intelligent gentleman, was so sceptical, that before coming down he said *"seeing* was *not* believing" *with him,* but that he must *feel* it before he would believe it – he became a beautiful example, and after being released, described his feelings to the audience. During these proceedings three more of the company sent themselves into the condition, by fixing their gaze and thoughts upon points in the room, according to what I had indicated in my lecture as sufficient to produce the sleep. I knew nothing of their acts or intentions until called upon by their friends to unlock them from the profound sleep into which they had fallen, and from which they could not succeed in arousing them.

I was equally successful in operating upon a number of strangers together at a private conversazione, given to the profession in London, in March 1842, sixteen out of eighteen [89%] having passed into the sleep, simply by maintaining a steady fixed stare and fixed act of attention, whilst gazing at the root of a chandelier. Most of these had never been so tried before. I never touched any one of them until their eyelids closed. Mr. Herbert Mayo, the eminent physiologist and surgeon, tested them, and ran a needle from the back to the palm of the hand of one patient without his (the patient) evincing the slightest consciousness of pain, or remembrance of it after awaking. Entrancing a fowl, by holding its bill to the floor or a table, so as to cause it to gaze at a chalk line or stripe of coloured paper placed before it, is also a familiar example in point. From these facts, and innumerable others which have occurred to myself and to those who have adopted my views and mode of operating; and also from the practices of the Fakirs of India, who, for religious purposes, have been accustomed for the last 2,400 years to throw themselves into the state of ecstatic trance by similar processes – viz., by each looking steadfastly at the point of his nose, or some other part of his own body, or at some inanimate or ideal [imaginary] object, as one of their gods, and fixing their undivided attention on the act – I say, inasmuch as similar results arise from *all* these *personal acts,* there can be no reason to doubt that the influence is essentially *subjective* or *personal,* and that the subsequent results are merely modified or intensified by others, by suggestions or impressions conveyed to the subjects through words spoken within their hearing, and other physical impressions acting on their organs of special sense. **The condition is essentially one of mental abstraction or concentration of attention, in which the powers of the mind are engrossed, if not entirely absorbed, with a single idea or train of thought, and concurrently rendered unconscious of, or indifferently conscious to, all other ideas or impressions. In this condition the imagination becomes so vivid as to invest with present reality whatever idea arises spontaneously in the mind, or is suggested to it by another person on whom their attention has become specially fixed; and the oftener these phenomena are excited, the more easily may they be reproduced through the laws of association and habit.** Moreover, patients who are naturally highly susceptible of such impressions may at length become so impressible as to be liable to lapse into the condition entirely through the force of imagination and fixed belief that some process is going forward elsewhere, which is competent to throw them into the state; and this may happen without any process whatever being in operation at the time. This is, no doubt, a grand source of fallacy with those who allege, through occasional coincidences of trials and results, that they possess the power of influencing patients at a distance, through mere volition or secret passes.

[Hypnotic Suggestion Considered]

It is an undoubted fact, that there is great difference in the susceptibility to the Mesmeric impression, some becoming rapidly and intensely affected, others slowly and feebly so. This want of uniformity in the results has been seized upon by sceptics as a warranty for their suspecting the whole phenomena manifested to be a tissue of collusion or illusion – whereas, when viewed in the light in which I advocate the science, that is, as the result of a *subjective* or *personal* influence, we ought naturally to expect as great difference in the results as there are differences in the mental and physical constitutions of the patients subjected to the processes. Upon this principle, therefore, I contend that the *variety* manifested by *different individuals* is the strongest proof of the *genuineness* of the phenomena. In the ordinary Mesmeric state, where the eyes are closed and the patient passes into that condition called **the double-conscious state – that is, a state in which the patient forgets, when aroused from the sleep, all which had occurred during that condition, but of which he recovers a perfect recollection when he passes into the sleep again** – it is generally found that the mind of the subject is very much in the same condition as in ordinary dreaming, every idea arising in the mind spontaneously, or suggested to it by words spoken in hearing, or by other impressions made upon his organs of special sense, being instantly accepted by him as truths, and invested by him with all the force of present reality. In this state the imagination seems to assume a supremacy over the reason, will, and natural functions of the organs of special sense, and the concentrated state of mind enables them readily to be imposed upon, and induced to act out their dreams, excited by such suggestions, precisely in the manner referred to by Dr. Abercrombie, in the case of the officer whom his companions could converse with in his sleep, and convince of anything; and whom they even conducted through the whole process of a duel, till the firing of the pistol awakened him by its report. On another occasion, being asleep on the locker of the cabin, he was made to believe that he had fallen overboard, and was told to save himself by swimming. He imitated the act of swimming, when they told him to dive for his life, as a shark was pursuing him, which he attempted so energetically that he threw himself from the locker, by which he bruised himself severely.

The sense in action may through suggestion be rendered inordinately active, or its natural function may be temporarily suspended by mental impressions strongly imprinted on the minds of the subjects by repeated and appropriate suggestions. In short, in this condition the mind seems ready to accept as truth the first suggestion; and, from its abstractive tendency, becomes so absorbed with that as to be dead, or comparatively indifferent, to all else during the dominance of that idea or train of thought. We see an analogous condition in individuals noted for absence of mind; indeed, in a less degree, it must have been observed by most people in their own persons, as they may have been so engaged in a train of thought as not to observe a passing friend, or have had any distinct apprehension of conversation going on around them.

With most patients, so long as they remain in that condition in which they can remember on awaking what had been said and done during the sleep, there remains a degree of reason and volition sufficient to enable them to distinguish true from false and merely suggested ideas, and to enable them, moreover, to resist complying with whatever they do not approve of There are some subjects, however, who, *even in this stage,* are so imaginative and abstractive, possessed of such easy credulity and passive obedience to the will of others, that they can be subjugated and controlled as those last referred to when in the *deeper* state; and indeed not a few of them can be so influenced and controlled by suggestions of others, whilst wide awake and remaining perfectly conscious. These were the subjects which used to manifest what were called by the Mesmerists the "vigilant or waking phenomena", and were precisely similar to what have been exhibited by Dr. Darling in Edinburgh, and lately in this quarter by his countryman and friend, Mr. Stone, under the new designation of "Electro-Biology".

[Electro-Biology Criticised]

It will be observed, that the processes resorted to by these Americans is merely a variety of my old process for inducing what I called the hypnotic or Mesmeric state. The zinc and copper are merely visible and tangible objects for aiding the patients in fixing their attention, and inducing that state of mental abstraction which is the real origin and essence of all that follows. I know, from experience, that any other object would be equally efficient, provided, the patients were impressed with that conviction. All in which their processes differ, therefore, from what I had been accustomed to do for more than nine years past is, in beginning, to make mental and physical impressions on the patients *before* the subjects close their eyes and pass into a state of sleep; and it will be shown presently that I had investigated the subject in *this* mode also, and published narratives of cases, in [*The Power of the Mind over the Body*] July 1846, precisely similar to those of Dr. Darling and Mr. Stone. I explained the phenomena differently, however, and when my *mental* theory has been propounded, shall leave it to others to decide which theory is preferable, the *mental* or the *electric.* The auricular or audible suggestions and other impressions resorted to by these experimentalists (for they speak aloud, within the hearing of the patient, the idea or act which they wish and intend to be manifested, or give some visible signal or a tangible impression, to excite ideas or actions in their subjects) are merely modes of influencing the minds of their patients, and of reflecting the habit of concentrated attention, superinduced by the first process, from one idea or purpose and fixing it on another; and the expression, by the experimentalist, of "all right", or a nod of his head, or other manoeuvre for dissipating the existing delusion, are merely **different modes of breaking down the previously existing ideas**, just as a tap upon the shoulder will restore to consciousness of all around the individual who was wrapt in mental contemplation as to have passed his friend without recognition, or been insensible to what was being said or done in his presence previously. Now, the repetition of these audible, visible, and tangible suggestions being requisite to insure the result, is a clear proof that the influence is *psychical* or *mental* in its nature, and that it is not a *physical* or *electric* influence, as they allege. Were it *electric,* there ought to be no more need for their auricular suggestions and manoeuvres to produce the results on their patients than there would be for such to insure the one side of a Leyden jar [a primitive battery] being charged negatively with electricity when the other is being charged positively, or for the attendant to speak aloud to the electric telegraph the message which he wishes it to convey. The few *occasional* examples adduced by them in which they allege that they can convey their behests to subjects *silently and unseen,* through *pure sympathy* and power of their will, I consider inadequate to sustain their hypothesis. At best they are but exceptional cases; and where I have had opportunities of testing such patients, I have soon been able to demonstrate the sources of fallacy which had misled the operators.

It is a well established physiological fact, that the moment the trunk of a nerve is divided, all sense and voluntary motion is abolished in parts supplied by such nerve beyond the point of section. Now, are we to believe that it could be possible that such a degree of sympathy could exist between different individuals as to enable one, by the exercise of his volition, or other silent and unseen manoeuvres, to force his own nervo-vital influence beyond his own organism, so as to control the acts of the other at a distance, even when miles apart, when he could not propel it a fraction of a line beyond the section of the nerve in his own limb (the divided ends of the nerve being in close apposition), so as to produce a voluntary movement of his own member?

[The Reichenbach Phenomena]
In July 1846, I published a little brochure, entitled "The Power of the Mind over the Body". The object of that work was to point out what appeared to me an important source of fallacy, which had been overlooked, or not sufficiently attended to, by Baron Reichenbach when instituting experiments to prove the existence of a new imponderable, which he has designated the Od, or Odyle force. I most readily admit that Baron Reichenbach's experiments were carefully conducted, and well contrived for determining *merely physical* facts; but there seemed to have been a want of due consideration given to the very important part which the *mind* of the *patient* plays in such experiments, in producing or modifying results, quite irrespectively of external influences. The only test or proof of this alleged new force was certain effects produced on the human nerves of some highly nervous subjects. Now, my experiments went to prove that precisely similar phenomena might be realised in such highly sensitive subjects as the Baron succeeded with as the mere result of sustained mental attention of the patient alone, changing the physical action of the part so regarded especially when done with the expectation of something being about to happen. These effects might be increased in intensity by the subject, or feeling anything drawn over a part, from the visible or tangible object aiding the subject in concentrating his mental attention, without the transmission of any occult or external influence, proceeding from the object or operator to the subject. Of this there can be no doubt, as the results of my experiments, which I shall now quote from the above work, will prove.

> With nearly all the patients I have tried, many of whom had never been hypnotised or Mesmerised, when drawing the magnet or other object slowly from the wrist to the points of the fingers, various effects were realised, such as a change of temperature, tingling, creeping, pricking, spasmodic twitching of muscles, catalepsy of the fingers, or arm, or both; and reversing the motion was generally followed by a change of symptoms, from the altered current of ideas thereby suggested. Moreover, if any idea of what might be expected existed in the mind previously, or was suggested orally, during the process, it was generally very speedily realised. The above patients being now requested to look aside, or a screen having been interposed, so as to prevent their seeing what was being done, and they were requested to describe their sensations during the repetition of the processes, similar phenomena were stated to be realised, even when there was nothing whatever done, beyond watching them, and noting their responses. They believed the processes were being repeated, and had their minds directed to the part, and thus the physical action was excited, so as actually to lead them to believe and describe their feelings as arising from *external* impressions. [*The Power of the Mind over the Body*, 1846]

Immediately after my little work on "The Power of the Mind over the Body" was published, Dr. Henry Holland – a very competent authority in such matters – wrote to me to say, that my experiments and comments were so satisfactory, to his mind, that he considered no farther refutation of Baron Reichenbach's speculations about the Od force was necessary. I certainly had been enabled clearly to prove that the *mind* of the patient *alone* was adequate to produce the effects attributed to odyle; and I had also been enabled to prove that, with such subjects, ideas *audibly suggested* by a second party could speedily produce the like results; but I have never yet seen any specific influence from *silent* willing, either when near or at a distance, *when all sources of fallacy were duly guarded against.* It is now nearly five years since that little work was published, and I am not aware that my objections to the validity of Reichenbach's alleged discovery have ever yet been satisfactorily answered. Dr. Mayo's odylometer, instead of opposing, actually furnishes additional proof in support of, my theory. Again I quote, from the above work:–

> A lady, upwards of fifty-six years of age, in youth a somnambulist, but now in perfect health, and wide awake, having been taken into a dark closet, and desired to look at the poles of the powerful horse shoe magnet of nine elements, and describe what she saw, declared, after looking a considerable time, that she saw nothing. However, after I told her to look attentively, and she would see fire come out of it, she speedily saw sparks, and presently it seemed to her to burst forth, as she had witnessed an artificial representation of the volcano of Mount Vesuvius at some public gardens. Without her knowledge, I closed down the lid of the trunk which contained the magnet, *but still the same appearances were described as visible.* By putting leading questions, and asking her to describe what she saw from *another* part of the closet (where there was nothing but bare walls), she went on describing various shades of most brilliant coruscations and flame, according to the leading questions I had put for the purpose of changing the fundamental ideas. On repeating the experiments, similar results were repeatedly realised by this patient. On taking this lady into the said closet, after the magnet had been removed to another part of the house, she still perceived the same visible appearances of light and flame, when there was nothing but the bare walls to produce them; and, two weeks after the magnet was removed, when she went into the closet by herself; the mere association of ideas was sufficient to cause her to realise a visible representation of the same light and flames. Indeed, such had been the case with her on entering the closet ever since the few first times she saw the light and flames. In like manner, when she was made to touch the poles of the magnet when wide awake, no manifestations of attraction took place between her hand and the magnet; but the moment the idea was suggested that she would be held fast by its powerful attraction, so that she would be utterly unable to separate her hands from it, such result was realised; and on separating it, by the suggestion of a new idea, and causing her to touch the *other* pole in like manner, predicating that *it* would *exert no attractive power* for the fingers or hand, such negative effects were at once manifested. I know this lady was incapable of trying to deceive myself or others present; but she was self-deceived and spell-bound by the predominance of a preconceived idea, and was not less surprised at the varying powers of the instrument than others who witnessed the results. [*The Power of the Mind over the Body*, 1846]

After detailing a number of experiments on patients in the waking condition, I adduced the following:–

> In like manner, several other patients whom I took into the dark closet could see nothing until told to look steadily at a certain point, and they would see flame and light of various colours proceeding from it, which predictions were speedily realised, whilst they were wide awake, and nothing but bare walls towards which to direct their eyes. Not only so, but I have moreover ascertained that, even in broad daylight, a strong mental impression is adequate to produce such delusions with certain individuals of a highly imaginative and concentrative turn of mind. This fact was beautifully illustrated in the case of a gentleman, twenty-four years of age, who had suffered severely from epilepsy for eleven years. When taken into the above closet, and tested as the latter, he likewise saw nothing till I suggested that he would see flame and light, after which prediction he very speedily saw it accordingly, not merely where the magnet was, but also from other parts of the room. Now this patient, and the last two referred to, when taken into the closet *after* the magnet had been a long time removed to a distant part of the house, still saw the flames and changing colours as before – a clear proof that the whole was a mental delusion, arising from an excited imagination on the point under consideration, changing physical action. The same gentleman, being made to look at the point of a piece of brass wire, could be made to imagine that he saw any sort of flame or colour indicated issuing from it, *even in broad daylight;* and when made to touch it with *a finger,* and being then told that he would find it impossible to draw it away, the mere idea was sufficient to paralyse his volition, the whole muscles became rigid, and he looked with astonishment at his condition; but the moment I said, *Now the attraction is gone, and his hand will separate,* such results followed. Moreover, now that his finger was a little withdrawn, by simply saying confidently that it would *now* be found that he could not touch the wire, as it would repel him, the idea once more paralysed his volition, and he again manifested his incapacity, and in spite of his anxious but misdirected efforts, there he remained fixed as a statue. On hinting that *now* the influence was suspended, the hand and arm became limber, when I told another person watching the experiment, that *now* he would find the hand irresistibly drawn to the wire, and such result was presently manifested. No one had touched this wire for hours. It was merely a piece of bent brass wire, which was lying loosely and projecting from the chimney piece. This power seems to have been understood by Virgil, when he said:–
>
> *Possunt, quia posse videntur.*
> ["They can because they believe they can." – *The Aenid*.]
>
> In like manner, having intimated to a friend the remarkable vividness of this patient's imagination, implicit belief, and credulity, which rendered him liable to believe that he had an ocular perception of an external change, according to whatever idea might be suggested to him by others, I requested this friend, when he went into the room, to look at the end of the above wire at the same time with the patient, and that the former should pretend to me, when asked what coloured flame he saw emanating from it, to give a new idea at each inquiry. By this mode the patient caught the ideas suggested, having no notion that he was deluded in the manner indicated. He left with the full conviction of the physical reality of all he had seen and described; and he has manifested like phenomena as frequently as he has been so tested.
>
> I have detailed the above case so much at length, because it is a very good type of a class of patients

to be met with, who readily become the dupes of suggested ideas, in the manner presently to be explained, without the least desire to deceive others, or the most distant idea that they are themselves deceived. I have proved all I have advanced by so many concurrent examples, with individuals of the utmost probity and competency to describe their feelings, that there can be no doubt of the facts.

But not only may patients in the waking state be made to believe that they see various forms and colours, and perceive variable and sensible impressions, and irresistible powers, drawing, repelling, or paralysing them, from a strong mental impression changing the physical action of the organ, or part usually engaged in the normal manifestation of such functions; but I have, moreover, ascertained that the same influence may be realised in respect to sound, smell, taste, heat, and cold – so that suggested ideas and concentration of inward consciousness are competent, with some individuals, to excite ideas not merely of hearing vague sounds, but particular tunes, the smell of particular odours, and to discriminate particular tastes, and feel heat or cold. All this, I have proved, may be realised with some excitable subjects when they were wide awake, and when there was neither actual sound, nor odour, nor taste in the situation or substances to which they referred; and by merely asking what tune, what odour, what animal, or what substance they perceived *now* (a mode of interrogation which naturally suggests the idea of change), I clearly proved that ideas may be thus excited in the minds of subjects totally different from those existing in my own at the time. The subjects with whom I made these experiments were worthy of implicit credit as to their integrity in describing their feelings and belief; and the whole results, therefore, are attributable to the remarkable reciprocal action of the mind and body upon each other, to which I have so often referred. Indeed, one of the most beautiful examples I have had of these "vigilant phenomena", in respect to *all* the senses, occurred in the case of a gentleman of high classical and mathematical attainments, as well as in general science. He had seen no experiments of the sort before I tested him. On finishing my round of experiments with him, he begged of me to explain the *rationale* of what had occurred. I requested him to read what I had written on the subject, which he perused with great attention, after which he expressed himself perfectly satisfied that I had hit upon the true solution of the problem. Indeed, he was so kind as to authorise me to refer anyone to him for a confirmation of the *rationale* I had given of the phenomena, as experienced by him in his own person, when wide awake, and in the bright light of day. [*The Power of the Mind over the Body*, 1846] – Pages 21-24.

[Braid's Meeting with Mr. Stone]

I may here observe, that when he was in Manchester, Mr. Stone requested a mutual friend to introduce him to me. At our interview I read to him the foregoing extract from my work, when he expressed his surprise that he had not before been aware of experiments so entirely similar to his own, having been made and published in this country. He admitted that my explanation was quite satisfactory where audible suggestions were required, but still wished to hold to the electric theory, as the only mode of explaining their alleged power of conveying their behests and feelings to patients silently and unseen, through pure sympathy or silent willing at a distance – phenomena, the actual existence of which I very much doubt. Again,

> The true cause of these "vigilant phenomena" is not a physical influence from without, but a mental delusion from within, which paralyses their reason and independent volition; so that, for the time being, they are mere puppets in the hands of another person, by whom they are irresistibly controlled, so that they can only see or hear, or taste, or feel, or act, in accordance with his will and direction. They have their whole attention fixed on what may be said or signified by this alleged superior power, and consequently perceive impressions through the excited state of the organs of sense called into operation, which they could not perceive in their ordinary condition. It may have been interesting enough to have demonstrated that the human mind could be so subjugated and controlled; but I do not consider the *continual repetition* of such experiments in the waking condition as at all proper, or free from the danger of throwing the faculties of the minds of such patients into a permanently morbid *condition*. – *The Power of the Mind over the Body,* Pages 33-34.[71]

The processes, however, when prudently and skilfully conducted are perfectly harmless, and are, moreover, capable of being turned to the happiest results in the relief and cure of several affections which are most intractable, or altogether incurable, by the ordinary modes of treatment, by the exhibition of medicine. In this manner we can excite or depress the state of sensation and circulation locally or generally, and consequently the function of any organ or part, in a most remarkable degree, according to the mode of procedure and mental suggestion resorted to in each individual case – so that, **in this way, morbid delusions and diseases may not only be excited but cured in many instances**, not merely as regards the faculties of the mind but also as regards the functions of the body. Whatever function can be paralysed

---

[71] Since this lecture was delivered, which was on the 26th March 1851, I have been much gratified by the perusal of two admirable lectures on the subject, by Professor J. Hughes Bennett of Edinburgh. In these lectures, that acute physiologist and accomplished physician advocates essentially similar views to those which I have so long contended for. Like a true philosopher, Dr. B. interrogated nature by experimental observation; and, in reference to the doctrine of *external influence* as the cause of the phenomena, he says, "I know of no series of well-ascertained facts capable of supporting such a doctrine." Regarding the ascertained facts, the Professor adds, that they "are highly important, and demand the careful consideration of the physiologist and medical practitioner". To the same effect are the following observations of Dr. Henry Holland of London, bearing date 26th April, 1851, addressed to me by that highly accomplished physician and able writer. After acknowledging receipt of a copy of a synopsis of this lecture, he says, "You take the true course in regard to both Mesmerists and biologists in keeping ever before you the main question, Is there *any* unknown influence, *communicated from A to B, by* which the latter attains a state and powers not otherwise attainable?

"This is the gist of the whole question; and I doubt not you are right in your conclusion, that there is no Mesmeric phenomenon (well verified, and free from all charge of *accident, mistake,* or *imposture*) which is not explicable by causes, normal or abnormal, within the Mesmerised individual himself.

"Your experiments," Dr. H. adds, "have done much, and by new methods, to elucidate and justify this conclusion; and they apply very explicitly also to this *biological branch of Mesmerism.*"

or perverted by a given mode of procedure, and suggestion, and manipulation, **may be invigorated and corrected by an opposite mode of management.** This is still more remarkably verified in patients who pass into the sleep.

[The Physical Reality of Suggested Phenomena]

I am as well aware as any sceptic can be, that many of the phenomena manifested by such subjects, both when asleep and in the waking condition, are capable of being feigned. Indeed, like the correspondent in *Chambers' Journal*, I set about the experimental investigation of the subject with the full conviction that there was imposture, and with the determination, moreover, if possible, to discover and expose the *trick*. With such evidence as presented itself before me, however, of the genuineness of the phenomena, as exhibited in parties known to me to be possessed of the strictest probity, and honour, and Christian principles, it became impossible for me, with a proper regard for candour and honour, to persist longer in a course of dogmatic scepticism. I therefore confessed that my former notions had been erroneous, and set about the farther investigation of the subject with the honest desire to arrive at truth. It is important to remark, however, that these vigilant phenomena prove that a strong fixed idea of determined scepticism may so possess the mind of an inquirer as to render him a totally unfit person to be a valid witness of what are matters of plain fact and observation to those who are not so enslaved by prejudice. His imagination and fixed conceit may be so powerful and engrossing that unconsciously he is forced to interpret the *ideas of his* own *mind* as the *facts,* instead of what is actually presented before him. This view of the subject throws important light upon the nature and value of evidence in cases where parties point-blank contradict each other when describing occurrences of which they have both been eye-witnesses. A strong mental impression or prejudice may have deceived one or more witnesses, without the slightest intention to misrepresent facts.

Chambers' correspondent has, to a certain extent, hit upon the true solution of the cause of these vigilant phenomena – viz., that it is a play upon the *will* of the patient, and the influence of sympathy and imitation upon certain individuals. This theory readily accounts for all the phenomena in which muscular motion is concerned; but it does not at all account for a much larger and more surprising class of phenomena – viz., suspending, intensifying, or perverting impressions addressed to any or all of the organs of special sense. These results are to be accounted for only by an appeal to the power of an over-excited and vivid imagination, and fixed idea changing physical action. **Those who suppose that the power of the imagination and sustained mental attention directed to any part of the body is a mere *mental* condition, without being accompanied by any change in the physical organism, labour under a grave mistake. Sustained mental attention directed to any part changes both the sensation and circulation of the part so regarded, and in a more marked degree according to the imagination and belief of the patient. From this cause the most grave and fatal diseases may be engendered, and by withdrawing the attention, and fixing the train of thought on some new object or pursuit, relief and cures may be effected in cases which would utterly fail without such management of the mind.** In support of this doctrine, I beg to refer to Dr. Holland's "Medical Notes and Reflections", where he treats of "the effects of mental attention on the bodily organs" with his usual ability.

Voluntary motion arises from a mandate of the *will* giving a special direction to the nervo-vital influence, so as to excite into action the class of muscles which naturally produce such motion, whilst their antagonists remain passive.

In these electro-biological experiments or vigilant phenomena, however, the suggestion of the operator excites a greater flow of nervous force into the class of muscles which produce the action *suggested* than the patient is able to throw into the opposite class. *Both* classes of muscles, therefore, are called strongly into action but the suggested idea being the *stronger,* there is no efficient voluntary motion, notwithstanding a great amount of nervous influence may be expended by the patient, as evinced by his rapid exhaustion. In this manner I lately caused a patient's hands to become involuntarily closed on a walking-stick, so that he could not relax his hold of the stick; and then, by saying aloud in his hearing, "I will now make it so heavy that it will be impossible for him to support its weight," the idea excited by this simple auricular suggestion was more than a match for his energetic but misdirected muscular efforts, for there he struggled, until at last he fell upon the floor, quite exhausted by his efforts to support his imaginary load. The patient assured us, after the experiment was over, that he firmly believed he saw a fifty-six pound weight put upon each end of the stick at points indicated and that he felt the weight increase at each addition, and that its weight at last became quite overpowering. It was obvious, from the condition of the patient, that he was quite as much exhausted by his efforts to support the imaginary weight as he could have been had it been real. Most people must have experienced a similar feeling and result from an attack of nightmare, during common sleep. The struggle and exhaustion are in both cases analogous. On the other hand, if the suggested idea and strongly fixed belief go along with the will of the patient, his volition may thereby be so much intensified as to enable him to lift a weight which he would be quite incapable of doing in his ordinary state. The history of cases of panic in an army from slight causes, and deeds of daring and achievements almost superhuman, during fits of enthusiasm, are examples in point on a large scale.

Neither a play upon the will, nor sympathy, nor imitation, can account for patients feeling insufferable heat or cold, or for having the organs of sight, hearing, smell, and taste paralysed, or so that the patient should be made to perceive impressions at variance with the ordinary effects of the exciting cause, according to the suggestions of the experimentalist. **A strongly fixed idea and vivid imagination, however, are well-known to be quite adequate to do so, as witnessed in monomania, delirium tremens, intoxication, and narcotism from opium, the hashish, and other drugs, as well as in various other morbid conditions. In all these states, it is a well ascertained fact, that ideas may become so vivid as to assume all the force of reality, and that whilst the individual so affected retains a certain amount of consciousness of all around, still he cannot emancipate himself from the erroneous impression, or that he may be so engrossed with the one idea as to be dead or indifferent for the nonce to all other impressions.**

[On Mesmeric Passes]

Before concluding this paper, I shall state my views regarding the nature and effects of what have been called Mesmeric passes. The passes have been divided into *contact* passes, in which the fingers of the operator are drawn gently over the part intended to be affected, and into non-contact passes, which consist in passing the hand over the part, near to, but not touching it, the fingers being extended and held apart, with a tremulous motion, so as to cause a slight agitation of the air in contact with the part operated upon. The Mesmerists alleged, that the effects realised arose from some occult or magnetic influence, or the odyle force of Baron Reichenbach, affecting the part in a particular manner. My researches, however, have led me to attribute it to the power which the mind of the patient possesses to change the physical action of the part to which it is strongly drawn and fixed by sensible impressions of an external nature, or by a steady fixed state of mental attention, by an effort of the patient's own will, especially if done with the expectation and confident belief of some change being about to happen. If, at the proper stage of the sleep, the impressions are directed to the organs of special sense, ideas will be excited in the mind of the patient in accordance with the special function of the organ to which the mind has been so directed; if to a part where there are muscles subjacent, it will excite the muscles into action, and probably such ideas also as usually occasion or precede such physical actions.

One of the most puzzling classes of phenomena which I had occasion to observe was the *reverse* results which seemed to arise from the *same sensible* impressions. Thus, contact passes, or agitating the air along the course of an arm or leg, would call the muscles into action and elevate the limb. This the Mesmerists called "Mesmerising passes"; and wafting the air across the extremity caused it to descend, and this they called "deMesmerising passes"; or agitating the air over one side of the head would cause the head to follow the hand of the operator first to the one side and then to the other; or darting a hand over the hand of a patient and suddenly withdrawing it, and repeating the operation, would cause the hand to rise and become cataleptic. This was set down by the Mesmerist as indubitable proof that there was an attraction between the hand of the operator and the patient's hand, which attracted it as the magnet does iron. I very soon perceived that, on first going into the sleep, patients had sufficient mobility to be affected by certain impressions, and that they would approach to or recede from impressions, according as they were agreeable or disagreeable in quality or intensity. Thus, soft music they would be delighted with, and approach to, whilst they would be painfully affected, and run from, loud or harsh music; and the same of odours, and impressions of heat and cold. I ascertained that titillating the skin, or agitating the air over the skin, would call into action the subjacent muscles, and thus you might flex the hand, and raise the arm; and by acting in a similar manner with the *opposite* class of muscles, the hand and fingers would become extended, and the arm fall. This seemed simple and comprehensible enough. But at length I ascertained that a class of muscles, having been called into action by such impressions, and allowed to remain a short time in the position assumed, the repetition of the like sensible impression on the same points through which it had produced the action, would now reduce it, thus producing, from the *same apparently exciting cause,* the very *reverse effects,* whether that had been a contact pass or a simple agitation of the air. I found, moreover, that my *will* had nothing to do with these results, as precisely the usual result would be realised whilst I was willing the reverse. These opposite effects from the same exciting cause puzzled and perplexed me vastly; but at last I arrived at a very simple solution of the apparent mystery. When the patient got into the proper stage of the sleep for manifesting these phenomena, I recalled to mind that consciousness and the will are so much adumbrated that the movements are instinctive or automatic, and hence the impression merely gives a tendency to motion, the direction and character of the motion being the *most natural motion under the circumstances which exist at the time.* Hence, if a muscle is passive, it will become active, and if active, it will become passive, from the same exciting cause. Thus, when an impression is made on the hand or arm when reposing on the lap, as it cannot descend it will rise, and become rigid; but by making a like impression on it after remaining in that condition for a little while, it will give a tendency to perform the most natural motion, which, in *this* instance, is to descend. If any obstacle be interposed to its rising or descending, and the impression be repeated, it will move laterally. **This same mode of exciting action by sensible impressions, and reversing results in the way described, may be confined to individual muscles, or classes of muscles, and in this way we may act on the muscles of expression, so as to** awaken any passion or emotion in the mind; the action of the muscles, which constitute the "Anatomy of Expression", suggesting the feeling to the mind of the entranced subject, as the idea, in the waking state, naturally calls such anatomy of expression into play. It is, therefore, a mere inversion of the sequence which ordinarily obtains between mental emotion and physical manifestations of such emotions. That there is nothing occult or specific in the pass with the hand is manifest from this, that a similar agitation of the air by the blast from a pair of bellows will produce precisely similar results as the like current of air from the wafting of the human hand, as I have proved to the entire satisfaction of hundreds of intelligent individuals.

A pass, therefore, as a visible or sensible impression, aids the patient in concentrating his mental attention to a given organ or part, and thus influences the function, through giving a special direction to a power residing within the patient's own frame; but it no more imparts a virtue of an occult nature from the operator to the patient, than the lens *produces* the light and heat which it makes visible and perceptible to the senses, through concentrating the luminous and calorific rays of the sun, and drawing them to a focus. Both the pass and the lens aid in concentrating and manifesting the respective influences; but neither the operator nor the lens is the source or origin of the power or influence so manifested.

The above is an explanation of what may be realised naturally in subjects without any previous training or auricular suggestions whatever. It is quite possible, however, to subvert the whole of these natural phenomena by a system of training, as follows:– Supposing that, with each touch or agitation of the air, the operator speaks aloud and predicts what should happen, the auricular suggestion may be so strong as to cause the *predicted* manifestation to be realised instead of what otherwise would have been the case; and thus, from this time forward, through the double conscious memory, the like impression on that part or organ of sense, will recall the previously associated idea and manifestation. We may, therefore, have an *artificial* as well as *natural* set of phenomena manifested, according to the mode of operating and intention of the operator.

It also merits notice that there are some subjects who, during the sleep, see through their partially closed eyelids. In the case of such subjects, if the operator gazes steadfastly at any part of their bodies, such as a leg or arm, the patient will immediately catch the suggestion, and imagine that a movement of the member looked at is wished to be made, and his docility will instantly incline him to obey the suggestion, as if it had been excited *by* a contact-pass, or any other stimulus applied directly to the part – i.e., if the member is down it will rise, or if up it will descend, or will move laterally if a mechanical obstacle is interposed to prevent it moving upwards or downwards. In like manner the remarkable tendency to sympathy and imitation in such patients, will induce them to observe and imitate every physical act of the operator, or other person to whom he has specially directed the patient's attention. Interpose a screen, however, and then make movements of the body extremities, and they will rely upon hearing, instead of sight, under these circumstances and will only be *occasionally* correct now in their imitation of physical acts; which is a clear proof that, in the other instances, they were directed by sight – *viz.*, seeing through the partially closed eyelids.

All these phenomena may be realised without the patient intending to play off any deception on others, or having any remembrance of the facts on coming out of the sleep.

[Criticism of Paranormal Claims]

I have never yet seen any phenomena during either the hypnotic or Mesmeric sleep, or during the state for manifesting vigilant phenomena, which were not in accordance with generally admitted physiological and psychological principles. The senses and mental powers may be torpified or quickened in an extraordinary degree; but I have never seen anything to warrant a belief that individuals could thereby become gifted with the power of reading through decidedly opaque bodies; acquire the faculty of knowing the meaning of language which they had never learned; and other transcendental phenomena, called by the Mesmerists the *higher* phenomena. The power of a strongly fixed attention, vivid imagination, and self-confidence, however, enables them to perform some extraordinary feats of phonic imitation, and writing and drawing by touch, without the use of their eyes; discovering parties who own certain articles worn by them, through the quickened sense of smell; overhearing conversation in a distant apartment, which they could not do in the waking condition; of recalling to mind things long forgotten when awake; and also of deducing conclusions, manifesting uncommon shrewdness, from premises suggested to them, or arising in their minds spontaneously from recollection of past events, to which they have directed their concentrated attention. These latter feats are precisely analogous to those manifested by the Celtic Seers, or Second-sight men, in the Highlands of Scotland. Their attention was so fixed, and their spirits so rapt in the subject of their deep contemplation, that they stood with staring eyes –"the eyes being open, but the sense shut" – similar to some somnambulists, and the shrewdness of some of their deductions was looked upon as the result of a sort of inspiration peculiar to that class of men.

Several important inferences may be drawn from what has been adduced regarding the power of the imagination, belief, and fixed act of attention, in changing and controlling physical action, and of the state of the body thus superinduced re-acting on the mind. It not only enables us to comprehend, upon scientific principles, the cause and cure of many diseases, where there has been no specific and adequate external physical agency to account for the results; but it also explains many phenomena which used to be attributed to demonology, witchcraft, ghost-seeing, being spell-bound, the power of the Obi women, who could cause their credulous victims to wither and die under their assumed malign power and maledictions; the power of charms, spells, and amulets, of Perkins' metallic tractors, the efficacy of galvanic rings, bread pills, and such like. It also explains the alleged clairvoyance of the Egyptian boys after looking steadfastly at an inky globule held in their hands, narratives of which are published by Lord Prudhoe and Mr. Lane. The revelations of Kelly, recorded daily for Dr. Dee, Warden of Manchester in the reign of Queen Elizabeth, and which were alleged to be revealed to him by a spirit whilst gazing into Dr. Dee's celebrated show-stone; the fortune-tellers, who exercise a similar mode of looking into futurity, by gazing into a glass egg; and the late revelations of the same sort, published at the end of Zadkiel's Almanac for this year, as to the revelations of the Angel in Lady Blessington's magic crystal, all come under the same category, being merely figments of *fancy,* excited by questions or otherwise, set down for visions seen, and answers audibly uttered, or written in visible characters before them by the said Angels. Whatever greatly excites and changes the existing train of thought and feeling, especially if done with faith and expectation, and fixed mental attention, will assuredly be followed by a change in the previously existing mental and physical condition of the subject.

We also thus acquire this salutary lesson, that, in order to have a healthy state of mind and body, it is requisite that *all* our faculties should be duly cultivated, and that the attention should not be devoted too long and exclusively to any *one* object or pursuit, as the latter course has a tendency to engender a morbid state of mind as well as of body. Hence the advantage of relaxation and amusements of various kinds, so long as they are pursued in reason and with moderation. We are also taught this important fact, that dogmatic scepticism, or prejudice, not only beclouds the reason, but also destroys or perverts the perceptive faculties. This truth seems to have been clearly perceived by Dugald Stewart, when he penned the following notable paragraph:– "Unlimited scepticism is equally the child of imbecility, as implicit credulity."

[Conclusion]

I shall conclude this essay by a very simple mode of illustration, as respects the different points of view in which the Mesmerists, the electro-biologists, and myself, stand toward each other in *theory,* by referring to the two theories of light contended for at the present time. Some believe in a positive emission from the sun of a subtle material, or imponderable influence, as the cause of light; whilst others deny this emission theory, and contend that light is produced by simple vibration excited by the sun, without any positive emission from that luminary. I may, therefore, be said to have adopted the *vibratory* theory, whilst the Mesmerists and electro-biologists contend for the *emission* theory. But my experiments have proved that the ordinary phenomena of Mesmerism may be realised through the subjective or personal mental and physical acts of the *patient alone;* whereas the proximity, acts, or influence of a *second* party, would be *indispensably* requisite for their production, if the theory of the Mesmerists were true. Moreover, my experiments have proved that audible, visible, or tangible suggestions of another person, whom the subject believes to possess such power over him, is requisite for the production of the *waking* phenomena; whereas no audible, visible, or tangible suggestion from a *second* party ought to be required to produce these phenomena, if the theory of the electro-biologists were true.

There is, therefore, both positive and negative proof in favour of my *mental* and *suggestive* theory, and in opposition to the magnetic, occult, or electric theories of the Mesmerists and electro-biologists. My theory, moreover, has this additional recommendation, that it is level to our comprehension, and adequate to account for all which is demonstrably true, without offering any violence to reason and common sense, or being at variance with generally admitted physiological and psychological principles. Under these circumstances, therefore, I trust that you will consider me entitled to your verdict in favour of my MENTAL THEORY.

Arlington House,
Oxford Street,
Manchester.[72]

---

[72] [A lengthy appendix on Dr. Ashburner's claims regarding odyle has been omitted as some of the content is reproduced elsewhere, and the remainder seemed of little relevance to the modern reader.]

Observations on Trance
or Human Hybernation
(1850)

by James Braid
M.R.C.S. Edinburgh, C.M.W.S., etc., etc.

"No affection, to which the animal frame is subject, is more remarkable than this.
(Catalepsy or Trance)
There is such an apparent extinction of every faculty essential to life,
that it is inconceivable how existence should go on during the continuance of the fit."
– Macnish

"*Ex Oriente Lux.*"
["From the Light of the Orientals."]

London:
John Churchill,
Prince's Street, Soho

Edinburgh:
Adam and Charles Black

1850

Preface

Some years ago I had a number of queries published in the medical journals, and also printed in a separate form for circulation, both at home and abroad, with the view of accumulating additional and accurate information regarding the curious points in Physiology treated of in this pamphlet. Through the kindness of my friend, George Swinton, Esq. of Edinburgh, and Sir [Charles Edward] Trevelyan, of the Treasury [and the East India Company], application was made to Sir Claude Martin Wade [a distinguished army officer of the East India Company] on my behalf, and a copy of the said queries was given to him; to which application Sir Claude kindly responded, by furnishing me with the valuable narrative now published, regarding what he was an eye-witness of when acting as Political Agent at the Court of Runjeet Singh, at Lahore [i.e., Maharaja Ranjit Singh, ruler of the Sikh state of Punjab]. The narrative bears internal evidence that Sir Claude was a most accurate observer, as well as a lucid writer. To all of those gentlemen I beg to tender my very best thanks for furnishing me with such a valuable document. **It was intended to have appeared in a new edition of my work on *Hypnotism;* but as the publication of that work must unavoidably be postponed for a short time longer**, I have thought it desirable to print the original information which I have obtained immediately, in a separate form, as it cannot fail to be most interesting to all scientific men; and *its* publication may, moreover, stimulate others to investigate and furnish additional evidence on the subject.

The second case, by an eye-witness of the facts, was furnished to me by a retired Major, who served as an officer for many years in India. He requested me not to publish his name, because he understood the Directors disliked that any official men in their service should be known to take a prominent part in anything so far out of the line of their special duties. However, after I had written my narrative of the transaction, from the facts which he had communicated to me, he was kind enough to hear it read over to him, in the presence of several mutual friends, when he pronounced it correct on *every* point. He assured us that he never could forget the circumstances of that transaction, in as much as the part which he took in it, and his dread, in the end, that the devotee must have perished in the enterprise, and he be thereby rendered liable to be indicted as accessory to his murder, had caused him greater anxiety and horror than all the actions and scenes of danger he had encountered during the whole of his military career.

If medical gentlemen residing in India would only take the trouble of investigating a few of these cases systematically and carefully, not merely with the view of guarding against all sources of collusion and fraud which might be perpetrated in such exhibitions, but also by weighing the body of the Fakeer before his being shut up or buried, and again on being exposed to view; and also by noting particularly the relative degree in which respiration and circulation become respectively affected, both as regards time and extent of change, by the voluntary processes of the Fakeer for inducing the Trance, we might very soon be in possession of all the information on the subject which we could desire. I should feel much obliged to any gentleman who would be so kind as to forward such information to me, and, in publishing, I should duly acknowledge the extent of my obligation to each individual who might entrust such information to my care.

It may here be requisite for me to explain, that by the term *Hypnotism,* or *Nervous Sleep,* which frequently occurs in the following pages, I mean a peculiar condition of the nervous system, into which it may be thrown by artificial contrivance, and which differs, in several respects, from common sleep or the waking condition. I do not allege that this condition is induced through the transmission of a magnetic or occult influence from my body into that of my patients; nor do I profess, by my processes, to produce the higher phenomena of the Mesmerists. My pretensions are of a much more humble character, and are all consistent with generally admitted principles in physiological and psychological science. Hypnotism might therefore not inaptly be designated, *Rational Mesmerism,* in contra-distinction to the *Transcendental Mesmerism* of the Mesmerists.[73]

Arlington House,
Oxford Street,
Manchester,
July, 1850.

---

[73] [Braid's long footnotes have been relocated to separate appendices for readability and aesthetic reasons, and to provide titles to highlight their content.]

Observations on Trance or Human Hybernation

[Introductory Remarks]
In the year 1845 I published some observations on the remarkable feats of the Fakeers of India, who had been represented as having acquired the power of suffering themselves to be buried alive, enclosed in bags, shut up in sealed boxes, or even of being buried for days or for weeks in common graves, and assuming their wonted activity on being released from their temporary confinement or sepulture. ['The Fakirs of India.' *Medical Times*, 1845; 12: 437]

Such extraordinary feats were naturally looked upon with suspicion, and believed to be a **species of deception**, accomplished entirely through collusion, and not at all *bona fide* transactions, such as alleged. Whilst I **think it highly probable that this is the true character of *many* of these alleged feats, still there are others which admit of no such explanation**. The difficulties of eluding detection in several carefully narrated cases, were evidently so great as to have rendered deception impossible; and it therefore becomes the duty of scientific men fairly to meet the difficulty, and to endeavour to arrive at a satisfactory solution of the phenomena on physiological principles.

On careful consideration of the whole phenomena narrated in connection with these cases, coupled with my experience of the powers of hypnotism, by which individuals can throw themselves into a state of catalepsy or trance, more or less profound, in which condition, like the hybernating animals, all the vital functions are reduced to the minimum of what is compatible with continued existence and restoration to their former activity, I arrived at the conclusion, that the individuals referred to accomplished these apparently impossible feats by throwing themselves into this state of temporary hybernation or trance, through suppressing the respiration and fixing the mind, just as was manifested by the well-attested case of Colonel Townsend in this country, and by many patients whom I have myself witnessed, who have acquired the like power in a minor degree.

[The Death-like Trance of Colonel Townsend]
The following is the narrative of Colonel Townsend's case, as recorded by the late Dr. [John] Cheyne of Dublin [physician-general to the forces in Ireland]; and, when we take into consideration the deservedly high estimation in which Dr. Cheyne was held, as a practical physician, possessed of high talents and scientific attainments, and the high character he bore as a Christian man and a gentleman, it is impossible to have had the Colonel's interesting and uncommon case attested and recorded more satisfactorily. Dr. Cheyne narrates the case as follows:–

> He could die or expire when he pleased, and yet, by an effort, or somehow, he could come to life again. He insisted so much upon us seeing the trial made, that we were at last forced to comply. We all three felt his pulse first; it was distinct, though small and thready [a fine or weak pulse], and his heart had its usual beating. He composed himself on his back, and lay in a still posture for some time; while I held his right hand, Dr. Baynard laid his hand on his heart, and Mr. Skrine held a clean looking-glass to his mouth. I found his pulse sink gradually, till at last I could not feel any, by the most exact and nice touch, Dr. Baynard could not feel the least motion in the heart, nor Mr. Skrine perceive the least soil of breath on the bright mirror he held to his mouth. Then each of us, by turns, examined his arm, heart, and breath, but could not, by the nicest scrutiny, discover the least symptom of life in him. We reasoned a long time about this odd appearance as well as we could, and, finding he still continued in that condition, we began to conclude that he had, indeed, carried the experiment too far; and at last we were satisfied that he was actually dead, and were just ready to leave him. This continued about half an hour. By nine in the morning, in autumn, as we were going away, we observed some motion about the body, and, upon examination, found his pulse and the motion of his heart gradually returning; he began to breathe heavily and speak softly. We were all astonished to the last degree at this unexpected change, and, after some further conversation with him, and among ourselves, went away fully satisfied as to all the particulars of this fact, but confounded and puzzled, and not able to form any rational scheme that might account for it.

In the "Dabistan", [*Dabistān-i Mazāhib*, a 17th century Persian religious text of a syncretistic nature] a learned work on the religious sects in India, translated a few years ago from the Persic, reference is made to the power acquired by various individuals of separating their souls from their bodies, as they style it, and resuming their wonted relations to each other again at will. One individual is specially referred to by name, who had attained the power of suppressing his breath for *three hours;* another who could do so for *twelve hours;* another who could do so for *two* DAYS; and Balik Natha, who attained to above a hundred years of age, could suppress his breath for A WEEK. Here, then, we have exactly similar phenomena exhibited by these Hindoos, as those recorded in the above case of Colonel Townsend; and the knowledge of these facts will prepare the reader, in some measure, for the reception of the still more astounding phenomena recorded in the following narratives.

Since the above-named period, I have lost no opportunity of accumulating additional evidence on the subject; and the result is, that I am now enabled to publish two valuable documents from eye-witnesses of the facts, which, together with the evidence we formerly possessed, must set the point at rest for ever as to the fact of the feats referred to having been *genuine phenomena.*

[Sir Claude M. Wade's Account]
Sir Claude M. Wade's narrative was accompanied by the following polite note:–

Edinburgh
September 13th 1845.

Sir Claude Wade presents compliments to Dr. Braid, and has much pleasure in enclosing, for his *free* use and information, in the form of a narrative, replies to the queries received from Dr. Braid, through Mr. George Swinton, regarding the Fakeer who buried himself alive at Lahore in 1837. Sir Claude regrets, that in consequence of his being constantly on the move, and unable to refer to his papers for information, he has only now found leisure to comply with Dr. Braid's application. Should any point be omitted in Sir C. Wade's account, he will be happy to supply the deficiency on a further application, addressed to his usual place of residence, Ryde, Isle of Wight.

To Dr. Braid, *etc., etc.*, Manchester.
REPLIES TO DR. BRAID'S QUERIES
REGARDING THE FAKEER WHO BURIED HIMSELF ALIVE AT LAHORE IN 1831.

I was present at the Court of Runjeet Singh [Maharajah of the Sikh kingdom of Punjab] when the Fakeer mentioned by the Honourable Captain Osborne was buried alive for six weeks; and, although I arrived a few hours after his actual interment, and did not, consequently, witness that part of the phenomenon, I had the testimony of Runjeet Singh himself, and others the most credible witnesses of his Court, to the truth of the Fakeer having been so buried before them; and, from my having myself been present when he was disinterred, and restored to a state of perfect vitality, in a position so close to him as to render any deception impossible, it is my firm belief that there was no collusion in producing the extraordinary feat which I have related. Captain Osborne's book is not at present before me, that I might refer to such parts of his account as devolve the authenticity of the fact on my authority. I will, therefore, briefly state what I saw, to enable others to judge of the weight due to my evidence, and whether any proofs of collusion can, in their opinion, be detected.

On the approach of the appointed time, according to invitation, I accompanied Runjeet Singh to the spot where the Fakeer had been buried. It was in a square building, called a *barra durra,* in the middle of one of the gardens, adjoining the palace at Lahore, with an open veranda around, having an enclosed room in the centre. On arriving there, Runjeet Singh, who was attended on the occasion by the whole of his Court, dismounting from his elephant, asked me to join him in examining the building to satisfy himself that it was closed as he had left it. We did so; there had been a door on each of the four sides of the room, three of which were perfectly closed with brick and mortar, the fourth had a strong door, which was also closed with mud up to the padlock, which was sealed with the private seal of Runjeet Singh in his own presence, when the Fakeer was interred. Indeed, the exterior of the building presented no aperture by which air could be admitted, or any communication held by which food could be conveyed to the Fakeer. I may also add, that the walls closing the doorway bore no mark whatever of having been recently disturbed or removed.

Runjeet Singh recognised the seal as the one which he had affixed, and as he was as sceptical as any European could be of the success of such an enterprise – to guard as far as possible against any collusion – he had placed two companies from his own personal escort near the building, from which four sentries were furnished and relieved every two hours, night and day, to guard the building from intrusion. At the same time, he ordered one of the principal officers of his Court to visit the place occasionally, and to report the result of his inspection to him, while he himself, or his Minister, kept the seal which closed the hole of the padlock, and the latter received the report, morning and evening, from the officer on guard.

After our examination we seated ourselves in the veranda opposite the door, while some of Runjeet Singh's people dug away the mud wall, and one of his officers broke the seal and opened the padlock. When the door was thrown open, nothing but a dark room was to be seen. Runjeet Singh and myself then entered it, in company with the servant of the Fakeer; and a light being brought, we descended about three feet below the floor of the room, into a sort of cell, where a wooden box, about four feet long by three broad, with a sloping roof, containing the Fakeer, was placed upright, the door of which had also a padlock and seal similar to that on the outside. On opening it we saw a figure enclosed in a bag of white linen, fastened by a string over the head – on the exposure of which a grand salute was fired, and the surrounding multitude came crowding to the door to see the spectacle. After they had gratified their curiosity, the Fakeer's servant, putting his arms into the box, took the figure out, and closing the door, placed it with its back against it, exactly as the Fakeer had been squatted (like a Hindoo idol) in the box itself.

Runjeet Singh and myself then descended into the cell, which was so small, that we were only able to sit on the ground in front of the body, and so close to it as to touch it with our hands and knees.

The servant then began pouring warm water over the figure; but, as my object was to see if any fraudulent practices could be detected, I proposed to Runjeet Singh to tear open the bag, and have a perfect view of the body before any means of resuscitation were employed. I accordingly did so; and may here remark, that the bag, when first seen by us, looked mildewed, as if it had been buried some time. The legs and arms of the body were shrivelled and stiff, the face full, the head reclining on the shoulder like that of a corpse. I then called to the medical gentleman who was attending me to come down and inspect the body, which he did, but could discover no pulsation in the heart, the temples, or the arm. There was, however, a heat about the region of the brain, which no other part of the body exhibited.[74]

The servant then recommenced bathing him with hot water, and gradually relaxing his arms and legs from the rigid state in which they were contracted, Runjeet Singh taking his right and I his left leg, to aid by friction in restoring them to their proper action; during which time the servant placed a hot wheaten cake, about an inch thick, on the top of the head – a process which he twice or thrice renewed. He then pulled out of his nostril, and ear, the wax and cotton with which they were stopped; and after great exertion opened his mouth by inserting the point of a knife between his teeth, and, while holding his jaw open with his left hand, drew the tongue forward with his right – in the course of which the tongue flew back several times to its curved position upwards, in which it had originally been, so as to close the gullet.

He then rubbed his eyelids with ghee (or clarified butter) for some seconds, until he succeeded in opening them, when the eyes appeared quite motionless and glazed. After the cake had been applied for the third time to the top of his head, the body was violently convulsed, the nostrils became inflated, when respiration ensued, and the limb began to assume a natural fullness; but the pulsation was still faintly perceptible. The servant then put some of the ghee on his tongue, and made him swallow it. A few minutes afterwards, the eyeballs became dilated, and recovered their natural colour, when the Fakeer, recognising Runjeet Singh sitting close to him, articulated, in a low, sepulchral tone, scarcely audible, "Do you believe me now?" Runjeet Singh replied in the affirmative, and invested the Fakeer with a pearl necklace and superb pair of gold bracelets, and pieces of silk and muslin, and shawls, forming what is called a *khelat*, such as is usually conferred by the Princes of India on persons of distinction.

From the time of the box being opened, to the recovery of the voice, not more than half an hour could have elapsed; and in another half-hour the Fakeer talked with myself and those about him freely, though feebly, like a sick person; and we then left him, convinced that there had been no fraud or collusion in the exhibition we had witnessed.[75]

I was present, also, when the Fakeer was summoned by Runjeet Singh from a considerable distance to Lahore, some months afterwards, again to bury himself alive before Captain Osborne and the officers of the late Sir William M'Naghton's mission in 1838; which, after the usual preparation, he offered to do for a few days, the term of Sir William's mission being nearly expired; but from the tenor of the doubts expressed, and some observations made by Captain Osborne as to keeping the key of the room in which he was to be buried in his own possession, the Fakeer, with the superstitious dread of an Indian, became evidently alarmed, and apprehensive that if once within Captain Osborne's power, he would not be allowed to escape. His refusal on that occasion will naturally induce a suspicion of the truth of the transaction which I witnessed; but to those well acquainted with the character of the natives of India, it will not be surprising that, where life and death were concerned, the Fakeer should have manifested a distrust of what to him appeared the mysterious intentions of a European who was a perfect stranger to him, while he was ready to repose implicit confidence in Runjeet Singh and others before whom he had exhibited. I am satisfied that he refused only from the cause I have mentioned, and that he would have done for me what he declined doing for Captain Osborne.

It had previously been observed, also, by Sir William M'Naghton and others of the party, truly, though jestingly, that if the Fakeer should not survive the trial to which he was required to submit, those who might instigate him to it would run the risk of being indicted for murder, which induced them to refrain from pressing the subject further.

I share entirely in the apparent incredibility of the fact of a man being buried alive, and surviving the trial for various periods of duration; but however incompatible with our knowledge of physiology, in the absence of any visible proof to the contrary, I am bound to declare my belief in the facts which I have represented, however impossible their existence may appear to others.[76]

---

[74] Might not this "heat about the region of the brain" have been caused by the warm water poured over the head imparting the greatest degree of heat to the part with which it came first in contact? – J. Braid.

[75] These feats of the Fakeers in no way invalidate the importance of the Gospel miracle of the resurrection of Christ. In the latter case, the transfixing of the heart by the soldier's spear was necessarily a mortal wound, from which recovery was impossible unless by a miracle.

[76] There may be some hypercritical, suspicious individuals ready to allege, as no direct declaration to the contrary has been recorded in the narrative, that some subterranean communication may have existed, so as to have afforded access to the Fakeer by accomplices during his imprisonment in the *barra durra*, and that without the possibility of their being detected by the guards surrounding the exterior of the building. When we reflect, however, on the fact, that the object of Runjeet Singh was not to prove, but to disprove, the possibility of the success of such an enterprise, it is impossible for us to imagine, with all the precautions narrated as having been adopted by him for guarding against deception exteriorly, that he should not have exercised equal scrutiny and care to guard against *subterranean*

> I took some pains to inquire into the mode by which such a result was effected, and was informed that it rested on the doctrine of the Hindoo physiologist, that *heat* constituted the self-existent principle of life, and that if the functions of the other elements were so far destroyed as to leave that one in its perfect purity, life could be sustained for considerable lengths of time independent of air, food, or any other means of sustenance. To produce such a state the patients are obliged to go through a very severe preparation; for a description of which, *vide* the enclosed note. (Unfortunately this note did not come to hand with the narrative. – James Braid)
>
> How far such means are calculated to produce such effects the physiologists will be better able to judge than I can pretend to do. I merely state what I saw and heard; and think, that when we consider the incredulity and ridicule, and actual persecution, with which some of the most wonderful discoveries of modern times have been regarded – *viz*., galvanism, Harvey's system of the circulation of the blood, Mesmerism, etc. etc.; that it is presumptuous in any of us to deny to the Hindoos the possible discovery or attainment of an art which has hitherto escaped the researches of European science.

Such, then, is the narrative of Sir C. M. Wade; and when we consider the high character of the author as a gentleman of honour, talents, and attainments of the highest order, and the searching, painstaking efforts displayed by him throughout the whole investigation, and his close proximity to the body of the Fakeer, and opportunity of observing minutely every point for himself, as well as the facilities, by his personal intercourse with Runjeet Singh and the whole of his Court, of gaining the most accurate information on every point, I conceive it is impossible to have had a more valuable or conclusive document for determining the fact, that no collusion or deception existed in the above case.

[Sir C.E. Trevelyan's Account]
The next case I shall adduce is one furnished to me by Sir C. E. Trevelyan, of the Treasury. He was not an eye-witness of the transaction, but the source of his information seems to be highly satisfactory. He says:–

> I perfectly well recollect, that when I was acting as political agent at Kotah, in 1829-30, the Rajah Rana's Vukeel [solicitor], (who was a very respectable, and, for a native Indian, a very truthful man) told me one day, when he happened to be with me on business, that he had been present that morning with the Rajah Rana at the digging up of a Fakeer, who had been buried, as well as I recollect, ten days; and that after his resurrection he was in good health, and when he had refreshed himself with eating and drinking, was quite himself again. The Vukeel also assured me, that there could be no deception, because the man had been buried in the Rajah Rana's presence, and a guard of trusty soldiers had been constantly stationed over the place until he was dug up.
>
> I also recollect that the commandant of my escort and the surgeon to the political agency were fully impressed with the belief that the facts of the case were as stated by the Vukeel. They obtained their information from the independent source of some of the Sepoys [Indian soldiers] of the escort, who were present at the digging up; and I received several additional particulars from this source, which I cannot now call to mind, except that the Sepoys stated it as a fact, that some Fakeers and others had a way of drawing in their breath, and thrusting their tongues back and clenching their fingers, which enabled them to subsist for a long time without food, and with very little air.
>
> I believe the man who was buried at Kotah to be the same person who is spoken of in "Boileau's Journal", and that he went from one native court to another to get money by a display of his powers.
>
> My own belief is that he really did remain without food, and with only so much air as could reach him in his box underground, for a period of ten days or thereabouts.

I feel deeply indebted to Sir C. Trevelyan for the above valuable testimony relative to this curious inquiry. The following case occurred under the eye of Lieut. A. Boileau, a British officer, and is recorded in his "Narrative of a Journey in Rajwarra, in 1835", and is that referred to above by Sir C.E. Trevelyan:-

> Just before our arrival at Jesulmer the Rawul had adopted a most singular expedient to obtain an heir to his throne, and the circumstances of the case are altogether so extraordinary that we should hardly have given them credence had they not occurred so immediately under our notice. We were told, soon after our coming, that a man had been buried alive, of his own free will, at the back of the tank close to our tents, and that he was to remain under ground for a whole month before the process of exhumation should take place. The prescribed

---

intrusion; without which security, all the external precautions would have been a gross absurdity In fact, such an oversight on a point regarding which the most simple individual would not readily suffer himself to be deceived, would have exposed Runjeet Singh, and the whole of his Court, to the suspicion of being accomplices of the Fakeer in the perpetration of a gross public imposture – a most improbable position for such a prince to place himself and his Court in, for such a purpose.

And again; that Runjeet Singh was sceptical up to the moment of the Fakeer's restoration, is obvious from the terms in which the Fakeer addressed him when he recovered his sight – "Do you believe me now?" The mildewed state of the bag, as remarked by Sir Claude M. Wade, at the time when the box was opened and the figure first exposed, was most conclusive as to its having been buried for some time.

Lieut. A. Boileau's case meets all the objections – for the cell, or grave, was lined with masonry, and large slabs of stone covered it, so as to render it impossible for the Fakeer to escape – *vide* page 19. Indeed at a subsequent interment of this Fakeer, besides all the precautions enumerated above as resorted to on that occasion, after the box containing the Fakeer was deposited in the cell, locked and sealed, earth was turned in and trodden down, so as completely to surround and cover the box; a crop of barley was sown over it; and a constant guard maintained on the spot. Moreover, twice during the period of interment Runjeet Singh had the body dug up, when it was found to be in exactly the same position as when interred, and in a state of apparently entirely suspended animation. At the expiration of this prolonged interment, the Fakeer recovered under the usual treatment.

period elapsed on the 1st of April, 1835, and in the forenoon of that day he was dug out alive, in the presence of Goshur Lal, one of the ministers who had also superintended his interment. The place in which he was buried is a small building of stone, about twelve feet long, and eight feet broad, built on the west edge of the large tank called Gurressie, so often mentioned. In the floor of the house was a hole, about three feet long, two and a half broad, and the same depth, or perhaps a yard deep, in which he was placed, in a sitting posture, sewed up in a linen shroud, with his knees doubled up towards the chin, his feet turned inward towards the stomach, and his hands also pointed inward towards the chest. The cell, or grave, *was lined with masonry,* and floored with many folds of woollen and other cloth, that the white ant, and such insects, should be the less able to molest him. *Two heavy slabs of stone, five or six feet long, several inches thick, and broad enough to cover the mouth of the grave, were then placed over him, so that he could not escape,* and, I believe, a little earth was plastered over the whole, so as to make the surface of the ground smooth and compact. *The door of the house was also built up, and people placed outside to mount guard during the whole month, so that no tricks might be played, nor deception practised.* (...) Lieut. Trevelyan and I set off together to see what might remain to be seen. The outer wall of the house door had been broken up, the covering of the grave removed, and the body lifted out in the presence of Goshur Lal. The moonshee [a language teacher] arrived in time to see the opening of the shroud, as above mentioned, and stated that he was taken out in a perfectly senseless state, with his eyes closed, his hands cramped and powerless, his stomach very much shrunken, and his teeth joined so fast together, that the bystanders were obliged to force open his mouth with an iron instrument, in order to pour a little water down his throat. Under this treatment he gradually recovered his senses, and was restored to the use of his limbs. (...) *He conversed with us* in a *low, gentle tone of voice, as if his animal functions were still in a very feeble state; but so far from appearing distressed in mind by the long interment from which he had fast been released he said* THAT WE MIGHT BURY HIM AGAIN FOR A TWELVEMONTH IF WE PLEASED!

He is rather a young man, about thirty years of age, and his native village is within five kos [5-15 miles] of Karnaul; but, instead of remaining at home, he generally travels about the country to Ajmer, Kotah, Indor, *etc.*, allowing himself to be buried for weeks or months by anyone who will pay him handsomely for the same. (...) This individual is said to have acquired by long practice the art of holding his breath for a considerable period, as during the time that one might count fifty, and gradually increasing at intervals to one hundred, two hundred, and so on, as the pearl-divers may be supposed to do. He is, moreover, said to have acquired the power of shutting his mouth, and at the same time stopping the interior opening of the nostrils with his tongue, which latter feat is at times practised as a means of suicide by the negro slaves in the West Indies, when suffering under the lash. (...) As a farther preparation for this long burial, the subject of the present experiment abstains from all solid food some days previous to interment, taking no other nourishment than milk, which is believed by the natives to pass off almost entirely by the urethra, so that he may not be inconvenienced by the contents of the stomach or bowels while pent up in his narrow grave.

[An Anonymous British Major's Account]

The next case I have to narrate, is, if possible still more conclusive, inasmuch as the devotee was buried in a common grave, within the military limits, exactly in the same manner as they buried the common soldiers – with this exception, that he had no coffin – in an open space, where the whole transaction was witnessed by thousands of Hindoos, who were anxiously watching to guard their sainted brother against foul play which might be inflicted on him by the Mussulman guards, who were appointed to do duty at his grave, so as to prevent the possibility of intrusion or collusion during the whole period of his interment. There were thus a fair field and no favour for the devotee; abundance of witnesses, and the contending interests and bitter religious antipathy existing between the two parties [Muslim and Hindu] at work, constituting them a *counter* guard, thereby rendering collusion or foul play in the transaction impossible.

The following is the narrative of the facts, as communicated to me by Major ——, a retired officer of the Honourable the East India Company's service. This gentleman requested me not to publish his name, lest he might incur the displeasure of the Directors, for having taken such a prominent part in a transaction so much beyond the line of his official duties. However, in order to give the greatest possible authenticity to the facts which he dared venture to do, under the circumstances, after I had written my narrative from the facts which he had communicated to me, he was so kind as to hear the whole read aloud in the presence of several mutual friends, when he pronounced my narrative correct on *every* point, and concluded with the remark, that the case made too deep an impression on his memory ever to be forgotten by him, from the fact of his having been personally so painfully implicated in the transaction.

Whilst staff-officer of a British military station in the Concon, in 1828, this gentleman had heard of some of these strange feats of Fakeers burying themselves alive in that neighbourhood, but took no interest in the reports, believing the whole alleged feats to be mere hoaxes or tricks. However, the following circumstance occurred, which proved to him the reality of certain individuals being veritably possessed of such extraordinary powers.

One day this officer was waited upon by a Brahmin [a member of the Indian priestly caste], who held the public office of Chowdrie. – The Chowdrie is a civil functionary who has the superintendence of Courts, and all public transactions or feats within his district; but he is subordinate to the staff-officer in regard to all which occurs within what is called the military limits or cantonments, so that, in all which appertains to the said localities he is, in the first place, obliged to obtain the sanction of the British officer in command. – The Chowdrie told the officer, that the object of his visit was to obtain his sanction for one of his sainted countrymen – who had come hither for the purpose of performing one of those feats above referred to – to bury himself for nine days within the military boundary. He moreover added, that an immense number of people had assembled from the neighbouring country to witness the holy man perform the said feat. To this the officer replied, that he did not believe any man was such a fool as to suffer himself to be buried alive for nine days, because in such case he must inevitably perish; and, having said so, he dismissed the Chowdrie abruptly, without complying with his request.

Shortly thereafter, however, the Chowdrie returned, to urge the officer to comply with the request of the Fakeer, assuring him that the holy man was proposing it in good faith, and was most anxious to be permitted to do so within the military limits, as affording better proof that there could be no collusion than if he did so elsewhere; he also added, that he had frequently done so before, and that his sanctity would save him on this as on former occasions. The Chowdrie even went so far as to say, that his sanctity had given him such power with God, that he could remain for any length of time he chose underground with perfect safety. At length the officer replied, "Well if the man is determined to bury himself, you shall have my sanction for him doing so within the military limits; but remember this, that I shall take care that *no trick shall be played, but that he shall be buried in good earnest;* and, the more certainly to secure this, his grave shall be surrounded the whole time by a guard of Mussulmans, so that no Hindoo shall approach it during his sepulture." With all this the Chowdrie was perfectly satisfied, seeming firm in his faith that the sanctity of the holy man was quite sufficient to save him during this extraordinary trial.

Hereupon the officer instantly gave instructions to an orderly to send a corporal to see the man fairly buried, and to set a sentry, to be relieved in the usual manner, to keep strict watch over the grave during the whole of the nine days, and to suffer no one even to approach the grave; and, the more certainly to secure this being faithfully accomplished, none but Mussulmans were to be deputed as guards.

In a few hours after these orders had been issued by the said officer, the corporal returned and announced to him, that, after certain proceedings on the part of the saint, and receiving many gifts from the assembled multitude, he laid himself down and passed into a particular condition, after which his followers wrapped his body in a covering called a "kumlee", and then laid him in a grave dug in the ordinary way and of the usual size, from three to four feet deep, and then turned in the earth upon his body. No coffin was used. On this being done, a Mussulman guard was placed, with orders to walk round the grave, and on no account to suffer anyone even to approach it.

Every two hours reports were brought to the officer or his orderly that fresh guards had been set to relieve those on duty, and that all remained as when the earth was thrown over the devotee. So invincible was the hatred of the Mussulman guards against the Hindoos, that they would not suffer any one of them even to approach the grave to get a particle of the sacred earth (a gift inestimable in their opinion) which covered the holy man, whom the Hindoos firmly believed would rise again on the ninth day, as predicted by him.

On the evening of the third day, when other active and important duties had entirely banished from his mind the condition of the buried Fakeer, the officer's attention was drawn to the subject by the person who came to report to him that the sentry had been relieved, and the "dead man all well", that was to say, remained as at the time he was buried, three days previously. On this announcement being made, the officer, whose faith was less vigorous than that of the Hindoos as to the sanctity of the devotee being able to save him under such circumstances, became alarmed, inasmuch as the feat having taken place with his sanction, within the military limits, and he having set a sentry over his grave, should the man be really dead, as he had no doubt must be the case ere then, he might be brought into trouble and arraigned as accessory to his murder, and lose his commission, with other dire consequences.

The officer, therefore, hurried home, and instantly sent for the Chowdrie, who applied to him for his sanction for the feat to take place within the military boundary, told him his doubts and fears, and urged the instant disinterment of the devotee. The Chowdrie hereupon begged to assure the officer that there was no cause whatever for alarm about the safety of the buried saint, as he had been frequently buried in the same manner, and added, that so great was his sanctity, that he would be perfectly safe, and certain to recover were he to remain in his grave for twelve months or for a hundred years, and he therefore urged upon the officer to allow him to remain in his grave for the full term of nine days, originally stipulated for. Military faith and courage, however, were by no means equal in this instance to that of the Brahmin, and the soldier quailed whilst this enthusiast stood firm, urging the full term of the feat to be exhausted before the exhumation should take place. The officer, however, would not consent to this, but insisted on the instant disinterment of the holy man; and, moreover, by way of self-defence, in case the worst of his fears should be realised, he ordered the Chowdrie, in case the devotee was found to be really dead, instantly to have his body carried beyond the military territory.

The more certainly to guard against all further mischance, my friend instantly ordered his horse and rode to the spot, that he might be an eye-witness of all the future proceedings. When he arrived at the place, he found the grave surrounded by an immense crowd of Hindoos, all anxiously waiting to witness the result of this exhumation or resurrection of their sainted brother. The Chowdrie having arrived also, orders were instantly given to remove the earth and drag forth the body of the holy man. To the horror of our military friend, forth it came, wrapped in its camel-hair coverlet, on removing which, he found the body cold and stiff as a mummy. When he had satisfied himself of this by personal examination, both by sight and touch, he felt assured that his fate was sealed, that his commission would be lost, and himself implicated in the murder of this religious enthusiast.

There was yet one hope, although to him apparently a forlorn one, that the Fakeer might be restored by the use of those means of restoration which two of the holy man's followers were about to apply, according to instructions which he had previously given to them. They began by rubbing some preparation over his head, eyes, and eye-brows, and also over the palms of the hands and soles of the feet, and were particularly assiduous of their application of it, and friction over the region of the heart. They had persevered in these attempts for about a quarter of an hour without the slightest apparent impression being made on the subject, and the Christian's hope was now completely extinguished. Not so that of the idolaters of the East. They plied their manipulations with unremitting assiduity, and presently were enabled to open the eyes. Still it was but the glassy look of the eyes of a corpse. By degrees, however, slight motion of the eyes was discernible, which increased until he could slowly move the head; and, after lengthened manipulations and pummelling about his chest, a visible heaving of the chest took place, and still later he was able to articulate a few words, to the unspeakable joy of the Christian master of ceremonies, as well as of the Hindoos and Brahmins assembled on the occasion.

In about an hour the Fakeer had pretty well recovered the use of his faculties, mental as well as physical, and the major left the field quite as much gratified to find he had escaped the loss of his commission, and the risk of being arraigned as accessory to the murder of this devotee, as the latter was to remain and receive the numerous presents and mutual congratulations of his admiring and adoring countrymen.

[Self-Hypnosis & Catalepsy]
I think the evidence afforded by these narratives proves, beyond doubt, that the individuals referred to possessed the power they represented themselves to have acquired, and performed the feats indicated *bona fide;* and that the true physiological explanation is that which I adverted to at the commencement of this paper; namely, that they were self-hypnotists, and that they were in a state of temporary hybernation, or trance, during which, although the lamp of life was burning slowly, still it *was* burning, otherwise death would have been the inevitable result.

It does not appear that this practice has been long known to exist, and it is rather a curious speculation to determine how it could have originated. The following ideas have occurred to me, and I think a quotation from the "Dabistan" furnishes the key to unlock this mystery:—

> It is an established custom amongst the Yogis (Fakeers) that, when malady overpowers them, they bury themselves. They are wont, also, with open eyes, to force their looks towards the middle of their eyebrows, until so looking they perceive the figure of a man; if this should appear without hands, feet, or any member, for each they have determined that the boundaries of their existence would be within so many years, months, or days. When they see the figure without a head, they know that there certainly remains very little of their life; on that account, having seen the prognostic, they bury themselves. (vol. ii. p. 138-139.)

Thus, then, they die voluntarily, in order that they may escape the ordinary pangs of dissolution; that is, they reduce themselves to **the deep state of self-hypnotism, which I have likened to trance or hybernation in man**, in which condition they are committed to their tombs or graves, as their final earthly resting-places. Now, it appears to me no very improbable supposition to allege, that accident had revealed to them the fact, that some of those who were thus buried might be restored to life after exhumation – the action of the air restoring respiration and circulation, on an *accidental disinterment of the body of someone thus interred;* and the fact once observed would encourage others to try how much *they* could accomplish in this way, as the newest and most striking achievement which they could perform in token of the divine origin and efficacy of *their religion over that of all others.*

We have the analogue to these feats of the Fakeers, not merely in the hybernating animals which periodically pass into the torpid [i.e., insensible and dormant] state, and which, consequently, in them, is looked on as a mere matter of course, and not at all to be wondered at; but we have it also occurring spontaneously, occasionally, in the human species, **in the disease called catalepsy, or trance**. Many cases of trance are upon record, in which the patients remained for considerable periods of time in a state of apparent death, during which preparations were being made for their interment, but who were restored before being buried; whilst there is no doubt of the fact, that, in many others, they had been consigned to their graves whilst yet alive – for, in some such instances, accidental circumstances have led to the opening of their graves, by which means they were released, and lived for years thereafter. In the latter cases, the feats of these Fakeers have been fully realised in all but the *intention* and *artificial contrivance* of the patients *inducing the condition;* and, in the former, had the subjects been actually interred, and their graves opened in proper time, the like results would have ensued.

Besides the numerous cases of trance already recorded, I have had the history of several others communicated to me, in two of which the patients remained in the horrible condition of hearing various remarks made about their death, and preparations were being made for their interment. All this they heard distinctly, without having the power of giving any indication that they were alive, until some accidental abrupt impression aroused them from their lethargy, and rescued them from their perilous situation. On one of these occasions, what most intensely affected the feelings of the entranced subject, as she afterwards communicated to my informant, was hearing a little sister, who came into the room where she was laid out for dead, exulting in the prospect, in consequence of her death, of getting possession of a necklace of the deceased.

In like manner, in cases of **catalepsy**, patients have been known to be alive, and still to remain for a great length of time in a state of insensibility and torpor of all the vital functions to an alarming degree, and to subsist for considerable periods of time without food. This was strikingly illustrated in the case of a patient of my late friend, Dr. John Mitchell of this city, of which he furnished me with the following report. The patient was a poor married woman, who was brought into the Manchester Royal Infirmary, and placed under his care. She remained in that institution in such an intense state of catalepsy, with her jaws locked, that she neither had *meat* nor *drink* for FOURTEEN DAYS, after which she became so much relieved, that she could be removed to her home, about seven miles in the country.

During the period this patient remained in the cataleptic state, the only visible signs of vitality were a *slight* degree of animal heat, and appearance of moisture from her breath when a mirror was held close to her face. Every variety of contrivance and torture was resorted to by various parties who saw her, for the purpose of testing the degree of her insensibility, and for determining whether she might not be an impostor, but without eliciting the slightest indication of activity of *any* of the senses.

A most important fact has since been communicated to me by this patient's friends – a fact which merits the most serious consideration of all who come in contact with such cases, *viz.*, that whilst she had no voluntary power to give indication, either by word or gesture, that she suffered from the said inflictions, nevertheless she *heard and understood all that was said and was proposed to be done, and suffered the most exquisite torture from various tests applied to her!!* A fact so important as this ought to be published in every journal throughout the civilised world; so that in future professional men might be thereby led to exercise greater discretion and mercy in their modes of applying tests to such patients. It may have been excusable to have done so when unaware that they might thereby be inflicting torture upon a helpless and passive human victim; but, after being made aware of this example to the contrary, they would be altogether inexcusable.[77]

The same discretion ought also to be extended to the modes of testing somnambules. There is no doubt whatever, that in certain stages of that condition, whether occurring spontaneously or induced by artificial contrivance, that some of these patients are perfectly insensible at the time of inflictions the most severe. However, if the means have been sufficiently severe to lacerate, or in any way destroy the tissues, the natural consequences of such inflictions necessarily manifest themselves after the patients are aroused. Thus, in a patient of my own, about whom I was first consulted for an attack of spontaneous somnambulism, besides violent pinchings of her flesh and skin, needles and pins were thrust under her nails, and so anxious was her father to determine whether she might not be imposing on them, as had been suggested to him by some *kind* friend, that he so pinched and bruised the roots of her nails as caused them subsequently to suppurate, and that without her giving the slightest indication of feeling pain at the moment of infliction, or during the sleep. When the poor girl awoke, she wondered what was the matter with her fingers, and what could have made them so painful. This patient was very soon cured of her natural somnambulism, simply by inducing a similar condition artificially by the mode which I designate *hypnotising*. On one occasion, when I had hypnotised her, I extracted one of her teeth without the slightest indication of her feeling pain, nor was she aware of it after she was awoke, until her father asked her to feel in her mouth. This patient has now been in the enjoyment of good health for several years, and has never been subject to spontaneous attacks of somnambulism since I first cured her by *hypnotism*.

[The Trance-Like Effects of Cannabis]

The phenomena realised by the use of ether and chloroform, in like manner, manifest similar states of anaesthesia more or less profound, according to the quantity exhibited and constitution of the patient, and have given a ready credence to phenomena realised by these means which had been by many pronounced cases of rank imposition when induced by Mesmeric or hypnotic methods. The peculiar conditions, also, induced by the use of *Bangue*, *Hashish*, and *Dawamesc* [cannabis-based drugs], in the East, all tend to illustrate certain conditions of the nervous system producible by artificial contrivances. Thus, a slight dose of these produces mental hallucination, with some degree of control over the train of thought – a sort of half-waking dream. As the effects advance, the imagination becomes more and more vivid, and a rapid succession of ideas passes through the mind, assuming all the force of present realities. At this stage, as

---

[77] Through the kindness of my excellent and truly worthy friend, the late Rev. Geoffrey Hornby, rector of Bury, I was informed, that this patient was still alive in 1845, and might be seen by me, if I wished to make personal inquiries regarding her state, beyond what he had kindly obtained for me. This I considered it better to avoid, for the following reasons: She had been insane for some time immediately before and after the cataleptic seizure, for which she was sent to the Infirmary, and was still in no very bright state of intellect. I therefore thought it just possible, that, were her mind strongly directed to these past painful occurrences, it might be the means of exciting another paroxysm of active insanity, for which I would be certain to get blamed, and to guard against such risk, I declined calling on her – a degree of caution which Mr. Hornby highly approved of.

well expressed by Dr. Carpenter, "The internal tempest becomes more and more violent; the torrent of disconnected ideas increases in power, so as completely to arrest the attention, and the mind is gradually withdrawn altogether from the contemplation of external realities being engrossed by the consciousness of its own internal workings. There is always preserved, however, a much greater amount of self-consciousness than exists in ordinary dreaming – the condition rather corresponding with that just referred to, in which the sleeper *knows* that he is dreaming. The succession of ideas has at first less of incoherence than in ordinary dreaming, the ideal events not departing so far from possible realities; and the disorder of the mind is at first manifested in errors of sense, in false convictions, or in the predominance of one or more extravagant ideas. These ideas and convictions are generally not altogether of an imaginary character, but are called up by external impressions, which are erroneously interpreted by the perceptive faculties. The error of perception is remarkably shown in regard to time and space; minutes seem hours, hours are prolonged into years, and at last all idea of time seems obliterated, and past and present are confounded together as in ordinary dreaming; and in like manner streets appear of an interminable length, and the people at the other end seem to be at a vast distance; still there is a certain consciousness of the deceptive nature of these illusions, which, if the dose be moderate, is never entirely lost.

The effect of a full dose, however, is at last to produce the complete withdrawal of the mind from any distinct comprehension of external things; the power of the will over the current of thought is in like manner suspended, and the condition of the mind becomes the same in all essential particulars with that of the ordinary dreamer, differing in this chiefly that the feelings are more strongly expressed, and that they still take their tone almost entirely from external impressions. Thus, says M. Moreau,

> It will be entirely dependent on the circumstances in which we are placed, the objects which strike the eyes, the words which fall on our ears, whether the most lively sentiments of gaiety or of sadness shall be produced, or passions of the most opposite nature shall be excited, sometimes with extraordinary violence; for irritation shall pass rapidly into rage, dislike to hatred, and the desire of vengeance and the calmest affection to the most transporting passion. Fear becomes terror, courage is developed into rashness which nothing checks, and which seems not to be conscious of danger, and the most unfounded doubt or suspicion becomes a certainty. The mind has a tendency to exaggerate everything. Those who make use of the hashish of the East profit by all the means which the dissolute manners of the East place at their disposal. It is in the midst of the harem, surrounded by their women, under the charm of music and of lascivious dances, executed by the Almees, that they enjoy the intoxicating Dawamesc; and with the aid of superstition, they find themselves almost transported to the scene of the numberless marvels which the Prophet has collected in his paradise.

A still more intense dose, however, reduces the patient to a state of profound narcotism, during which painless operations may be performed, as narrated by Mr. Urquhart in his "Pillars of Hercules", "Travels in Morocco in 1848". He says on this point,

> In a very short time he (the patient) becomes so insensible that he seems intoxicated or deprived of life. Then, according as the case may be, the operations are performed, of amputations, etc., and the cause of the malady is removed. Subsequently, the tissues are brought together by sutures, and liniments are employed. After some days the patient is restored to health, without having felt, during the operations, the least pain.

Such is our daily experience of the anaesthetic effects of chloroform during surgical operations; and in India the experience of Dr. Esdaile has proved Mesmerism equally potent with the population of the East for like purposes. Indeed it has been proved so in many cases in this country, but I still think that chloroform is the more certain and speedy agent for effecting such purpose in this country; and perfectly safe, provided care is taken to procure pure chloroform, and to administer it with due caution.[78] All the above recited phenomena are, in many cases, as genuine and as truly the result of the hypnotic or Mesmeric processes, as when induced by the ingestion into the stomach or through the lungs of the medicinal agents referred to, and I believe **the great cause of opposition which has been offered to the acceptance of the truth of the genuine phenomena of hypnotism and Mesmerism, has arisen from the extravagance of the Mesmerists, who have contended for the reality of clairvoyance in some of their patients**, such as seeing through opaque bodies, and investing them with gifts and graces of omniscience, omnipresence, Mesmeric intuition, and universal knowledge – pretensions alike a mockery of the human understanding, as they are opposed to all the known laws of physical science.

[Critique of Paranormal Theories]
In support of the above sentiments I gladly avail myself of the following quotation, from an article in *Fraser's Magazine* for July, 1845 (page 3), by a most acute observer and forcible and clever writer. When writing regarding the feats of the Pythoness [the ancient Greek oracle at Delphi], the author says:–

> Now we take it that the Pythoness, not by the *objective* operation of magnetism *from without,* but by the *subjective* or *personal* influence of *internal* agencies, was enabled intensely to concentrate her conceptive

---
[78] [See appendix (originally a lengthy footnote) 'On Cannabis'.]

faculties (aided by the workings of her perceptive powers which had drank in certain transactions of the outer world, and stored them up in her memory), from the thousand influences which must ever be at work around her in her waking state, and concentrate them upon a given purpose; whether it were to forecast the probable duration of a man's life or the fall of a kingdom. **By throwing herself into the nervous sleep described by Mr. Braid (and we mean to show how common this has been practised from the earliest ages down to the present time), she becomes, as it were, isolated from the external world, her whole attention is abstracted from external influences and transactions, and intensely concentrated in the** *world within herself.* In this condition the memory is almost supernaturally vivid; she remembers circumstances in the character of the man's life, and remarkable vicissitudes in the history of the kingdom; she reasons logically from the *petitio principii* [i.e., "question begging"] to the rational conclusion; all the material *facts* in both cases (that of the man and that of the kingdom) pass in review before her; she weighs them with scrupulous nicety, in combination and in their relative bearings, and she arrives at a conclusion which surprises everybody because it is so much more accurate and positive than any which could have been attained by faculties distracted and disturbed by the ever-varying and constantly-succeeding events of the outer world. And this is what the Mesmerists call clairvoyance! At this rate the sublime imagination of Homer himself would be looked upon as the gift of a magician rather than the gift of nature – a piece of witchcraft rather than a concomitant of true genius.[79]

When, to the following circumstances recounted in these acute observations, we add the aids which the patients draw from the exalted state of smell, hearing, feeling, heat, and cold, whereby they are enabled readily to perceive impressions bearing on the subject in which they are for the time interested, which would be inappreciable to them in their ordinary waking condition, together with the amazing quickness with which they catch suggestions from questions asked, or observations made within the range of their quickened hearing at the proper stage of the sleep, and **the acuteness of the reasoning power, quickened memory, and vivid imagination in that state of mental concentration, excitement, and self-confidence, we can easily perceive why they may be enabled intellectually to arrive at striking results occasionally, far beyond the waking capabilities of the same individuals**; just as extraordinary feats are accomplished occasionally in dreams (even without many of the above recited aids), of which we have many interesting and undoubted examples recorded. **Nor should we overlook the tendency of the human mind in those with a great love of the marvellous, to interpret the slightest approach to a correspondence in their replies into a literal description of their own mental impressions (as many do in interpreting ordinary dreams), and even, unintentionally, to give slight aids to the sleeper, who is very quick to drink in and profitably to digest the slightest suggestion, such as even from the tone of voice of parties around; as is every day done to a considerable extent, and with wonderful success in many cases by those wide-awake clairvoyants** *called fortune tellers.* **In the one case as in the other, questions put suggest corresponding answers, and these again suggest fresh questions, and the tone of voice, looks and gestures of parties engaged in this sort of "Canning's game", (at which he undertook to tell,** *at twenty guesses,* **anything which anyone should** *think* **of) form wonderful assistance in ultimately arriving at an apparently satisfactory result. That an exaltation of functions or faculties which we all possess in a minor degree when awake, may take place during this sleep in the manner explained, I readily admit; but they do not amount to anything like the extent and minuteness of detail to warrant such conclusions as the Mesmerists contend for. If true and unaided and vigorous as they allege their powers to be, the answers ought** *always* **to be** *right,* **whereas, it is notorious that they are far** *oftener wrong* **than** *right.* **The results of carefully tested cases seem to warrant no such conclusion as that of a patient being able veritably to see through decidedly opaque bodies. All the patients possessed of such** *alleged* **powers, when tested with the rigour which I adopted, or suggested as requisite for guarding against all sources of fallacy which occurred to my mind, have** *always* **decidedly failed; and I quite concur in opinion with the formerly quoted acute writer in** *Fraser,* **as expressed by him in the following pithy paragraph – "To insist upon it that a person can see through a thousand brick walls between London and Gravesend, who cannot read plain print covered by only a few sheets of writing paper within a few inches of his nose, is an insult to the understanding."[80]**

[Animal Hibernation]

In cases of asphyxia from hanging or drowning, if the action of the lungs is entirely suspended whilst the heart's action continues in some degree, in general, in a very few minutes, the patient is irrecoverably dead. There are well-attested cases on record, however, in which patients have been recovered after submersion for three quarters of an hour. In these cases, which are not numerous, of course, respiration must have been suspended from the moment of submersion, and it is believed their recovery has been due to a state of

---

[79] The article from which I have made the above extract, and another in the June number of *Fraser* for 1844, entitled, "Animal Magnetism and Neuro-hypnotism", were both published anonymously. They were justly esteemed two of the ablest, most clever, and agreeable articles which had appeared on the subject; and I think it is much to be regretted that they have not, long ere now, been published in a separate form. The real author of these clever articles was Robert S. Sowler, Esq., Barrister-at-law, of Manchester.

[80] [See appendix (originally a lengthy footnote) 'On Sensory Hyperacuity in Hypnotism'.]

syncope or faint (which consists in an entire suspension of the heart's action) having taken place *before* submersion.

In cases of syncope [loss of consciousness from lack of oxygen], without submersion, patients may remain for a few seconds, or a few minutes, or for some hours, in a state of apparent death, the body being pale and powerless, and the action of the heart and lungs being apparently entirely suspended. Some few cases are recorded where this has continued for several days; but in such cases, I believe, respiration, and circulation, and vital action have not been totally arrested, but going on feebly and imperceptibly, as in cases of intense hybernation or trance.

The term *hybernation* has been adopted to designate that peculiar state of torpor or profound sleep into which some warm-blooded as well as coldblooded animals are liable periodically to fall, and to which it seems as natural and regular in its *access* as common sleep is to all other creatures. They generally pass into this condition in autumn, and continue in it, entirely without food, during the winter months; hence the designation, *hybernation,* or winter sleep.

It seems quite obvious that temperature plays an important part in relation to this condition; for it has been proved that hybernation may be prevented by keeping these creatures in an artificially elevated temperature; and, even when they have passed into the state, that they may be aroused from it, at any time, by *artificial* heat, as well as by the genial warmth of spring.

In warm-blooded animals which hybernate completely, such as the marmot, the power of generating heat is so feeble, that the temperature of their bodies follows pretty nearly that of the surrounding air; so that, at a temperature a little below the freezing point, the thermometer placed within the body falls to 35° [Fahrenheit, or 1.7° Celsius], and may remain at this point for some time, without apparent injury to the animal, as it recovers when subjected to a higher temperature. It is thus obvious, that the vital properties of the tissues had been preserved during this state of arrest or depression of their usual vital activity; but when long subjected to a much more intense degree of cold, it has been found that there is not merely a temporary suspension of activity, but that total loss of life is the result.

During hybernation, all the vital functions are proportionally depressed below the natural standard. The pulse is reduced to one-tenth its usual number of beats, and the breathing to about one-thirtieth the number of respirations, whilst it is accomplished with very little perceptible heaving or enlargement of the chest. Now the activity of respiration and quantity of carbonic acid gas eliminated in a given time being the surest test of the general activity with which the vital functions are progressing, it thus becomes obvious that they must all be greatly depressed during this condition; and that, consequently, the disintegration and waste of tissue must be going on at a very slow rate compared with that of the normal active condition. Such is actually found to be the case, and, consequently, these creatures, when in that state, can subsist for a great length of time without food, merely consuming a portion of their own tissues, and that at a very slow rate. They are thus enabled to live without food for a period far beyond what could possibly happen with them during the active state of their existence.

When in an *intense* state of hybernation, moreover, sensibility is so depressed as seems completely to lock up all the senses; but, when in a less intense degree, there is merely diminished sensibility.

Even in the coldblooded animals, the activity of the functions and demand for oxygen are less at low than at higher temperatures, as has been beautifully shown by the experiments of Dr. Edwards. Thus, during winter, as I have myself frequently witnessed, frogs can live and move under the ice without the necessity of coming to the surface to breathe, the *aerated* water surrounding their bodies being sufficient to produce that change on their blood through the skin, requisite to sustain the demands of their feeble life at that low temperature; but, when the season advances, with the increased temperature the activity of the animal ensues, when it becomes indispensable that it shall be permitted to come to the surface to breathe occasionally; and if prevented from doing so after the heat has become considerable, the creature speedily dies. As remarked by Dr. Carpenter, page 369 of his "Manual of Physiology" – "When the temperature of the reptile is raised, by external heat, to the level of that of the mammal, its need for respiration increases, owing to the augmented waste of its tissues. When, on the other hand, the warm-blooded mammal is reduced, in the state of hybernation, to the level of the cold-blooded reptile, the waste of its tissues diminishes to such an extent as to require but a very small exertion of the respiratory process to get rid of the carbonic acid, which is one of its chief products."[81]

As the tear and wear of the tissues, then, and consequent demand for food to supply this waste, are in exact ratio with the activity of the vital functions; and, as we have seen, these are so wonderfully depressed during complete hybernation, as to enable the creatures to subsist for *many months* on their own tissue, *entirely without food,* with a pulse at one-tenth its usual number of beats, and respiration reduced to one-thirtieth its usual frequency, both of which being still cognisable to the human senses, we need be the less surprised that **the Fakeer, who has acquired the power, by artificial contrivance and *long training as a religious exercise,* of throwing himself into such an intense state of hybernation, or trance**, that neither the beating of the pulse nor of the heart, nor the process of respiration can be detected by the nicest scrutiny, should be enabled to subsist without food several days, or even for six weeks, as has been

---

[81] [See appendix (originally a lengthy footnote) 'On Migration & Hybernation'.]

represented to have happened in the case narrated by Sir Claude Martin Wade. Still, there must, of necessity, be a limit to this state of abstinence, even during the state of human hybernation, as the available supply of fat and other tissues would at length become exhausted, when death must inevitably ensue, if not warded off by a suitable supply of food in due time. Whilst we may readily believe it possible, therefore, for the Fakeer to have existed in the state of trance or human hybernation, for the space of six weeks without food, the allegation of the Chowdrie to my friend the major, that the individual to whom he referred would be perfectly safe and certain to recover, were he to be left in the condition for twelve months, or for a *hundred years,* must be looked upon as a mere fiction of his fervid imagination and unbounded religious faith. All hybernating animals, however corpulent they may have been when they passed into the state of hybernation, are found to be quite emaciated when they come out of it; and we have no reason to suppose that it could be otherwise with man, when placed under similar circumstances.

Perhaps there could not be a more interesting proof adduced in point, as regards the relation which subsists between the amount of tear and wear of tissue in a given time, and the degree of vital activity, than was afforded in the experiment with the humble bee, which is recorded to have eliminated more carbonic acid in *one* hour, when in a state of excitement, incident to its recent capture, than it did in *twenty-four* hours subsequently, when in a state of quiescence. This experiment, moreover, proves, that as great a degree of increase in waste of tissue in a given time may result from excessive excitement and muscular effort beyond that of a state of ordinary repose, as this latter exceeds that more profound repose and inactivity realised during complete hybernation.

Moreover, we have remarkable instances of protracted fasting during disease. Thus Macnish, in his chapter on Protracted Sleep, cites an instance of a patient who remained *eight* days without food or drink; and of another who, on one occasion, *"slept three weeks",* and who, during that period, "took not a particle of either food or drink; nothing could arouse him, even for a moment; yet his sleep seemed to be calm and natural!" In his chapter on Catalepsy, also, he refers to the case of a Polish soldier, who fell into that condition from terror, and who remained for *twenty days* without nourishment.

[Cases of Human Phenomena]
Whilst this pamphlet was going through the press, I was favoured with the following narrative of a case of trance, which occurred some years ago in a patient of John Woods, Esq., surgeon, Newry, and which he has kindly furnished to me for publication. Mr. Woods writes:–

> The case of the young lady, Miss P. C., related to you by my esteemed friend, Mr. Waddell, was one of hysteria, terminating in trance of *four days' duration.* It was not caused by her hearing of the death of her father, or any unpleasant news; her father was dead some years at the time of her illness. She laboured under chlorosis ["green sickness", a kind of anaemia], and, in consequence of this and her complexion being naturally very fair and pale, with white flaxen hair, she had a very corpse-like appearance. Her pulse, which was quick and chlorotic before the trance commenced, became soft and slow. Her breathing, although slow and weak, was always quite perceptible. She would open her eyes when pulled and shook by the arms, and then close them and fall asleep again. It was with great difficulty that she was forced to swallow a few teaspoonsful of drink for three or four days; and any person looking at her without feeling her pulse, and examining her closely, would say she was dead. Although I, her only medical attendant at the time, and her friends could not but feel very uneasy and anxious about her, yet we always entertained hopes of her recovery, which did not take place suddenly, as we learn that the greater number of cases of trance do, but gradually; leaving her very weak for some time, and, as well as I remember, totally unconscious of anything that occurred during its continuance.

About twenty years ago my friend Dr. Jarrold, of this city, attended a gentleman forty-four years of age, who fell into a state of trance, in which he continued for a whole week. During this period the Doctor watched him closely, and informs me that the vital processes were reduced to such a low ebb, that he had no expectation of his patient's recovery; the pulse being scarcely perceptible, and the respiration faint, and repeated only about *once in three-quarters of a minute.* After continuing in this state for a *week,* without swallowing a particle of food or drink, he awoke from his trance, and called for *beef steaks,* when the Doctor had the pleasure of seeing him make a hearty meal. He recovered from this affliction, and lived a year thereafter, when he died from a different disease.

The following narrative of another case I give *verbatim* from a letter of the patient's sister, furnished by her to me for publication. The lady writes:– "She and my eldest sister walked to church, scarcely a mile through the fields from their house. Without giving any intimation of feeling unwell, she dropped down in a faint. She was carried out of church to the manse, and though every possible means we tried to restore her to consciousness, *she lay from Sabbath mid-day till Wednesday evening, without giving any sign of life.* It was exactly a fortnight from the day she fainted before she opened her eyes; but from the fourth day she gave occasionally signs that she knew what was said to her." She adds that two medical men attended this patient throughout her illness, one of whom remained with her on the night when a crisis seemed to be approaching, of which she says:– "Little hopes they had that it would terminate so favourably"; by which it appears that they expected her death at the period when she revived. She took no food during the fortnight she remained in the trance.

In an early number of "The Philosophical Transactions", Dr. Oliver has given an account of **one of the greatest sleepers on record**. The patient was Samuel Chilton, of Tinsbury, near Bath. He was a labourer, twenty-five years of age, not fat, but muscular, with dark brown hair. In 1694, he fell asleep, and **slept for a month**, when he awoke, and went about his work as usual. During this period, he partook of food set beside him, and had the usual evacuations, without awaking. In 1696, he again fell asleep, and continued in it for seventeen weeks, during the *last six* of which *he ate nothing.* During the former period, therefore, he was in the sleep waking condition, during which there is present a certain degree of consciousness and voluntary power, resembling those animals which sleep most of the winter, but rouse up sufficiently, occasionally, to enable them to feel hunger, and satisfy the craving for food, which they do by partaking of a portion of what they had stored up for themselves during the preceding autumn. During the latter period, however, like the animals which hybernate completely, he must have survived entirely by consuming a portion of his own tissues. It is much to be regretted that no mention is made as to the extent of emaciation which took place during the latter six weeks, when he eat *nothing,* because in all cases of long protracted fasting, whether the patient is asleep or awake, we may be quite certain that some collusion is going on by which food is clandestinely obtained by the faster, if there is not some perceptible wasting of the body of the faster. To believe the contrary, would be to admit an impossibility – namely, that we might abstract continually from a given quantity, without diminishing the original amount.

Samuel Chilton again fell asleep in 1697, and **slept for six months**. His habits, in respect to food, during this period, are not recorded. Many extraordinary and cruel inflictions were perpetrated on his person during these periods, for the purpose of gratifying the curious, and enabling them to determine whether he had any feeling, or whether he might not be an impostor. He gave no indication of feeling pain at the time, nor does he seem to have had any recollection whatever of these inductions when he awoke.

In the *Medical Gazette* for 1835, page 264, Dr. Sloan narrates the case of **John Brown, aged 65, who became imprisoned in a coal-pit in Ayrshire**, on the 8th of October, 1835, by the falling in of a portion of the roof. He had gone to work without breakfast, had no food with him, and only a quarter of an ounce of tobacco. On the 31st of the same month he was discovered alive, having thus **existed *upwards of twenty-three days without food.*** He had also been *entirely without water for the last thirteen days,* having lain down at some distance from some water, and become so weak that he could not move from the spot on which he lay. He was of course emaciated in the greatest degree; but he was conscious when taken out of the pit, and the following day was able to give a detailed and distinct narrative of his sufferings. He died on the fourth day after his release from the coal pit. [Reported in *The Scotsman* newspaper, 7th November, 1835]

In the same volume of the *Medical Gazette,* Dr. Thornhill, of Darlaston, Staffordshire, gives the history of eight men and a boy, all of whom were imprisoned in a coal-pit for *eight days, entirely without food,* and with only a very little water. *All of them recovered* and with the exception of the boy, who subsequently got burnt to death, they were all alive, and in the enjoyment of tolerable health, twenty-two years after the above imprisonment in the coal-pit. Sickness and excessive thirst were the symptoms they complained most of.

These are remarkable proofs of the capabilities of the human body for enduring starvation in the active state of existence, and may tend to make us consider it the less surprising at the length of time the Fakeers can remain without food in their state of self-induced human hybernation. I believe the case of John Brown is the most prolonged instance on record in which a person in such circumstances has subsisted entirely without food.

But again, besides the brown and polar bears, which are well-known to sleep profoundly and without food for many months every winter like other hybernating animals, we have instances in our own country of sheep surviving for several weeks under wreaths of snow, when entirely deprived of food; and the fat pig recorded by Martell as having been overwhelmed by a slip of earth, is a still more remarkable instance in point, as it lived in this situation 160 days without food, and was found to have diminished in weight in that time 120 lbs.; being, as well observed by Dr. Lion Playfair, "an instance quite analogous to the state of hybernation".

I am well aware that there were individuals in this country, as well as elsewhere, who hastily published observations, from limited data, pronouncing the whole of these feats of the Fakeers as mere Hindoo tricks; and, consequently, who will now feel themselves bound, in self-defence, to stand by their former verdicts. I know human nature too well to expect to extort a confession of conviction to the contrary from such individuals, by any amount of evidence which could possibly be adduced, even if they were permitted to be eye-witnesses of the facts themselves. To all unprejudiced persons, however, possessed of minds capable of weighing the force of evidence – for "unlimited scepticism is equally the child of imbecility, as implicit credulity" – I think the original proof which I have been enabled to bring forward in addition to what we formerly possessed on the subject, must be sufficient to prove the *bona fide* nature of some of these feats of the Fakeers, and, consequently, that human hybernation (or a state analogous to that of hybernation in the lower animals) is a physiological fact, and is capable of being induced by artificial contrivance, as well as of occurring spontaneously occasionally in the condition designated *catalepsy* or *trance.*

[Three Conclusions Drawn]
Three very important inferences may be deduced from what has been said, namely,

1st That great discretion ought to be used in applying tests for the purpose of determining the extent of torpor of the senses which may exist in any particular case, because it is quite possible that the patient may suffer intensely from such inflictions, without being able, at the time, to give any sensible sign of doing so, from the existence of a complete paralysis of all voluntary power; such as occurred in the case of Dr. Mitchell's patient, and in many others who recovered after having been considered dead, and who declared that they heard and understood all that was said regarding them, and the preparations, which were making for their interment, without having the power to give any indication that they were alive, until some accidental, abrupt impression aroused them from their lethargy, and rescued them from their perilous situations.

2nd, That all tests which would produce laceration or permanent injury of tissue, should be avoided, even in that class of patients in whom loss of feeling is complete, or who remember nothing of it afterwards, because, although not felt by the patient at the time of infliction, nor remembered afterwards, whether the state of loss of feeling may be the consequence of spontaneous trance, or anaesthesia induced by hypnotism, Mesmerism, chloroform, hashish, or any other narcotic, such inflictions are certain to manifest their natural baneful influence on the patient, after he is restored to the normal state of sensation – as was evinced in the case of the natural somnambulist to which I alluded.

3rd, And the third inference is of still greater importance; namely, that in all cases of trance, and indeed in *every case of death,* no patient ought to be interred until there have been indubitable signs of decomposition of the body, because, without this appearance, there is no certain sign of death – and nothing could be more horrible, either to the survivors, or to the apparently dead, than the idea of themselves or friends being buried alive, not as the Fakeers, with the hope of being released at a stipulated period, but with the certainty that there was no hope of their escape from the grave to which they had been consigned.

The late Miss Beswick, of this city, from the circumstance of having had a brother who made a very narrow escape from being buried alive, became so alarmed that she might run the hazard of being so herself, as induced her to bequeath a large sum to the late Mr. White and his heirs, on the express condition that her body should not be buried, and hence it has been mummified, and subsequently presented to the Manchester Natural History Museum, where it may be seen by the curious.

[Hypnotic Therapy Restores Menstruation]
A very natural inquiry here forces itself upon the mind of every intelligent individual – namely, what is the best mode of **treating cases of catalepsy or trance**, so as to ward off the danger of being placed in such a painful and perilous situation as those adverted to. In reply to this, I beg leave to remark, that it is well-known that most of these cases have occurred in females; that they are closely allied to hysteria; and that they have an ultimate relation to irregularities in the female functions. Now, the catamenial function, and various morbid phenomena connected therewith, are so **remarkably under the control of the hypnotic mode of treatment**, that there can be no doubt whatever of its superiority over all other methods in the treatment of such afflictions. If any other functional derangement exists which could be benefited specially by any other established mode of treatment – by the exhibition of medicines – I would by no means object to their exhibition; but, I maintain that the re-establishment of the catamenia by hypnotism is more certainly realised by this method alone than by any other; and, in proof of this, I beg leave to subjoin the following case, in addition to others which have long ago occurred to me, and have already been published.

In July, 1849, I was called to attend Mrs.——, thirty years of age, married, and the mother of three children. She had suffered from attacks of epilepsy for four years, for which she had been under the care of several medical men. The attacks became a little less frequent for some time, but again increased in frequency and severity, until, at the period when I was consulted, notwithstanding she was under the constant care of a physician, and was taking medicine prescribed by him repeatedly every day, still she was getting worse, so that she had as many as twenty-eight fits daily, besides what occurred during the night, when her attendants were asleep. The day before I first operated on her, she had thirteen violent fits in the space of eight hours; and, when I first saw her, she was jaw-locked, as a sequel to one of these epileptic attacks. Her friends told me, that whenever this state of locked-jaw occurred, they were never able to open her mouth for many hours, however much force they might apply to effect it. They were, therefore, not a little surprised to observe that, by one of my usual processes for reducing the cataleptic state of muscles during hypnotism or Mesmerism, I was enabled, in a *few seconds,* to unlock her jaws and open her mouth, without the slightest difficulty or force. This patient was speedily thrown into the hypnotic condition by *my* usual method, and the result of my first operation, which was not more than of a quarter of an hour's duration, was this – that the patient had only *four* fits in eight hours, instead of the thirteen which she had during the corresponding period on the day previous.

This patient was operated on by me twice each day subsequently, and on the fourth day the catamenia, which had been absent for several months, re-appeared, and, in the course of a week, the fits were almost entirely arrested. Indeed, from that period, she had only three fits, and these were brought on by causes of considerable mental excitement. The catamenia recurred regularly for the next six months, and the results realised from the use of hypnotism, when they again became suspended, beautifully and conclusively illustrate the value of this mode of treatment in such affections.

At six successive periods I had occasion to resort to hypnotism, for this purpose, and in *every* instance with *entire success,* by a *single operation of from ten to eleven minutes each.* Moreover, I ascertained that this important result could be effected without either touch or pass, but by mental concentration and direction, and management of the circulation alone. On two or three other occasions, when I hypnotised this patient for neuralgic or rheumatic pain in a leg or arm, through the mode of managing and directing the influence, the pains were immediately removed, without exciting any visible manifestation on *any* special organ or function.

[Further Cases of Hypnotic Therapy]

Hypnotism is, therefore, not only a most efficient, but also a perfectly safe mode of treating various affections, by those who understand its practical application, and how to control and direct its power: and here I shall adduce a few examples in point.

The first day I visited the epileptic patient, whose case I have already narrated, her mother, who was fifty-four years of age, and the mother of a numerous family, told me she had been grievously afflicted with headaches, so that she had not known what it was to have been entirely free from headache for the previous *fourteen years.* She stated, moreover, that she suffered from pain and smarting of her eyes, and that her sight had become so affected, that she could not then see to read a sign across the street. I recommended her to try the effect of hypnotism, which I believed calculated to afford her relief for *both* affections. To this she readily consented, and, to her great delight and surprise, on being aroused from the first hypnotic sleep, she found herself *quite free from headache, for the first time for fourteen years.* Next day I found she had a slight return of headache, and, for a few days thereafter, less and less of it daily, during which period I hypnotised her daily, and, in the course of one week, the headaches were entirely gone, and never returned since, unless for a short time occasionally, as will occur to anyone; and the pain and smarting which she formerly felt in her eyes, also entirely disappeared, and her sight became greatly improved, and has continued so ever since.

In August, 1849, I called on the above patient with my friend Professor Shaw, who was anxious to witness the effects of hypnotism, and she happened to live near his residence, and was known to me as a trust-worthy person. She told me that she had been severely afflicted, during the previous night, with diarrhoea, and that she had had six calls within the last two hours. I told her that I could soon relieve her by putting her into the hypnotic state. Notwithstanding the great benefit which had been realised from it, both in her own case and that of her daughter, she seemed quite sceptical as to the power of hypnotism affording any relief to her present affection. I thought otherwise, however, and consequently she submitted to the operation, and on being aroused from the sleep, all the griping and feeling of sickness at stomach were gone, and she had no return of the complaint subsequently.

Three days after the above occurrence I was sent for, in consequence of my former patient, the epileptic daughter, having been seized in the same manner as her mother had been three days previously, and they were anxious to know whether I could afford as speedy and effectual relief to her, by the same means, as I had done to the mother. I operated on her accordingly, in the manner calculated to produce this effect, and with equal success as in the case of the mother, all the unpleasant symptoms being gone when I aroused her, and there was no return of them subsequently.

In July, 1849, when visiting a child, the mother of whom was forty years of age, and had had nine healthy children, the mother stated that she herself had been tormented for four days with the most disgusting smell. The impression had arisen from her going into the house of a relative whose body had been kept till it was in a state of advanced decomposition. From the moment the impression was made on her olfactory nerves on entering the house of the deceased, she had never been able to get rid of it, whether within doors, or in the open air, notwithstanding she had resorted to the use of all sorts of fragrant scents, to sal volatile [smelling salts], to snuff, and even to the fumes of tobacco and burning lucifer-matches [an early, toxic, brand of match], and every other contrivance she could think of. Still all had proved in vain, the disgusting odour being still as vivid as the first moment of its impression. **The patient, therefore, was glad to try any method I might suggest, and consequently I threw her into the hypnotic state, during which I kept her mind constantly dwelling on the idea of fragrant odour, by exciting the idea in the mind through auricular and muscular suggestion, according to the principles laid down in my writings on hypnotism. I took care to awake her with the mind actively engaged with these agreeable ideas, and the result was, that the moment she was aroused from the sleep, she exclaimed with delight, that she *now* enjoyed a smell as *delightful* as the former had been disgusting. From that moment this patient was never again annoyed with the disgusting odour, not even when, on several**

occasions, she attempted, by way of experiment, to recall it. Can there be any ground to doubt the value and power of hypnotism in such a case as this?

On the 28th of March, 1843, I was requested by a philanthropic gentleman (the individual here referred to was the late Hon. and Rev. William Herbert, Dean of Manchester) to extend my charitable sympathy to a poor woman of the name of Barber, and by the power of hypnotism to relieve her of a severe rheumatic affection, from which she had been suffering for several months. She was forty-four years of age, and a most pitiable object, suffering severely from pulmonary affection, as well as from rheumatism. With the latter affection she became afflicted about the beginning of winter; about the end of December, 1842, she had been entirely confined to her bed for five weeks, after which she was able to get up; but the flexors of the legs and toes were so contracted that she could not extend them, and it was with great pain, as well as with difficulty, that she crawled about her apartment. Her hands, wrists, and fingers, were also much affected; so that she was very helpless. Her pain was not only severe, but unremitting either by day or by night. After being hypnotised the first time, during which I endeavoured to regulate the irregular condition of the muscles, she was enabled to straighten her legs and toes, and move her wrist and fingers, could walk with great freedom, and expressed herself almost entirely free from pain both of legs and arms before I left her house. After *five* operations, as is well-known to many, she was so well as to be able either to walk or run across her room, and even to step on a chair, with either foot first, without assistance. I operated on her thirteen times altogether, and she remained, to my certain knowledge, free from rheumatism up to the end of December, 1848, and I have reason to believe had no other attack of it subsequently, as I heard nothing farther of her, and she had my assurance, as well as that of the late Dean, that I was willing to give her any farther assistance of the sort she might require at any time, as an act of charity.

[Braid's use of Self-Hypnosis for Rheumatic Pain]
It is commonly said that seeing is believing, but feeling is the very truth. I shall, therefore, give the result of my experience of hypnotism in my own person. In the middle of September, 1844, I suffered from a most severe attack of rheumatism, implicating the left side of the neck and chest, and the left arm. At first the pain was moderately severe, and I took some medicine to remove it; but, instead of this, it became more and more violent, and had tormented me for three days, and was so excruciating, that it entirely deprived me of sleep for *three nights successively,* and on the last of the three nights I could not remain in any one posture for five minutes, from the severity of the pain. On the forenoon of the next day, whilst visiting my patients, every jolt of the carriage I could only compare to several sharp instruments being thrust through my shoulder, neck, and chest. A full inspiration was attended with stabbing pain, such as is experienced in pleurisy. When I returned home for dinner I could neither turn my head, lift my arm, nor draw a breath, without suffering extreme pain. In this condition I resolved to try the effects of hypnotism. I requested two friends, who were present, and who both understood the system, to watch the effects, and arouse me when I had passed sufficiently into the condition; and, with their assurance that they would give strict attention to their charge, I sat down and hypnotised myself, extending the extremities. At the expiration of *nine minutes* they aroused me, and, to my agreeable surprise, *I was quite free from pain, being able to move in any way with perfect ease.* I say *agreeably* surprised, on this account; I had seen like results with many patients; but it is one thing to *hear of pain,* and another to *feel it.* My suffering was so exquisite that I could not imagine anyone else ever suffered so intensely as myself on that occasion; and, therefore, I merely expected a mitigation, so that I was truly agreeably surprised to *find* myself *quite free from pain.* I continued quite easy all the afternoon, slept comfortably all night, and the following morning felt a little *stiffness,* but *no pain.* A week thereafter I had a slight return, which I removed by *hypnotising* myself *once more;* and I have remained quite free from rheumatism ever since, now nearly six years. Was there the slightest room to doubt the value and efficacy of hypnotism in this case?

[Hypnotic Therapy in a Severe Case of Tonic Spasm]
I shall only give one more case here in confirmation of the value of hypnotism as a therapeutic agent in certain forms of disease, and a more interesting example in point could not well be met with.

In the beginning of spring, 1849, a young lady, about fourteen years of age, was brought to me from Armagh, in Ireland, for a case of permanent tonic spasm of the left hand and wrist, of four months' standing. She had been attended by two eminent professional gentlemen from her first seizure, and from the high character they bear I doubt not but they exhausted the whole resources of our art in her behalf. Still with all this the case remained as bad as ever, or rather getting worse by lapse of time. The spasm never relaxed either by night or day, asleep or awake; and when I first examined her, no force I was capable of exerting made any impression on it, so firmly was the hand locked. I hypnotised her, and on the third day, whilst in the sleep, I was enabled to unlock her hand, and in a few days she could use it in tying her bonnet, and in feeding herself; and very soon was quite well, and has continued free from any attack of the sort ever since. She neither had internal medicine nor external application from me, to aid in this happy result; and therefore there is no room to doubt the value and efficacy of hypnotism in treating this interesting case, as the change was effected so speedily as to place hypnotism and the cure in the obvious relation of cause and effect.

[Concluding Remarks on Hypnotic Therapy]

Nothing can be more preposterous and presumptuous than continually to hear professional men who have had no *practical* experience of this mode of treating disease, presuming to dogmatise, condemning it on mere *theoretical* grounds, and setting up their *theoretical* and preconceived notions as of force to countervail the results of the *actual practical* experience of those who have studied the subject for years with the greatest care and attention. In all other matters practical experience, as well as scientific knowledge, is deemed requisite to constitute an individual an authority upon a given subject, and why not also upon this? Such sceptics allege that inasmuch as some of the phenomena realised by hypnotism or Mesmerism have a strong *similarity* to certain forms of hysteria, that it must be a great delusion to suppose that we can cure a disease by inducing a state *so like it*. Have I not already stated the fact that I cured a case of natural somnambulism very speedily by inducing an *analogous* state by the process which I call hypnotising? I was equally successful in curing sleep-walking in a near relative of my own, by hypnotism. He was accustomed to rise in his sleep, and talk, and walk in this state, so as to cause considerable anxiety for his safety, but after being hypnotised a few times this tendency vanished, and has not recurred for many years past.

Here, then, we have spontaneous somnambulism by day, and sleep-walking and talking by night, *both* cured by inducing an *analogous* condition by *artificial* contrivance. **In many cases, inducing an *analogous,* whilst it is *not* an *identical* condition, seems to be the most speedy and certain mode of curing various affections – as for example, a solution of nitrate of silver applied to the eyes in cases of chronic ophthalmis. Some cases again are more benefited by an *opposite* mode of treatment; and I hold it to be the duty of every medical man to adopt whatever mode of treatment experience has proved to be most speedy and certain in curing his patient, provided it is also a perfectly safe method. At all events, I am warranted to speak most confidently, as the result of considerable extent of practice in *both* modes of treatment, and that without the slightest desire of holding up hypnotism as a panacea or universal remedy, that, when judiciously applied, it is capable of being made one of the most efficient modes of treating various forms of hysteria, spinal irritation, spinal distortion[82], epilepsy, and many other nervous disorders, including neuralgic and rheumatic pains, which are well-known to be most intractable according to the ordinary medical modes of treating them.**

In the little *brochure* which I published in 1846, on "The Power of the Mind over the Body", abundance of evidence was adduced to prove that, even In the wide-waking condition, a constant fixed attention of the mind concentrated on any part of the body, or on any special organ or function, would change the physical action of the part so regarded; and the more so if the mind was fully persuaded of the certainty of such result being realised. In a certain stage of the hypnotic sleep there is a greater degree of mental concentration, and a greater vividness of the imagination in those who pass into the second-conscious state of the sleep, and a greater general mobility of the system accordingly, and thus we obtain the effects in a proportionally more speedy, intense, and certain degree than in the waking condition; and thus, by inducing a *new* and *altered* action, we get rid of the previously existing *morbid* action.

Remarkable and important, therefore, as the phenomena which I contend for as producible by hypnotism are, it must at once be obvious to every candid and intelligent member of the profession, that they violate no established law and recognised principle in physiological and psychological science.

Arlington House,
Oxford Street,
Manchester,
July, 1850.

---

[82] [See appendix (originally a lengthy footnote) 'A Case of Spinal Distortion'.]

Appendix:
On Cannabis

Mr. [David] Urquhart [a British diplomat and writer], in the narrative of his travels in Morocco, in 1848, has furnished many additional interesting remarks regarding the hashish, from which I extract the following. He says:–

> It appears as the *potomantes* of the Indus, the *gelotaphylis* of Bactria, the *achemenes* of the Persians, the *ophisnu* of Ethiopia, the *nepenthes* of the Greeks. The apparently contradictory qualities ascribed to these may all be found in the hashish. Like the *ophisnu*, it recalls consciousness of the past, and inordinate fear; on account of which it was given as a punishment to those who had committed sacrilege; but above all it brings, too, that forgetfulness for which Helen administered to Telemachus the *nepenthes* [in Homer's *Odyssey*], and which, no doubt, she had learned in Egypt. Equally does it become a poison which absorbs all others. It will explain the incantations of Circe, and the mysteries of the cave of Trophonius. When taken without suspicion, its effects would appear as the workings within themselves of the divinity. It goes some way to account for the long endurance of a religious imposture, so slightly wove and so incessantly rebelled against. Here was a means at the disposal of the priest, diviner, and thaumaturgist, and beyond all appeals to the mere imagination. The epithets which the Hindoos apply to their *Bangue* might equally serve for the *hashish* – "assuager" of sorrow", "increaser of pleasure", "cementer of friendship", "laughter-mover". *Bangue*, however, when often repeated, is followed by catalepsy, or that insensibility which enables the body to be moulded into any position, like a Dutch jointed-doll, in which the limbs are made in the position in which they are placed; and this state will continue for many hours.

It appears that Mr. Urquhart had much difficulty in arriving at any certain mode of obtaining the preparation, but still remained convinced that there was such a plant as *produced* it. At length he observes:–

> At Tangier, I observed a diminutive pipe, about the size of a thimble; I asked what kind of tobacco they were smoking. I was answered *kef* (literally, enjoyment) – it was the hashish. I found that it was also taken inwardly. Either the leaves are swallowed with water, after being crushed, or it is prepared, and boiled with sugar, or honey, and butter, like horehound [an English herb], a great variety of seeds and spices entering into the composition, which is thus said to vary in its effects, and to be gifted also with medicinal powers. This preparation is [called] the *majoun*. Its effects were described as those of the laughing gas, except that, instead of a few minutes, it lasts for many hours. Some cry, some laugh, some fall into drowsy listlessness; some are rendered talkative and funny. They see visions, imagine themselves reduced to poverty, or become emperors and commanders of armies, the natural disposition predominating in the derangement. Men under its influence were pointed out to me in the streets. Everything that one hears of it has the air of fable; and I should have been inclined to treat it as such, but for the evidence of my own senses.

Mr. Urquhart was evidently a thorough investigator, and went to work in the best possible manner for arriving at the truth regarding the preparation and properties of this famous medicine, as the following quotation will prove. He says:–

> Finding that I could not understand from description either the mode of preparing it, or the effects, I determined to get those who were accustomed to make it to bring the materials, and prepare it before me, and then to try it myself, and on as many others as I could. I was so engaged for a week after my return to Rabat, for I had successively the three most noted confectioners to try their skill against each other. They have not a regular or uniform process, and the *majoun* is consequently of very unequal strength and efficacy. Our first attempts were failures. The first proof of the success of our preparation was in the case of a young English clergyman, to whom some of it had been given as a sweetmeat. Some hours passed without any visible effects, when a musician, who had the faculty of strangely distorting his features, came in, dressed as a mummer. The Englishman took him for the devil, and a most laughable scene ensued. Next morning, on enquiries after his health, he said he had slept soundly and agreeably as the windows and doors were bolted. Later in the day, the effect disappeared entirely, and he seemed to recollect the circumstances with a composed pleasure, describing various things that had never happened.

Its effects upon himself are thus narrated:–

> The first time I took it was about seven in the morning, and in an hour and a half afterwards I perceived a heaviness of the head, wandering of the mind, and an apprehension that I was going to faint. I thence passed into a state of half-trance, from which I awoke suddenly, and much refreshed. The impression was that of wandering out of myself. I had two beings, and there were two distinct, yet concurrent trains of ideas. Images came floating before me – not the figures of a dream, but those that seem to play before the eye when it Is closed, and with those figures were strangely mixed the sounds of a guitar, that was being played in the adjoining room; the sounds seemed to cluster in and pass away with the figures on the retina. The music of the wretched performance was heavenly, and seemed to proceed from a full orchestra, and to be reverberated through long halls of mountains. These figures and sounds were again connected with metaphysical

reflections, which also, like the sounds, clustered themselves into trains of thought, which seemed to take form before my eyes, and weave themselves with the colour, and sounds. I was following a train of reasoning; new points would occur, and concurrently there was a figure before me, throwing out corresponding shoots like a zinc tree; and, then, as the moving figures re-appeared or as the sounds caught my ear, the other classes of figures came out distinctly, and danced through each other. The reasonings were long and elaborate; and, though the impression of having gone through them remains, every effort has been in vain to recall them.

Such, then, is the interesting description of Mr. Urquhart's personal experience of the effects of the hashish.

There is no reasonable ground to doubt that the *Cannabis Sativa* or *Cannabis Indica,* or Indian hemp, is the chief ingredient in the *Hashish* or *Bangue.* Like all vegetable preparations, much will depend on the condition of the plant at the time it is preserved, and the mode of its preparation, and other ingredients with which it may be combined, as to the actual results realised from its use; and also not a little on the constitution of the patients, mental as well as physical, to whom it is exhibited.

The general effects on man, as stated by Dr. O'Shaughnessy, from his own observations (at Calcutta), are alleviation of pain (mostly), remarkable increase of appetite, unequivocal aphrodisia, and great mental cheerfulness. Its more violent effects were delirium of a peculiar kind, and a cataleptic state. These effects are so remarkable that I shall quote some cases (says Dr. Pereira, from whose "Elements of Materia Medica" pages 1097, 1098, I make this quotation) by way of illustration.

> "At 2 p.m. a grain of the resin of hemp was given to a rheumatic patient. At 4 p.m. he was very talkative sang, called loudly for an extra supply of food, and declared himself in perfect health. At 6 p.m. he was asleep. At 8 p.m. he was found insensible, but breathing with perfect regularity, his pulse and skin natural, and the pupils freely contractile on the approach of light. Happening by chance to lift up the patient's arm – the professional reader will judge of my astonishment," observes Dr. O'Shaughnessy, "when I found that it remained in the posture in which I placed it. It required but a very brief examination of the limbs to find that the patient had, by the influence of this narcotic, been thrown into that strange and most extraordinary of all nervous conditions, into that state which so few have seen, and the existence of which so many still discredit – the genuine *catalepsy* of the nosologist. We raised him to a sitting posture, and placed his arms and limbs in every imaginable attitude. A waxen figure could not be more pliant or more stationary in each position no matter how contrary to the natural influence of gravity on the part. To all impressions he was meanwhile almost insensible. He continued in this state till 1 a.m., when consciousness and voluntary motion quickly returned.
>
> "Another patient who had taken the same dose fell asleep, but was roused by the noise in the ward. He seemed vastly amazed at the strange aspect of the statue-like attitudes in which the first patient had been placed. On a sudden he uttered a loud peal of laughter, and exclaimed that four spirits were springing with his bed into the air. In vain we attempted to pacify him; his laughter became momentarily more and more uncontrollable. We now observed that the limbs were rather rigid, and in a few minutes more his arms and legs could be bent, and would remain in any desired position. He was removed to a separate room, where he soon became tranquil, his limbs in less than an hour gained their natural condition, and in two hours he experienced himself well and excessively hungry."

Dr. Royle, in his "Illustrations of the Botany of the Himalayan Mountains", page 334, suggests that the hemp may have been the "assuager of grief", or the *nepenthes (νηπενθες)* of which Homer speaks; and, as already said in this note, it is known in India as the "increaser of pleasure", the "exciter of desire", the "cementer of friendship", the "laughter mover", *etc. etc.*

Some imagine that it is through the influence of a *large* dose of hashish that the Fakeers accomplish the above-recorded feats of suffering themselves to be reduced to a dormant state for various periods of duration; but I think a state of self-induced trance, or human hybernation, producible at will by artificial contrivance, as I have elsewhere explained, is a far more rational solution of the phenomena.

Appendix:
On Sensory Hyperacuity in Hypnotism

In proof of the wonderful exaltation of the natural faculties which may be realised at a proper stage of the nervous sleep, I beg to call the reader's attention to the following facts, which I have proved in the most satisfactory manner.

I have frequently proved the sense of smell to be so acute in some hypnotic patients, as enabled them readily to detect, in the midst of a large company, any person familiarly known to them; or the owner of any glove, although a stranger to the sleeper, could in like manner be readily detected *by smell,* the patient first smelling at the glove, and then setting off round the room, and unhesitatingly and unerringly presenting the glove to the proper owner, and that without touching him or her; but, if the nostrils were stopped, the clairvoyant faculty instantly ceased, and was recovered the moment the nostrils were unstopped.

In like manner the sense of touch, and the muscular sense, have been so remarkably quickened as to enable persons to write with great neatness during the sleep, without the use of their eyes, as when a large broad book was interposed between their eyes and the paper – a far more certain test than any mode of blindfolding with bandages or masks. With all this precaution some patients would write neatly, crossing the t's and dotting the i's and would even go back a line, strike out a word or letter, and write the correction in the proper place. I had one patient who could go back, and correct with accuracy, the writing on the whole of a page of note-paper; but, if the paper were moved from its relative position on the table, all the corrections would be on the wrong points of the paper, but correct as regarded their position in space in relation with the table, i.e., if the paper had been moved *upwards* the corrections would be so much *below* the line, or if it had been moved *downwards* they would be so much *above* the line; and if to the *right*, or *left,* the correction would be so much wrong in the *opposite* direction. Curiously enough, sometimes this patient took his ideas of relative position from the *upper left hand corner* of the paper, and, on *these* occasions, it did not matter for the paper being moved to another part of the table, as that did not disarrange the association, which he had made in his muscular sense. He always, in those instances, felt at the corner of the paper, and then went on inserting all the corrections in their proper places. I once saw him do this even to the double dotting a vowel in a German word at the bottom of the page – a feat which greatly astonished his German master, who was present at the time. Still, with all this I have never seen any patient in this condition of sleep write *as well without* the use of the eyes as they were capable of doing when awake with the aid of ordinary vision; but there are some patients who have the use of their eyes during the sleep, that is, *seeing through their partially closed* eyelids, and if not tested in the manner I have indicated, but only by blindfolding them, they are very apt to contrive to displace the bandages or masks, so as to see from under them, when they may read or write much better than when in the wide waking condition, to the utter astonishment of those who do not comprehend that the natural organ of vision, the eye, is the real clairvoyant instrument in such cases.

Again, the quickness of hearing and accuracy of the muscular sense, together with their self-confidence and tendency to sympathy and imitation, enables them to perform feats of phonic imitation which are truly astounding, and of which there can be no mistake. Many patients will thus readily repeat accurately what is spoken in any language; and they may also be able to sing correctly and simultaneously both words and music of songs in any language, which they had never heard before – i.e. they catch the words as well as music so instantaneously as to accompany the other singer, as if both had been previously equally familiar with both words and music. In this manner a patient of mine who, when awake, knew not the grammar even of her own language, and who had very little knowledge of music, was enabled to follow Mdlle. Jenny Lind [a world-famous soprano] correctly in songs in different languages, giving both words and music *so correctly and simultaneously with Jenny Lind,* that two parties in the room could not for some time imagine that there were two voices, so perfectly did they accord, both in musical tone and vocal pronunciation of Swiss, German, and Italian songs. She was equally successful in accompanying Mdlle. Lind in one of her extemporaneous effusions, which was a long and an extremely difficult, elaborate, chromatic exercise, which the celebrated cantatrice [opera singer] tried by way of taxing the powers of the somnambulist to the utmost. When awake the girl durst not even attempt to do anything of the sort; and after all, wonderful as it was, it was only *phonic imitation,* for she did not understand the meaning of a single word of the foreign language which she had uttered so correctly, either when asleep or when awake.

All these phenomena, therefore, wonderful though they be, are only exaggerations or exaltations of functions or faculties which are possessed by all of us in a less degree in the ordinary or waking condition. They do not, however, amount to universal lucidity, or thought-reading, or *community of ideas* with those with whom they are *en rapport,* for, whilst exaltation of her natural faculties of *vocal phonic imitation* enabled the somnambulist girl to imitate correctly the words and music enunciated by Mdlle. Jenny Lind, she understood not one word of the language they uttered, nor could she have imitated Mdlle. Jenny Lind's accompaniment on the pianoforte for a single bar – these being arbitrary arrangements only to be acquired by training and practice.

Appendix:
On Migration & Hybernation

The power, and propensity, and instinct for migration has been given to certain classes of animals as a means of preserving their lives, by inducing them to roam to those climates most congenial to their feelings, whilst affording an abundant supply of appropriate food. When the season becomes cold, and the supply of food scarce, they congregate and fly to warmer climes, from which to return again the following spring. The class of animal which hybernate, being physically incapable of such locomotive power, must necessarily have perished for lack of food had their demands for it continued equal during winter to what it would have been in the ordinary state of activity of their vital functions. Hybernation, therefore, seems to be one of those wonderful and wise ordinations of Providence for preserving the lives of these creatures during the winter months, by reducing their vital processes to such a low ebb that their lives can be sustained at the minimum expenditure, and which demand can be supplied from the absorption of the fat with which their bodies had become loaded from the abundant supply of food enjoyed by them during the preceding autumn. The whole of that fat, and of the food required to produce it, would not have been adequate to have sustained these creatures during the winter months had they been in a state of ordinary activity; but, by being reduced to this state of torpor and inactivity, the expenditure of tissue is correspondingly small; and thus the means and the end are made beautifully to harmonise with each other. In fact, in animals which do not hybernate, a greatly increased amount of food is required during the intense cold of winter to keep up the temperature of their bodies to an adequate degree beyond what is required for the like purpose in a similar period during the warm season.

But, again, there are other creatures which have not the power of migrating from climes too intensely hot for the normal exercise of their physical functions, and the lives of these animals are preserved through a stage of torpor superinduced by the want of sufficient moisture – their bodies being dried up from excessive heat. This is the case with snails, which are said to have been revived by a little water being thrown on them after having remained in a dry and torpid state for fifteen years. The *vibris tritici* [a species of worm] has also been restored after perfect torpitude and apparent death for five years and eight months, by merely soaking it in water. Some small microscopic animals have been apparently killed and revived again a dozen times by drying and then applying moisture to them. This is remarkably verified In the case of the wheel-animalcule [the *rotifer*, a microscopic creature]. And Spallanzani states, that some animalculi have been recovered by moisture after a torpor of twenty-seven years. According to Humboldt, again, some large animals are thrown into a similar state from want of moisture. Such, he states, to be the case with the alligator and boa-constrictor during the dry season in the plains of Venezuela, and with other animals elsewhere. It thus appears that the Almighty has decreed to manifest His boundless wisdom and power by accomplishing the preservation of His creatures by analogous effects produced by the two extremes (within certain limits) of heat and cold.

The conservative powers of nature, manifested by an arrest or temporary suspension of *vital activity,* superinduced through excessive heat or cold, as above described, is not confined to the animal kingdom. It is also displayed in a remarkable manner in the vegetable kingdom. The almost universal sterility of winter, in cold climates, is familiar to everyone who looks abroad over the face of nature, and contrasts it with the rich verdure and bloom of spring and summer; and in hot climates, again, at certain seasons, the face of nature is equally barren and withered from excessive heat. It is well-known that the seeds of various plants may remain almost an indefinite period in a state of dormant vitality, superinduced through aridity and seclusion from air, and yet be capable of renewing all their vital actions when sufficient moisture, heat, and air are again supplied to them. Thus, there have been undoubted instances in which the grains of wheat and peas taken from the wrappers of Egyptian mummies have germinated and produced grain different from the present produce of the country, although they must have been so preserved for at least three thousand years. It is therefore impossible for us to set any limit to the period of duration to which this dormant vitality of seeds and germs might be extended, provided they were securely secluded from those circumstances which are well-known to expose them to decay or to call their vital properties into activity.

In like manner the mosses and liverworts do not suffer permanently from being, to all appearance, completely dead, dried up, and withered by heat; but revive and vegetate actively so soon as they are thoroughly moistened. Instances are recorded in which mosses have been restored to active life by a sufficient supply of moisture after they had been preserved and completely dried up for years in a herbarium.

> There is a *lycopodium* (club-moss) inhabiting Peru. which, when dried up for want of moisture, folds its leaves and contracts into a ball; and in this state, apparently quite devoid of animation, it is blown hither and thither along the surface by the wind. As soon, however, as it reaches a moist situation, it sends down its roots into the soil, and unfolds to the atmosphere its leaves, which, from a dingy brown speedily change to the bright green of active vegetation. The *anastatica* (rose of Jericho) [known as the "resurrection plant"] is the subject of similar transformations; contracting into a ball, when dried up by the burning sun and parching air; being detached by the wind from the spot where its slender root had fixed it, and rolled over the plains to indefinite

distances; and then, when exposed to moisture, unfolding its leaves, and opening its rose-like flower, as if roused from sleep. There is a blue water-lily, abounding in several of the canals at Alexandria, which, at certain seasons, becomes so dry, that their beds are burnt as hard as bricks by the action of the sun, so as to be fit for use as carriage-roads; yet the plants do not thereby lose their vitality; for when the water is again admitted, they resume their growth with redoubled vigour. – Dr. Carpenter's *Manual of Physiology,* page 91.

Appendix:
Hypnotic Therapy for Spinal Distortion

Apropos of spinal distortion, I should do great injustice to a most talented and meritorious member of my profession, were I not to record the following facts:– About eighteen months ago, a metropolitan surgeon, of high mental attainments, called on me with a letter of introduction from a mutual friend. A principal object of inquiry with him was to obtain a knowledge of my views of hypnotism and Mesmerism. I consequently explained and exhibited to him my views of hypnotism, and especially its applicability to the successful treatment of various forms of disease. The better to illustrate its influence to this gentleman, I also operated several times on himself. This same individual was lately in attendance on a family in which there were two daughters severely afflicted with spinal curvature. The elder daughter was sixteen years of age, and had been under constant treatment for this affection for nearly six years. Under the care of one gentleman, celebrated for his treatment of spinal affections, this young lady had been made to recline night and day for *sixteen months;* during which period she was subjected to the counter extension of pulleys and weights attached to her body, extending from under the chin, and both arms, and opposed to those were others attached to both ankles. This patient was also made to pull a rope and lift a weight appended to it, with one arm, *three hundred times each day,* for four years, besides other gymnastic exercises; but still she got worse, not withstanding this prolonged use of the *procrustean bed,* and other appliances enumerated to boot. The advice of professional gentlemen in the metropolis, eminent for their reputed skill in the treatment of such affections, was had recourse to; amongst others, that of *the most* eminent for his reputed skill in joint and spine affections. By the advice thus obtained, various complicated and expensive mechanical apparatus were obtained and persevered with for upwards of *four years more;* but the result was that instead of improvement, there was a decided and rapid progression of the complaint for the worse. The younger sister, now fourteen years of age, had also become affected, and had been subjected to constant treatment from the first moment she was discovered to be so. She had persisted in treatment for *three* years, but without the slightest improvement; on the contrary, she had rapidly lapsed into a state of distressing and complicated distortion of both sides of the chest. At this stage of the complaint the parents became painfully convinced of the utter hopelessness of benefit from further perseverance in a similar course of treatment, as it had been commenced with when the deformity was so slight as to be quite invisible when the patients were dressed; whereas, they had at length attained to a most distressing extent of deformity. As remarked in the mother's first letter to me, notwithstanding all the means used, "and reclining *a great deal,* the deformity has continued slowly but *most surely to gain ground,* till It is now *very extensive.* The instrument (she adds) holds the figure wonderfully well, but when that is removed there is evidently *less and less strength in the weaker muscles to do the duty for themselves."*

At this stage of the complaint the surgeon above referred to lent the mother my work on hypnotism, and expressed himself convinced that the hypnotic mode of treatment was likely to be more successful than any other with her daughters. This gentleman, had he been selfishly inclined, might have retained the two patients under his own care, as he had the entire confidence of the family, and might have urged that I had personally communicated to him a theoretical knowledge of my hypnotic mode of treatment; but, with a rare degree of liberality and kind humane feeling, he expressed himself fully convinced that hypnotism was likely to do them more good than any other mode of treatment, and alleged, moreover, that I must more thoroughly understand its *practical* application than those who had only studied my method theoretically. The consequence was, that the two young ladies were brought to Manchester, and put under my personal superintendence. I think it only an act of justice to the individual who acted thus nobly and generously and humanely to his patients, to announce his name, *viz.,* J.J.G. Wilkinson, Esq., surgeon, Hampstead, London. [A successful author, who subsequently praised Braid's work in his writing.]

Whilst this pamphlet was passing through the press, the mother of these ladies, a most acute and talented person, arrived in Manchester, to place her two daughters under my care. My first hypnotic operation with them was on the 10th instant, when both patients were rendered cataleptic, but on being aroused they had a perfect recollection of all which had occurred in the room during their sleep. Next morning they were again operated on, when they were not only rendered cataleptic, but also talked, and wrote, and exhibited mental emotions through muscular excitation, of all which they remembered nothing when awake, but on being sent to sleep again they remembered every particular – thus manifesting double-consciousness [i.e., "artificial somnambulism" characterised by reversible amnesia]. In the evening of that day I had the steel apparatus removed before operating on my patients, because I then intended to turn to account, in rectifying the spinal distortion, the peculiar susceptibility [these are two *unusually* responsive subjects] which had been induced in my patients by the two previous operations.

The instant the apparatus was removed, the result of the erroneous mode of treatment which they had been pursuing manifested itself; for there was no muscular power to support the body in the proper position; and the falling down and distortion of *both* patients was most painful to witness, the more so as they were two most intelligent and sensitive girls. The falling in or contraction of the left side, and projection of the right shoulder, in the elder sister, were most painful to look upon; and the *double* curvature of the younger sister, although of shorter duration, was still more appalling to witness. Having hypnotised these patients, and called a cataleptiform degree of energy into the morbidly weakened muscles, and thus brought the body into a more favourable position, it is impossible for me to describe the astonishment of the mother and the ladies' maid of the patients, when they witnessed the power which the patient had so speedily acquired of supporting themselves, during the sleep, in this improved position – far superior even to the position in which they were ordinarily supported by the mechanical apparatus. Their surprise was still greater, however, when they found that after the patients were aroused they still retained an increased degree of power, by which they were enabled to support themselves so well by voluntary effort, which they had not had the power of doing for a long period previously. The mother exclaimed, that much as she expected from what she had heard, both from Mr. Wilkinson and myself, still what she now witnessed far exceeded her most sanguine expectations; and added, that she only wished that all medical men, and all others who had relatives suffering from such affliction, could only witness what she had then seen, as It was utterly impossible for anyone to resist the force of such ocular demonstration as she had then had presented to her, regarding the value and power of hypnotism in the treatment of such affections.

Twice each day these operations were repeated, and with such marked improvement, that without the slightest inconvenience, in less than a week, they could walk about from half an hour to three-quarters after the operations, without the apparatus or any support from stays, with perfect ease, supporting themselves by muscular effort alone, and in a better position than the instruments afforded; whereas before my operations, they durst not remain a single minute in the erect posture without their mechanical apparatus. The gratification of the patients and their mother is unbounded, from my success with them having so far exceeded their most sanguine expectations in both cases. **In short, hypnotism is by far the *most rational* as well *as most successful* mode of treating such complaints, because it infuses increased vigour into the weak muscles, which, increased by each repetition of the process, to a considerable extent persists after the patient is awake.** Moreover, by cataleptiformly fixing certain muscles, and preventing the expansion of corresponding regions of the chest, the formerly collapsed or depressed portions of the chest and lungs are brought into play, and thereby expanded; whereas the mechanical supports now applied, unless when there is positive disease of the bones of the spine, are worse than *useless,* for this reason, because they *waste by compression,* or *weaken by inaction,* muscles which naturally ought to give due support and form to the human figure; so that, as well expressed by the mother of these patients, as quoted above, when the instruments are removed, there is evidently *less and less strength in the weaker muscles to do the duty for themselves"*. In all cases of spinal distortion which are capable of cure or amelioration – and almost all cases are so at an early stage – there is no reason to doubt that hypnotism, when properly directed, is quite capable of arresting, or of entirely curing, cases of spinal curvature; and it is, moreover, a far more agreeable, safe, and less expensive method than that which requires the aid of so much mechanical apparatus, and so much confinement of the patients to the recumbent posture.

After I had attended these patients for a week, the mother called my attention to the contracted state of her elder daughter's arms, both of which she had been unable to extend fully for upwards of four years. The right fore-arm I ascertained could not be extended beyond an angle of about 55° with the humerus; the left was considerably less contracted. The malposition had been induced by the position in which her arms had been held so long during her first sixteen months' recumbent posture, I immediately acted on the right arm so as to ensure the cataleptiform state of the extensor muscles, and on arousing the patient a few minutes thereafter, it was ascertained that she could then extend the arm completely by her own voluntary effort; and by then operating on the left arm, an equally satisfactory result ensued. **All this may appear very marvellous to those who are unacquainted with the extraordinary power acquired by us over the muscular system during the hypnotic state. Let them judge of this power by the following fact, detailed by Dr. Carpenter in his article on sleep in the "Cyclopaedia of Anatomy and Physiology". He there says, "We have seen one of Mr. Braid's hypnotised subjects, a man remarkable for the poverty of his muscular development, lift a twenty-eight pound weight upon his little finger alone, and even swing it round his head." I may add to the above important fact, that the said individual had not, for six years, been able to lift with impunity more than fourteen pounds when in the waking condition; and yet, on another occasion, I saw him in the sleep lift as high as his knee, on the last joint of his forefinger, a fifty-six pound weight. Such increased muscular power, then, being infused into morbidly weak muscles, an increased power persists in them after they come out of the sleep ; and this accumulating by each repetition of the process, readily accounts for the satisfactory results realised, upon the principle of an improved system of training.** Nor should I omit to add, that morbidly contracted muscles can be as speedily reduced to a natural condition by appropriate management during the hypnotic state. [See the various accounts throughout this text.]

"On Mesmerism & Chemical Anaesthesia": Letter (1849)

To the Editor of the *British Record of Obstetric Medicine & Surgery*.

My dear Sir,

In your *Record* for the 1st current, I observe a lecture on Ether and Chloroform by Dr. Tyler. On perusing the said lecture, I was sorry to find that the learned author was one of those zealous partisans who cannot content themselves with advocating a cause on its own independent and intrinsic merits but must needs resort to coarse and illiberal attacks upon those who adopt any rival method. Actuated by this principle, Dr. Tyler seems to have thought that he could not do sufficient justice to his favourite anaesthetics, without having a fling at Mesmerists and Mesmerism; and, in his ardent zeal, has not scrupled to advance most erroneous statements and illiberal sentiments. For the cause of truth and of suffering humanity, therefore, may I crave a little space, in your pages for the purpose of correcting the erroneous impressions which Dr. Tyler's observations are calculated to make, on the minds of those who are personally ignorant of the real powers and value of what is commonly called Mesmerism? Dr. T.'s observations having been addressed to his pupils, renders them the more reprehensible.

In limine, [at the outset] I beg leave to observe, that, **strictly speaking, I am not a Mesmerist, inasmuch as I differ from the Mesmerists in my mode of *explaining* the phenomena, as also in respect to the *extent* of the *genuine* phenomena.** I do not pretend to produce clairvoyance by my processes, nor any other phenomena which do not admit of explanation, on generally admitted physiological and psychological principles. But that certain remarkable physiological effects can be produced on man and brutes by certain processes resorted to by the Mesmerists and myself, and that by this means many diseases may be cured, without medicine, which are most obstinate or altogether incurable by ordinary medical means, I am as certain of from personal experience, as I am of my own existence. Moreover, as to the reality of the *ordinary* and *useful* phenomena of Mesmerism, instead of being refuted, they are actually confirmed by the phenomena realised during the use of ether and chloroform. Phenomena formerly declared impossible are now common every-day occurrences. Had Dr. Tyler contented himself with declaring his belief that ether and chloroform were decidedly superior to Mesmerism for inducing the state of anaesthesia requisite for surgical and obstetric purposes, from their being more speedily and generally successful in producing the requisite intensity of effects, it would have been a statement which no one could reasonably have found fault with. In fact, it would have been in exact accordance with my published opinion on the subject, as it appeared in The Medical Times for the 27th February, 1847, in my paper entitled "On the relative value of Mesmeric and Hypnotic Coma, and Ethereal Narcotism, for the mitigation or entire prevention of pain, incident to surgical operations." I had tried *both* methods, and had found hypnotism quite sufficient to suspend pain entirely during some *minor* operations in *my own* practice, and I had no doubt, from the published reports which I had read, that it had been used successfully by others in many *capital* operations. Still I was well aware that comparatively few subjects, in this country, could be reduced to the requisite intensity for such purposes, and even in those where it succeeded, that it would take up so much time as must prove a barrier to its general adoption for such purposes, especially now that ether and chloroform are ascertained to be so speedy and certain in their effects, and capable of narcotising every human being to whom a sufficient dose is given.

Still, whilst I readily yield the palm to ether and chloroform for *surgical* and *obstetric* purposes, I feel quite confident that they will never prove so extensively useful as Mesmerism and hypnotism for the cure of a large class of diseases in which this mode of treatment has been proved to have been eminently successful; and that in diseases, too, which are most obstinate, or altogether incurable by ordinary medical means. It is with the view, therefore, of preventing suffering humanity from being deprived of this important boon, and valuable adjunct to ordinary medical means in suitable cases, by parties being misled by Dr. Tyler's erroneous statements that I have entered on this discussion.

Dr. Tyler says, "Shortly before the application of ether was mooted as an assuager of pain, a last desperate and dying effort of the Mesmerists was made to bring Mesmerism into fashion. Books were published on its powers, and innumerable cases detailed where it was *said* painful operations had been performed during the Mesmeric sleep, without suffering on the part of the patient. We know that men of undoubted talents advocated the practice of Mesmerism, and not only lent their energies, but, in some instances, sacrificed their private interests, for the sake of propagating what the majority of the profession looked upon as a delusion, or, as some might express it, "*arrant humbug*".

In the first place, Dr. Tyler here wishes to set forth that the practice of Mesmerism was all but extinct "shortly before the application of ether", that is, about two years ago. Now either Dr. Tyler must be profoundly ignorant on the subject, or else he must intentionally have published what he knew was not true, in order to disparage Mesmerism; for the fact is notorious to all who know anything of the subject, **that the Mesmeric and hypnotic practice had never been so widely diffused, and so successfully used for the relief and cure of disease, as well as for annulling the pain of surgical operations, as at the very time when Dr. Tyler alleges the Mesmerists were making "a last desperate but dying effort" to *bring it "into fashion"*. Not only was this the case in Great Britain, and a great part of Europe and America, but in our possessions in the Far East, at Calcutta, it was being practised by Dr. Esdaile with a degree of success which had never been realised at any period, or in any other part of the habitable globe.**

But again, Dr. Tyler admits the reality of pain having been annulled by ether and chloroform. He gives full credit to the details of others on the point, but when he refers to the published statements of the "innumerable cases" of similar effects having been realised through Mesmerism, he makes use of the phrase, "it was said", no doubt wishing it to be inferred that such statements about the success of Mesmerism are *untrue*. Permit me to ask Dr. Tyler whether the "men of undoubted talents who advocated the practice of Mesmerism," were not, many of them at least, as veracious and worthy of credit as Dr. Tyler himself? And if some of them sacrificed their private interests for the sake of propagating Mesmerism, *after they had investigated the truth and worth of it*, was this not a more satisfactory proof in its favour than the pooh poohs, and sneers, and shrugging of the shoulders, and expressions of "arrant humbug", and other opprobrious terms applied to it by uninquiring dogmatic sceptics?

Dr. Tyler farther states, "Certain it is that three months after the advent of sulphuric ether in these countries, Mesmerism was no more; its former worshippers submitted to their untimely fate. Never was a victory more triumphant, or a defeat more complete than the rise of anaesthesia and the fall of Mesmerism."

By these remarks Dr. Tyler wishes to make it be believed that Mesmerism is no more; that it has been fairly and irrecoverably asphyxiated by ether and chloroform; that it has been dead – irrecoverably dead and buried for the last two years, and, consequently, that he and its other opponents may now gloat over the untimely and sudden death, and final extermination, of the hated thing. I beg leave, however, to ask whether the erroneous statements set forth in the above extracts from Dr. Tyler's lecture were put forth by him in ignorance of the true state of the case, or with the intention of wilfully misrepresenting it?

Whatever were his motives and intentions, there can be no doubt but he has grossly misrepresented the true state of the case, for not only are Mesmerism and hypnotism extensively practised, *at the present time, in the British dominions* – for proof of which I beg to refer to Sandby's "Mesmerism and its Opponents", lately published, and to *The Zoist*, published quarterly – but so successfully has it been prosecuted in India by Dr. Esdaile, that one of the first public duties which devolved on Lord Dalhousie on his arrival at Calcutta, last spring, as Governor-General of India, was to investigate the claims and pretensions of Mesmerism, and the high favour in which it was held by the most influential natives there, who presented a memorial to the new Governor-General, setting forth *the great good realised by the Mesmeric Hospital*, which had been appointed at Calcutta by his predecessor, for one year, and which they *craved as a boon*, might be *permanently* re-established, to be supported by their own public subscriptions. On inquiry, Lord Dalhousie (one of the most clear-headed and intellectual men of the age) was so well satisfied with the public benefits which had resulted from the Mesmeric practice at the Hospital, that he not only complied with the prayer of the petition, to re-establish the Mesmeric Hospital, but, moreover, appointed Dr. Esdaile to have the superintendence of it, and, as a reward for his past energy in prosecuting *this* inquiry, and as an encouragement for his future exertions, he appointed him to the honourable and lucrative situation of being one of the Presidency Surgeons, – a certain guarantee to fame and fortune. These are significant and *publicly recorded facts*, which neither the sophistry nor bold assertions of Dr. Tyler and his aiders and abettors can gainsay. Do these facts look as if Mesmerism was all "*arrant humbug*", or that the rise of ether and chloroform was the fall of Mesmerism, or that three months after the discovery of ether "Mesmerism was no more"?

I by no means wish to hold up Mesmerism or hypnotism as a panacea or universal remedy, for I believe in no UNIVERSAL remedy in the treatment of disease, but I am equally confident in their great value, in certain forms of diseased action, when properly and skilfully used, and, consequently, I have recourse to this method *in suitable cases*, in the same manner as I prescribe medicines, and other ordinary medical appliances, where they are particularly indicated, and with these facts before him I trust Dr. Tyler is a more humane man than to wish to persist in raising a prejudice against an important mode of treating diseases which we cannot treat with anything like the same success by ordinary medical means.

I remain, my Dear Sir,

Yours, very faithfully,

James Braid.

3, St. Peter's Square,
Manchester.

"On Esdaile & Hypnotic Anaesthetic":
Letter to The Medical Times (1847)

> This small study could be considered to show, at best, either 30% or 60% "success" for Esdaile's Mesmeric anaesthesia, depending on whether subjects who *acted* as if suffering pain but *denied* feeling pain can be counted as positive outcomes. However, this is *not* a high success rate and conceivably within the potential range of a placebo anaesthetic. Either way it probably does *not* prove the efficacy of Esdaile's *specific* method, but probably *does* suggest, as now seems likely, that *non-specific* factors (as found in placebo control group outcomes) might be expected to reduce pain.

Facts & Observations
as to the relative Value of Mesmeric and Hypnotic Coma, and Ethereal Narcotism,
for the Mitigation or entire Prevention of Pain during Surgical Operations.
James Braid, M.R.C.S.E., etc.

Time works wonders: it is the great reformer. Never was this more strikingly displayed than in the revolution which has recently manifested itself in professional faith and practice, as to the possibility and eligibility of suspending consciousness by artificial contrivance during surgical operations. But a very few years ago, those who contended for the *possibility* of inducing such a condition by Mesmeric or hypnotic processes were, by the great majority of the profession, looked upon as credulous fools or arrant impostors. The patients who had been so operated on, and were represented as having been thus saved from physical and mental suffering, were most mercilessly assailed as arrant rogues who ought not to be trusted. It was contended, in the face of their most solemn asseverations to the contrary, that they *must* have felt pain, but, by constraint at the time, had managed to conceal exhibiting any physical manifestation of suffering, and, when aroused, for some sinister purpose, mendaciously denied the fact. Nay, there were not wanting even men of high standing in the profession who, in their rabid hostility to the new doctrine, went so far as to become the apologists of "cruelty to animals"; contending that the agony inflicted by the surgeon's knife acted as a *salutary stimulus*. Had such an absurd and cruel opinion not been openly avowed, and put upon record at the moment it was uttered, it could hardly have been believed possible that any intelligent member of the profession should have promulgated such a revolting doctrine – a doctrine, too, so much at variance with experience, as well as opposed to the dictates of humanity; for is it not well-known to every practical surgeon, that the shock sustained by the nervous system is generally the greatest cause of mortality, subsequent to accidents and surgical operations?

No sooner, however, was the discovery of our transatlantic brethren made known in this country, that, by the inhalation of the fumes of ether, consciousness, could be suspended, and that thus the pain of surgical operations might be mitigated or entirely prevented, than it was at once eagerly resorted to by the very individuals who were most zealous in their opposition, and most loud in their declarations of scepticism, as to the truth or *worth* of inducing a similar immunity from suffering by the former method. And let it be specially observed, that the evidence for the efficacy of the *former* method was precisely of the same character, and equally strong as that which sustains the latter, namely, the physical condition of the patients during the operations, and their personal testimony afterwards, as to their partial or entire freedom from pain during such operations. Now, however, medical men have become so humble and credulous, and, withal, so imbued with Christian charity, as to believe and admit that, after all, it is just possible that patients themselves may be the best judges as to the amount of pain felt by them during severe surgical operations and other physical inflictions; and, moreover, that it may be possible for such individuals to speak the truth.

It is undoubtedly true, that there were not a few members of the profession who were beginning to have a glimpse of the truth – who were perceiving that they had been too rash in their sweeping expressions of scepticism in respect to the Mesmeric phenomena, and their practical importance – who were yielding to the pressure from without, and accumulation of evidence on the point, as to the power of certain Mesmeric or hypnotic processes effecting this happy immunity from suffering during surgical operations.

The remarkable success of Dr. Esdaile, in India, was well calculated to arrest attention; and in an able article on the subject, in the *British and Foreign Review*, for October last, the author avows, as the result of a dispassionate consideration of the amount of evidence on the subject, together with the known influence of certain processes on the nervous system, that the time has arrived when it is the *duty* of the medical profession to test the matter fully and fairly.

Inasmuch as this subject has been fairly tested last September, at Calcutta, before a committee appointed for the purpose, by the Government, I have thought it might be interesting to many of your readers to have the results of the investigation laid before them, so that they may compare the said results with those of the operations performed during the ethereal narcotism, so many interesting examples of which have lately appeared in The Medical Times. The satisfactory results of the latter mode, when properly managed, are now attested by the experience of medical men throughout the length and breadth of Great Britain, as well as America; and it is therefore now established beyond a doubt, to the entire conviction of every unprejudiced and intelligent member of the profession. Indeed there seems at the present time to be a perfect enthusiasm and rivalry amongst medical men of every condition, as to who shall prove the most zealous patrons of this novelty. This may partly arise from the fact that here is something they can see, and feel, and smell, as the *cause* of the peculiar condition induced by the ether; but is it not probable there may be not a few who manifest their zeal for advancing the new method as a rival to the former method, which they had so vehemently and reasonably opposed? May there not, moreover, be many who, wise in their generation, think the best mode of hiding their former delinquency and unreasonable dogmatical opposition, is to make a retreat under the shelter of the noise, and turmoil and fumes, attending on this ethereal visitant? Be the cause what it may, it is of comparative insignificance, so long as suffering humanity profits by change.

Having personally tried *both* methods, and satisfied myself of their respective powers for suspending consciousness, and thus saving patients both from the dread and suffering of surgical operations, I beg leave to offer a few remarks on what appears to me to be their relative merits; I presume it will no longer be contended that the anguish of body and mental dread of the knife are desirable, either as respects the patient or operator. My own experience of hypnotism, or Mesmerism was this, that in many cases of highly susceptible subjects, by proper management, they could be reduced to such condition as would enable them to undergo severe surgical operations without their manifesting the slightest symptoms of consciousness or pain during the sleep or nervous coma; and they would have no recollection of such awaking; that, in other cases, they might manifest physical indications of suffering pain during the artificially-induced sleep, but have no recollection of it after awaking; and that, in other cases there might be consciousness of what was being done whilst little or no pain was experienced by them. It always appeared to me, however, that a great drawback existed to these processes becoming generally available for such purposes, from the great length of time which was required in many cases to render the patients susceptible of going so deep into the sleep as is requisite to secure a complete immunity from pain, and especially so if they went into the sleep with the idea on their minds that the operation was to be performed there and then. In most cases it must have been necessary to put the patient repeatedly into the sleep, and to conceal from him the particular time when the operation was really intended to be performed – leading the patient, in fact, to expect it was to be done on *some future day.* Then, again, a considerable number of those who are susceptible of the influence to an extent sufficient for the cure of disease would not, even *with all the above precautions,* be readily reduced into the profound unconscious state requisite to ensure complete immunity from pain during surgical operations.

Such was my personal experience, and for these reasons I considered Mesmerism and hypnotism far less available for such purposes with British subjects, than for the relief and cure of various forms of disease. The success of Dr. Esdaile, however, with Hindoos and Mohamedans, seems to have been very great; but still the objection as to the length of time required would be felt to be a serious inconvenience even with such subjects, compared with the rapidity with which the desired ethereal narcotism can be induced. Many individuals, for example, are not possessed of those physical and mental qualities requisite to secure entire success by the hypnotic and Mesmeric processes; and comparatively few could be reduced into the state, provided they chose to resist complying with the conditions required. They are much in the position of the person who may have any quantity of wine or spirits set before him without becoming intoxicated, provided he effectually resists drinking them. If they are conveyed into his stomach, however, in sufficient quantity, intoxication is sure to follow, however much he might have attempted to resist their ingestion. Just so is it with the fumes of ether: we have the power of narcotising patients by this agency, will they or nill they; drunkards, however, seem to be affected with difficulty by the ether. This is the great recommendation of the ether method then, its greater rapidity in inducing the required coma, and the greater number of patients who may be thus rendered entirely unconscious, than by the Mesmeric or hypnotic processes. In such cases, however, as can be readily sent deep enough into sleep by these processes, I should decidedly prefer this method, as the patient is less likely to experience after-inconvenience from Mesmeric coma than from inhaling the offensive, narcotising fumes of sulphuric ether. Moreover, certain states of constitution or of general health will contraindicate the application of the ether; and experience has shown that considerable difference exists as to the susceptibility of different subjects to its influence, some becoming highly excited and hilarious, whilst the majority are speedily rendered comatose.

But to return to Dr. Esdaile's operations performed during Mesmeric coma. It is well-known to your readers that the doctor published a book last summer, detailing his great success [i.e., *Mesmerism in India, and its Practical Application in Surgery and Medicine,* 1846], of which cases you published a considerable number in The Medical Times. I shall not, therefore, now advert to the cases published in that volume, but confine any remarks and quotations to the cases operated on by him in presence of the committee above referred to, as your readers must feel assured they were not likely to afford the new heresy any special favour; and the following names will be sufficient guarantee as to the respectability and fitness of the individuals for the task imposed upon them by the Governor:–

The committee consisted of James Atkinson, Inspector-General of Hospitals, as chairman; Evelyn N. Gordon; D. Stewart, Presidency Surgeon; James Hulme; J. Jackson, Surgeon to the Native Hospital; A. Rodgers; W. B. O'Shaughnessy, M.D., F.R.S., secretary to the committee. The second, fourth, and sixth gentlemen named are high officials in the Honourable East India Company's service. I believe they are judges. The preliminary arrangements having been agreed upon, the committee assembled at the hospital on the 7th of September, 1846, when Dr. W. B. O'Shaughnessy was requested to act as secretary, record each day's proceedings, and keep minutes of the cases. It was also agreed that the minutes of each day should be read at the next meeting in Dr. Esdaile's presence, and that the meetings should take place at half-past seven a.m.

The committee accordingly assembled on fourteen successive days, and had under their consideration ten surgical cases taken by Dr. Esdaile from the general wards of the native hospitals, all needing operations of more or less severity. These cases are given in outline in the journal, and any remarkable phenomena exhibited are farther recorded minutely in the statement of each day's proceedings. From the facts elicited by these cases, the committee deduced the following conclusions, as in their opinion being strictly warranted by the premises:–

> The patients treated were all native males, from eighteen to forty years old, Hindoos and Mahomedans [i.e., Hindus and Muslims]; in all conditions of general health, from extreme emaciation to ordinary strength. Their diseases are specified in the annexed table:–

No.	Name	Age	Admitted	Disease	Duration
1	Cheedham	40	September 7	Double hydrocele. [Accumulation of fluid in the scrotum.]	Several months.
2	Bissonath	20	September 7	Tumour of scrotum.	Several months.
3	Nilmoney	45	September 7	Tumour of scrotum.	Several months.
4	Neechul	35	September 7	Phymosis.	Several months.
5	Deeloo	40	September 7	Double hydrocele.	Three years.
6	Jahiroodeen	33	September 7	Hypertrophy of penis.	Two years.
7	Dohmun	40	September 10	Hypertrophy of scrotum.	Several months.
8	Ramchund	18	September 13	Hypertrophy of scrotum.	Two years.
9	Hyder Khan	30	September 16	Mortification of leg.	Fifteen days.
10	Murali Doss	30	September 14	Hypertrophy of scrotum.	Six years.
				(Signed) W. B. O'Shaughnessy, Secretary	

Dr. Esdaile had stipulated that he should only operate on natives and that he should have the sole management or medical charge of the hospital wards set apart for his patients to be submitted to operation during the Mesmeric coma; that he should have for his own subordinate hospital establishment, those employed by him as Mesmerisers in Hooghly; and that there should be a daily sitting of the committee. The committee assented to these conditions, and made arrangements for three apartments being at Dr. Esdaile's disposal: one as a committee and operating room, the other two rooms provided with three beds each for the accommodation of the patients. The doors of these rooms opened into the committee-room and into each other, so that the committee could either enter these sleeping wards, or observe the appearance and conduct of the patients from their own room, as they might incline. Here, then, every precaution had been taken to guard against error or deception.

> The Mesmerisers employed by Dr. Esdaile were young men, Hindoos and Mahomedans, from fourteen to thirty years of age, most of them compounders and dressers from the Hooghly Hospital. To each patient a separate Mesmeriser was assigned. The room in which they operated was darkened, but from time to time the committee were enabled to witness, through small apertures made in the door panels, the manner in which the processes were carried on. Profound silence was observed. The processes were continued for about two hours each day in ten cases, for eight hours in one case in one day, and for six hours, in another case, without interruption. Three cases of the ten, Bissonath, Deeloo, and Neechul, were dismissed without satisfactory effect; Bissonath suffering from slight cough, which Dr. Esdaile considered to render the Mesmeric manipulation inefficient; Deeloo, on the fifth day, for having taken spirits; and Neechul having resisted the Mesmeric processes during eleven days without conclusive result. [That gives a 30% combined drop-out/failure rate at the outset of treatment.] In seven cases, in a period varying from one to seven sittings, deep sleep followed the processes above described.

I have considered it unnecessary to give their Mesmerising processes in detail, but I beg the reader's special attention to the following description of the peculiar character of the sleep thus induced, which I shall transcribe verbatim from the report:–

> This sleep, in its most perfect state, differed from ordinary natural sleep, as follows. The individual could not be aroused by loud noises, the pupils were insensible to light; and great, and in some cases apparently perfect,

insensibility to pain was witnessed on burning, pinching, and cutting the skin and other sensitive organs. This sleep, in its general character, differed from that which would be produced by narcotic drugs, in the quickness with which, in eight out of ten cases, the patient was awoke, after certain transverse passes and fanning by the Mesmeriser, and blowing upon the face and on the eyes; in the natural condition of the pupils of the eye and the conjunctivae in all the cases after awaking, in the absence of stertorous breathing, and of subsequent delirium or hallucination, and of many other symptoms familiar to medical observers, which are produced by alcoholic liquors, opium, hemp, and other narcotic drugs. It is right, however, to add that in two cases the patients showed much confusion and disinclination to answer, and complained of giddiness for some time after being suddenly aroused.

Here then, we have proof of careful observation and minute record of facts, as well as clear and accurate deductions, both as to the reality and peculiarity of the sleep thus induced.

In seven cases (thus continued) surgical operations were performed, in the state of sleep above described.

In the ease of Nilmoney Dutt, there was not the slightest indication of the operation having been felt by the patient. It consisted in the removal of tumour. It lasted four minutes. The patient's hands or legs were not held. He did not move, or groan, or his countenance change; and, when awoke after the operation, he declared he had no recollection of what had occurred.

In another case, Hyder Khan, an emaciated man, suffering from mortification of the leg, amputation of the thigh was performed, and no sign of its causing pain was evinced.

In a third case, Murali Doss (the operation he underwent being very severe), moved his body and arms, breathing in gasps, but his countenance underwent little change, and the features expressed no suffering; and, on awaking, he declared he knew of nothing having been done to him during his sleep.

A case of tapping one side of a double hydrocele is passed over as insignificant and inconclusive, although apparently painless, for the operation was repeated on the other side while the patient was awake, with the same result. The operation, too, is one daily borne without material suffering by numerous patients in all our hospitals.

In the three other cases observed by the committee, during the performance of operations in the state of sleep above described, various phenomena were witnessed, which require to be specially pointed out. While the patients did not open their eyes, or utter articulate sounds, or require to be held, there were vague and convulsive movements of the upper limbs, writhing of the body, distortion of the features, giving the face a hideous expression of suppressed agony; the respiration became heaving, with deep sighs. There were, in short, all the signs of intense pain which a dumb person undergoing operation might be expected to exhibit, except resistance to the operator.

But in all these cases, without exception, after the operation was completed, the patients expressed no knowledge or recollection of what had occurred, denied having dreamed, and complained of no pain till their attention was directed to the place where the operation was performed.

It, therefore, becomes a question whether the writhings and distorted features, in the three cases above described, are to be regarded as proof that the operations occasioned at the time the actual agony of which such symptoms are the usual evidence, or whether they were mere "instinctive movements" (reflex or automatic movements) as Dr. Esdaile represents them. But our province is only to record facts, and not to enter upon that of the physiologist or the metaphysician.

The general result arrived, at then, on the question of pain during the Mesmeric surgical operations we witnessed, amounts to this, that in three cases there is no proof whatever that any pain was suffered, and that in the three other cases *the manifestations of pain during the operations are opposed by the positive statement of the patients that no pain was experienced.*

The following table shows the curious fact that, in the three cases in which there was no evidence of pain, the pulse rose remarkably during the operation. But in the cases in which there were the [behavioural] symptoms of pain, described in paragraph 20, the pulse continued exactly the same before and during the operations.

Patient	Disease	State of Pulse			Operation
		Before	During	Immediately After	
Nilmoney	Tumour.	84	124	Natural.	Apparently painless.
Nilmoney	Dressing changed on September 12.	80	108	Natural.	Apparently painless.
Dohmun	Tumour.	72	72	Natural.	Doubtful.
Jahiroodeen	Excision of thickened prepuce.	60	60	Natural.	Doubtful.
Ramchund	Tumour.	68	68	Natural.	Doubtful.
Hyder Khan	Amputation of thigh.	108	112	100	Apparently painless.
Murali Doss	Tumour.	68	108	72	Apparently painless.

This acceleration of the pulse, in cases which showed no evidence of suffering pain during the operation, whilst it remained unaltered in those cases which were accompanied with writhing and distortion of features, seems to have puzzled and perplexed both Dr. Esdaile and the committee, as it may many others, who would naturally have expected the very opposite results. The fact is very easily explained, however, and the solution of this apparent anomaly will at once suggest itself to all who have read my little treatise on Hypnotism [*Neurypnology*, 1843] with attention. In the former cases the stimulus of the knife has excited a greater or lesser degree of rigid catalepsy, which is always attended with acceleration of pulse, generally in the ratio of the intensity of the rigidity (and it also suspends motion); whilst in the latter cases, accompanied by distortion of features and jactitation [i.e., restless agitation] of the limbs, there being no rigidity of muscles to obstruct the transmission of blood through the limbs, there would not necessarily be any acceleration of the pulse, unless from mental emotion. The tranquillity of the pulse in these cases, therefore, was the surest possible indication that the patients spoke the truth in declaring that they had felt no pain. The jactitation of the limbs, and convulsive movements of the muscles of the face, in the latter, as well as the rigidity in the former cases, might all arise as reflex or automatic actions, of which the brain might take no cognizance, as is well-known to every physiologist, and is daily witnessed during the second conscious state [i.e., artificial somnambulism] of nervous sleep.

Dr. Esdaile considered much less blood was lost by patients who were operated on during the Mesmeric sleep; but three of the four medical members of the committee expressed as their opinion, that there was no material difference observable. Neither did the medical members consider that the after-treatment of the patients was in any degree ameliorated, or the cure accelerated, by the operation having been performed in the Mesmeric sleep.[83]

The following is the only case to which the committee attached any importance to renewing the dressings of sores during the sleep:–

> In Ramchund, an examination of the wound, of a peculiarly painful nature, was required (dressing) involving two separate incisions; just as the first was completed (it lasted about a quarter of a minute, and caused writhing of the body and distortion of the face) he awoke, and, on proceeding to the second step, he shouted aloud in pain and terror, and struggled so violently that the operator could not proceed.

This seems pretty conclusive evidence, that whilst he was a person of keen feelings, the induced sleep had saved him much suffering during the first incision. It also tends to support the truth of his statement, as to having suffered no pain when *first* operated on, on the 13th of September. It strikingly proves, moreover, the superiority of sleep thus induced for such purposes from that induced by an opiate, as the following case will show:–

> The committee, having adjourned to the Native Hospital, inspected No. 4, Neechul, upon whom Dr. Jackson operated, removing the hypertrophied prepuce [foreskin] at one stroke.
> *Ninety* drops of laudanum had been administered half an hour previously, and the patient was sound sleep when operated on: pulse 90.
> At the moment of operating, he shouted aloud, struggled violently, drew up his legs, and kicked hard: pulse rose to 120; he continued to struggle for several minutes.

In paragraph twenty-seven, the committee express a similar opinion to that which I have already stated as my own conviction, respecting the great length of time required destroying its general applicability in surgical practice. They say:–

> The uncertainty of the time required in producing the intense condition of the Mesmeric sleep, in the majority of the cases now under notice, appeared very unfavourable to the general introduction of Mesmeric manipulations in the practice of surgery, especially in hospitals. But Dr. Esdaile states positively, that by frequently changing the Mesmerisers, and performing the manipulations without interruption, the same results may possibly be produced in one day, which would, in the manner pursued before the committee, have been necessarily extended over several days. In the cases of Hyder Khan and Murali Doss, several Mesmerisers were successively employed, and the result seemed to the committee corroborative of Dr. Esdaile's statement.
> The committee farther apprehend that a serious practical obstacle to the universally useful application of Mesmeric processes exists in the resistance to the sleep, which, Dr. Esdaile acknowledges, is given by cough, by pain, by mental excitement, by fever, and by the sinking state of the vital system induced by protracted and dangerous diseases.

I can state, as the result of my own experience, that patients with restless and excitable minds are generally, if not always, difficult to be reduced into a deep state of nervous sleep. In cases of fever, so long as it is possible to arouse and arrest the attention of the patient, he may be affected; I have failed, however, with one of the most susceptible subjects I ever met with, when in a state of such profound delirium from fever that the attention could not be arrested and fixed: a clear proof that hypnotism is as much a mental as a physical influence.

The fears expressed in paragraph 30, that the repetition of the processes may bring the nervous systems of patients into a morbidly impressible condition, which might render them liable to numerous nervous maladies, I feel assured, from very extensive experience, is a groundless fear, *provided the patients*

---

[83] [That is, by comparison with no anaesthetic; there might have been more difference if Mesmeric subjects were compared with patients under chemical anaesthetic.]

are treated with care and judgement. In the whole course of my experience I have met with no such untoward result, although I have hypnotised some patients daily for several months successively.

I most heartily concur in the just tribute of praise awarded to Dr. Esdaile in the concluding paragraph of the committee's report:–

> The committee are unanimously of opinion that great credit is due to Dr. Esdaile for the zeal, ability, and boldness with which he has taken up and pursued this inquiry.

They further add:–

> His sphere, however, has been hitherto limited, but the committee hope that his further investigation may be extended to medical as well as surgical cases, to European as well as native patients, and to the elucidation of the several questions which have been adverted to in the course of this report.

In the Deputy Governor's reply to the above report, he says:–

> So far has the possibility of rendering the most serious surgical operations painless to the subject of them been, in his honour's opinion (it was written by the secretary), established by the late experiments performed under the eye of a committee appointed for the purpose, as to render it incumbent on the Government to afford to the meritorious and zealous officer by whom the subject was first brought to its notice, such assistance as may facilitate his investigations, and enable him to prosecute his interesting experiments under the most favourable and promising circumstances.
>
> With this view his honour has determined, with the sanction of the Supreme Government, to place Dr. Esdaile for one year in charge of a small experimental hospital, in some favourable situation in Calcutta, in order that he may, as recommended by the committee, extend his investigations to the applicability of this alleged agency to all descriptions of cases, medical as well as surgical, and all classes of patients, European as well as native. Dr. Esdaile will be directed to encourage the resort to his hospital of all respectable persons desirous of satisfying themselves of the nature and effects of his experiments, especially medical and scientific individuals in or out of the service. Medical officers of the presidency are also to be appointed as "visitors", to inspect the proceedings of Dr. Esdaile, and report thereon to the Government, but without interfering with the doctor's proceedings.

Here, then, we have an example of the most judicious, praiseworthy, and enlightened conduct, both on the part of the Government and the committee, which has ever been recorded, in connection with this highly interesting inquiry. It is conduct not only deserving of all praise, but also worthy of universal imitation. Extending the inquiry and treatment to medical cases, I feel confident, is a movement in the right direction, as it may be rendered of far more avail for the relief and cure of disease, than for suspending the anguish of painful surgical operations; and the latter application is the less important now that we can achieve the like purpose so much more generally and rapidly by ethereal narcotism. That the latter process may also be used with advantage in the treatment of various forms of disease I have no doubt. Indeed I have been in the habit of using the fumes of ether for such purposes, in my own practice, for the last thirty years. Still I feel well assured, from what I know of both methods, that whilst the ethereal narcotism is likely to prove most available for preventing pain during surgical operations, it will never be rendered so available for the relief and cure of disease as Mesmerism and hypnotism, when the latter are judiciously and skilfully managed. I presume it is scarcely necessary for me to add, what must be apparent to every reflecting person, that practical experience is as requisite for the successful treatment of disease by hypnotism or Mesmerism, as by any other mode of cure.

In *theory* I entirely differ from Dr. Esdaile. He is a Mesmerist – that is, he believes in the transmission of some peculiar occult influence from the operator to the patient, as the cause of the subsequent phenomena. He has entirely failed, however, in adducing any new or additional evidence in support of this position, which had not been adduced before by European Mesmerists; with which opinions I am entirely at issue for reasons which are well-known to your readers, from my previous contributions to The Medical Times. In these papers I have illustrated and explained, as the ground of my dissent from the occult influence theory, that all the well-ascertained phenomena of Mesmerism can be equally, readily, and more satisfactorily explained, without the aid of any occult or exoteric influence. It is gratifying to me to be able to add, in support of my opinion on this point, that since the publication of my observations "On the Power of the Mind over the Body", I have had the honour to receive numerous letters from some of the most eminent members of the profession and of general science, expressive of their entire concurrence with my views of the nature and cause and extent of Mesmeric phenomena generally; and also of my mode of explaining the extraordinary phenomena adduced by Baron Reichenbach, as proof of a "*new imponderable*". On this last point I have only met with one or two dissentients, and these were parties who were previously strongly committed to the mystical notions of the Mesmerists.

Dr. Carpenter, in the third edition of his "Principles of Human Physiology" – one of the most perfect and valuable works on physiology extant – has fully admitted the reality and peculiarity of all the Mesmeric phenomena which I contend for. He says to that extent he considers they have "as just a title to the attention of the scientific physiologist as that which is possessed by any other class of well-established facts". Dr. Carpenter was present at a private *conversazione* at my house, when he had an opportunity of investigating the phenomena most minutely; and the lucid manner in which he has described the nature and modes of educing the genuine manifestations does him infinite credit. In respect to my mode of operating, he has done me the honour to say, at page 757, that he "considers that this curious class of phenomena cannot be better prosecuted than by that method [i.e. Braid's hypnotism]."

I have thus endeavoured, to the best of my ability, to submit to your readers a candid estimate of the relative value of hypnotism, Mesmerism, and ethereal narcotism, for the relief and cure of disease, as well as for suspending consciousness, and thus relieving or entirely preventing pain during surgical operations. I shall be glad if my public endeavours may in any degree tend to the advancement of what seems to be so well calculated to promise amelioration to suffering humanity.

3, St. Peter's Square,
Manchester.
January 30th [1847].

[A long postscript on the use of chemical anaesthetic follows which has been omitted from this edition, as being of no discernable relevance to hypnotism.]

[Braid, "Facts and Observations as to the Relative Value of Mesmeric and Hypnotic Coma and Ethereal Narcotism, for the Mitigation or entire Prevention of Pain during Surgical Operations", *Medical Times*, 13th February, 1847, vol. XV, 1846-47, pp. 381-382; continued vol. XVI., 27th February, 1847: 10-11.]

The Power of the Mind over the Body
(1846)

Editor's Preface
Donald Robertson

This is a short booklet by Braid, written in response to a widely-read book by the eminent Viennese chemist, Baron von Reichenbach, translated into English in 1846 by Dr. William Gregory, professor of medicine at Edinburgh University, under the title *Abstract of Physical Researches* (1846). Reichenbach argues for the existence of an invisible energy, similar to animal magnetism, which he calls "od" (and others termed "odyl", or "odylic" force) after the Norse god Odin.

Reichenbach's work had attracted interest on account of the experiments he reports which appear to show that subjects would respond physically and psychologically to supposedly magnetic objects. Braid proceeds to reproduce identical effects by means of concentrated attention and various forms of suggestion, conclusively *debunking* the claims of Reichenbach.

Many of these experiments were conducted in the "waking state" without any use of a hypnotic induction, and seem to have contributed to Braid's increasing emphasis upon the role of suggestion in his later writings on hypnotism, and an increasingly sceptical attitude toward the claims of Mesmerism and similar techniques, which Braid was progressively gathering more and more evidence against.

The Power of the Mind over the Body

[Introductory Remarks]
Few publications have lately issued from the press so well calculated to excite general interest and inquiry, as Baron von Reichenbach's *Researches on Magnetism*. The high reputation of the author, as well as that of his learned translator and annotator, Professor Gregory, who has furnished a condensed view of the subject in an English Dress [*Abstract of Physical Researches*, 1846], were all calculated to produce an effect – the greater, because the subject discussed was represented as bringing under our notice "a new imponderable", through which we should realise a clear and satisfactory solution of many problems in the mental and physical constitution of man, which had puzzled and perplexed alike the savage and the sage from the earliest ages.

The vast interest which the above-named brochure has created is evinced by the extent to which it has been quoted, referred to, and reviewed in our numerous periodicals. Nor is it devoid of interest to observe the various awards of these different authorities. Thus, one quotes at great length, and not only with seriousness sets down the whole as fully established, but, moreover, with much self-complacency exults in the proof thereby adduced of the correctness of all the most extreme views he and other Mesmerists may have promulgated on certain points of this keenly debated science; whilst another writes a clever burlesque article holding up the whole speculation as worthy only of unsparing ridicule. Between these two extremes, again, we have every grade of approval or scepticism.

On the first announcement of Dr. Gregory's abstract of Baron Reichenbach's *Researches on Magnetism*, I lost no time in procuring a copy, which I perused with intense interest. I had not proceeded far, however, when my experience with hypnotic patients enabled me to perceive a source of fallacy, of which the Baron must either have been ignorant, or which he had entirely overlooked. From whatever cause this oversight had arisen, I felt confident that, however carefully and perseveringly he had prosecuted his experiments, and however well-calculated they had been for determining mere physical facts, still no reliance could be placed upon the accuracy of conclusions drawn from premises assumed as true, where especial care had not been taken to guard against the source of fallacy to which I refer – *viz.*, the important influence of the mental part of the process, which is in active operation with patients during such experiments. I therefore resolved to repeat his experiments, paying the strictest attention to this point; and, as I had anticipated, the results were quite opposed to the conclusions of Baron Reichenbach. It is with considerable diffidence that I venture to publish an opinion opposed to such high authority; but I shall briefly state the grounds of my own opinion, and leave it to others to repeat the experiments, and determine which opinion is nearer the truth. The observations which I have to submit may, moreover, prove suggestive to others, and enable them not only to avoid sources of fallacy with which I am familiar, but may also lead to the detection of many which may have escaped my own observation.

[Sensations due to Suggestion not Subtle Energy]
The great aim of Baron Reichenbach's researches in this department of science has been to establish the existence of a new imponderable, and to determine its qualities and powers in reference to matter and other forces, vital and inanimate. It unfortunately happens, however, that the only test of this alleged new force (with one solitary exception, and that as I thought by no means a satisfactory one) is the human nerve; and not only so, but it is further admitted that its existence can only be demonstrated by certain impressions imparted to, or experienced by, a comparatively small number of highly sensitive and nervous subjects. **But it is an undoubted fact that with many individuals, and especially of the highly nervous, and imaginative, and abstractive classes, a strong direction of inward consciousness to any part of the body, especially if attended with the expectation or belief of something being about to happen, is quite sufficient to change the physical action of the part, and to produce such impressions from this cause alone, as Baron Reichenbach attributes to his new force. Thus every variety of feeling may be excited from an internal or mental cause – such as heat or cold, pricking, creeping, tingling, spasmodic twitching of muscles, catalepsy, a feeling of attraction or repulsion, sights of every form or hue, odours, tastes, and sounds, in endless variety, and so on, according as accident or intention may have suggested. Moreover, the oftener such impressions have been excited, the more readily may they be reproduced, under similar circumstances, through the laws of association and habit.** Such being the fact, it must consequently be obvious to every intelligent and unprejudiced person, that no implicit reliance can be placed on the human nerve, as a test of this new power in producing effects from external impressions or influences, when precisely the same phenomena may arise from an internal or mental influence, when no external agency whatever is in operation.

[Braid's Initial Experiments]
In order to guard against this source of fallacy, therefore, I considered it would be the best mode to throw patients into the nervous sleep, and then operate on such of them as I knew had no use of

their eyes during the sleep (for some patients have), and to take accurate notice of the results when a magnet capable of lifting fourteen pounds was drawn over the hand and other parts of the body without contact, after the manner described as performed by Baron Reichenbach in his experiments.

I experimented accordingly, and the results were, that **in no instance was there the slightest effect manifested, unless when the magnet was brought so near as to enable the patient to feel the abstraction [i.e., loss] of heat, (producing a sensation of cold), when a feeling of discomfort was manifested, with a disposition to move the hand, or head, or face, as the case might be, from the offending cause**. This indication was precisely the same when the armature was attached, as when the magnet was open; and in both cases, if I suffered the magnet to touch the patient, instantly the part was hurriedly withdrawn, as I have always seen manifested during the primary stage of hypnotism, when the patients were touched with any cold object. Now, inasmuch as patients in this condition, generally, if not always, manifest their perceptions of external impressions by the most natural movements, unless the natural law has been subverted by some preconceived notion or suggested idea to the contrary, and as I have operated with similar results upon a considerable number of patients, we have thus satisfactory proof that there was no real attractive power of a magnetic or other nature, tending to draw the patient, or any of his members, so as to cause an adhesion between his body and the magnet, as between the latter and iron, as Baron Reichenbach had alleged. I conclude, therefore, that the phenomena of apparent attraction manifested in his cases were **due entirely to a mental influence**; and I shall presently prove that this is quite adequate to the production of such effects.

[Account of Reichenbach's Theory & Observations]

But I must now give an extract, so as to state Baron Reichenbach's views, as expressed in Professor Gregory's abstract.

> Magnets of 10 lbs. supporting power, when drawn along the body, without contact, produce certain sensations in a certain proportion of human beings. Occasionally, out of twenty, three, or four sensitive individuals are found [15-20%]; and in one case, out of twenty-two females examined by the author eighteen were found sensitive [82%].
>
> The sensation is rather unpleasant than agreeable, and is like an aura: in some cases warm, in others cool; or it may be a pricking, or the sensation of the creeping of insects on the skin; sometimes headache comes on rapidly. These effects occur when the patient does not see the magnet, nor know what is doing; they occur both in males and females, though more frequently in females; they are sometimes seen in strong, healthy people, but oftener in those whose health, though good, is not so vigorous, and in what are called nervous persons. Children are frequently found to be sensitive. Persons affected with spasmodic diseases, those who suffer from epilepsy, catalepsy, chorea, paralysis, and hysteria, are particularly sensitive. Lunatics and somnambulists are uniformly sensitive. The magnet is consequently an agent capable of affecting the living body. The object of the author is to solve some of the disputed questions, and to bring a number of phenomena under fixed physical laws.
>
> Healthy sensitive subjects observe nothing farther than the sensations above noticed, and experience no inconvenience from the approach of magnets; but the diseased sensitive subjects experience different sensations, often disagreeable, and occasionally giving rise to fainting, to attacks of catalepsy, and to spasms so violent that they might possibly endanger life. In such cases, which generally include somnambulists, there occurs an extra-ordinary acuteness of the senses; smell and taste, for example, become astonishingly delicate and acute; many kinds of food become intolerable, and the perfumes most agreeable at other times become offensive. The patients hear and understand what is spoken three or four rooms off, and their vision is often so irritable, that, on the one hand, they cannot endure the sun's light, or that of a fire; while, on the other, they are able, in very dark rooms, to distinguish, not only the outlines, but also the colours of objects, where healthy people cannot distinguish anything at all. Up to this point, however strange the phenomena, there is nothing which may not be easily conceived, since animals and men differ very much in the acuteness of the senses, as is daily experienced.

Having met with a patient, Mlle. Nowotny, who was subject to catalepsy, who possessed such a high degree of acuteness of the senses, that "she could not endure the daylight, and in a dark night perceived her room as well lighted as it appeared to others in the twilight, so that she could quite well distinguish colours"; from a consideration of this circumstance, and remembering that the aurora borealis appears to be a phenomenon connected with terrestrial magnetism, or electro-magnetism, it occurred to the Baron "that possibly a patient of such acuteness of vision might see some luminous phenomenon about the magnet".

"The first experiment was performed by the patient's father;" no doubt by the suggestion of the Baron, and with the idea conveyed to him that some luminous appearance was likely to be discovered by the patient. It would be interesting to know whether the patient had not also been led, by some means, to understand the object of the inquiry, as such expectation, according to my own experience with such subjects, was quite adequate to the production of the expected phenomenon; and, moreover, once realised, it would be liable to recur ever after, under the same combination of circumstances.

> In profound darkness, a horse shoe magnet of nine elements, capable of carrying 80 lbs., was presented to the patient, the armature being removed; and she saw a distinct and continued luminous appearance, which

uniformly disappeared, when the armature was applied.

The second experiment was made on her recovery from a cataleptic attack, when the excitability of her senses was greatest. She saw two luminous objects, one at each pole, (the magnet was open) which disappeared on joining the poles, and reappeared on removing the armature. At the moment of breaking contact, the light was somewhat stronger. The appearance was the same at both poles, without any apparent tendency to unite. Next to the metal, she described a luminous vapour, surrounded by rays, which rays were in constant shooting motion, lengthening and shortening themselves incessantly, and presenting, as she said, a singularly beautiful appearance. There was no resemblance to an ordinary fire; the colour of the light was pure white, sometimes mixed with iridescent colours.

The next patient "was far more sensitive to the magnet than the former". She declared that, at the moment the armature was withdrawn, she had seen fire rise from the magnet, the height of a small hand, white, but mixed with red and blue.

Mlle. Maix. – As often as the armature was removed from a large magnet, in the dark, she instantly saw the luminous appearance above the poles, about a hand-breadth in height. But when affected with spasms, she was more sensitive, and the phenomenon increased in her eyes amazingly. She not only now saw the magnetic light at the poles much larger than before, but she also perceived currents of light proceeding from the whole external surface of the magnet, weaker than at the poles, but leaving in her eyes a dazzling impression, which did not for a long time disappear.

Mlle. Barbara Reichel saw the magnetic light not only in the dark, but also in such a twilight as permitted the author to distinguish objects, and to arrange and alter the experiments. The more intense the darkness, the brighter and larger she saw the emanations; the more sharp and defined their outline, and the more distinct the play of colours.

In the dark she saw the magnet giving out light, when shut, as well as when open, with this difference, that in the former case there were no points where the light appeared concentrated; but all the edges, joints, and corners of the magnet gave out short flame-like lights, uniform in size, and in a constant undulatory motion. From the large magnet these were about as long as the thickness of a little finger; when the armature was removed, however, the light was concentrated at the two poles, from which the flames arose to about the height of eight inches and a half, rather broader than the bar.

At each depression, where two plates of the magnet were laid together, there appeared smaller flames ending in point-like sparks on the edges and corner.

These small flames appeared blue, the chief light was white below, yellow higher up, then red and green at top. It was not motionless, but flickered and undulated, or contracted by starts continually, with an appearance as of rays shooting forth. There was no appearance of mutual attraction, or mutual tendency towards each other of the flames, or from one pole to the other; and as in the case of Mlle. Nowotny both poles presented the same appearance.

Mlle. Reichel was tested with a straight magnet. At the pole pointing to the north, or negative end of the magnet, the flame was larger than at the opposite end; it was sometimes undulating, sometimes starting, and shot out rays as in the horse shoe magnet; it was red below, blue in the middle, green at top.

[Contradictions in Reported Phenomena]

In order to enable the reader to form a correct estimate of what is represented in these several narratives, I have quoted the more important parts verbatim; and by comparing the results recorded by the different patients, no one can fail to be struck with the remarkable discrepancy in their description of what has been alleged as a physical fact. All expected, as I presume, to see light, and they saw light or flames accordingly; but let us remark another result: Mlle. Nowotny, in her most sensitive state, saw luminous vapour surrounded by rays which were in a constant shooting motion. "The colour of the light was nearly pure white, sometimes mixed with iridescent colours." The appearance was the same at both poles; the length of the flames, about one-half or three-fourths of an inch. Mlle. Maix, in her ordinary state, saw flames (from the same magnet I presume) a hand breadth in height, and when in the more sensitive state they were much larger; and she now saw currents of flame proceeding from the whole external surface of the magnet, but weaker than at the poles.

Mlle. B. Reichel saw the magnet giving out light, not only when open, but also when closed. When open, the flames from the poles were about eight inches high, those at the joining of the plates of the magnet about a finger's breadth in length. "These small flames appeared blue, the chief light was white below, yellow higher up, then red, and green at top." As with the others, both poles seemed to have given out similar appearances of light and flame. This same patient being experimented on with the above straight bar magnet, about a foot and a half long, we are told that, "at the pole pointing to north, or negative end of the magnet, the flame was larger than at the opposite end"; and we are further told that, "it was red below, blue in the middle, and green at the top". When we advance to the flames seen to be given out by crystals, from the human hand, and other forms of matter, we have equally discordant descriptions as to colour and size of the flames as seen by different sensitive subjects. Now, to my mind, these discordant statements, as to the colour of the flames, are quite fatal to the notion of such representations proving a physical fact; and in an especial manner is that remark applicable to the statement of Mlle. Reichel, who not only saw the colour different which was emanating from a straight bar magnet from that of the horseshoe variety, but also described the size of the flame as larger from the north pole of the straight bar magnet than from the other end, whereas it was always seen by her, as well as by others, to be the same size at both poles of a horse shoe magnet. If there be a physical reality in these alleged flames and colours, there ought to be no discrepancies of this sort; and the fact of such discordant statements having been made will tend to prepare the mind of the reader for the solution of the problem which I have now to submit.

[Braid's Psycho-physiological Explanation]

In prosecuting the inquiry, Baron Reichenbach considered he had not only proved the existence of this new force, which produced all the physical effects enumerated, with streams of light from the poles, and the power of attracting the human body, and adhering to it, as steel to the magnet – I say he alleged that he had established such a force, not only as residing in the magnet, in addition to the ordinary magnetic force but, moreover, that it was found **equally active in crystals**, where it existed quite pure and distinct from ordinary magnetism. He also now ascertained that his subjects could discover "that from the finger points of healthy men, fiery bundles of light streamed forth, exactly as from the poles of magnets and of crystals visible to the sensitive". **He alleges, moreover, that he had proved that where it was passive, it could be excited into activity by the sun's rays, by the moon's rays, by starlight, by heat, by chemical or mechanical action, and finally, that this luminous or phosphorescent appearance, and certain other peculiar properties, might be discovered by the highly sensitive in almost every place, and from nearly every object or form of matter, solid or fluid, animate or inanimate. Also, that it could be conducted through all other matter, and that all substances, not naturally actively charged with it, could be so temporarily, by proximity and contact of those which were actively charged.**

I have already stated the wonderful power of the human mind, when inward consciousness is strongly directed to any part of a sensitive person, in changing physical action, and leading the subject to attribute to an external cause what may have arisen entirely from an internal or mental cause. It has also been stated that, when I resorted to a mode of operating which rendered the subjects more highly sensitive to external influences, and at the same time was calculated to obviate any source of fallacy, as to mental emotion or expectation being directed to the part from their seeing what was being done, the results were in direct opposition to what was represented as having been realised by the Baron. I have particularly adverted to this in respect to the alleged attraction of the magnet for the human frame; I have proved it to be equally so in respect to the human hand, and crystals, etc., where all sources of fallacy are guarded against. In my experience, moreover, with such cases, no light or flames have been perceived by patients either from the poles of a magnet, crystals, the points of the fingers, or other substance, unless the patients have been previously penetrated with some idea of the sort, or have been plied with such questions as were calculated to excite notions, when various answers were given accordingly, and when in the sleep, there appeared an equal aptitude to see something when neither magnet nor fingers were in the direction indicated, as when they were – **a clear proof that the impressions were entirely imaginary, or mental in their origin.**

[Braid's "Placebo" Experiments]

I shall now proceed to detail the results of experiments with patients when wide awake, and when they had an opportunity of seeing what was being done, and expected something to happen; and also when the same patients saw nothing of what was doing, but supposed I was operating, and consequently expected something to occur.

With nearly all the patients I have tried, many of whom had never been hypnotised or Mesmerised, when drawing the magnet or other object slowly from the wrist to the points of the fingers, **various effects were realised**, such as a change of temperature, tingling, creeping, pricking, spasmodic twitching, catalepsy of the fingers, or arm, or both; and reversing the motion was generally followed by a change of symptoms, from the altered current of ideas thereby suggested. Moreover, if any idea of what might be expected existed in the mind previously, or was suggested orally, during the process, it was generally very speedily realised. The above patients being now requested to look aside, or a **screen having been interposed**, so as to prevent their seeing what was being done, and they were requested to describe their sensations during the repetition of the processes, **similar phenomena were stated to be realised, even when there was nothing whatever done**, beyond watching them, and noting their responses. They believed the processes were being repeated, and had their minds directed to the part, and thus the physical action was excited, so as actually to lead them to believe and describe their feelings as arising from external impressions.

The above fact was most remarkably evinced in a young gentleman, twenty-one years of age. I first operated in this manner on his right hand, by drawing a powerful horseshoe magnet over the hand, without contact, whilst the armature was attached. He immediately observed a sensation of cold follow the course of the magnet. I reversed the passes, and he felt it less cold, but he felt no attraction between his hand and the magnet. I then removed the cross-bar, and tried the effect with both poles alternatively, but still there was no change in the effect, and decidedly no proof of attraction between his hand and the magnet. In the afternoon of the same day I desired him to look aside and hold his hat between his eyes and his hand, and observe the effects when I operated on him, whilst he could not see my proceedings. He very soon described a recurrence of the same sort of sensations as those he felt in the morning, but they speedily became more intense and extended up the arm, producing rigidity of the member. In the course of two minutes this feeling attacked the other arm, and to some extent the whole body, and he was, moreover, seized with a fit of involuntary laughter, like that of hysteria, which continued for several minutes – in fact, until I put an end to the experiment. His first remark was, "Now this experiment clearly proves that there must be some intimate connection between mineral magnetism and Mesmerism, for I was most strangely affected, and could not possibly resist laughing during the extraordinary sensations with which my whole body was seized, as you drew the magnet over my hand and arm." I replied that I drew a very different conclusion from the experiments, as I **had never used the magnet at all**, nor held it, nor anything else, near to him; and that the whole proved the truth of my position as to the extraordinary power of mind over the body, and how mental impressions could change physical action.

I operated on two other gentlemen the same day, who were much older, and with decidedly marked effects in both, though less so than in the last case. The experiment being tried with a lady of fifty-six years of age, by drawing a gold pencil-case slowly from the wrist to the finger ends, a creeping, twitching sensation was felt, which increased until it became very unpleasant, and excited a drawing, crampy feeling in the fingers of that hand. On causing her to look aside, watch, and describe her feelings during my subsequent operations, the results were similar, and that whilst I had done nothing; and the whole, therefore, was attributable to the power of the mind in changing the physical action.

Another interesting case of a married lady I experimented with in presence of her husband, is as follows. I requested her to place her hand on the table, with the palm upwards, so situated as to enable her to observe the process I was about to resort to. I had previously remarked, that by my drawing something slowly over the hand, without contact, whilst the patient concentrated her attention on the process, that she would experience some peculiar sensations in consequence. I took a pair of her scissors, and drew the bowl of the handle, slowly from the wrist downwards. I had only done so a few times, when she felt a creeping, chilly sensation, which was immediately followed by a spasmodic twitching of the muscles, so as to toss the hand from the table, as the members of a prepared frog are agitated when galvanised. I next desired her to place her other hand on the table, in like manner, but placed so, that by turning her head in the opposite direction, she might not see what was being done, and to watch her sensations in that hand, and tell us the result. In about the same length of time, similar phenomena were manifested, as with the other hand, although in this instance I had done nothing whatever, and was not near her hand. I now desired her to watch what happened to her hand, when I predicated that she would feel it become cold, and the result was as predicted, and *vice versa*, predicating that she would feel it become intensely hot, such was realised. When I desired her to think of the tip of her nose, the predicated result either of heat or cold, was speedily realised in that part.

Another lady, twenty-eight years of age, being operated on in the same manner, whilst looking at my proceedings, in the course of half-a-minute, described the sensation as that of the blood rushing into the fingers; and when the motion of my pencil-case was from below, upwards, the sensation was that of the current of blood being reversed, but less rapid in its motion. On resuming the downward direction, the original feeling recurred, still more powerfully than at first. This lady being requested now to look aside, whilst I operated, realised similar sensations, and that whilst I was doing nothing.

The husband of this lady, twenty-eight and a half years of age, came into the room, shortly after the above experiment was finished. She was very desirous of my trying the effect upon him, as he was in perfect health. I requested him to extend his right arm laterally, and let it rest on a chair with the palm upwards, to turn his head in the opposite direction, so that he might not see what I was doing, and to concentrate his attention on the feelings which might arise, during my process. In about half-a-minute he felt an aura like a breath of air passing along the hand; in a little after, a slight pricking, and presently a feeling passed along the arm, as far as the elbow, which he described as similar to that of being slightly electrified. All this, while I had been doing nothing, beyond watching what might be realised. I then desired him to tell me what he felt *Now* – speaking in such a tone of voice, as was calculated to lead him to believe I was operating in some different manner. The result was that the former sensations ceased; but, when I requested him once more, to tell me what he felt now, the former sensations recurred. I then whispered to his wife, but in a tone sufficiently loud to be overheard by him, observe now, and you will find his fingers begin to draw, and his hand will become clenched, – see how the little finger begins to move, and such was the case; see the next one also going in like manner, and such effects followed; and finally, the entire hand closed firmly, with a very unpleasant drawing motion of the whole flexor muscles of the fore-arm. I did nothing whatever to this patient until the fingers were nearly closed, when I touched the palm of his hand with the point of my finger, which caused it to close more rapidly and firmly. After it had remained so for a short time, I blew upon the hand, which dissipated the previously existing mental impression, and instantly the hand became relaxed. The high respectability and intelligence of this gentleman rendered his testimony very valuable; and especially so, when he was not only wide awake, but had never been either Mesmerised, hypnotised, or so tested before.

Another gentleman, twenty-one years of age, was tried by drawing a gold pencil-case along the palm of the hand, without contact. At the fourth traction, he looking at the part and my process, he described a cold aura following the course of the pencil, then a pricking, and after a few more courses, he described it as rather a warm pricking sensation; such as that experienced from the sun's rays concentrated on the skin by a lens. By reversing the passes, from the points of the fingers towards the wrist, the aura was changed, and he described the sensation as that of forcing back the blood in the veins, when they are much distended. I then proposed to experiment on his other hand, whilst his head was held aside, when similar sensations were realised, although on this occasion I had done nothing – the whole results having arisen from his own concentration of inward consciousness, changing the physical action of the part, and recalling his former association of ideas in reference to the other hand. **I thereupon explained to him the law, (for he was a very acute young gentleman) which seemed to obtain in the production of such phenomena, and desired him to satisfy himself of the fact, by concentrating his attention on the upper part of his foot, and watching the result. Here, also, he experienced similar sensations to arise, even whilst he was aware that I was doing nothing; but the effects took place less rapidly than was the case in the former experiments with his hands.** [Braid thus shows that the "placebo" effect does not depend upon *deception* but that suggestion may occur with the subject's knowledge and co-operation.] It is also worthy of remark, that this gentleman experienced very severe headache to result from these experiments, which, however, I was enabled very speedily to remove by another process.

A lady thirty years of age was requested to hold out her right hand over the arm of an easy-chair, whilst she turned her head to the left, to prevent her from seeing what I was doing, and to watch and describe to me the feelings she experienced in the hand during my process, which was to be performed without contact. She very soon felt a pricking in the point of the third finger, which increased in intensity, and at length extended up the arm. I then asked her how her thumb felt, and presently the same feeling was transferred to it; and when asked to attend to the middle of the forearm, in like manner the feeling was presently perceived there. All the time I had been doing nothing; the whole was the result of her own mind acting on her hand and arm. I now took the large magnet, and allowed her to watch me drawing it slowly over the hand, when the feeling was much as before, only that she felt the cold from the steel when brought very near to the skin. It was precisely the same when closed as when opened, and the same sensations occurred when the north pole alone was approximated, or the south alone, or both together. She experienced no sense of attraction between her hand and the magnet from either pole, nor from both combined. I now requested this lady to keep a steady gaze upon the poles of the large horseshoe magnet, and tell me if she saw anything, (the room was not darkened nor was the light strong) but nothing was visible. I then told her to look steadily, and she would see flame or fire come out of the poles. In a little after this announcement she started, and said, "Now I see it, it is red; how strange my eyes feel," and instantly she passed into the hypnotic state. This lady had been repeatedly hypnotised. I now took the opportunity of testing her as to the alleged power of the magnet to attract her hand when asleep, but, as in the other cases, the results were quite the contrary; the cold of the magnet (and of either pole alike) caused her to withdraw her hand the moment it touched her. I now requested her to tell me what she saw (she being still in the sleep). She said she still saw the red light. I desired her to put her finger to the place where she saw it. This she declined to do, being afraid that it would burn her. I thereupon assured her that it would not burn her, upon which she pointed to the same place where the magnet was held before she went into the sleep, instead of to where it was now held, which was near to her face, but towards the opposite side of the chair. This lady does not see from under her closed eyelids when hypnotised, as some patients do; and the evidence her testimony affords in support of my opinion upon this subject is very conclusive, as she is a lady of very superior mental attainments, and one whose testimony merits unlimited confidence.

I beg to call particular attention to the fact, that in this latter case, as with the fifth of the vigilant [non-hypnotised] cases narrated, the first experiments were tried without any magnet or other object being pointed at or drawn over them, and still the mental influence was quite sufficient to change the physical action, and produce decided and characteristic effects, where there could be no influence from without, of the nature alleged by Baron Reichenbach and the Mesmerists.

A lady, upwards of fifty-six years of age, in perfect health, and wide awake, having been taken into a dark closet, and desired to look at the poles of the powerful horse shoe magnet of nine elements, and describe what she saw, declared, after looking a considerable time, that she saw nothing. However, after I told her to look attentively, and she would see fire come out of it, she speedily saw sparks, and presently it seemed to her to burst forth, as she had witnessed an artificial representation of the volcano of Mount Vesuvius at some public gardens. Without her knowledge, I closed down the lid of the trunk which contained the magnet, but still the same appearances were described as visible. By putting leading questions, and asking her to describe what she saw from another part of the closet, (where there was nothing but bare walls) she went on describing various shades of most brilliant coruscations and flame, according to the leading questions I had put for the purpose of changing the fundamental ideas. On repeating the experiments, similar results were repeatedly realised by this patient. On taking this lady into the said closet after the magnet had been removed to another part of the house, she still perceived the same visible appearances of light and flame when there was nothing but the bare walls to produce them; and, two weeks after the magnet was removed, when she went into the closet by herself, the mere association of ideas was sufficient to cause her to realise a visible representation of the same light and flames. Indeed such had been the case with her on entering the closet ever since the first few times she saw the light and flames. In like manner, when she was made to touch the poles of the magnet when wide awake, no manifestations of attraction took place between her hand and the magnet, but the moment the idea was suggested that she would be held fast by its powerful attraction, so that she would be utterly unable to separate her hands from it, such result was realised; and, on separating it, by the suggestion of a new idea, and causing her to touch the other pole in like manner, predicating that it would exert no attractive power for the fingers or hand, such negative effects were at once manifested. I know this lady was incapable of trying to deceive myself, or others present; but **she was self-deceived and spell-bound by the predominance of a pre-conceived idea**, and was not less surprised at the varying powers of the instrument than others who witnessed the results.

Similar phenomena were manifested by this patient when she was requested to place a finger or hand in contact with a table, or any other inanimate object – the results being either negative, or irresistibly attractive, or repulsive, according to the ideas suggested; and that without any passes or manipulations on any part. Moreover, these results occurred whilst I was willing the very opposite effects might arise from those she had heard me predicate. The results always corresponded with the mental impression or belief of the patient, and might have been just as readily suggested by a pass or silent signal, to which she had attached a particular idea, as by vocal enunciation.

In like manner several other patients whom I took into the **dark closet** could see nothing, until told to look steadily at a certain point and they would see flame and light of varying colours proceeding from it, which predictions were speedily realised, whilst they were wide awake, and with nothing but bare walls towards which to direct their eyes. Not only so, but I have, moreover, ascertained, that, even in broad daylight, a strong mental impression is adequate to produce such delusions with certain individuals of a highly imaginative and concentrative turn of mind. This fact was beautifully illustrated in the case of a gentleman, twenty-four years of age, (who had suffered severely from epilepsy, for eleven years, notwithstanding the persevering use of medicine of various sorts, prescribed by many of the most able members of the profession, but who is recovering very satisfactorily under the hypnotic treatment) when taken into the above closet and tested as the latter. He likewise saw nothing till I suggested that he would see flame and light, after which predication he very speedily saw them accordingly, not merely where the magnet was, but also from other parts of the apartment. Now, this patient, and the last two referred to, when taken into the closet after the magnet had been a long time removed to a distant part of the house, still saw the flames, and changing colours as before – a clear proof that the whole was a mental delusion arising from an excited imagination, on the point under consideration, changing physical action. The same gentleman being made to look at the point of a piece of brass wire [brass is non ferrous, i.e., *non-magnetic*], could be made to imagine that he saw any sort of flame or colour indicated issuing from it, even in broad daylight; and when made to touch it with a finger, and then told he would find it impossible to draw it away, the mere idea was sufficient to paralyse his volition, the whole muscles became rigid and he looked with astonishment at his condition; but the moment I said now the attraction is gone, and his hand will separate, such results followed. Moreover, now that his finger was a little withdrawn, **by simply saying confidently** that it would now be found that he could not touch the wire, as it would repel him, the idea once more paralysed his volition, and he again manifested his incapacity, and in spite of his anxious, but misdirected efforts, there he remained fixed as a statue. On hinting that now the influence was suspended, the hand and arm became limber, when I told another person watching the experiment that now he would find the hand irresistibly drawn to the wire; and such result was presently manifested. No one had touched this wire for hours; it was merely a piece of bent brass wire which was lying loosely and projecting from the chimney-piece. This power seems to have been understood by Virgil when he said – "*Possunt, quia posse videntur.*" ["They can because they believe they can."]

In like manner having intimated to a friend the remarkable vividness of this patient's imagination, implicit belief, and credulity, which rendered him liable to believe that he had an ocular perception of an external change, according to whatever idea might be suggested to him by others, I requested this friend, when we went into the room, to look at the end of the above wire at the same time with the patient, and that the former should pretend to me, when asked what coloured flame she saw emanating from it, to give a new idea at each inquiry. By this mode the patient caught the ideas suggested, having no notion that he was deluded in the way indicated. He left with the full conviction of the physical reality of all he had seen and described; and he has manifested like phenomena as frequently as he has been so tested.

I have detailed the above case so much at length, because it is a very good type of a class of patients to be met with, who readily become the dupes of suggestions, in the manner presently to be explained, without the least desire to deceive others, or the most distant idea that they are themselves deceived. I have proved all I have advanced by so many concurrent examples, with individuals of the utmost probity and competency to describe their feelings, that there can be no doubt of the facts.

But not only may patients, in the waking state, be made to believe that they see various forms and colours, and perceive variable sensible impressions and irresistible powers, drawing, repelling, or paralysing them, from a strong mental impression changing the physical action of the organ or part usually engaged in the normal manifestation of such function; but I have, moreover, ascertained that the same influence may be realised in respect to sound, smell, taste, heat, and cold – so that **suggested ideas and concentration of consciousness** are competent, with some individuals, to excite ideas, not merely of hearing vague sounds, but particular tunes, the smell of particular odours, and to discriminate particular tastes, and feel heat or cold. **All this I have proved may be realised with some excitable subjects when they were wide awake**; and when there was neither actual sound, nor odour, nor taste, in the situations and substances to which they were referred; and by merely asking what tune, what colour, what animal, or what substance, they perceived now, I clearly proved that ideas were thus excited in the minds of subjects totally different from those existing in my own at the time. The subjects with whom I made these experiments were worthy of implicit credit as to their integrity in describing their feelings and belief; and the whole results, therefore, are attributable to the remarkable **reciprocal actions of the mind and body** on each other, to which I have so often referred.[84] Indeed, one of the most beautiful examples I have had of these "**vigilant phenomena**", in respect to all the senses, occurred in the case of a gentleman of high classical and mathematical attainments, as well as in general science. He had seen no experiments of the sort before I tested himself.[85] **On finishing my round of experiments with him, he begged of me to explain the rationale of what had occurred. I requested him to read what I had written on the subject, which he perused with great attention; after which he expressed himself perfectly satisfied that I had hit upon the true solution of the problem. Indeed, he was so kind as to authorise me to refer anyone to him for a confirmation of the rationale I had given of the phenomena, as experienced by him in his own person when wide awake, and in the bright light of day.**

It is stated by Baron Reichenbach that the sensitive can uniformly detect water which has had the magnetic current passed through it, by having an open magnet brought over and in contact with the opposite sides of the glass in which the water is contained. I have tried this experiment in such a manner as was calculated to guard against various sources of fallacy which I knew were likely to mislead the unwary; such as the varied tone of voice or look of the experimentalist, when investigating the subject, and trying to elicit from the patient his candid opinion as to the qualities of each glass of water. The results were, that none of the patients tried could detect either by smell, taste, or any other sensible effect, any difference between the magnetised and the unmagnetised water. At each trial I made use of four similar glasses, filled to the same height, two of which, by the contact to the glass of a powerful magnet for a minute or two, were magnetised, the other two not magnetised. The patients were all first tested in this way when awake, and then when asleep. Magnetising by passes, or breathing on the water, I should not consider a fair experiment, and for this reason, that the halitus [vapour] of the breath, or from the skin, might very readily be detected by a highly sensitive patient, by smell, and probably also by taste. I have met with a patient who could very readily detect water so treated from that which had not, and I ascertained that she did so by smell.

The extreme acuteness of the organs of special sense, under certain circumstances, is well illustrated in certain states of disease, and by what is realised in the feats of some savage tribes. They appear quite as exalted as anything I have met with, in the hypnotic or Mesmeric state; and which has been sufficient to enable me to account, on natural principles, for what others have attributed to some new faculty or sense developed by their processes, and distinct from the ordinary organs of sense.

However, I have never met with any case of accurate thought-reading, where the patients could generally and accurately interpret my unexpressed thoughts and desires regarding him, without some sensible sign to indicate my ideas to him; but, as already stated, I feel confident that there are many, who, from their excited and concentrated state of mind, and quickened senses, will catch ideas far more quickly than in the ordinary condition, who may be thus imposed upon, and excited to act by means of impressions received through the senses, which would entirely escape them in the ordinary condition.

[Considerations on Magnetism]

In consequence of the statement made in the third section, of the tranquillising effect of causing highly sensitive patients to lie with the head towards the north, and the extreme discomfort of other directions of the body, in reference to the magnetic meridian, I had a patient who had been long an extreme sufferer, and in whose welfare I felt the deepest interest, to submit to the trouble of such a change in the position of her bed, but, I am sorry to say, it was followed by no beneficial effect.

---

[84] For remarkable examples of the extent, to which mental impression is capable of changing physical action, I beg to refer to my papers in The Medical Times for December 1844, and January and February 1845. It is particularly gratifying to be able to refer, in confirmation of most of the views I advocate, to Dr. Holland's "Medical Notes and Reflections" – one of the most masterly works I ever read, which I had the pleasure of perusing for the first time in June 1845.

Ten days ago I had the gratification to receive from this gentleman a letter, expressing his entire concurrence with my published views of Mesmeric phenomena generally; and in respect to my comments and experiments in opposition to the views of Reichenbach, he considers them so satisfactory and conclusive that "no further contradiction is necessary". I have also had similar testimony in favour of my views from many other gentlemen of high talents and attainments.

Farazi, the Persian necromancer's answer to Firuz Shah, is also quite corroborative of my views. When asked how it was possible for him to bring a person immediately to that spot, who was known to be at the time 800 or 900 miles distant, he replied that "he could not bring her in person, but could produce such a likeness of her that he could swear to her being his own wife" – Late Right Hon. Sir Gore Ousley's "Biographical Notices of Persian Poets".

[85] [See appendix (originally a lengthy footnote) 'On Muscular Suggestion'.]

I am perfectly aware that the results of a single case are not competent to refute what has been alleged, as proved by a number of others. However, I have stated my fact on the point; and, whilst I readily admit my firm conviction that, with sensitive patients, who, from whatever cause they may have imbibed notions that certain directions of the body, either when asleep or awake, might be followed by feelings of physical as well as mental discomfort, the mere idea would be adequate to the production of such effects; still, I do not believe there is any adequate physical cause for such results, merely as regards the polarity of the earth and human frame. The following are the grounds for this opinion. The constituent parts of the human frame are all dia-magnetic, that is, under the magnetic influence, they have a tendency to assume the equatorial axis, instead of the polar direction; and it therefore appears to me extremely improbable that a combination of dia-magnetics should, merely in consequence of their combination, become invested with the very opposite qualities of the constituent parts. To say the least of it, this would be at variance with all which has yet been ascertained of such powers on the inanimate, physical, and chemical world. It therefore appears to me, that the peculiarities referred to by Baron Reichenbach, under this head, are more likely to have arisen from a mental than a physical cause.

A few days after the above paragraph was written, I read it to a most intelligent friend, who told me, that she had just received a letter from her brother, who had been attending some lectures by **Professor [Michael] Faraday**, and kindly offered to send me an extract from his letter, corroborative of what I had read to her. The following is the extract which I received the following morning, and is particularly gratifying, coming as it does from the very highest authority we have on this subject. "I have been greatly interested lately with a course of lectures by Faraday on Electricity and Magnetism, which, I am sorry to say, is just concluded. You will no doubt be gratified to learn that, in common with the whole human race, you are a magnet! with this peculiarity only, that if you were suspended by the middle, you would point East and West, instead of North and South – with which interesting fact, I leave you to your meditations!"

That some of Baron Reichenbach's patients should have manifested the power of seeing luminous emanations in the dark, over the graves of the dead, more especially of those recently buried, I think admits of a more probable explanation than that propounded by the Baron. **We know that during certain stages of decay of vegetable and animal matter, a phosphorescent appearance is manifested in the dark to ordinary vision, and, of course, it must be still more so to the highly sensitive.** But there is another result of such organic decay still more powerfully felt by all, namely, its disagreeable odour. Few can escape the recognition of this, even in the bright light of day. Again, we are so much in the habit of associating visible or tangible forms with impressions which are conveyed to our minds through any of the organs of sense, that the blind are in the habit of expressing themselves as seeing such and such persons, whom they recognise approaching, merely by the sound of their voices, or tread of their steps, and so on.

In like manner a smell of any sort suggests corresponding ideas; and I have found hypnotic patients who recognised individuals of their acquaintance quite readily by smell, who always said, when asked how they knew who was present, "I see him or her," and, when the nostrils were stopped, thought the party had gone away. The sympathy which exists between the eyes and the nose is well proved by a strong light producing sneezing; and the converse of this is very natural, that a strong impression on the olfactory nerves might excite in the mind of a highly sensitive and imaginative person the idea of some visible appearance. This will account for the ghost-story quite as readily as the theory of the Baron, and will be found more generally available, as few people are so constituted as to be able to pass through such places without being painfully reminded, through their olfactory organs, that they are treading on the mortal remains of friends departed.

[Aura Photography Refuted]

But I may be met with the objection to my arguments by an appeal which has been made to the Daguerreotype [a primitive photographic technique] (a purely physical fact) – which could not be influenced by mind – for an experiment has been recorded by Baron Reichenbach, where, by the mere exposure of a sensitive plate in a box with a magnet, all light being excluded, an impression had been made, as if it had been exposed to the full influence of light, which did not happen when another plate was so confined without the magnet. It appeared to me that such an important deduction ought not to have been arrived at, from one or two experiments of such a ticklish nature; and more especially so, when the iodised plates were so long kept before being exposed to the mercurial vapour; for it was natural to expect some chemical change might take place with them irrespective of light. I have repeated these experiments with nine plates, prepared at different times with the greatest care by Mr. Akers, the patentee of the Manchester photographic gallery, (one of the most correct professors of his art) and the experiments varied so as to guard against error, by mutual correction. The experiments have been tried by close and free exposure of three plates to the poles of a powerful horseshoe magnet, (originally of 80 lbs. lifting power, but somewhat reduced from use) and of another three similarly situated, only with two sheets of black paper interposed so as to intercept the rays of light, if any were emitted from the magnetic poles, and another was enclosed in a box at a distance from the magnet, and all kept from 66 to 74 hours; but in no instance was there any appearance of them having been acted on by light – the only change being such chemical changes as generally arise from keeping prepared plates for some time before being exposed to mercury. The latter process was also performed by Mr. Akers for the purpose of insuring greater accuracy from his daily practice of the art. Two other plates were enclosed in a camera and exposed at such a distance as must have given a picture of the poles of the magnet, and flames issuing from them – for the camera was adjusted to 4½ times the distance of ordinary light, and one left 66 the other 35½ hours – but no such indications manifested themselves. I think, therefore, that I am warranted to conclude that no light, capable of affecting an iodised plate, is given out at the poles of magnets, as alleged from the experiments referred to by Baron Reichenbach.[86]

Having thus far investigated Baron Reichenbach's speculations, and proved the major propositions to be erroneous, as respects proving the phenomena he refers to as resulting from a "new imponderable", I consider it unnecessary to prosecute the subject in the minor details. I may, however, remark that I can readily imagine, from the exalted sensibility of particular individuals, and their highly concentrative state of mind, that they may be competent to detect electric, calorific, and physical qualities of objects, which would escape the observations of themselves and others, when in the ordinary and less sensitive condition. And, again, whilst I deny that we have any satisfactory proof of this new imponderable, passing from the operator to the patient, as alleged, during the processes of the Mesmerists, still I readily admit that the operator, for the reasons already assigned, of mental impression changing physical action, is very likely to feel an aura in his finger ends, the position, action, and mental direction, all tending to excite in them turgescence [i.e., slight swelling and warmth] and increased sensibility. I can also easily conceive, that the passes, through their physical, electrical, and other effects, tending to draw the patient's attention to particular parts, thus exciting their functions, and withdrawing it from others, thereby depressing their functions, and especially if the patient expects such results to ensue from such processes, are very likely to be followed by such results, irrespective of any special influence being transmitted from the operator to the patient, of the nature alleged by Baron Reichenbach and others.

The Mesmerists, who have entertained the notion that the sleep and other phenomena occurring during their processes arose from a magnetic fluid, or some special influence issuing from their persons, and passing into that of the patient, of course hail these speculations of Baron Reichenbach as demonstrative proof of the correctness of their theory of Mesmerism. Some of their patients having declared that they saw blue or variegated sparks passing from the fingers of the operator, when making passes in Mesmerising a patient, water, or other inanimate object; or that they saw a blue fluid, or one of still brighter hue, issuing from the eyes of the operator and darting towards them, when gazing fixedly for the purpose of Mesmerising; or that they perceived a luminous halo surrounding the head of a person engaged in deep thought, must have felt gratified by the announcement, considering it well calculated to confirm in their minds, the notion of the physical entity of the agent. But, when those patients have further described that when the operator has been engaged in silently willing, for example, that a patient should be made to come towards him, there is seen by the patient, a stream of something passing from the head of the operator to that of the patient, like a rope, and that he not only sees this, but feels its influence as a rope, or innumerable threads drawing him irresistibly towards the operator, the entity must now appear fully confirmed. But again, when some of these subjects become, at length, so accomplished and susceptible as to be able to perceive these visible appearances in the wide waking state, it cannot be wondered at that those whose long cherished opinions lay in that direction, should jump to the conclusion that now the point is fully and satisfactorily settled. Under such a combination of circumstances, individuals may be excused for overlooking what to others is a very obvious source of fallacy, – *viz.* **the tendency of a continued fixed gaze to confuse the vision, and of a fixed idea and expectation to confuse and bewilder the mind.**

It is well-known that the undue excitement of an organ disturbs the normal functions of such organ; and that in a state of fever, delirium tremens, and various morbid states of the nervous system, and even in the healthy state during dreaming, the patient imagines that he feels, and sees, or hears all sorts of forms, colours, sounds, *etc.* We do not, on that account, subscribe our belief in the reality of the objects, or peculiar attributes he has seen, heard, or felt, or the imaginary feats he has accomplished. In this case we estimate the phenomena as mental and morbid delusions; and such I apprehend ought to be our conclusion in reference to these extraordinary and startling allegations.

[Self-Hypnosis & Yoga]
Inasmuch as patients can throw themselves into the nervous sleep, and manifest all the usual phenomena of Mesmerism, through their own unaided efforts, as I have so repeatedly proved by causing them to maintain a steady fixed gaze at any point, concentrating their whole mental energies on the idea of the object looked at; or that the same may arise by the patient looking at the point of his own finger, or as the Magi of Persia and Yogi of India have practised for the last 2,400 years, for religious purposes, throwing themselves into their ecstatic trances by each maintaining a steady fixed gaze at the tip of his own nose; it is obvious that there is no need for an exoteric influence to produce the phenomena of Mesmerism. The agency may be entirely personal or subjective, and in such cases as I have illustrated by extracts from Ward's "History of the Hindoos" and the "Dabistan" [*Dabistān-i Mazāhib*, a 17th century Persian religious text], through certain associations of ideas,

---

[86] Mr. Dancer, the optician, kindly lent me apparatus, and saw and approved of my arrangements, as well adapted for the purpose.

such self-Mesmerised patients can see and imagine as great, or indeed far greater wonders than are recounted by our most successful Mesmerists of modern times, with the additional aid of their alleged Mesmeric fluid. In proof of this I beg to refer to my paper in The Medical Times, page 272, vol. xi. The great object in all these processes is to induce a habit of abstraction or concentration of attention, in which the subject is entirely absorbed with one idea, or train of ideas, whilst he is unconscious of, or indifferently conscious to, every other object, purpose, or action.[87]

[Further Experiments with Suggestion]
I had long been familiar with the fact, that during a certain stage of hypnotism, patients may be made to give various manifestations, or declarations of their feelings and emotions, according to previously existing ideas, or suggestions imparted to them during the sleep; and, moreover, that such associations once formed, were liable to recur ever after, under a similar combination of circumstances. As occurs in ordinary dreaming, they seem generally at once to adopt the idea as a reality, without taking the trouble of reasoning on the subject as to the probability of such ideas being only imaginary; and their extreme mobility in the hypnotic state at a certain stage renders them prompt with their corresponding physical response. In proof of this, and how readily those inattentive to these facts may misapprehend what they see realised in such cases, I beg to submit the following interesting illustration. When in London lately, I had the pleasure of calling upon an eminent and excellent physician, who is in the habit of using Mesmerism in his practice, in suitable cases, just as he uses any other remedy. He spoke of the extraordinary effects which he had experienced from the use of magnets applied during the Mesmeric state, and kindly offered to illustrate the fact on a patient who had been asleep all the time I was in the room, and in that stage, during which I felt assured she could overhear every word of our conversation. He told me, that when he put the magnet into her hands, it would produce catalepsy of the hands and arms, and such was the result. He wafted the hands and the catalepsy ceased. He said that a mere touch of the magnet on a limb, would stiffen it, and such he proved to be the fact.

    I now told him, that I had got a little instrument in my pocket, which although far less than his, I felt assured would prove quite as powerful, and I offered to prove this by operating on the same patient, whom I had never seen before, and who was in the Mesmeric state when I entered the room. My instrument was about three inches long, the thickness of a quill, with a ring attached to the end of it. I told him that when put into her hands, he would find it catalepsise both hands and arms as his had done, and such was the result. Having reduced this by wafting, I took my instrument from her, and again returned it, in another position, and told him it would now have the very reverse effect – that she would not be able to hold it, and that although I closed her hands on it, they would open, and that it would drop out of them, and such was the case – to the great surprise of my worthy friend, who now desired to be informed what I had done to the instrument to invest it with this new and apposite power. This I declined doing for the present; but I promised to do so, when he had seen some further proofs of its remarkable powers. I now told him that a touch with it, on either extremity would cause the extremity to rise and become cataleptic, and such was the result; that a second touch on the same point would reduce the rigidity, and cause it to fall, and such again was proved to be the fact. After a variety of other experiments, every one of which proved precisely as I had predicted, she was aroused. I now applied the ring of my instrument on the third finger of the right hand, from which it was suspended, and told the doctor, that when it was so suspended, it would send her to sleep. To this he replied, "It never will," but I again told him that I felt confident that it would send her to sleep. We then were silent, and very speedily she was once more asleep. Having aroused her, I put the instrument on the second finger of her left hand, and told the doctor that it would be found she could *Not* go to sleep, when it was placed there. He said he thought she would, and he sat steadily gazing at her [to induce Mesmerism], but I said firmly and confidently that she would not. After a considerable time the doctor asked her if she did not feel sleepy, to which she replied "not at all"; "could you rise and walk?", when she told him she could. **I then requested her to look at the point of the fore-finger of her right hand, which I told the doctor would send her to sleep, and such was the result; and, after being aroused, I desired her to keep a steady gaze at the nail of the thumb of the left hand which could send her to sleep in like manner, and such proved to be the fact.**

---

[87] From careful observation, I feel convinced that the principal differences between nervous and common sleep, consist in the state or condition of the mind, and the physical effects which flow therefrom. In proof of this and the proposition above referred to, I beg to refer to the fact that I never yet succeeded in hypnotising an idiot; for the very obvious reason that there was not a sufficient amount of intelligence to enable me to fix their attention. However, I have frequently succeeded in inducing the sleep in ordinary cases of insanity, and monomania, and in several instances with decided advantage. In some by restoring refreshing sleep which had been long absent, in others by exciting in their minds during the sleep, antagonist ideas to those which constituted their chief delusion. Fixing the attention through visual sensation, as specially indicated in my little treatise on Hypnotism [*Neurypnology*, 1843], is the most rapid and certain mode of inducing the state of nervous sleep, but the patient may be affected, as the blind are, by closing the eyes and keeping his mind fixed on some imaginary object or idea. After the impressibility has been stamped on subjects which are naturally highly susceptible, they become liable to be affected entirely through mental impression, belief, and habit – that is to say, they will become affected from any visible process which they believe intended and capable of producing the effect, or even where no process whatever is in operation, if they only imagine something is being done at a distance to throw them into the sleep, they will become affected through the mere force of this mental impression and belief. This seems to be a grand source of fallacy with many who allege that they can affect patients at a distance, through mere volition, or secret passes, occasional coincidences being exalted by them into a positive law.

Having repaired to another room, I explained to the doctor the real nature and powers of my little and apparently magical instrument – that it was nothing more than my portmanteau key and ring, and that what had imparted to it such apparently varied powers was merely the predictions which the patient had overheard me make to him, acting upon her in the peculiar state of the nervous sleep, as irresistible impulses to be affected, according to the results she had heard me predict. Had I predicted that she would see any flame, or colour, or form, or substance, animate or inanimate, I know from experience that such would have been realised, and responded to by her; and that, not from any desire on her part to impose upon others, but because she was self-deceived, the vividness of her imagination in that state, inducing her to believe as real, what were only the figments of fancy, suggested to her mind by the remarks of others. The **power of suggestions** of this sort also, in paralysing or energising muscular power is truly astounding; and may all arise in perfect good faith with **almost all patients who have passed into the second conscious state, and with some, during the first conscious stage; and with some weak-minded, or highly imaginative or credulous and concentrative people, even in the waking condition.** The latter constitutes that class of subjects who manifest what are called the **"vigilant phenomena"**. The true cause of these "vigilant phenomena" is not a physical influence from without, but a mental delusion from within, which paralyses their reason, and independent volition, so that for the time being they are mere puppets in the hands of another person by whom they are irresistibly controlled, so that they can only see, or hear, or taste, or feel, or act, in accordance with his will and direction. They have their whole attention fixed on what may be said or signified by this alleged superior power, and consequently perceive impressions through the excited state of the organs of sense, called into operation which they could not perceive in their ordinary condition; and this sort of clairvoyance or thought-reading, the Mesmerists attribute to some special influence, such as the new imponderable of Reichenbach. So soon as patients can be made to believe that in the waking state, the evidence of their senses is more trust-worthy than mere idea or suggested impressions; and that they can really exercise their own independent powers in opposition to the alleged power of the will of another, **through his auricular suggestions** or passes, and other manoeuvres, it will instantly be found that the spell is broken, and that rational beings can no longer be magnetically tied together, or to chairs, or tables, or the floor; or made to see an object of every colour and hue, or metamorphosed into every nature, form, or creature, the operator may incline and indite. It may have been interesting enough to have demonstrated that the human mind could be so subjugated and controlled; but, as I have formerly said, and now repeat, **I do not consider the continual repetition of such experiments in the waking state, as at all proper, or free from the danger of throwing the faculties of the mind of such subjects into a permanently morbid condition.**

[Conclusion: The Power of the Mind]

It would be inconsistent with the scope of this paper to enter into an elaborate detail of my views as to the philosophical explanation of the modes of exciting and varying certain trains of ideas, and their consequent manifestations during the nervous sleep. The inquiry is not only curious, but also one of great interest, in respect to the power of the mind in controlling physical action, and of physical impressions in reacting on the mind. I have given a pretty ample discussion on these topics in **a second edition of my little work on hypnotism, now preparing for the press**, to which I beg leave to refer those who feel desirous of prosecuting the inquiry, and particularly those who desire to do so for curative purposes.

In conclusion, I beg particularly to remark, that, whilst my experiments and observations are opposed to the theoretical notions of Baron Reichenbach and the Mesmerists, in all the more important points, they directly confirm the reality of the facts, as to the power which we possess of artificially producing certain phenomena by certain processes; as also of intensifying aspects which arise in a minor degree, spontaneously, or by the patient's own unaided efforts. They allege that the exciting cause is the impulsion into the body of the patient from without of a portion of this new force; whilst I attribute it to a subjective or personal influence, namely, that of **the mind and body of the patient acting and re-acting on each other in a particular manner, from an intense concentration of inward consciousness on one idea, or train of ideas, which may, to a certain extent, be controlled and directed by others.** The latter power [of hypnotising others], however, merely arises from the mental and physical impressions producing still greater concentration of the patient's attention in a particular direction; that is to say, by concentrating their attention to the point over which they see anything drawn, or upon which a mechanical, calorific, frigorific, or electric impression is made, whereby a greater supply of nervous influence, blood, and vital action, is drawn to the part from the physical and mental resources of the patient himself, and not from the person or substance exciting those physical impressions. They enable the patient more effectually to concentrate his own vital powers, and thus to energise function; **on the same principle as a patient afflicted with anaesthesia, or loss of feeling, is able to hold an object in his hand whilst he looks at it, but will allow it to drop when his eyes are averted.**

It is worthy of particular remark, that my researches prove the power of concentration of attention, as not only capable of changing physical action, so as to make some patients, in the wide-waking state, imagine that they see and feel from an external influence what is due entirely to an internal or mental cause; but I have extended the researches, so as to prove, that the same law

obtains in respect to all the other organs of special sense, and different functions of the body. My theoretical views, therefore, instead of diminishing, rather enhance the value of this power as a means of cure. They strikingly prove how much may be achieved by proper attention to, and direction of, this power of the human mind over the physical frame, and *vice versa*, in ameliorating the ills which flesh is heir to. I beg further to remark, in support of my views, that in the experiments of Baron Reichenbach, and the Mesmerists generally, all which I have endeavoured to prove as requisite for the production of the phenomena referred to, is necessarily brought into play during their processes, in super-addition to their alleged Mesmeric fluid, or new force: of the latter, therefore, under such circumstances, I maintain that we have, as yet, no direct and satisfactory proof; and it is unphilosophical to attribute to a new and extraneous force what can be readily accounted for from the independent physical and psychical powers of the patient, which must necessarily be in active operation, along with their processes, and alleged new imponderable.[88]

---

[88] [Here, as elsewhere, Braid appears to be referring to the principle of parsimony or Occam's razor, in scientific method, which holds that entities, such as Reichenbach or the Mesmerists' new forces, should not be multiplied without necessity.]

Appendix:
On Muscular Suggestion

[Braid begins in the body of the text: 'Indeed, one of the most beautiful examples I have had of these "**vigilant phenomena**", in respect to all the senses, occurred in the case of a gentleman of high classical and mathematical attainments, as well as in general science. He had seen no experiments of the sort before I tested himself.']

When testing this gentleman, by requesting him to listen attentively and tell me what tune he heard from an object held near to, but not in close contact with his ear (it was merely a pencil case), he named a well-known *cheerful* tune. Without saying a single word, I applied the finger and thumb of my other hand so as slightly to corrugate the integuments of the forehead [i.e., making him frown], when he instantly said, "The tune is changed; it is Roslin Castle now." [This is probably the mournful, Scottish folk tune to which Robert Burns had set his song 'The Gloomy night is gath'ring fast.'] On my separating the fingers and thumb, so as to expand the integuments, he answered, that the music was lively again. These changes took place from the grave to the gay and *vice versa,* as often as I made the corresponding changes on the integuments. If I named any particular tune which he would hear, without touching him, he immediately thought he heard the tune I had named.

In like manner, having asked him to tell me what *smell* he felt when the pencil case was held to the nose, (it was a gold pencil case, and therefore could have had neither smell nor taste), he named an odour, but the moment I corrugated the integuments of the forehead, as before named, it changed for something disagreeable, and *vice versa* as often as such changes in the "Anatomy of Expression" were made. Similar delusions took place likewise in respect to taste, when he was requested to tell me what *taste* the pencil case had under different circumstances, being agreeable with the expanded and elevated state of the integuments, and the reverse when they were contracted or depressed. Visual spectra, in like manner, could be rendered agreeable or disagreeable, bright or sombre, according to similar changes in the physical frame. The philosophical explanation of all this I have entered into pretty fully in my forthcoming treatise on hypnotism or nervous sleep; and it is on these principles that I have endeavoured to account, in a very simple and natural manner, for the excitation of the phenomena of Mesmero-phrenology as they have been called, by touching certain parts of the scalp during Mesmeric sleep, where all sources of fallacy are guarded against from auricular suggestion or previous knowledge of phrenology. According to my apprehension, exciting these phenomena in such manner, many of which are extremely interesting and beautiful, neither proves nor disproves the doctrines of phrenology, but just leaves that subject where we found it.

"Observations on Mesmeric & Hypnotic Phenomena": Letter to *The Medical Times* (1844)

I have great pleasure in answering the "questions in hypnotism" proposed by "a Subscriber", in your 232nd number [of *The Medical Times*]. Numerous private letters intimate that my late communications have excited considerable interest, and I shall therefore add a few additional remarks by way of answering their queries, and also with the view of explaining some of the more interesting points which were not embraced in what I have already published.

I have frequently hypnotised *insane* patients, and with marked advantage; but hitherto I never could succeed in inducing sleep in a *decidedly fatuous* [i.e., mentally handicapped] case. This I attribute to the great difficulty of arresting their attention; and after numerous and prolonged trials, being unwilling to waste more time, I have abandoned them, although it is highly probable that a continuance of the means might have ultimately succeeded. I am therefore unable to speak from personal experience as to what might have been the result of hypnotism on a decidedly fatuous person, but for the benefit of your correspondent I shall transcribe the following case of Mesmeric somnambulism from the learned and truly interesting work of J.C. Colquhoun, Esq., "Isis Revelata". It is recorded at page 74 of vol. ii.

> In the same article from which I have extracted the preceding account of the two young magnetisers the author mentions that, at Landau, he once magnetised a lady of about thirty years of age who had been fatuous from her birth. She belonged to an opulent and distinguished family, who had used every possible means to endeavour to restore her intellect, but without success. When placed in a state of somnambulism, she conversed upon various matters with great propriety: she was no longer the same being; a person who saw her for the first time would never have suspected that she was deficient in mental energy. Her parents, who were present, were astonished, wept for joy and exclaimed "Ah! Why is she not always a somnambulist?

As to your correspondent's last queries whether I have tried the effects of nitrous oxide [laughing gas], and whether I consider it might be hazardous – I beg to state that I have never tried such experiments, and therefore, any opinion I could offer would be mere conjecture. However, I am by no means inclined either to try or recommend such experiments, because I am quite certain that hypnotism alone, as I apply and recommend it, is not only *a safe, but also a most valuable remedy for a class of diseases which resist all ordinary means*, and are, therefore, considered the "*opprobrium medicorum*" ["shame of the doctors", a disease for which no cure has been found]. I am consequently unwilling to hazard the reputation of hypnotism, but associating it with any doubtful allies. Were an untoward event to happen, especially in my hands, from any experiments instituted to gratify idle curiosity, or the mere love of science, it might be turned to the prejudice of what, in itself, is both harmless and valuable when properly used. The propriety of such caution will be apparent when we look to the prejudice which has been excited against Mesmerism by such untoward accidents as have lately happened, where the patients could not be aroused for hours, or even for several days. I am glad to be able to say such accidents ought not to happen *from hypnotism*, for I have never had a case which I could not arouse in two minutes. In this respect, as well as in its more certain and speedy induction of sleep, hypnotism is decidedly preferable to Mesmerism as a therapeutic agent.

In my communication in *The Medical Times* of 13th January last, my object was to point out certain sources of fallacy, likely to mislead the Mesmerists in respect to the marvels of clairvoyance, which they have recorded from time to time. Everyone knows the extraordinary marvels lately recorded in this way of the boy Cooke, at Deptford. I addressed a few queries to his master (who was the Mesmeriser in this case) which he most obligingly answered, and authorised me to make what use of I pleased. From these answers, compared with the sources of fallacy pointed out in the above paper, it was quite clear that there were no real clairvoyant powers exhibited by Cooke, all which appeared to Mr. Smith and others as such, being attributable to the condition I had explained in the above paper. The case itself was a valuable proof of the extraordinary influence which had been effected on the mental and physical functions by the Mesmeric processes; but the erroneous views arising from the supposed marvels of clairvoyance, have furnished a handle to sceptics to throw a doubt on the veracity and good faith of the parties most nearly and painfully interested in it.

In your 216th number, I made allusion to the remarkable fact of the influence of contact, during hypnotism, in exciting memory. Thus, at page 75, "A patient may be unable to answer the most simple question, on a subject with which he is quite familiar; but touch any part of his person with finger, or any inanimate substance, or cause him to place one of his own hands or fingers in contact with any other part of his own body, and immediately he will be able to reply correctly." The Mesmerists might be inclined to attribute this to a mental influence passing from the operator when he touched the patient, but then the fact of the patient's *own* touch or any mechanical contact being established by a person coming into the room, without knowing the question proposed, having the same effect, is quite fatal to such an inference. At page

148 of my work on hypnotism, I stated that the phrenologists' point "eventuality" [on the forehead] I had strong grounds for believing to be the chief seat of memory. **I was led into this error** from finding that patients, when touched on that point, could always answer correctly any question about past events, although unable to do so *without* such contact. The circumstance now noted, however, proves I was so far in error, as **contact *with any part of the body* would have produced similar results.** Whether it is by partially arousing the patient, and thus bringing him nearer to the waking condition, or by merely mechanically arousing and fixing or concentrating the attention in one direction, instead of the mind being allowed to wander uncontrolled, and incapable of fixing itself definitively on any subject, whilst addressed only through the organ of hearing, (or both combined) may admit of some doubt. It throws much light on the supposed special influence of the "rapport" of the Mesmerists, however; as it proves the attention may thus be excited to receive impressions to which it would otherwise be quite dormant. [This technique can be seen as a precursor of Freud's early "pressure technique".]

There is also a stage when there seems to be an extraordinary revivification of the memory, so that there is a lively remembrance of what had been long forgotten during the waking condition; and the power of imagination pointed out in my former paper, gives to these remembrances of past impressions, all the force and vividness of present realities. May this not have proved a special source of error in cases of supposed clairvoyance and intuition? [This seems to be one of several passages where Braid hints at the apparent use of hypnosis to recover forgotten memory.]

Another most probable ground of error arises from the interesting state of double consciousness, the existence of which I have proved in almost every case in which I have tested for it. By double consciousness I mean that there is a stage of sleep, when a patient may be taught anything, and be able to repeat it with verbal accuracy as often as in that stage again, whilst he may have no idea either of the subject or the words when in the waking condition. [Double consciousness, or "split consciousness", is therefore a state of profound hypnosis accompanied by *reversible* amnesia.] This is quite analogous to what is recorded of natural somnambulists; but it was some time before I discovered the exact stage for eliciting it, and I had consequently recorded this as a remarkable difference between natural and artificially induced somnambulism. The following are interesting examples of this condition. The detail of the first case is also most interesting, as illustrating the power of hypnotism in curing an obstinate disease.

Mr. Jones, eighteen years of age, applied to me at the beginning of last winter. About two years previously he had been attacked by a powerful dog, and was thrown violently on the ground which hurt his back considerably, and alarmed him greatly, although there was no wound inflicted on his person by the teeth of the dog. Shortly after this he was attacked with fits of an epileptic character, which went on increasing in frequency and severity, in defiance of the medical treatment prescribed. Previously to applying to me he had frequently been out of one fit into another, for whole nights together, and had some times six or seven attacks in a day besides. His sleep was thus quite destroyed – sometimes eight or nine nights passed entirely without sleep. When Mr. Jones first applied to me, I hypnotised him in the ordinary [i.e., cataleptic] mode, but without apparent improvement. I now prescribed medicines for him *in addition* to the hypnotism, but without benefit. He was, therefore, sent into the country, but returned without improvement. On the 6th of January last I resolved to try hypnotism alone, and *in that mode calculated to depress the circulation* [i.e., the relaxed state], and immediately the beneficial effects were most manifest. The first night he had no fit, next day only one, and from that day they declined both in force and frequency. On the fifth night he had a slight attack, and none since, being a respite of more than ten weeks. [Notably, in this case, Braid implies that the cure depended upon the induction of a relaxed state antagonistic to anxiety, pre-empting Wolpe's use of reciprocal inhibition in behaviour therapy.] In order to test the extent of the double consciousness in this case, before he entered the room, I wrote a letter to him, and having explained my intention to a scientific friend (without the patient's knowledge), in the presence of my friend, after the patient was asleep, I read over the note, requesting him to repeat it after me, which after the second reading he did, *with verbal accuracy*, excepting the date, which he placed *after*, instead of *before*, the month. I considered this of no material consequence, and therefore deposited the letter in a drawer, and in a little time after aroused the patient, who remembered nothing of what had been done, said, or heard during his sleep. The following day, after being asleep and passed into the same stage as the previous day, the letter was taken out of the drawer, and held at a distance by one gentleman, whilst myself and another who was present the day previous, listened attentively to hear what he would say, when asked to repeat the letter he had from the day before. He repeated it *with verbal accuracy*. Shortly after he was aroused, when I asked if he remembered anything of what had been said or done during his sleep, he remembered nothing. I then asked if he received a letter from me the day before, to which he replied in the negative, and moreover added that he had never in his life received a letter from me. I told him that during his sleep he had admitted so, and even repeated its contents. He looked surprised at this, and could only be made to believe I was not hoaxing him by the other two gentlemen assuring him it was true. I then gave him the letter to read, and told him he had repeated the very words he now read, as a letter which he had received from me the day before. To this he replied, that as we all said so he was bound to believe us, but that to him it appeared a very strange affair, as he had not the slightest recollection of anything of the kind. After he had returned the letter to me, I requested him to repeat it now that he had read it whilst awake; but he could not repeat a single line, only a few of the leading words, and the general purport of the letter. He never saw the letter from that moment; but on every occasion when asleep since, he has repeated it with verbal accuracy, but remembers nothing of it when awake. About two weeks after the first trial, when he was asleep, I requested him to write me a copy of the said letter, which he did whilst a book was held betwixt his eyes and the paper. Of course he wrote, as he and other patients always do, under hypnotism, and as pointed out in my communication of the 13th January last, by feeling. The following are the original and copy which differ only in two unimportant words:—

> Sir, I am glad to inform you that you will have not more fits. Your case is a good proof of the power and use of hypnotism, and your sister's case also proves this equally well. – I remain, Sir, your obedient Servant,
> James Braid
> Manchester, 18th Jan. 1844"

> (Copy.)
> Sir, I am very glad to inform you that you will have no more fits. Your case is a good proof of the power and use of hypnotism, and your sister's proves this equally well. – I remain, Dear Sir, your obedient Servant,
> James Braid
> Manchester 18th Jan. 1844

Mr. Jones called on me on the 11th March, after an absence of five weeks. He was quite well, and when hypnotised, repeated the above letter with verbal accuracy, but remembered nothing of it after being aroused. His sister, who was speedily cured of spinal irritation by hypnotism, manifested double consciousness also.

Of course such experiments would be of no value, unless performed on patients on whose veracity we could repose the most implicit confidence; but I have now repeated them on so many patients of both sexes, with like results, and on individuals on whose veracity I can confidently rely, that there can be no doubt of the fact. Here there is another grand source of fallacy regarding investigations into clairvoyance and Mesmeric intuition. I have myself taught patients Greek, Latin, French, and Italian in this way, which they remembered quite correctly when again hypnotised, but of which they were quite ignorant when awake. Their great faculty for imitation while hypnotised, renders them very quick in catching the pronunciation; and the memory – that is, this double conscious, or second memory – seems to be very powerful.

It, therefore, seems highly probable that much of what has been considered Mesmeric intuition may be nothing more than the extraordinary conditions of memory referred to; at one stage revivifying waking impressions long forgotten, and at another this second, or double conscious memory, enabling them to remember impressions and ideas excited during this artificial sleep, of which they have never had any knowledge during the waking condition. Let these facts be kept in view, together with the extraordinary acuteness of the senses formerly pointed out, which enables them to detect physical changes, and conditions, and remarks, which all around (judging from the state of the senses in the normal condition) imagine to be impossible, and the power of detecting disease and prescribing for such, in this condition, may be far less marvellous than has hitherto been represented. In short, they may have acquired their knowledge through hints and observations dropt in their presence at different times, and of which neither the patients nor operators were aware when the impressions were made. **As to patients, under such circumstances, predicting particular crises, especially spasmodic seizures, in their own individual cases, I think it highly probable that** *such predications produced the results* **– results which might not have happened, but for the impressions left by those predications.** [Pre-empting modern cognitive therapy, Braid attributes hysterical attacks to negative beliefs, i.e., self-fulfilling prophecies.] **Many may be ready to admit this as regards a patient, who, in the vigilant state, has heard such oracular predictions regarding his future conditions. They may be ready to admit that imagination and memory might powerfully influence such patients, whilst they would deny the possibility of the somnolent patient being affected in a similar manner by such predictions. It is a well-known fact, that many people can, before going to bed, determine to awake at an unusual hour (for them) in the morning, and shall awake almost to the minute. Now, it is quite as difficult to account for** *this* **result, as to suppose that during the state of somnambulism, an impression may be made upon the mind which shall become manifest at a fixed time, in the** *waking condition*. In fact, many experiments are recorded confirmatory of this latter result – cases where patients have been made to promise whilst asleep, to perform some particular act, or go to some particular place at a time agreed on by both parties, and whilst the patients have entirely forgotten the circumstances when aroused, *they have had a vivid recollection of them when the particular period arrived*, and have performed their promises with care and punctuality. [A phenomenon now termed "post-hypnotic suggestion."]

It is important to remark, that in the double consciousness we have a most beautiful provision, under Providence, to protect patients against the villainy which might be perpetrated against them by parties getting them to sign deeds, *etc.*, whilst in this state; for although quite unconscious of this when awake, so soon as again rendered somnambulic, they would recollect all, and be able to give evidence against the perpetrators of such villainy.

When we consider the length of time the investigations have been prosecuted and the numbers engaged in it, I think every one must be struck with the small number of apparently satisfactory cases of clairvoyance which have been recorded. Comparatively few have met with them in their own practice. Then there is the acknowledged uncertainty of success, even the most clairvoyant patients being generally oftener wrong than right; whereas, were the answers from the true perception, they ought always to be right. Then there is vagueness of their replies, which are generally given in such prophetic language as may admit of different interpretations.

I think it is much to be desired that a series of experiments were instituted before an intelligent and respectable committee, who, fully aware of these various sources of fallacy, might investigate cases so as to ascertain what of the higher phenomena of the Mesmerists may be real, and what erroneous. Of course experiments of this sort should be performed on *fresh subjects*, who should only be experimented on before the said committee, and thus the decision of such committee should set the matter at rest. It must thus arrest much of the prejudice which at present exists against a valuable curative means, owing to the alleged mysterious agency, and omniscient and omnipotent powers of this agency, as hitherto propounded by the Mesmerists; for, I strongly suspect the extreme difficulty of the subject, and the numerous sources of error I have referred to, and which might be readily overlooked by those blinded by their attachment to a fascinating and mysterious theory, have led them to a belief in much more than can be fairly and truly realised by the volition – the unaided volition and simple contact of the operator. In such investigation, however, it would be quite requisite that the parties engaged in it should be as much as possible free from prejudice, candid and intelligent. Moreover, without considerable knowledge of *this* subject, they could be no more competent to test and form a correct estimate of what they witnessed (because of their knowledge of physiology and its phenomena in the normal state) than he who from being familiar with the common rules of arithmetic, should be, therefore, deemed a competent judge of the solutions of the most abstruse mathematical problems. In every other department of science, a thorough knowledge of *all* the states and conditions is considered necessary to warrant a person to give an opinion to be relied on; but, in the investigation of Mesmeric phenomena, this pre-requisite qualification has been entirely and most unaccountably overlooked; and hence the conflicting statements which we continually meet with. Truth is sure ultimately to prevail, and the sooner we can determine what is true from what is erroneous, the better, whether it may accord with, or be opposed to, our preconceived notions and prejudices. I hope the proposal by the editor of *The Critic*, of forming such committee in the metropolis, may be carried into effect.

In my work on Hypnotism [*Neurypnology*, 1843] I have expressed the difficulty of accounting for the remarkable effects of a current of air in arousing dormant senses, and reducing the cataleptiform state, and I solicited information on this intricate point from any readers of that work. No one having ventured to hazard an opinion I beg to state what has since occurred to me as the cause.

In the normal state, whether, whilst awake or passing into natural sleep, the attention is dissipated or diffused to a greater or lesser extent over the *whole* of the mental and physical functions, but, during a certain stage of hypnotism, there is a tendency to intense concentration of the attention to whatever function is called into action, and hence all the others merge rapidly into a deep state of torpor, ultimately far greater than what happens during natural sleep. Thus, only one function is active at any one time, and hence intensely active; and the rousing into activity of any dormant function must consequently be equivalent to suspending the one previously in action.

Moreover the impressibility of the sense of heat and cold *becomes exalted* whilst common sensation [the sense of touch] is *depressed*, so that whilst a limb may be insensible to pricking or pinching, it shall be slightly sensible to transitions of temperature so as to enable patients to perceive objects without natural contact. They are thus enabled, like the blind, to move about during their sleep without running against the furniture of an apartment however much disarranged. In this condition a waft of air directed against an elevated and rigid limb, by acting on the increased sensibility to heat and cold, instantly draws the attention to the function of the skin, withdraws it from the muscular sense, and thus the rigid muscles yield, and the member falls from its own gravity. The intense concentration of the *vis nervosa* [nervous energy] on muscular action, which had energised and heightened this to the condition of cataleptiform rigidity, is thus arrested, a new direction given to it, and a correspondingly intense state of the ventricular function, or sensibility to pricking and pinching, as well as heat and cold, is the result of this simple waft of air. A current of air being directed against any of the other organs of sense arouses their sensibility for the same reason – namely, that it directs the attention entirely to the function of the particular organs, which consequently becomes highly exalted, whilst that formerly in action is suspended.

When the patient has lapsed into that state in which the sense of heat and cold, as well as common feeling has become suspended, then those changes can be less efficiently and less rapidly effected. In this case the patient should be wafted over the face with cool air till partially aroused, when he may be acted on in the manner, and with results similar to those pointed out in the stage which has just been described. It ought never to be forgotten that during this condition the *patient acts under a peculiar state of consciousness and volition subject to definite laws, although when awake, he may remember nothing of what he had done.* Even at the risk of being deemed tautological, I beg to repeat that the peculiarity I refer to is the great docility and tendency to imitation; vivid imagination and concentration of the whole attention the subject in hand; and also the extreme acuteness of any of the organs of special sense when called into action. The consequence of all this is, that the patients perceive and obey the will of those present, by impressions on the senses which could not be perceived during the waking condition; and the intense concentration of the attention to the particular function in action, energises it to an extraordinary degree.

In the *Dublin University Magazine* for this month, I observe some remarks on the opinions and practice set forth in my work on hypnotism. I beg to thank the author of the paper for the handsome manner in which he has noticed my labours in this field of inquiry. Like many others he alleges that I am naturally a powerful magnetizer, and that whilst I am holding an object for the patient to gaze at, I am unconsciously Mesmerising him by the influence of my will and physical frame; and he adds, that were I to throw aside my lancet case, and Mesmerise by the hand only, he has no doubt but I would produce effects which would surprise myself. In reply to this, I beg to state that, on innumerable occasions, I have operated by the ordinary Mesmerising processes – including thumbing and staring, singly and combined; pointing; passes, near and at a little distance; willing the effect in the most intense manner, and at other times willing the patient should *not* sleep, but I have never witnessed an *essential* difference in the results. Nor could the patients themselves discern any, unless that my ordinary mode was more rapid and intense. We produce varieties by different processes, undoubtedly; and it seems to me that the great error with most experimenters has arisen from their not discriminating betwixt a *mere variety*, and *a distinct, or separate principle*. My ordinary mode of operating is decidedly the most rapid and intense, and the varieties which are afterwards elicited, I imagine, depend on the different modes of acting on the mind and body through impressions on the organs of sense. I have never myself produced an effect by *unaided volition*, and some of the most eminent Mesmerists now make the same admission. Nor have I ever met with a case of decided clairvoyance or Mesmeric intuition; but all the other phenomena of the Mesmerists, and such as can be made available in the cure of disease, I can produce with much greater certainty and celerity by my own processes than by theirs; and I have tried both methods fairly. The author of the paper referred to not only alleges that I *unconsciously* Mesmerise my patients during my hypnotising processes, but he also attributes much of the benefit which patients derive from their ordinary medical attendants, to a transmission of a Mesmeric influence passing, unperceived, from the body of the physician, to that of his patient, from their proximity during professional visits.

That a patient may derive much benefit from the *personal* attendance of a judicious and intelligent medical man, irrespective of the more natural effects of the medicines he may prescribe, I am quite ready to admit; but, instead of attributing this to a *Mesmeric* process, I consider it arises from the cheering influence of hope and confidence, which his presence, and manner, and conversation, may have inspired into the mind of his patient. [We now refer to the "non-specific" (or placebo) psychotherapeutic effects of mere attention from a sympathetic therapist.]

In like manner, the perusal of a letter may excite or depress the person who reads it, according to the purport of its contents; and, if received immediately before sitting down to a meal, for which he had a keen appetite, it may instantly destroy his appetite. Here, then, is a physical effect produced by a mental emotion. Is this the result of magnetism – and, if so, how comes it so to act that no such effect took place from the *mere proximity of the letter, but only for the perusal of its contents?*

As an additional illustration, I shall here quote from your own pages a most graphic and judicious reference to the importance of psychical medicine.

> The generality of medical men attach too exclusive an importance to the efficacy of the mere drug. They deal with people as if there were nothing psychical in them. If their diagnosis be correct, they write their prescription, and there is a stop to their operations. If part of the frame be diseased, there is no reason why the whole should not combine against the enemy. Faith saves physically as well as morally: and to lull the trembling mind to ease, is to stay the heart's rapid pulsations, to allay the blood's fever, and to stop life in its quickening flight, with strengthened wings, from the human tenement.

That the nervous sleep may be induced by the personal acts of the patient [i.e., by *self*-hypnosis], irrespective of any influence, either of a mental or physical nature, from another individual, I have abundant proof. I shall relate the particulars of three cases, all of whom hypnotised themselves, *for the first time*, at a distance of forty miles from where I was during the proceedings, and of whose intentions I knew nothing; indeed, one was a young lady whom I never saw in my life, and over whom I could not, therefore, be presumed to have any control. She proposed to hypnotise herself by a fixed stare, and abstraction of the attention. My family, who were present, urged her *not* to try such an experiment, but she reclined her head on her hand, as if fatigued, and in a very short time, to their surprise, they found she was decidedly hypnotised. The other was a young gentleman about twenty years of age, who, by a fixed stare at a point in the ceiling, speedily hypnotised himself. At a second trial, he lapsed so profoundly into the condition, and not being aroused at the proper stage, nor any of the parties present understanding how to manage it properly, that two hours elapsed before he was restored to the waking condition. I have since operated on this gentleman, but I aroused him in a few seconds, which I accomplished by observing the progress of the case, and not suffering it to go too far. The third was a gentleman about thirty-five years of age, healthy and energetic, who hypnotised himself by gazing at a point of the ceiling of his own room, and having elevated his legs and arms, those present soon ascertained that they were rigidly cataleptiform. He has repeatedly done this since, with like results. I could adduce abundance of cases similar to these, and I would ask whose magnetic influence of volition produced the results?

But, moreover, it is well known that there are many natural somnambulists, who become so in despite of their own will, as well as that of their friends. The same may be said of cases of catalepsy, which arise spontaneously in the course of disease. Now, as they frequently occur when no one is present with such patients, I would ask whose volition or magnetic influence is the efficient cause in *such* cases? As already stated, that it is quite possible to produce varieties in the effects, by varying the processes resorted to for acting on the mind and body, I am quite ready to admit; and am equally well convinced that it is possible to act powerfully on many people by exciting their imagination, and leading them to believe that by personal contact and passes, they are being acted on *by some mysterious agency*; but, philosophically considered, they are mere varieties of the same principle. It is still objective, or personal influence, and would not become efficient unless by the patient's belief, or compliance with certain conditions.

As many imagine that *excitement of the circulation* [usually associated with the rigid cataleptic state] is a *necessary* consequence of being thrown into the hypnotic, or Mesmeric state, I shall offer a few remarks in refutation of this erroneous notion. It may be made *either to excite or depress the force and frequency of the heart's action, according to the mode of management*. As a proof of its influence in *depressing* the circulation, and *promoting perspiration*, and *reducing febrile action* [i.e., fever], I shall record the result of its application in three cases of severe *scarlatina anginosa* [i.e., scarlet fever]. On the 15th Dec. 1843, I was requested to visit the family of Mr. C. I found his eldest son, who was fourteen years of age, suffering from an intense attack of *scarlatina anginosa*. The throat was much ulcerated, the rash partially visible, pulse about 150 strokes a minute, intense headache, considerable delirium, and a pungently hot and dry skin. His sister, four years of age, was in a very similar condition, only the pulse was a few beats a minute slower. I hypnotised both, and on arousing them, the mother, well aware of the difficulty of producing perspiration in such cases, was extremely surprised to *find both patients bathed in perspiration*. The pulse of the eldest, I found was reduced to 110, and that of the younger to 118; the headache and delirium almost gone; and the child, who had slept none for two nights, and was with difficulty kept in bed, in a quarter of an hour fell into a sound sleep, from which she did not awake for two hours. I prescribed the ordinary treatment in all other respects. The following day I found both patients with perspirable skins, the pulse of the eldest below 100, the sister's a little higher, and every other symptom satisfactory. I hypnotised them again on that and the following day, and nothing could be more satisfactory than the result, the convalescence being rapid for such severe cases of that disease; and there was much less extensive desquamation [i.e., flaking of the skin] than usual in such cases. A week after, a third member of the family, six years of age, was seized with the disease, and displayed similar symptoms to the others just recorded. I treated this patient in the same manner, and with like results; namely, the immediate reduction of the pulse, and flow of perspiration, with relief of headache. The case went on so much the same as the two last, that I deem it unnecessary to say more than that her convalescence was equally satisfactory.

I could easily adduce additional cases of an intensely febrile character, where an equally remarkable reduction of the pulse, and relief from headache immediately followed the operation of hypnotism, whilst the patient was made to recline and the muscular system was kept relaxed during the sleep, but I deem it unnecessary. The above were the first cases of *scarlatina* in which I had tried hypnotism, and I could not but feel gratified to find its extraordinary influence on the capillary circulation, so as to produce a profuse perspiration in a few minutes, in an intense case of such a disease. In fact, the force of the disease was instantly broken; and, from being a formidable disease, by this simple process it was reduced to a mild and manageable affection.[89]

---

[89] [Braid, "Observations on Mesmeric and Hypnotic Phenomena", The Medical Times, 13th April 1844 & 20th April 1844, vol. x., 1844, pp. 31-32 and 47-49.]

"On Thomas Wakley & John Elliotson":
Letter to *The Medical Times* (1844)

> **Editor's Preface**
> This short letter is Braid's response to the notorious argument between Thomas Wakley, editor of *The Lancet* and one of Mesmerism's staunchest critics, and John Elliotson, editor of *The Zoist*, and the pre-eminent British Mesmerist. Braid occupies a kind of *via media* between the two extremes represented by these authors. Whereas Elliotson believed the effects of Mesmerism were real and due to a genuine invisible force ("animal magnetism"), Wakley thought the effects were bogus and due merely to deception, *i.e.*, that the whole thing was false. Braid concludes, as the French Academy of Sciences imply in their early reports on Mesmerism, that the effects of Mesmerism are real enough, but that they are due to normal physical and psychological causes, such as attention and suggestion, rather than any paranormal force emanating from the Mesmerist. To make this distinction clear, Braid abandoned the terminology of Mesmer and coined the name "neuro-hypnotism" for his own method.

Sir,

I now forward the contribution which I promised at the conclusion of my last communication. I trust my remarks may tend to remove some erroneous notions which have prevailed, and which have tended, in no small degree, to keep up unwarrantable prejudices against the introduction of a most important mode of treating various intractable diseases.

The credulity alone of the marvellous in some of its friends, and the inveterate hostility of its opponents, have been equally prejudicial to Mesmerism. Each party has drawn conclusions too hurriedly, and from too narrow a field of observation; and opinions, and prejudices once promulgated have been contended for in many instances, with a zeal and pertinacity inconsistent with all true philosophical inquiry. Could a more eminent example of this be adduced than Mr. Wakley's experiments and observations in reference to the Okeys afford? [The Okey sisters were two young girls, suffering from epilepsy, who were used by Elliotson as his main demonstration subjects.] Dr. Elliotson had set forth that certain metals had the power of Mesmerising patients, whilst others had no such influence, and he offered to allow Mr. Wakley to operate on the Misses Okey to prove this. Mr. Wakley operated with the *non*-Mesmerising metal, whilst the patient was led to *believe* he was operating with the *Mesmerising one,* and *she fell asleep* again. He operated next with the *Mesmerising* metal, *whilst the patient believed it to be the OTHER, and no sleep resulted.* Now, this was a well-contrived and well conducted experiment to prove *whether the metals really possessed such opposite influences*, and the experiments clearly proved that Dr. Elliotson had been in error in regard to his *theory*; but then Mr. Wakley promulgated an equally erroneous, and far more heartless one, in publishing to the world, and reiterating and glorifying in it *that the patients were imposters*; and that, consequently, *all Mesmeric phenomena were unmitigated imposture.* My paper will illustrate the subject, and prove that the legitimate inference which should have been drawn from these experiments, was the extraordinary power of imagination, sympathy, and habit over those previously impressed. As recorded in page 61 of my work on Hypnotism [*Neurypnology*, 1843], "I have varied my experiments in every possible form, and clearly proved the power of imagination *over those previously impressed*, as the patients have become hypnotised (the term I use instead of Mesmerised) or not by the same appliance, according to the result which they previously expected."

Again, the circumstances detailed by Dr. Smethurst in your last number, are well calculated to give a handle to sceptics; but granting that the whole of what he witnessed that night was gross imposition from beginning to end, he is by no means thus warranted to draw his rash conclusions, that therefore, "Thus ends, I trust, at least in these parts, Mesmerism, a thing too contemptible in itself to engage the attention of any but such as the Great Wizard of the North [John Henry Anderson, a famous stage magician] or a pantomimic actor."

I would beg to remind this gentleman and others of the same temperament, that neither the theoretical errors, the extreme credulity, or ignorance, or intended imposture of a few of its professors can *now* stop – and the greater the pity if they *could* stop – the progress of such important investigations as Mesmerism and hypnotism, the objects of which are the development of modes of acting, by which we can exercise such a powerful control over the nervous system, and through it over the whole body, producing remarkable phenomena, and which may be turned to such useful purposes in the cure of disease, as may be readily demonstrated to the conviction of every candid and intelligent mind. Even the French commission of 1784 bore testimony *to the reality of the phenomena.* What they disputed was Mesmer's power of proving to them the existence of a magnetic fluid as the *cause* of the phenomena. They vaguely attributed the phenomena to the influence of the imagination, instead of to that of a magnetic fluid as alleged by Mesmer.

This was the real extent of their condemnation, which has been so constantly and triumphantly referred to in opposition to the pretensions of Mesmerism.

Again, the second French commission prosecuted the inquiry for five years, and drew up a report of the whole with great care, which was read to the Academy in 1831. After a variety of references to particular phenomena which followed certain experiments, and bearing testimony to its curative powers, as demonstrated in cases so treated in their presence, they recorded the following important remarks:- "Considered as a cause of certain physiological phenomena, or as a therapeutic remedy, magnetism ought to be allowed a place within the circle of the medical sciences; and, consequently, physicians only should practise it, or superintend its use, as in the northern countries. Your committee have communicated, in their report, facts of sufficient importance to entitle them to think that the Academy ought to encourage the investigation into the subject of animal magnetism, as a very curious branch of psychology and natural history."

When it is considered that these opinions were given *after five years' investigation*, and that the report was signed by Bourdois de la Motte, President Fouquier, Gueneau de Mussy, Guersent, Husson, Itard, J.J. Leroux, Marc, and Thillaye, it ought to put to shame those who presumptuously venture to pronounce an opposite opinion upon and condemn what they have never had opportunity, or taken pains, practically, to understand. Is it not notorious, that the great opponents of Mesmerism and hypnotism are *those who never studied it practically*, or who *have done so in the most superficial manner*, whilst those who were most violently opposed to it *through theory and book knowledge only*, have soon become convinced of the reality of the phenomena upon personal and careful investigation? I myself am of the latter class, and whoever will investigate the subject with an honest desire to arrive at truth, cannot long remain in doubt as to the reality and extraordinary nature of the phenomena, whatever difficulty he may experience in ascertaining the true cause of them. I would earnestly recommend all who engage in this study to endeavour as much as possible, to separate *facts* from *theories* – to study each apart. Let each individual conduct experiments for himself in the different modes recommended, and with an honest desire to arrive at truth, and there can be no doubt but he will soon be convinced, that by artificial contrivance the nervous system can be thrown into a new condition, which may be rendered eminently useful in the cure of disease. It appears to me that the knowledge of this fact, and the best modes of applying the agency, is of far more consequence than disputing about theoretical quibbles, which may never be determined to the satisfaction of all parties, as to the *modus operandi* of the means by which we produce our results.

I remain, Sir, your most obedient servant,

James Braid, M.R.C.S. Edin., etc.

3, St. Peter's Square,
Manchester.
16th December 1843.[90]

---

[90] ["Mr. Braid on Mesmerism", from The Medical Times, 6th January 1844, vol. ix., p. 203.]

"On Muscular Suggestion": Braid's Letters on Phreno-Hypnotism (1843-1844)

Editor's Preface
Donald Robertson

In a series of letters published immediately after *Neurypnology* (1843), Braid elaborates upon his theory of "phreno-hypnotism". It had become fashionable at this time for Mesmerism and phrenology to be combined into a theory known as Phreno-Mesmerism. Phreno-Mesmerism held that the vital force of the Mesmerist could be channelled into the body of the subject by touching specific regions of the scalp, in such a way as to affect the function of (supposed) regions of the brain, or "phrenological organs".

Braid carried out a number of small experiments which suggested an alternative explanation of the observed effects of phreno-Mesmerism. He found evidence to suggest that subjects in hypnosis or Mesmerism could become particularly sensitive to touch, and that the muscles of their body tended to contract when touched in this way. Braid felt that this led to changes in muscle tone, facial expression and body posture, sometimes quite subtle, which evoked subjective feelings, such as powerful emotional responses, by mental association. That is, normally our desires and emotions give rise to typical movements or facial expressions. By physically manipulating the body so as to create these same changes, the process could be reversed, and the emotions arise as the *effect* of their typical physical expressions. Braid refers to the "anatomy of expression", the physical language of emotion. He appeals to the philosopher Dugald Stewart's "law of sympathetic imitation", as a simple explanation of how physical states can evoke associated emotional reactions. In the *Experimental Inquiry* (1844) on phrenology here, and later in his *Observations on Trance* (1850), Braid uses the term "*muscular suggestion*" to denote the mechanism, which appears to have been more central to his therapeutic method, throughout his career, than the use of auditory (verbal) suggestion, common in modern hypnotherapy.

Braid even realises that the manipulation of the body in this way is a familiar notion to many actors, who realise that adopting physical mannerisms and facial expressions, etc., may help them to experience certain emotions associated with the role they are enacting. Decades after Braid's death, this notion was developed even further by Stanislavski in his system for training actors.

In these letters, Braid also speaks of *three* stages of hypnotism, instead of two, writing, 'There are three stages of sensation in the hypnotic condition.'

First (Conscious) Stage: Increased Awareness & Muscular Pliancy

According to Braid's article, the first stage is "characterised by increased sensibility, docility, and pliancy, so that any part readily yields or moves in the direction of the force applied, and will remain in the position in which it is placed". He says this is 'the condition called pliant catalepsy'.

Second (Conscious) Stage: Increased Awareness & Slight Catalepsy

"The second stage is that where there is increased sensibility and slight rigidity, with a tendency to contraction in the muscles immediately subjacent to the points touched or titillated." Braid states that this is the 'proper stage for exciting the manifestations' of phreno-hypnotism described in his approach.

He states that the technique of muscular suggestion used in this stage may be described as employing the "*direct* mode" as "it results from the stimulus being applied directly to the particular muscles to be roused".

Third (Torpid) Stage: Decreased Awareness & Rigid Catalepsy

"The third stage is that where there is rigidity of all the muscles, or rigid catalepsy, with *diminished* tactual sensibility. In this case, the patient may be pricked or pinched with little or no feeling; but continued gentle pressure or friction will *reduce the rigidity* in the *subjacent muscles*, and the member will be gradually drawn in the opposite direction, in consequence of the continued undiminished action of their antagonists."

In the third stage, "it will be found that the manifestations are inverted, those regions of the head corresponding to the animal propensities in the *second* stage, exciting the moral sentiments in the third stage, and *vice versa*; and the same with the extremities."

Hence, the technique of muscular suggestion in this stage may be called "the *in*direct mode", because "the motion is excited by *reducing the power of the antagonist* muscles".

In this stage, one side of the body may be "reduced" to the second stage so that opposite responses may be evoked in different sides of the body by the same manipulations.

Observations on the Phenomena of Phreno-Mesmerism (1843)

By Mr. James Braid, Surgeon, Manchester.
(From *The Medical Times* of November 11th, 1843.)
To the Editor of *The Medical Times*.

Sir,

In the preface of my work on "Hypnotism, or Nervous Sleep", lately published, I promised to institute a farther series of experiments on the phenomena of Phreno-Mesmerism, and to publish the results. Judging from the rapid sale of my book (nearly eight hundred copies having been disposed of in a few months) that the subject of Hypnotism and Mesmerism is now commanding general attention, both from the public and the profession, I feel anxious to redeem the pledge referred to as soon as possible, and know no better mode of doing so than by publishing the results in your liberal and widely diffused journal. Your inserting my paper at your earliest convenience will oblige, Sir, your most obedient Servant,

James Braid, M.R.C.S.E., etc.
3 St Peter's Square,
Manchester.
4th November, 1843.

The power we acquire during Mesmeric, hypnotic, or nervous sleep, of exciting the passions, emotions, and mental manifestations, through impressions made on different parts of the body, has produced much speculation as to the cause from whence it springs:

1st, Some [Phreno-Mesmerists] have attributed it to the *will* of the *operator*, exercising a direct influence on the nervous system of the patient, and thus affecting the bodies and minds of both similarly and simultaneously, or singly, according to the volition of the operator;

2nd, Others [Phreno-Mesmerists], to a magnetic medium transmitted from the operator, and stimulating the organ, or portion of the brain, directly subjacent, or from a distance, through what they call the poles of the particular cerebral organs;

3rd, Others [sceptics], to previous knowledge of phrenology, suggesting the idea to the mind when any particular organ was touched [i.e., expectation], or to a system of training whereby any mental idea might be excited in the mind of the patient, through arbitrary association with *any* part of the body [i.e., conditioning];

4th, In the sixth chapter of my work, entitled, "Neurypnology, or the Rationale of Nervous Sleep considered in relation with Animal Magnetism", lately published [1843], I endeavoured to reduce it to the laws of sympathy and association [in accord with the philosophy of Dugald Stewart], connected with automatic muscular action (that is, by titillating certain combinations of nerves, corresponding muscles were called into action), and to show that this muscular action renovated the past feelings with which it was ordinarily associated during the waking condition, in the active manifestation of the various emotions and propensities of the mind. [In *Observations on Trance* (1850), Braid calls this notion "muscular suggestion".]

Some of the highest authorities (Dr. Elliotson included) both as to Phrenology and Mesmerism, admit, that the same manifestations result from contact, or pointing over the previously excited parts of their patients, whether the operator knows or is ignorant of the part acted on; whether he wills or does not will any particular manifestation; whether he is a sceptic, and may be supposed to *will a contrary result*, or is a person entirely ignorant of Phrenology. Moreover, in some of my experiments, recorded at pages 141-3 of the above work, I proved, that by asking a patient to point to a particular organ, he would generally be wrong in respect to the organ named; but that the points pressed on gave their ordinary manifestations, even whilst the mind of the patient was directed to a different emotion or propensity. I therefore consider these facts are quite sufficient to refute the *first* theory [i.e., a kind of telepathy or telekinesis].

The facts also resulting from patients manipulating their own heads, as just stated, I consider sufficient proof that the excitation did not arise from any influence, either mental or physical, passing from those present to the patient, as their *own* contact produced the results. Moreover, the manifestations in most instances were entirely different from the ideas existing in the mind of the person who requested the patient to touch such and such organs or points of his body; and the like results are found to arise from any similar mechanical contact, in whatever manner it is brought into apposition with the patient, or from other impressions, such as electricity, galvanism, heat or cold, pulling a hair, *etc.* And, again, by allowing patients to pass into the *third* stage of sensation (which I shall immediately explain) before manipulating, it will be found that the manifestations are inverted, those regions of the head corresponding to the animal propensities in the *second* stage, exciting the moral sentiments in the third stage, and *vice versa*; and the same with the extremities. Or a still more interesting experiment may be performed thus:– Allow the patient to pass into the *third* stage, then reduce one side to the second stage before manipulation, and it will be found that the *opposite* manifestations will be educed from the relative points of the two sides of the head, trunk, and extremities. I consider these facts are quite at variance with the *second* theory [i.e., magnetism].

In respect to the *third*, that the phenomena *might* be excited by previous knowledge of Phrenology, or by a system of training, so as to establish artificial and arbitrary associations, I never could entertain a doubt, knowing as I do the extreme docility of patients, and the acuteness of the senses and mental functions at a certain state of hypnotism. I directed especial attention to these points so long ago as December, 1841. However, such a system I consider arbitrary and artificial, in contradistinction to the fourth, which I call the *natural* mode. I call that the *natural* mode, because it requires no training, but arises from the anatomical relations of the physical frame. In most patients the phenomena will come out more promptly, or more prominently, after having been previously excited, as all functions may become more facile from habit; but still the phenomena referred to *may* be excited at *first* trial, and *without* training, verbal prompting, or previous knowledge, to direct as to what is expected, *provided the manipulations are instituted at the proper stage*.

At page 146 of my work on "Neurypnology", after giving particular directions for eliciting the manifestations, I stated my views thus:

> Whispering, or talking, should be carefully avoided by all present, so as to leave Nature to manifest herself in her own way, influenced only by the stimulus conveyed through the nerves of touch exciting to automatic muscular action. We all know that during common sleep a person unconsciously changes from an uncomfortable position to one which is agreeable. This is a sort of instinctive action, and, as already explained, I think it highly probable, that by thus calling into action muscles which are naturally so exerted in manifesting any given emotion or propensity, they may, by reflection, thereby rouse that portion of the brain, the activity of which usually excites the motion. In this case, there would be an inversion of the ordinary sequence, what is naturally the consequence becoming the cause of cerebral and mental excitation. The following hypothesis will illustrate my meaning. It is easy to imagine that putting a pen or pencil in the hand might excite the idea of writing or drawing; or that stimulating the gastrocnemius, which raises us on our toes, might naturally enough suggest to the mind the idea of dancing, without any other suggestion to that effect than what arises from the attitude and activity of the muscles, naturally and necessarily brought into play whilst exercising such functions. However, I would very much doubt the probability of stimulation of the muscles of the leg exciting the idea of writing, or that putting a pen or pencil in the hand would excite the idea of dancing, without previous concert and arrangement to that effect. It is upon the same principle, as I imagine, that during the dreamy state of hypnotism, by stimulating the *sterno-mastoid* muscle, which causes an inclination of the head, the idea of friendship and shaking of hands is excited in the mind; and when the *trapezius* is excited at the same time, the greater lateral inclination of the head manifests still greater attachment, or "adhesiveness". Pressure on the vertex, by calling into action all the muscles requisite to sustain the body in the erect position, excites the idea of "unyielding firmness", etc., etc.

In following out this idea, I immediately found that my conjecture was correct, and that **the same phenomena might be excited through the muscles of the trunk and extremities, as through those of the head and face.** Thus, in patients who had never seen experiments of the kind, and who had no knowledge of anatomy and physiology, I succeeded at once in eliciting any manifestation I chose, by titillating the integuments so as to call into action the combination of muscles required. Thus, the pectoral and anterior portion of the deltoid, by elevating the arm and bringing it forwards, excites the idea of friendship, and the subject will lean against and clasp any person or thing near him. The central and posterior portions of the deltoid, by elevating and drawing back the arms, as if preparing to give a blow, excite the idea of combativeness. With many, clenching the fists will have the same effect, especially if the arms are correspondingly elevated. Titillating a little below the *axilla*, by stimulating the *pectoralis* and *latissimus dorsi* to contract, draws the arm to the side, and thus excites cautiousness, fear, or terror. The lower point of the sternum produces stooping, sighing, compassion, and benevolence; the *recti* muscles of the back excite the erect position with the feeling of firmness and self-esteem; the flexors of the fore-arm, the desire to grasp and appropriate to self all which comes in his way; the extensors the reverse, or conscientiousness and restoration; the larynx, the desire to sing or talk and so on in respect to the functions of other organs, or combinations of muscular actions.

I shall now give such instructions as may enable any expert experimentalist, well acquainted with anatomy, and who wishes to test this fairly, to prove the correctness of my views. In order to insure this success, however, it is of the utmost importance to pay particular attention to the *different stages of sensation during hypnotism*, which I am now about to explain.

There are three stages of sensation in the hypnotic condition (the term I prefer, to designate the peculiar sleep referred to), **the first characterised by increased sensibility, docility, and pliancy, so that**

any part readily yields or moves in the direction of the force applied, and will remain in the position in which it is placed. This is the condition called pliant catalepsy. The second stage is that where there is increased sensibility and slight rigidity, with a tendency to contraction in the muscles immediately subjacent to the points touched or titillated. The third stage is that where there is rigidity of all the muscles, or rigid catalepsy, with *diminished* tactual sensibility. In this case, the patient may be pricked or pinched with little or no feeling; but continued gentle pressure or friction will *reduce the rigidity* in the *subjacent muscles*, and the member will be gradually drawn in the opposite direction, in consequence of the continued undiminished action of their antagonists. The *second* condition is the proper stage for exciting the manifestations above referred to; and the operations, if skilfully conducted, are almost certain to be followed by the anticipated results, and will thus verify the correctness of what I have already advanced, and what was also referred to at pages 95, 96, 97, and elsewhere, of my treatise on Hypnotism.

The operation by which motion is excited during the *second* stage, may be called the *direct* mode; that during the *third*, the *in*direct, because, in the latter case, the motion is excited by *reducing the power of the antagonist* muscles, whereas, in the former, it results from the stimulus being applied directly to the particular muscles to be roused.

As the phenomena can be excited equally readily from the head and face, trunk and extremities, through automatic muscular action renovating past feelings, according to the ordinary laws of association, or from arbitrary associations, by contact with any part of the body, it appears to me, that they neither prove nor disprove the doctrine of Phrenology, or the allocation of different functions to separate organs in the brain. However, the situation of the sympathetic groups in the head, which I shall immediately explain, if taken at the *second* stage of sensation, corresponds with the three principal locations and divisions into animal propensities, moral sentiments, and intellectual faculties.

The fact of the opposite manifestations resulting from manipulating the head in the *third* stage, to what we realise during the *second*, clearly proves, that the results do not arise from a stimulus conveyed *directly*, from the point of contact, to the *subjacent portion of the brain*; but, as the effects on the muscles are inverted, so ought the points manipulated to be changed to produce the intended results. Now, this is precisely what happens – the *same muscular action* being excited from *opposite points*, both in the head, trunk, and extremities, in the one stage and in the other. Still, however, the same mental feeling is excited along with this muscular action, however *the latter has been excited*; and this, I think, is strongly corroborative of my theory.

A familiar example of the influence of muscular expression or action reacting on the mind, may be realised by any sensitive person, *even during the waking condition*. Let him assume, and endeavour to maintain, any particular expression or attitude, and he will very soon experience that a corresponding condition of mind is thereby engendered. Now, such being the case during the *waking* condition, when the faculties of the mind are so much dissipated and diffused by impressions on the various senses, we can readily understand why the influence should be so much more energetic during Hypnotism, the peculiar features of which are high sensibility, with the whole energies of the mind concentrated on the particular emotion excited. It is no doubt, in a great measure, owing to the same cause, that our greatest actors and actresses have become so profoundly penetrated by touching scenes as to shed floods of tears during their impersonations of character – the just conception of the character first producing appropriate physical action, and this again reacting on the mind in the extraordinary manner which was manifested in [Sarah] Siddons and [Eliza] O'Neil [two distinguished actresses].

Whilst others, from experiments in this department, have been multiplying phrenological organs to an amazing extent, the result of my researches tends rather to classify and curtail them. Thus, in the second stage, I find that the lateral portions of the head correspond with the flexors of the upper extremities – the anterior portion exciting flexion and movement of the fingers and hand, and the movement of hand and arm being increased in extent and energy by calling additional muscles of the shoulder and trunk into activity, as we proceed backwards. This portion, therefore, represents the animal propensities – the prehensile or selfish principle. The whole of the central and coronal region (excepting the vertex) corresponds to the opposite class of muscles, and the opposite condition of the mind – the relaxing, extensile, and distributive or benevolent tendency, respect and regard for others. In other words, the extensors represent the moral faculties, the flexors, the animal propensities and selfish principle; and, in the head, during the second stage of sensation, the central and coronal region represents the former, and the lateral regions correspond to the latter. The intermediate space seems to rouse partially *both* classes of muscles, and gives a mixed or varying character to the emotions, according as the one or the other predominates. This is [the founder of phrenology, Franz Joseph] Gall's region for Wit, Ideality, Caution, and Love of Approbation. The forehead excites an appearance of attention, observation, and reflection; but beyond this, and the different degrees of sensibility of different parts giving more or less promptness and energy to the various emotions and propensities, all appears to me to be inconclusive as far as illustrated by manipulating patients during the nervous sleep.

I shall now advert to one of the most remarkable circumstances connected with these

investigations; namely, the influence of contact in exulting memory. Thus, a patient may be unable to answer the most simple question, on a subject with which he is quite familiar; but touch any part of his person, either with a finger or any inanimate substance, or cause him to place one of his own hands or fingers in contact with some other part of his own body, and immediately he will be able to reply correctly. There are many patients with whom this may be repeated any number of times with the like results. It appears to me to be merely mechanically arousing and fixing or concentrating the attention in *one* direction, instead of the mind wandering uncontrolled and incapable of fixing itself definitively on any subject whilst addressed only through the organ of hearing. [Braid here appears to prefigure the "pressure technique" of memory recovery adopted by Sigmund Freud.]

Analogous to this is another curious fact, that most patients, from having contact established with almost *any* part of the body, whilst the mind is actively engaged by *any* idea or emotion, may have it prolonged, almost indefinitely, by maintaining the contact with which it has been thus associated. We have familiar examples of the influence of contact or muscular action in fixing attention and aiding memory in the waking condition, furnished by the many deep thinkers who are in the habit of pressing a finger or hand against different parts of the body, generally the forehead, or pinching or rubbing some part when engaged in deep study. Others, again, will seize hold of a button or thread, and, deprived of this, feel unqualified for the task most easy with such aid – as exemplified in Sir Walter Scott's victory over his rival schoolfellow, and the case of the lawyer, the thread of whose discourse was thus broken. It was also well exemplified by the blind man at Stirling, who could repeat any verse, or any chapter of the Bible, whilst twirling a key on his thumb, but was quite at fault if deprived of his key. [Here Braid alludes to an early example of the concept known as a conditioned "trigger", "cue" or "anchor" in modern hypnotherapy.]

Mr. H. G. Atkinson has lately promulgated some novel views, under what he calls "the functions of the cerebellum", and thus explained in No. 202 of *The Medical Times*:–

> That portion of the cerebellum nearest the ear, gives the disposition to muscular action; next to which, and about half way between the ear and the occiput, on the top of the cerebellum, *muscular sense* – a power conveying the sense of resistance, and the state of the muscles; beneath which is *muscular power* – giving force and strength; and in the centre are what are termed the physico-functional powers – a group of organs giving the sense of physical pain and pleasure, temperature, and having relation to the general condition of the body, and its secretions, Amativeness, etc. The part nearest the centre giving the sense of pain; the sense of temperature being nearer to the ear, and Amativeness beneath.

I have tried Mr. Atkinson's experiments with my patients, but I account for the results differently. Thus, the first I consider is merely an extension of the prehensile and appropriate group of muscular actions referable to the lateral parts of the head, as already explained; the second, an extension of the intermediate region, where both extensors and flexors are partially excited, corresponding with Ideality, Cautiousness, Love of Approbation, *etc.*, in the anterior region; the third, by stimulating the posterior *recti* muscles, which excite Firmness and Self-Esteem, of course gives the appearance of energy; and the fourth, corresponding with the softer and kindlier feelings, under the influence of the relaxing and distributive class of muscles, which represent the moral sentiments, will account for the last group. Such have been the conclusions to which I have come from personal observations on this point. Mr. A. is evidently a gentleman of great intelligence, and one who has devoted much pains to the investigation of Mesmeric phenomena; and his observations on this point, therefore, deserve the careful attention of others engaged in similar inquiries.

The investigations of the phenomena of Hypnotism and Mesmerism are not only curious, but most important, as daily experience amply proves to me, in the rapid relief and cure, by this mode of treatment, of diseases which had resisted all the ordinary and most approved methods. I shall defer some farther observations on other important points to a future opportunity having already, I fear, encroached too much on your valuable columns.

Letter from Mr. Simpson (1844)
On Hypnotism, and Mr. Braid's Theory of Phreno-Mesmeric Manifestations

To the Editor of *The Phrenological Journal*. [1st June 1844]

Dear Sir,

Happening to be in Manchester in March last, I had the pleasure of forming the acquaintance of Mr. James Braid, an eminent surgeon there; who, as is well-known to Mesmerists and phreno-Mesmerists, has gained no inconsiderable celebrity by certain discoveries, alleged to have been made by him, of the nature and cause of the Mesmeric sleep, and published, with his proofs, in a small volume, entitled, "Neurypnology, or the Rationale of Nervous Sleep", called also by him "Hypnotism", "considered in relation with Animal Magnetism, and illustrated by numerous Cases of its successful application in the Relief and Cure of Disease." As I had read, with great interest, Mr. Braid's work, and the summary of his views in your Number of January last, I considered myself fortunate in obtaining personal communication with him.

I have to acknowledge much courtesy and attention received from Mr. Braid, and the greatest assiduity on his part, in introducing me to his most instructive cases, and candidly and clearly submitting to me the proofs of his theory.

Mr. Braid holds that there is at least analogy, if not identity, between the Mesmeric sleep as induced by others, and the hypnotic sleep, as he certainly more philosophically calls it, as induced by himself.[91] This sleep, he alleges, is the result of an exhausted irritability in the motor nerves, and fatigue in the muscles, of the eyes; in which condition the eyes close. Nothing more is required than that the patient shall stare steadily at an object, animate or inanimate – the better if a short way above the head – till the exhaustion takes place. It is conditioned that the patient shall concentrate his thoughts on the fixed object, and yield himself implicitly to the operation. The nervous system is thrown into a new condition; and if the arms and legs be raised, the pulse speedily becomes greatly accelerated, and the limbs, in a short time, will become quite rigid and involuntarily fixed. It is also found that all the organs of special sense, except sight, but including heat and cold, and muscular motion or resistance, are, *at first*, much exalted, and have extreme sensibility. After a certain period, this exaltation of function is followed by a state of depression, far greater than the torpor of natural sleep. From this state of torpor of the senses and rigidity of the muscles, the patient may be *instantly* brought back to the state of exalted sensibility, and of extreme mobility of muscle, by *a current of air* directed against the organ or organs wished to be recalled to action. By mere repose this effect will in time take place. Mr. Braid was long puzzled to explain this effect of a current of air: a theory has recently occurred to him, which I shall presently notice.

I witnessed the results, now briefly described, but more fully in Mr. Braid's work and article above alluded to,[92] in a number of Mr. Braid's patients of both sexes, and had no doubt whatever of their reality. **Several of the patients were requested by him to throw *themselves* into the hypnotic state, without any operation of his; which they did by gazing steadily for a very few seconds upon a fixed object. Nay, more, if the object gazed at was another patient's eyes, the two persons could hypnotise each other. This, also, I saw done repeatedly.** From this reciprocal result, and likewise from the phenomenon of self-hypnotism, Mr. Braid concludes, as he appears entitled to do, that the nervous sleep of his patients, whatever be its nature, is not produced by any influence, magnetic or other, passing from one person to another. This is an immense point gained, if gained it be; for at one step it gets beyond the mystery and magic of Mesmerism, and finishes "Animal Magnetism".

Mr. Braid informed me – indeed, has stated in his work – that he has entirely *separated* Hypnotism from Animal Magnetism. By this I understood him to mean, that he investigates the former by its own facts, and independently of the controversy on the subject of Mesmerism. He does not, however, say that the Mesmeric and hypnotic states are essentially and intrinsically different, and does not hold that they are. The effects, as witnessed by me, left me without a doubt that they are one and the same, only that Hypnotism is the more brief, and decidedly the more certain, method of producing what has been called the Mesmeric sleep. The discovery of the cause, at least the *commencement*, of the hypnotic state, in the affection of the motor nerves and muscles of the eyes – which may come to be classed with those brilliant feats of science, which, in a moment, unlock a store of Nature's secrets, and give an immense onward move to human knowledge – this observation is Mr. Braid's own, safe from either envy or dishonesty, whatever may be its consequential value.

It was during a Mesmeric experiment conducted by M. Lafontaine – to which, in his then incredulity and disdain, he was almost dragged by a friend – that this idea occurred to Mr. Braid. The

---

[91] [See the appendix, originally a lengthy footnote.]
[92] See also his papers in The Medical Times of 6th and 13th January, and 13th and 20th April, 1844.

steady fixation of the patient's eyes suggested it; and that fixation, which was believed to be for the reception of an influence from the eyes of the Mesmeriser, but which is followed by the same effect when the object is something inanimate, not even *held* by another person, the very mode and occasion of the discovery are, to my mind, a proof that, by and through M. Lafontaine's patient's fixed gaze, and not by any influence passing from M. Lafontaine, the said patient was *hypnotised* in Mr. Braid's sense, not *Mesmerised* in M. Lafontaine's; the actual state being, however, the same in both senses.

Mr. Braid exhibited a number of his cases to me both in Manchester and its neighbourhood, and left me convinced of the identity of the Mesmeric and hypnotic states. The new consciousness, to be forgotten on waking up – the cataleptic state of the limbs – the insensibility to pain – and the obedience of the faculties of the patient to the impressions made upon them by the operator, were, as far as I could judge, the same in the hypnotised as in the Mesmerised patient. I saw no case of clairvoyance, introvision [the supposed ability to see inside other people's bodies and thereby diagnose disease, i.e., "x-ray vision"], or reading with the eyes bandaged, in Mr. Braid's hands. He himself is incredulous as to the reality, at least the alleged nature, of these phenomena; and some others, especially introvision, as it is called, he imputes to the exalted sensibility of the sense of smell. **I saw a boy in the hypnotic state restore to several persons, in a crowded room, each their own glove, which he previously applied to his nose. He followed me, like a questing hound, till he found me in a corner, and presented my glove. Mr. Braid showed me some instances of the increased sensibility of the sense of hearing, in which the slightest whisper was heard and answered at the distance of a large room. The effects, too, of the currents of air were very striking; the perception of them seemed most acute; and he thinks that the passes and attractions of the Mesmerists owe their effect to modifying the air in contact with the body of the patient, and producing a stream or current.**

The same boy who, in a large party, restored my glove by its odour, walked through and through the company and furniture, even the footstools, without touching any object whatever; from extreme sensibility, as Mr. Braid thought, to the state of the air around his body. The blind are believed to acquire some degree of the same power. This sensibility to the most evanescent impressions on certain senses, accounts, on natural laws, in Mr. Braid's opinion, for much of the mysterious influence of the Mesmerists. To verify this opinion, which seems very reasonable, would require a more extended and minute course of observation than my short visit permitted me to make.

Mr. Braid, I observed above, has ventured a rationale of the current of air. This he did in a paper read by him a few weeks ago [April 1844], with great effect, to a meeting of some of the most scientific men of Manchester, in the theatre of the Royal Institution, and reported in the *Manchester Times,* and also, less fully in *The Medical Times* of 18th May. The theory is ingenious, and I am happy to give it a place in my letter.

> At one stage of Hypnotism there is a great exaltation of the functions of all the organs of sense, sight excepted, and at another all these may be reduced to a state of *extreme torpor*. During the latter condition, a simple waft of wind may restore any part from the *extreme of torpor* to the *highest state of excitation*. Thus the arm may be extended, and in process of time the muscular activity shall have reduced the limb to that state of rigidity called the cataleptic state; so that it is not only held up as it were involuntarily, but will offer prodigious resistance before it can be depressed; nay, may actually be so unyielding that it could not be flexed without the application of such force as might endanger the integrity of the tissues. The arm shall also be insensible to pricking or pinching; but the moment a waft of wind is directed against it, the rigidity ceases, down drops the arm, and the skin is instantly highly sensitive to the slightest infliction. This extraordinary influence of a current of air puzzled and perplexed me exceedingly. I solicited information on the point from all quarters, but no one hazarded an explanation of the cause of the phenomenon. However, I have very lately arrived at what I believe to be the true *rationale* of the matter; which is this. I have already explained that it is the peculiar feature of Hypnotism for the *whole* energy of the *vis nervosa* to be concentrated on the function in action, so that exciting another function is equivalent to suspending the one previously in action. Now, by elevating the arm, the *attention* is directed and concentrated on *muscular effort*, the tone of the muscles increases till a state of cataleptiform rigidity is induced, the pressure of the rigid muscles on the arteries and nerves interrupts the free circulation in the member; but while the sensation to pricking and pinching diminishes, that of heat and cold, if it does not increase, at least diminishes less rapidly. Again, by pressure applied to the arm or hand, you offer resistance to the rigid muscles of the arm and shoulder, *and thus you stimulate them to still greater activity*; but a waft of wind acts on the sense of heat and cold, which is a function of the skin; and as only one function is energetically active at the same time during Hypnotism, directing the attention to the *skin* is equivalent to *suspending that of muscular action*, and, consequently, *down drops the arm from its own gravity*. This is quite analogous to what happens when a person drops anything from his hand *by being suddenly startled*. The same explanation accounts for the effects of a waft of wind against any of the dormant organs of sense, the attention being thereby directed to the function of the organs acted upon. It is never to be overlooked that at this [primary, or "conscious" and "mobile"] stage of the sleep the acts are voluntary acts, although unremembered by the subjects when awake; and that they are regulated in their actions by the ordinary laws of sensation and association of ideas, as in the waking condition, with this difference, that the quickness of their perceptions, and tendency to concentrate their attention entirely to individual acts, instead of the more diffusive tendency of the waking condition, give an energy and promptness to their actions almost equal to the force of instinct which we

observe in the lower animals. When, however, the patient has been allowed to lapse into the deep stage, when the sense of heat and cold, as well as sensibility to pricking and pinching, is gone, these transitions are effected with much more difficulty. The patient then requires continued wafting for a considerable time, more particularly over the face. The rigidity only yields gradually. Without especial attention being given to the *opposite* conditions and phenomena at the different stages of Hypnotism, it is impossible for anyone to test the subject correctly, or to comprehend what he really witnesses.

Having thus briefly described what I saw of the hypnotic state itself, I beg now to add what I shall call, for distinction, **the phreno-hypnotic phenomena which I witnessed; in other words, the excitement of mental manifestations by the operator. In this field Mr. Braid has made another discovery, quite as striking as that of tracing the commencement, if not the cause, of the hypnotic sleep to the motor nerves and muscles of the eyes. He has observed that, in the exalted hypnotic sleep, certain of the mental faculties can be called into manifestation, by touching, or, as he calls it, titillating, *other* parts of the body besides the head. Founding on the known fact that the trunk and limbs, as well as the face, pathognomically [i.e., symptomatically] express the various feelings, Mr. Braid thought that the operation might be reversed, and the emotions be excited by stimulating the parts of the body which appear to respond to them; in other words, that, as the cord must have two ends, one in the brain and the other in the corporeal muscles – the foundation of what Sir Charles Bell calls the anatomy of expression – stimulus applied to either end would produce the same effect.**

That I may not misstate Mr. Braid's views, I will again quote from his recent essay, which, of course, sets forth his latest and most matured experience.

> The idea occurred to me, that, by titillating certain combinations of nerves, and thus exciting into activity certain combination of muscles, by a sort of inversion of the ordinary sequence, we might thus, through muscular action, suggest to the mind the idea which ordinarily preceded and excited the muscular action. This, then, would be a mere inversion of the ordinary sequence, the attitude and muscular expression of our *own* body suggesting the idea to our *own* minds, just as the effect is produced through the eyes by looking at anyone pantomimically expressing any given passion or emotion. It is long since it was observed, that anyone, in the waking state, while assuming and endeavouring to maintain the attitude of expression of any passion or emotion, will soon experience a corresponding condition of mind engendered thereby. By a series of experiments, this theoretical view seems to be borne out; as I have found that stimulating into activity any class of muscles, either in the head, trunk, or extremities, speedily engenders the ideas with which they are ordinarily associated in the waking condition. Thus, putting a pen or pencil into the hand excites the desire to write or draw; moving the fingers or hand, as if sewing, gives the idea of sewing; approximating the palms of the hand gives the idea of devotion; clenching the fist, the idea of fighting; stimulating the muscles of the back, pride and firmness; and so on. This, however, is best illustrated by experiment, and I shall now proceed to do so, and have no doubt of enabling you readily to comprehend the subject in this way, in the course of a few minutes.

[The committee report on Braid's reading of his essay adds,]

> Mr. Braid having now finished his paper, stated that an experiment would illustrate the matter so much more readily, that he should, no doubt, make his views on the latter part of his subject be comprehended in a few minutes. He then directed a young lady, who was present for the purpose, to hypnotise herself; which she did very readily, by holding up and looking at one finger. It was necessary to explain, he said, that, at a certain stage of sensation, the muscles subjacent to any point titillated instantly had a tendency to contract; or any point touched, the patient had a tendency to lean against; and the tendency to self-balancing, so remarkable in somnambulic patients, called into action certain associated combinations of muscles; and that this action created the idea in the mind of the patient. He then commenced his experiments. On his touching the muscles of the back, the patient rose and assumed an air of self-importance. The hands having approached each other (apparently accidentally), the position of them seemed to have given the patient the idea of devotion, and she slowly and gracefully sank upon her knees. – Though this was not intended, it seemed to give much satisfaction, as illustrating the impression Mr. Braid had been seeking to convey in his paper. The muscles of the interior of the arm being touched, caused a clasping of the hands, and the patient seized hold of the operator's handkerchief: the back of the arm being touched, an opposite tendency was displayed, and the patient seemed disposed to restore. A point in the interior of the shoulder being touched, which naturally caused the patient to elevate the arm and bring it forwards, she immediately evinced a disposition to lean against the operator. Touching the posterior and top parts of the shoulder on the opposite or left side of the patient, she opened her hand, evincing a disposition, on that side, to guard the operator from some imaginary assailant. The opposite feelings thus brought into action by touching different muscles, Mr. Braid said, had not their origin in a wish to be friendly merely; and in proof of this, he placed the patient on the other side of him, when she leaned with her right arm against the chairman, clasping his arm, and when Mr. Braid approached her on the other side, she struck at him. The points of contact were reversed, and the patient clasped the operator, and evinced a disposition to use the opposite arm in defending him against the chairman. A touch on the middle of the chest, caused a stooping tendency in the patient, a distressed state of the respiration, and a strong emotion of compassion; and the patient laid hold of some of her own clothes, as if to give them to some distressed object. The next point of contact was behind the shoulders, and the patient's feelings seemed instantly reversed; a feeling of selfishness seemed to be predominant, accompanied with manifestations of great self-consequence. Various points of the head were touched, and the operator's finger being placed at the

top of the head, the patient assumed an appearance of great firmness. A part of the head a little more backward being touched, the patient's head was thrown more backwards, and the countenance displayed the appearance of great self-importance. Points more laterally situated being touched, vanity and self-admiration were manifested. On a point of the head a little anterior to the centre being touched, the patient sank down on her knees in a solemn devotional manner; and combining this touch with one a little more laterally, a more animated appearance was given to the countenance, and the patient unclasped her hands and tossed them about, as in an animated state of devotion. The first point of contact being combined with one more laterally situated, an appearance of extreme ecstasy was produced. After exhibiting many others of these phenomena, which seemed to bear out very fully, and to the satisfaction of the audience, the theory which he had propounded, Mr. Braid remarked, that he considered no experiments which had yet been made of this kind had either proved or disproved the doctrine of Phrenology, which had as yet been left in much the same state as it was found by them. [Report of a lecture to the Royal Institution in Manchester, April 1844.]

I can bear testimony to the truth of the above results; for I saw the stimulants tried, not on one, but on several subjects of both sexes. I was allowed to try the experiment myself, and received blows or caresses, as I stimulated the outside or the inside of the arms; nay, was encircled adhesively with one arm, which I had touched on the inside, while the other, touched on the outside, struck out at anyone near on that side; and, on changing my place with another person, that person was caressed and I most impartially beaten. This singular proof of the *duplicity* of all the organs and functions of the muscular frame, as well as of the brain, has been observed by others; especially by Dr. Elliotson, in one of whose patients I saw it realised by the most distinct antagonist-action, as in Mr. Braid's subjects. I would here remark, that what I saw was confined to effects or results. I did not see the *cause* of these responses; and must not forget to say, that, in imputing them to association of certain ideas or feelings with certain muscular movements, Mr. Braid has only assumed, not proved, the *modus operandi*. The anatomy of expression, which he adopts, is more tangible than association; and that is certainly by nervous communication.

With one conclusion to which Mr. Braid comes, I cannot, after the most careful consideration, agree; namely that Hypnotism, or, what is the same thing, Mesmerism, has done nothing in the way of confirming the organology of Phrenology. I cannot part with so direct and powerful an aid to the science, so slightly, I would almost say indifferently, as Mr. Braid has done in the last five lines of the extract above quoted. My difference from Mr. Braid is on the following grounds:–

First, All the feelings whose manifestations he called forth by muscular titillation, were those which Phrenology has distinguished as primitive by the size of the organs in the brain. I saw Self-Esteem, Veneration, Benevolence, Adhesiveness, Combativeness, Destructiveness, Secretiveness, and Acquisitiveness, successively, in marked manifestation under the muscular process.

Secondly, The same faculties were brought out by touching the head over their recognised organs in the brain, and, as can bear witness, considerably more unequivocally and distinctively.

Thirdly, I cannot see why the fact that the manifestations instantly obey the direct touch over their organs in the brain should in the least be weakened, because, inversely, the brain may be excited by touching the muscles of expression. Mr. Braid does not aver that the muscles are the *seats* of the emotions. The brain must be concerned even in this reverse indirect appeal to it. If so, what has Mr. Braid done, but most ingeniously confirmed the *pathognomy* of Phrenology, discovered muscular regions which respond pathognomically to the organs of the brain, and to which, on his own showing, the *brain* responds? Has he not thus materially added to the proofs of Phrenology, instead of merely leaving them as they were?

Fourthly, Not only were the responses, to my observation, more precise, when the head was touched in the situations of the cerebral organs of the eight feelings enumerated, but these eight were apparently all the feelings that Mr. Braid could excite muscularly. Others, however, were called forth when their organs in the brain were touched, and invariably in the recognised localities. For example, the repulsiveness of Self-Esteem was roused by touching the back on the spine, immediately below the shoulder-blades; and the feeling was also excited by touching the situation of its recognised organ in the head. But the coquettish manner of Love of Approbation could by no muscular touch, that was tried be called forth; yet it instantly appeared when the organ on each side of Self-Esteem in the head was appealed to. In one lady's case, I secretly concerted with Mr. Braid, that, when I said "centre", he should touch Self-Esteem, and "sides", Love of Approbation, both on the head. This we alternated a dozen of times, with the most amusing change, from hauteur to vanity, that a phrenologist could have wished to see. Tune, Time, Colour, Ideality, Caution, were not called forth by the muscular, but could be by the cerebral appeal. Now, even supposing that precise localities in the muscular frame shall in process of time be discovered, to the stimulating of which each and all of these feelings shall respond, still, as the feelings ultimately vibrate in the brain, where this takes place must be in the very localities ascertained by Phrenology, seeing that at *that* end of the cord, so to speak, the response is unequivocal; each kind of response being limited to the bounds of its own previously ascertained organ.

To my mind, the organology of Phrenology receives much confirmation, if by touching over the previously observed organs the manifestations are brought out; although it may be also true that the same manifestations can be brought out by touching other parts of the body. We do not question the localisation of its proper propensity in the cerebellum, because its specific feeling can be excited in other localities.

Neither is the evidence weakened by the fact, of which I saw several proofs in Mr. Braid's hands, that the ideas conveyed *in words* will rouse the feelings to a very great degree in the different organs. We know that this is true in the waking state; hence the danger of corrupting books or conversation. I saw different feelings – always, be it marked, the primitive faculties of Phrenology – called forth in Mr. Braid's subjects, who were, beyond all doubt, deeply hypnotic at the time. When he whistled a waltz, a lady in the sleep began to move in waltz measure with uncommon grace; when he sang, she sang; and, stimulated *by his words*, she made a fierce attack upon me to rob me, attempting to plunder my pockets, and possessing herself of something belonging to me – which, by an appeal, still in words, to her Conscientiousness and Shame, she was made to restore, with a flood of tears. I shall never forget that lady; she was in a superior rank in life, residing some miles out of Manchester; and I was introduced to her and her family by Mr. Braid, who paid her a non-professional visit, in the hope that she would consent to be hypnotised for my gratification. She most cheerfully and obligingly complied. Naturally a beautiful and elegant young woman, her movements and attitudes, in the exaltation of the hypnotic sleep, exceeded, in gracefulness and expressive power, anything I ever witnessed in the most accomplished displays of the stage. I was before aware, for I had seen several instances in Edinburgh and London, and one in Mr. Braid's own hands, that very ordinary looking persons can be rendered beautiful, and always graceful, in the nervous sleep – proving how much beauty depends upon expression; but the case now described presented a series of studies for the sculptor, painter, or actor, of the most exquisite kind. This young lady expressed no feeling that is not recognised by Phrenology, whether excited by touching the organs on the head, or the muscles, or by calling up the ideas by words; and when precision in manifestation was wanted, recourse was always had to the brain direct. One example I recall. As she joined her palms and sank gracefully on her knees, in answer to the muscular appeal to Veneration immediately under the breast-bone or sternum, the ingredient of rapturous ecstasy was added to her expression – and how? By touching the organs of Hope, Ideality, and Wonder, *on the head*. The attitude and expression became heavenly. In an instant, a touch on the spine roused her from her knees, and changed her whole demeanour to a strut of proud defiance. Another was given to the organ of Love of Approbation, on the head, when she bowed and moved her hands from side to side with an air of coquetry, with "nods, and becks, and wreathed smiles", from which the greatest adept in genteel comedy might have taken a lesson. The waltz easily followed when music was given her, and her dancing movements were perfect.

One observation made by Mr. Braid, if true, would, I freely admit, upset all my above arguments for Phreno-Hypnotism, namely, that, in the third or rigid and torpid stage of Hypnotism, the manifestations are reversed – the lower organs bringing out the higher manifestations, and *vice versa*. This is vastly too important to be lightly averred. We must see a hundred unequivocal instances of it, before we can subscribe to it. Now, I did not see one; and when it is recollected that the third stage is the stage of torpor, I should rather expect that *no* manifestations can be brought out in that stage at all. Nothing perplexed me more than this thesis of Mr. Braid's, and I am not sure that I understand it yet. Experiments, "*decies, deciesque, repetita*", are called for on this by far the boldest of Mr. Braid's propositions, and the greatest of his discoveries, if discovered it shall be, which, with great deference to him, I cannot imagine it ever will. On his own theory of suggesting ideas or feelings by stimulating certain muscles, the notion of inversion seems an absolute inconsistency.

I have to repeat my great obligations to Mr. Braid for much pleasure, and no small instruction. I witnessed some gratifying applications of Hypnotism to disease, saw marked improvement, and conversed with several cured patients, who described to me their interesting experience. But into that branch of the subject, as not suited for your Journal, I will not enter.

I am, yours, *etc.*,

James Simpson

Northumberland Street,
Edinburgh.
1st June 1844.

[Appendix]

In his *Neurypnology*, p. 21, Mr. Braid says:–

> For a considerable time I was of opinion that the phenomena induced by my mode of operating and that of Mesmerisers were identical; and, so far as I have yet personally seen, I still consider the condition of the nervous system induced by both modes to be at least analogous. (...) However, from what the Mesmerisers state as to effects which they can produce in certain cases, there seem to be differences sufficient to warrant the conclusion that they ought to be considered as distinct agencies.
>
> These effects, which he has never been able to produce by his mode, he states to be, "such as, telling the time on a watch held behind the head, or placed on the pit of the stomach; reading closed letters, or a shut

book; perceiving what is doing miles off; having the power of perceiving the nature and cure of the diseases of others, although uneducated in medical science; Mesmerising patients at miles' distance, without the knowledge or belief in the patient that any such operation is intended". It appears from a paper lately read by Mr. Braid at the Royal Institution in Manchester (quoted in a subsequent part of this article), that he has not yet seen reason to believe in the reality of any such feats as these.

There ought, in my opinion to be far stronger evidence, and a more extensive series of experiments, and those subjected to more searching scrutiny than hitherto, before being received as facts; for to me it appears far more probable that the narrators have been deceived than that the Almighty would ever delegate to man such dangerous prerogatives and powers – powers which are quite inconsistent with the security and harmony of society in the present state of our existence.

He referred, in support of this opinion, to the small number of satisfactory cases which had been met with of the kind, compared with the length of time over which they were spread, and the number of the investigators.

Then, again there is the acknowledged uncertainty of even the most clairvoyant patients, for in general they are oftener wrong than right; whereas answers from true perception ought always to be right. Nor should we overlook the fact that most of their answers are given in very vague language, which may admit of very different interpretations. Moreover, in every case of supposed clairvoyance which I have had an opportunity of investigating closely, I have been enabled to convince the parties that they had been deceived, and that the whole was explainable on principles which I shall immediately point out, and a want of the knowledge of which I believe has been the chief source of error in those inquiries. Until cases are investigated with due attention to these sources of fallacy, no implicit confidence should be given to the results recorded. For example, General Green of Philadelphia, a man of great talents and observation, honoured me with a call last summer. He believed his daughter highly clairvoyant, and she was represented as such by her Mesmeriser; but I very soon convinced him they had been mistaken. In like manner, the satisfaction of many with the late case of the boy Cooke, at Deptford, who was represented as highly clairvoyant, all arose from their ignorance of the sources of error I am about to explain, as a letter from the boy's master, compared with my paper in The Medical Times of 13th January last, clearly proves. In another case, published in the *Phreno-Magnet*, I wrote to the operator, requesting him to repeat the experiment, with *certain precautions I had suggested*, and offered L.5 [i.e., five pounds, a substantial sum of money] as a reward to his patient if successful, or to the patient of any of his Mesmeric friends who had met with such marvels; but although it was offered – not as a bet, involving risk to them, but as a reward – and I offered them any number of trials, if the first proved unsuccessful; while five months have elapsed, still the money has not been demanded.

He also appealed to a late investigation, made with precautions he had referred to, which had proved one of the most noted cases of clairvoyance to be a complete delusion. He said:–

Amongst the sources of error which should be kept in view whilst investigating the subject of clairvoyance, community of feeling, and Mesmeric intuition – the remarks apply equally to hypnotism as Mesmerism – the following are the most important:– The extreme exaltation of function, at a certain stage, of the organs of special sense, which enables them to perceive, through the ordinary media, impressions so faint that they could not be perceived in the waking condition; second the extreme docility and sympathy, which gives a tendency to imitate the actions of others; third, the extraordinary revivification of memory at a certain stage of the sleep, which enables them to remember things long forgotten in the waking condition; fourth, the remarkable effect of contact or touch in arousing memory; fifth, the remarkable condition of double consciousness, or double personality; sixth, the vivid state of the imagination, which instantly invests every idea suggested, or remembrance of past impressions, with the attributes of present realities.

On these and other grounds in the sequel, I should humbly hold that the states [of hypnotism and Mesmerism] are identical, not merely analogous.

Remarks on Mr. Simpson's Letter on Hypnotism (1844)

Published in the *Phrenological Journal* for July, 1844.

By Mr. James Braid, Surgeon, Manchester.

(From *The Medical Times*, No. 258, 31st August, 1844.)

To the Editor of *The Medical Times*,

Sir,

In the last number of the *Edinburgh Phrenological Journal*, I observe an elaborate and clever article by James Simpson, Esq., advocate, on my views and practice in Hypnotism, as personally witnessed by him during his late visit to Manchester. The article, as a whole, does great credit to the perceptive, reflective, and descriptive powers of its learned author. Few could have done so much, and so lucidly with the opportunities he enjoyed; but it was not to be expected that he should have mastered the *whole* subject at once; and I am desirous, through your pages, of correcting the two chief errors into which he has fallen, especially as they relate to a department on which I contributed a paper in your 216th Number. [*Observations on the Phenomena of Phreno-Mesmerism* (1843)]

The points to which I refer, are the different modes of exciting the mental manifestations during the nervous sleep. In your 216th Number, I stated three different theories which had been advanced by others, namely,

1st, That they arose from the *unexpressed will* of the operator exciting the ideas and propensities in the patients, from the power of the latter to read the secret thoughts and desires of the former;

2nd, That they arose from a magnetic or peculiar stimulus passing *directly* from the finger of the operator *through the skull*, and stimulating the *portion of brain immediately subjacent to the point of contact*;

3rd, Arbitrary association, by a system of training, or to previous knowledge of Phrenology.

I then adduced, what appeared to me, arguments sufficient to prove the untenableness of the first two theories; and, whilst I admitted the possibility or probability of the third, still I held it to be an arbitrary and artificial system, compared to that which I have adopted, as the most natural and simple of all which have yet been propounded, because arising from the anatomical relations of the physical frame. I endeavoured to explain the whole on the laws of sympathy, and association of ideas, connected with automatic muscular motion, which I shall presently explain briefly.[93]

It is necessary here to explain, that, at what I call the *second stage* of sensation during Hypnotism, the muscles subjacent to any point titillated instantly have a tendency to contract, or the patient manifests a tendency to *lean against* the point touched; and then the tendency to self-balancing, so remarkable in somnambulic patients, calls into action certain associated combinations of muscles; and, finally, as already explained, such muscular action or attitude creates or excites a corresponding idea in the mind of the patient, through the laws of sympathy and association.

In illustrating the above proposition to Mr. Simpson, I confined my examples to a few of the more leading and prominent feelings, believing *that* to be the mode calculated for *most* rapidly conveying to him my views of my subject. I find, however, at page 269, that he erroneously alleges that the eight he there names were "apparently *all* the feelings that Mr. Braid could excite muscularly". In reply to this, I beg to state, that, in addition to the eight referred to, Nos. 2, 9, 11, 12, 17, 18, 19, 20, 21, 22, 32, 33, may be excited by *muscular action only*; and any of the others, by proposing a leading question, *combined with contact with any part of the body*.

The other point on which Mr. S. is at fault, he refers to at page 271, namely, the *inversion* of the results obtained by manipulating the respective points during the *third* stage of sensation, from what are

---

[93] We omit the explanation, as it has already been repeatedly given in this volume [in the previous letters]. By stimulating the muscles of expression of various emotions, Mr. Braid, as our readers will remember, excites in the mind those feelings which usually precede the muscular actions. With respect to some of the cerebral organs excited by touching the head over them, the theory appears not inapplicable; but in the case of such organs as Veneration, Benevolence, Conscientiousness, Imitation, Tune, and Constructiveness, it is difficult to see in what manner excitement of the muscles over these can rouse the faculties.

We take this opportunity of expressing our obligation to Mr. Braid, for the ready kindness with which he lately exhibited to us several interesting hypnotic cases in and near Manchester. The phenomena exhibited were of the kind which Mr. Simpson has graphically described in our July number. In particular, we saw the "reversed manifestations" when Mr. Braid touched the head over the organ excited, as well as when he touched the muscles of expression, while the patient was in what he stated to be the third stage of Hypnotism. – [Editor of the Phrenological Journal.]

realised during the second stage. His misapprehension here has arisen entirely from *not having made himself master of my definitions of these two stages*, which I shall now quote from page 75 of your 216th Number:–

> The *second* stage is that where there is increased sensibility and slight rigidity, with a tendency to contraction in the muscles immediately subjacent to the point touched or titillated. The *third* stage is that where there is rigidity of all the muscles, or *rigid* catalepsy, with *diminished* tactual sensibility. In this stage, the patient may be pricked or pinched with little or no feeling, but continued gentle pressure or friction will *reduce the rigidity in the subjacent muscles*, and the member will gradually be drawn in the *opposite* direction, in consequence of the continued undiminished action of *their antagonists*.

The emotion excited by operating during the *second* stage, may be called the *direct* mode; that during the *third*, the *indirect*, because the latter is excited by *reducing the power of the antagonist muscles*, whereas, in the former, it is from the stimulus being applied *directly* to the particular muscles to be excited.

The fact of the opposite manifestations resulting from manipulating the head in the *third* stage, to what we realise during the *second* clearly proves that the results do not arise from a stimulus conveyed DIRECTLY *from the point of contact to the* **SUBJACENT PORTION OF BRAIN; but as the effects on the muscles are inverted (or reversed), so ought the points manipulated to be changed (or reversed), to produce the intended results. Now, this is precisely what happens – the *same muscular action being excited from opposite points*, both in the head, trunk, and extremities, in the one stage, from what happens in the other. Still, however, the mental feeling is excited along with this muscular action, *however the latter has been excited*; and this is, I think, strongly corroborative of my theory.**

I trust these remarks are sufficiently plain to make it obvious to anyone, that my having stated that, "in the third or rigid and torpid stage of Hypnotism, the manifestations are reversed – the lower organs bringing out the higher manifestations, and *vice versa*," – involves no inconsistency, neither does it warrant the inference at page 272, "On his own theory of suggesting ideas or feelings by stimulating certain muscles, the notion of inversion seems an absolute inconsistency." The arguments quoted in the last paragraph, are sufficiently explicit to clear up this point in my favour; and, in proof of the facility with which this may be demonstrated, I may remark, that on the first patient I operated on (after reading Mr. Simpson's paper), I called the attention of a friend to his remarks, and demonstrated to him the *inversion* both on the head, trunk, and extremities; **nay, I even exhibited the opposite manifestations on the opposite sides of the body at the same time, by manipulating alternately the *same relative points in opposite sides of the head, trunk, or extremities*.** This, of course, was done by permitting the whole frame to pass into the *third* stage, and then rousing only one-half till it was in the *second* stage. In the evening of the same day, I illustrated the same practical facts to the entire satisfaction of Mr. Scott, a practical phrenologist, well-known both to Mr. Simpson and to Mr. Cox, editor of the *Phrenological Journal*. The experiments in this latter case were performed on two patients who had never been so tested before, and who had never even seen or heard of such experiments; nor was there any auricular suggestion given as to what might be expected.

But, moreover, there is a particular state of the *reflective*, as well as of the *perceptive, faculties, requisite to insure the success of these experiments*. Thus, for some time after passing into the sleep, the memory and judgement are sufficiently active to enable the subject to reason on the natural instinctive tendency of the perceptions, and to control or direct his actions accordingly. In this state, the subject will remember, after being aroused, all that has happened; and, during such stage, the attempts to excite mental manifestations will generally fail, unless with such as are quite in accordance with the *will of the subject*. When, however, the subject lapses into the deeper stage – during which he will *not* remember, when awake, *what had been done or said* – the reason seems also to be less active; whereas the imagination has become more vivid, and the consequence is, that he obeys the dictates of *instinct* rather than of reason and reflection. Every idea now suggested partakes of all the attributes of present reality; and, accordingly, the subject acts as during a fit of monomania, being entirely absorbed in some particular contemplation, or in the execution of some special act; and hence the remarkable vigour and precision of such acts. Of course, those subjects – and there are many such – who do not pass into this deeper stage, cannot properly exhibit these manifestations which are so characteristically and beautifully done by those in the deeper stage.

I shall, however, give an additional illustration, which, I think, cannot fail to make anyone comprehend my meaning, both as to *how* and *why* certain attitudes are produced in the *reverse* order, in the *third* stage, from what is realised by the application of the same means during the *second* stage. Let us suppose a spring fixed perpendicularly, with two cords, passing over two pulleys, placed to the right and left; and that one end of each cord is made fast to the point of the spring and the other to scales for receiving weights. The two scales being loaded with weights, and equipoised, of course the spring will maintain its perpendicular position; but, if additional weight is put into the *right-hand* scale, the spring will assume a corresponding inclination, from the greater or additional weight drawing the spring in that direction. But, supposing that, instead of loading the *right*-hand scale with this *additional* weight, an equal amount *had been taken out of the left*-hand scale, there would still have been the same loss of equipoise – an equal amount of inclination of the spring from the perpendicular; and this change would still have been in the *same direction*, as happened in the *former* experiment, namely, to the *right*. There would thus have been produced the *same amount, and the same direction, in both experiments*; but the former I call the *direct* mode, because it arises from an *addition* of force on the right, *drawing* the spring in *that* direction; and the latter I call *indirect*, because, in this case, it arises from a *diminution* of the *antagonist* power, or that on the left, *permitting* it to be drawn in the *opposite* direction.

Remembering the opposite results, mental and physical, which arise from manipulating patients at these two different stages, and the modification which is characteristic of what I call the *first* stage; and keeping in view, also, the important fact, that these different stages *gradually merge into each other*, and, consequently, that it is only when the *exact nick of time is hit for manipulating, we can insure the successful and characteristic manifestation of the feelings* at first trials, we are furnished with a pretty rational solution of the cause why so many patients had been manipulated or handled, for so many years, without the characteristic feelings having been excited and recorded, as has happened within these last three years, when manipulations have been made, and patiently persevered in, with the hope of eliciting them.

There can be no doubt of the power we possess of rousing the various feelings and mental manifestations, during Hypnotism, through muscular excitation only, through the laws of sympathy and association of ideas. But, in this manner, the *same* muscular motion may excite *different* feelings and ideas in the minds of *different* patients, according to their previous occupation and habits in respect to such physical efforts; *e.g.* – set the subject to the exercise of moving his hand and arm with a rotatory motion, as if turning something, and then put the question, "What are you doing?" I know, from experience, that the answer will be in accordance with the usual ideas and occupation with which such motion is associated in such an individual's mind, during the waking condition. Thus, an Italian boy would think he was grinding an organ; a cook, that she was winding her jack or coffee-mill; a blacksmith, that he was turning a grind-stone, or some other wheel he was accustomed to drive; a reeler, that she was winding; a person, accustomed to turn an organ for psalmody, would be inspired with devotional feeling; another, accustomed to playing or hearing waltzes on the same instrument, would think of dancing; and so on. It thus plainly appears that, through the laws of sympathy and association, connected with muscular action, you may excite various feelings from the same point, according to circumstances. On this ground, therefore, I still consider that none of the experiments hitherto instituted give any decided proofs, of themselves alone, either *for* or *against* Phrenology, or the existence of separate organs in the brain, for the manifestation of each of the mental functions. However, as it is the peculiar feature of this excitable state of the nervous system, that the mind should manifest itself as entirely absorbed in whatever individual passion or emotion it may be directed to, it appears to me to be quite possible to institute a series of experiments which might determine the relative powers or intensities of the feelings and propensities, which, being afterwards compared with the phrenological indications and known character of the subjects, would be a more decided test for or against Phrenology than any hitherto applied. I intend, shortly, to perform such a set of experiments, with every possible precaution to guard against deception. They shall be performed before a number of respectable and intelligent gentlemen, when a faithful and minute record shall be taken for publication. This appears to me to be the only mode of determining this question in a satisfactory manner. The discrimination of what is true from what is erroneous, is my sole object in entering upon the inquiry; and my motto shall be,

"Nothing conceal,
Nor set down aught in malice."[94]

I remain, Sir, your most obedient servant,

James Braid, M.R.C.S. Edin., etc.

3 St. Peter's Square,
Manchester.
17th July 1844.

---

[94] [Braid made good on this promise a year later, in the article entitled 'Experimental Inquiry to determine whether Hypnotic and Mesmeric Manifestations can be adduced in proof of Phrenology' (1844).]

Experimental Inquiry (1844)

Experimental inquiry to determine whether Hypnotic and Mesmeric Manifestations can be adduced in proof of Phrenology

> **Editor's Preface**
> To be clear, in this experiment, Braid used *five* subjects who were examined before a group of physicians, scientists, and other educated men. The phrenologist William Bally was asked to predict the strength of thirteen separate emotional responses by examining their scalps to measure the size of the primary "phrenological organs", recording his assessment on written evaluation forms which were kept hidden from the other experimenters until the end. The other experimenters apparently also attempted to predict the strength of the responses based on educated guesses about the subjects' personalities, *without* the aid of phrenology. Subjects were then hypnotised in a separate room and given the verbal suggestion that they would experience each given emotion in turn while a ring (acting as a trigger) was placed on one of their fingers. The thirteen suggested emotional responses were observed and rated for intensity by the group of observers, using written evaluation forms. These were then compared with Bally's predictions to determine how accurate phrenology had been as a means of gauging the capacity for different responses. The outcome was deemed *negative*: that phrenology had failed to accurately predict the given response in the majority of cases. Braid states that in one case there was no correspondence whatsoever, and that in none of the other cases did Bally predict more than four out of thirteen [31%] responses correctly. By contrast, the other experimenters had apparently made *more accurate* estimates *without* phrenological assessment. Phrenology, in this case, proved an unreliable means of predicting emotional responses compared with mere common sense observations.

By James Braid, M.R.C.S.E., Manchester.

(From *The Medical Times*, No. 271, 30th November 1844, vol. xi, pp. 181-182.)

In a paper in The Medical Times (No. 258) ['Remarks on Mr. Simpson's Letter on Hypnotism' (1844)], I intimated my intention of instituting a series of experiments, on a plan which I considered better calculated for testing Phrenology than any which had been applied during the hypnotic Mesmeric sleep. I shall now very briefly detail the result of the experiments performed for that purpose.

In the above paper, I explained the reasons which led me to consider that none of the experiments which had been performed for this purpose, during the Mesmeric or hypnotic conditions, should be held as proof either *for* or *against* Phrenology. I especially contended for this, on the ground of the undoubted fact, that, through the laws of sympathy and association, it was quite possible to excite *various and opposite feelings from the same points,* according to circumstances.

In *The Medical Times* for the 13th of January, 1844, **I explained, as one of the peculiar features of the excitability of the nervous system induced by Hypnotism, that the mind is liable to manifest itself as entirely absorbed in whatever individual passion or emotion it may be directed to; and, moreover, that an idea being excited in the mind, *associated with contact with* ANY *part of the body,* whether head, trunk, or extremities – by *continuing such contact* the mind might be riveted, for an almost indefinite length of time, *to the same train of ideas,* which would work themselves up into more and more vivid manifestation, according to the length of time afforded for that purpose.** It thus appeared to me, that, by availing ourselves of these peculiarities, we might very readily determine the *relative forces of the different emotions and propensities.* For example, by **exciting the various passions and emotions in succession, through auricular [verbal] suggestion, and by fixing each new idea by mechanical contact with the *same point* of the patient.** As the *suggestion and fixation of the ideas* would be *the same in all,* provided an equal length of time was allowed for each to develop the force of its manifestation, any *difference* in the *relative force* could only be attributable, on phrenological principles, to a corresponding difference in original development as regards size, or to greater or lesser activity of the respective organs, arising from the degree of exercise of corresponding portions of the brain. Then, again, by comparing the *relative forces* of the *manifestations realised by such experiments,* with the *known character* of the individual, provided they both coincided; by again comparing them with what a practical phrenologist should determine, *simply from the cranial developments,* as to what *ought* to be the character of such individual; if the latter was found to correspond with the former, then would Hypnotism be a proof *in favour of* Phrenology; but, if *they differed,* it would prove just as much *the contrary.*

On the 3rd of August, 1844, in the presence of a number of scientific friends, including Sir [Thomas] Willshire [a distinguished military officer], Bart.; Mr. Jewett, of Oxford; Capt. Thomas Brown; Mr. Sowler, barrister (of this town), *etc.*, *etc.*, after explaining my views and intended mode of proceeding, we commenced as follows:– We had the heads of five patients examined by Mr. [William] Bally, an eminent phrenologist of this town, and the relative forces or values of the phrenological developments of each carefully noted on his printed forms. Each of the subjects was then hypnotised separately, in another room, in the presence of the gentlemen already referred to, when all the leading emotions, denoted by phrenological organs, were excited successively, in the following manner, the resulting manifestations of each being carefully noted.

I considered that putting a ring on the same finger or thumb of a patient, was the most convenient and least objectionable mode of fixing the ideas suggested. This, therefore, was the mode of procedure. On each occasion I spoke aloud to this effect:– "Now, gentlemen, the moment I place this ring on his (or her) finger or thumb (as the case might be), you will observe that he (or she) will think of *devotion*"; at the same time putting the ring on the finger or thumb indicated. **Immediately the emotion was manifested; and, having afforded it a certain time to develop itself, its *relative force* was determined on, and accurately noted on a blank form. The ring being removed, the patient, who had been kneeling, now arose; and another idea was then excited and fixed in the mind in the same manner.** This new idea having been allowed time to develop itself in the same manner, and its relative force determined and recorded as in the former case, we passed on to others, until, in this manner, we had tested all the emotions and propensities which we deemed of most importance. The same plan was adopted with all the **five subjects**.

Our next object was to compare the results obtained by this process, with Mr. Bally's phrenological record. I must not omit to add, that the forms on which Mr. Bally had recorded the relative values of the organs, previous to the patients being hypnotised, had been put aside, so that we might not be biased in our estimate of the manifestations by our knowledge of the *phrenological development*. **On comparing the two records, the result was certainly unfavourable to Phrenology; for in no instance did the manifestations accord with the value or force set upon the several organs, in more than four out of thirteen leading characteristics [i.e., Bally's phrenological predictions were accurate *less* than 31% of the time]; whilst, in one case, there was no coincidence whatever – proving, at all events, to our minds, that Phrenology can gain no corroborative aid either from Mesmerism or Hypnotism. The manifestations were quite as characteristic when excited by *auricular* suggestion as by muscular suggestion, or manipulating either the head, trunk, or extremities.**

On comparing the *known characters*[95] of the above individuals, with what was developed and recorded of them during hypnotism, there was a remarkable coincidence. Similar results have also been realised in several other patients whom I have tested in the same manner, since. Nor is it at all surprising that such should have been the case, and that Phrenology should not derive any direct and decided support from Hypnotism and Mesmerism, as had been anticipated. In the latter condition, even granting the organology of phrenologists to be strictly true, the hypnotic and Mesmeric manifestations will accord rather with the *acquired energy and activity* than with the *mere size* of particular organs, or separate portions of the brain. On the contrary, Phrenology merely contemplates the estimating what *ought* to be the value of certain tendencies by the *size* of the organs which answer to them. Moreover, although it is true that a muscle increases considerably and visibly in *size* by exercise, it does not follow that separate organs of the brain must increase in the same ratio (or in any ratio at all), with particular qualities of the mind.

Mere *size* is not sufficient to determine the *force* of function. Much of the perfection and force of function may depend on the *perfection of structure,* arising from practice and habit, giving greater proclivity to act in a particular manner. I am aware that instances are referred to, where extraordinary corresponding changes have taken place in the form of the head, in individuals who have been actively engaged in new pursuits; but I suspect that such constitute the *exceptions, not the rule.* I believe that great changes may take place in the moral and intellectual powers, without any appreciable corresponding change being manifested in the external form of the skull. For example, every one knows that a moderate sized eye may be as useful for correct vision as a very large one; and it is also an undoubted fact, that the eye may be greatly improved in *accuracy of function by practice, and consequent greater concentration of the powers,* but who will maintain that there is thus induced a positive and appreciable enlargement in the *size* of the *organ of vision?*

No one will dispute that the brain is the organ of the mind; nor will any dispute the power of moral and religious training in changing character, whether they hold that the mind manifests its powers through the brain as a *series* of *distinct organs,* or parts, adapted for *separate* purposes, or as a *single organ,* and consequently as a servant of all work. In whichever mode this is to be viewed, experience proves that there are antagonist powers and principles in our nature, and that it is indispensably requisite that we should endeavour to "cease to do evil," in order that we may "learn to do well". Whether corresponding changes in the *size* of the *brain,* and *form* of the *skull,* take place *pari passu* [in parallel] with such changes in the mental and moral condition, I do not pretend to be competent to decide; but, as already stated, I strongly suspect

---

[95] In a note which we have received from Mr. Braid, he says:– "I formed my opinion of the 'characters' partly from personal knowledge, and partly from inquiries at the relatives and most intimate friends of the individuals." He has sent us the developments, and estimates of the strength of the manifestations, which latter, he says, are noted in accordance with the opinion of the majority of those present; but their publication does not seem to be necessary. – [Editor of *Phrenological Journal*.]

that great changes may take place in the moral and intellectual powers and tendencies, without any *appreciable* corresponding changes being manifested in the external form of the skull.

This, then, seems to be the true position and relation between the two sciences. Phrenology professes to determine character, according to the relative *sizes* of particular parts of the brain, and not according to the different *degrees of activity* of these parts, *independently of size*. The latter is an extent of refinement to which it does not pretend to have attained The manifestations realised by **Mesmerism and Hypnotism, on the contrary, display the *energy acquired from habit or practice*, as well as (or rather than) the *original proclivity* to particular trains of thought and action. However well adapted, therefore, the latter mode may be for determining the relative force of the existing tendencies (and, therefore, might be useful as an adjuvant to Phrenology), if taken alone, it is calculated rather to *oppose* than *corroborate* the deductions from mere cranial development.** Thus, granting, for the sake of argument, that all the separate organs of phrenologists were satisfactorily established, the *extreme activity* of one function or propensity, *superinduced by habit and practice,* and the dormancy or sluggishness of others *from want of exercise, might, or, rather, most probably would,* give manifestations quite at variance with existing development, estimated by the *relative size of the different organs.*

This very circumstance, however, proves that Hypnotism or Mesmerism might be made a valuable adjuvant, for enabling the phrenologist to estimate character more correctly and certainly than by Phrenology only. He would thus, at once, be furnished with a key for determining how far habit, practice, and other concurring circumstances, have been at work *in aiding or counteracting original predisposition.* This has always been a very difficult point for phrenologists to determine; perhaps it has been the greatest difficulty they have had to contend with. I would, therefore, recommend them to avail themselves of Hypnotism or Mesmerism, as valuable auxiliaries for this purpose; but, if they seek for more from them, I suspect that they will find, that **the genuine manifestations brought out by Hypnotism or Mesmerism *are more likely to contradict than to support Phrenology.***

In conducting the experiments detailed in this paper, the greatest care was taken to guard against every source of fallacy. I should be glad if others would repeat them, *with equal care,* on a greater number of patients, and record the results. The method indicated is so simple and obvious, that anyone having time and inclination for prosecuting the inquiry farther, may very easily do so. I beg, however, to offer one parting remark, which, if not strictly attended to, will render such experiments utterly worthless. **The auricular suggestions must be given in every instance in the same form of words, excepting the indispensable change of the name of the new emotion to be excited, and also, as nearly as possible, *in the same tone of voice*. If a different degree of *force* of *utterance* is used in any instance, it will, in a considerable degree, modify the character of the subsequent result.** And no whispering or hints should be given, as to the degree of force which may be expected to manifest itself in any instance. Neither should they know, before being hypnotised, the relative value of their phrenological developments.

Neurypnology: The Rationale of Nervous Sleep
(1843)

NEURYPNOLOGY

OR THE
RATIONALE OF NERVOUS SLEEP
CONSIDERED IN RELATION WITH
ANIMAL MAGNETISM

ILLUSTRATED BY
NUMEROUS CASES OF ITS SUCCESSFUL APPLICATION
IN THE RELIEF AND CURE OF DISEASE

BY

JAMES BRAID, M.R.C.S., C.M.W.S., ETC.

"Unlimited scepticism is equally the child of imbecility as implicit credulity."
– Dugald Stewart.

JOHN CHURCHILL, PRINCES STREET, SOHO, LONDON
ADAM AND CHARLES BLACK, EDINBURGH
1843

Original Dedication
to
Charles Anderson, M.D., F.R.C.S. Ed., *etc.*

[Anderson was the surgeon to whom Braid had been apprenticed on graduation from Edinburgh University and a founding member of the prestigious Wernerian Natural History Society, of which Braid became a corresponding member.]

My dear Sir,

Inclination as well as duty induces me to dedicate this work to you: that I may publicly express the lively sense of gratitude I entertain for the many opportunities enjoyed during my apprenticeship with yourself and your late father, of acquiring a practical as well as theoretical knowledge of my profession; of becoming familiar with your comprehensive views of disease, and their happy application in practice; for the personal kindness shown me during my pupilage; and for the uninterrupted friendship which has ever since existed betwixt us.

I am aware that you are not practically acquainted with the subject of this treatise, but your intimate knowledge of general science renders you eminently qualified for prosecuting the subject with success; and permit me to assure you, that its value as a curative power, for an intractable class of diseases, renders it well worthy of your best attention.

Believe me,

    My dear Sir,

        Most faithfully yours,

            James Braid.

3 St. Peter's Square,
Manchester.
June 2nd, 1843.

Editor's Preface
Donald Robertson

It is difficult to read Braid's *Neurypnology* and fully grasp his meaning without realising that he envisages, in this text, a model of hypnotism which comprises two 'consecutive' stages, which merge into each other in degrees, and can be modified by suggestion, expectation, habit, and other factors, such that either one can be turned into its opposite.

First Stage: **Sensory Excitation & Muscular Mobility**
A state of mental abstraction, or concentration, induced by fixed gaze on an unexciting external object, which is accompanied by consciousness (sensibility) and increased sensitivity of all the special senses except vision (hyperacuity). Subject recalls everything that they experience. The body's muscles are pliant and mobile.
Second Stage: **Sensory Torpor & Muscular Catalepsy**
By progressive stages, the first stage merges into a state of sensory torpor, or insensibility, accompanied by gradual loss of consciousness and amnesia, approaching a state resembling sleep. The muscles become generally rigid and involuntarily cataleptic. However, the body may be thrown into the opposite state by physical manipulation or suggestion.

The following changes have been made for the sake of clarification, as Braid's work is notoriously difficult to read. Key passages and terms have been placed in **bold** type. Several of Braid's lengthy footnotes, which read like small essays in themselves, have been moved from the body of the text into appendices where they can be more easily perused.

Section headings have been added; where possible these were based on Braid's own table of contents. However, new titles were invented for the chapters and appendices. Minor changes to the punctuation and formatting have been made for the sake of readability. Many comments have been included in square brackets to help clarify Braid's meaning.

Author's Preface

The circumstances which led me to engage in the investigation of hypnotism, are detailed in the introduction to this little work; in the first part of the treatise I have endeavoured to give the results at which I arrived, in most instances sketching the route by which I travelled, and stating the inferences drawn from the various incidents which occurred in the course of my progress. Having furnished the data from which I drew my conclusions, the reader is thus prepared to determine, whether, on any occasion, I have come to these conclusions without what he would consider sufficient evidence, and in such case can institute additional experiments to any extent he may judge requisite. One circumstance, however, I may remark. **From a fear of being misled, I have requested the most sceptical individuals I knew, both professional and merely scientific men, to scrutinize all my experiments in the most critical manner; and have also induced some of my most intelligent and respected friends to submit to the operations, in the hope that I might thus more certainly guard against being deceived.**[96] The results I now submit to the public, and to the kind and candid consideration of my professional brethren, whom I should wish to investigate the subject coolly, and with an honest desire to arrive at truth. Having myself been sceptical, I can make every reasonable allowance for others; on this point I fully subscribe to the propriety of the remark of Treviranus, the celebrated botanist, when speaking of Mesmerism. He says, (I quote from memory,) "I have seen much which I would not have believed on your telling; and in all reason, therefore, I can neither hope nor wish that you should believe on mine."

It is quite natural for any man to prefer the evidence of his own senses to that of all others, and I think no one who has the opportunity of examining the phenomena for himself should neglect to do so. However, there are some circumstances which ought to be particularly borne in mind, or very erroneous opinions may be formed by the uninitiated, from what is actually witnessed.

[1.] First, there is a remarkable difference in the degree of susceptibility of different individuals to the hypnotic influence, some becoming rapidly and intensely affected, others slowly and feebly so. This is only analogous to what we experience in regard to the effects of medicines on different individuals, and especially as regards wine, spirits, and opium, and nitrous oxide. Whilst this is a recognised fact, as regards the latter, it appears to me somewhat surprising to find many, and even professional men too, who seem to expect as much uniformity ought to obtain, in regard to the phenomena during hypnotism, as if we were operating on inanimate matter. On the contrary, they ought to be ready to admit that a variety might be expected to arise, even in the same individual, according to the physical and mental condition of the patient at the moment the operation is performed.

[2.] The next most important point for consideration is, the fact of all the phenomena being consecutive. We have thus the extremes of insensibility, and exalted sensibility, of rigidity and mobility, at different stages, and these **merging into each other by the most imperceptible gradations, or in the most abrupt manner, according to the mode of treating the patient. It is no unusual thing for different parties to be testing, or calling for tests, for the *opposite conditions,* at the *same instant of time.* These, of course, are incompatible, but, at a certain stage, the transitions from torpor of all the senses, and cataleptiform rigidity, to the most exalted sensibility, and flaccidity of muscle, may be effected almost with the celerity of thought, even by so slight a cause as a breath of air directed against the part.** If left at rest it will speedily merge back again, and thus those unacquainted with such peculiarities, will be continually liable to think they discover discrepancies, which, however, only originate from their imperfect knowledge of the subject; just as an unskilful manipulator will be ready to suppose, from his different results, that the observations of other chemists have been erroneous.

[3.] The third point meriting especial attention is the condition of the *mind* at different stages. As results from opium, so also from hypnotism. At one stage it gives an extraordinary power of concentration of thought, or disposition to rapt contemplation, whereas, at another stage, the discursive, or imaginative faculties are excited into full play, and thus the most expanded, bright, and glowing scenes and images are presented to the fervid imagination. Such effects are quite analogous to those described as resulting from the use of opium, and detailed by the late Sir Humphry Davy, as experienced in his own person, from the inhalation of the nitrous oxide. "I thus felt a sense of tangible extension, highly pleasurable in every limb, my visible impressions were dazzling and apparently magnified. I heard distinctly every sound in the room, and was perfectly aware of my situation. By degrees, as the pleasurable sensation increased, I lost all connection with external things; trains of vivid visible images rapidly passed through my mind. I existed in a world of newly connected and newly modified ideas."[97] It must also be borne in mind, that **these opposite *mental* conditions** may glide into each other by the most imperceptible degrees, or by the most abrupt transitions, according to the modes of management, and thus

---

[96] [That Braid did so is a fact, substantiated by the existence of many such reports in various publications.]
[97] [See Appendix I, note I.]

consciousness or unconsciousness, sound sleep, dreaming, or somnambulism, will result, according as sensations or ideas predominate, or are equally vivid. See Hibbert's *Philosophy of Apparitions.* At a certain stage the same abruptness of transition may be realised in the mental phenomena, as were referred to in the last paragraph, in respect to the *physical,* and from equally slight causes. I presume it is from this cause that the phrenological manifestation may be so readily and characteristically exhibited at this period. [In Chapter 7] I have stated that, were it not that I should consider it an unnecessary waste of time to prosecute the inquiry [into phrenology] farther, after the amount of evidence obtained by myself, and others, I had no doubt but I might soon obtain any number of additional cases I might desire. In proof of this, I may remark, that since that period, I was induced one day to try some fresh subjects, when I succeeded in eliciting the manifestations in the most satisfactory manner in the case of a man of forty-five years of age, and in three other male subjects upwards of twenty years of age.

Of the latter, under the excitation of [the "phrenological organs" named] constructiveness and ideality, one wrote, and the other drew patterns, and neither of them had seen such experiments, nor expected to be so tested, nor remembered what happened. The same day I also manipulated three females, one 45 years of age, a young lady of nineteen, and a girl, all of whom exhibited the manifestations quite distinctly. Another day, to satisfy a number of intellectual friends, I hypnotised three of their personal friends, two of whom were entire strangers to me, and were quite sceptical as to the possibility of my being able to affect them at all. They all exhibited the manifestations most distinctly, two of them in a remarkable degree, and to the extent of twenty manifestations at first trial. Under "conscientiousness", one restored a reticule she had stolen, and burst into a flood of tears at the thought of her delinquency. The friends were alarmed at the intensity of her emotion, but by changing the point of contact, I had her changed from the grave to the gay in a few seconds. A few days after, I had other two cases, and I feel assured that in most of the twelve cases here referred to the parties knew nothing of phrenology, and that not one of them could with certainty point to two of their own organs. I may also add, they were all tested before competent and observant witnesses, who can testify there was no prompting by anyone.

It appears quite evident, that **whatever images or mental emotions or thoughts have been excited in the mind during nervous sleep, are generally liable to recur, or be renovated and manifested when the patient is again placed under similar circumstances**. Notwithstanding the apparent conclusiveness of the cases recorded, that there exists a *natural* connection betwixt certain localities touched and the peculiar manifestations which follow, in order to determine this question in the most decided manner, it is my intention to institute a series of experiments on fresh patients, in order **to ascertain to what extent it may be practicable, by arbitrary association, to excite the *opposite* tendencies from the *same* points**; also, whether they can be exhibited in the same striking and natural manner by *both* methods, or by which points they can be elicited with the greatest facility and fidelity to natural expression.

There will thus be both positive and negative proof to aid us in determining, whether there is any natural and necessary connection existing betwixt the points manipulated, and the manifestations excited; or whether it may depend entirely upon associations which have originated from some partial knowledge of phrenology, from arbitrary arrangements, or accidental circumstances or causes which have been entirely overlooked or forgotten; and which afterwards produce the results from **"that ultimate law of the mind, which ordains, that the repetition of a definite sensation shall be followed by a renovation of the past feelings with which it was before associated"**. (Hibbert, page 316.) I am induced to adopt this course, from my anxiety to remove every possible source of error as to the cause of the original manifestation, and from the recollection of the remarkable circumstance of **the woman who, during natural somnambulism, could repeat correctly large portions of the Hebrew Bible, and other books, in languages she had never studied, and was perfectly ignorant of when awake, but which was at length discovered to have been acquired from hearing a clergyman, with whom she resided when a girl, reading them aloud to himself; and also of some patients whilst labouring under disease remembering languages long forgotten.** I wish to ascertain whether any such accidental circumstance may have been the cause of the remarkable manifestations arising in the minds of patients when first manipulated. Whatever are the results of my farther inquiry shall be carefully noted and published, as **my object is neither to prove nor disprove the truth of phrenology, but to establish the value of hypnotism**, and determine how best to apply it, as a means of meliorating the mental, and moral, and physical condition of man.

That **during the nervous sleep, there is the power of exciting patients to manifest the passions and emotions, and certain mental functions, in a more striking manner than the same individuals are capable of in the *waking* condition**, no one can doubt who has seen much of these experiments. And it can in no way alter the importance of hypnotism, as a curative power, and extraordinary means of controlling and directing mental functions, in a particular manner, by a simple association of impressions, whether we thus act on the brain as a *single* organ, or as a combination of separate organs; or whether the primary associations have originated from a special organic connection, or from some accidental and unknown cause, or from preconcerted arrangement and arbitrary association.

In such operations as particularly require the use of the eyes, I have never seen patients in the hypnotic state perform what they attempted with the same celerity and accuracy as they were capable of doing when awake, and with the aid of sight. In short, I have never witnessed any phenomena which were not reconcilable with the notion that they arose from the abnormal exaltation or depression of sensations and ideas, or to their being thrown into unusual and varied ratios by the processes resorted to.

Having heard it reported, that by establishing a connection betwixt two patients by a chain or string, that manipulating one would manifest the same phenomena in both, I tried the experiment, but with the precaution that the patients should be in separate rooms, so that the one could not hear, nor feel, from the motion of the air, what the other was doing. I formed the connection by a cord in some cases, and in others by a copper wire, and had parties stationed where they could observe the movements of both at the same time. We could discover no such sympathetic influence as is asserted to have been realised by others.

The experiments recorded [in Chapter 7] of my having caused patients to **hypnotise, manipulate, and rouse themselves, (by simply desiring them to rub their own eyes,) and which produced results precisely the same as when done by anyone else,** seem to me the most decisive proof possible that the whole results from the mind and body of the patients acting and re-acting on each other, and that it has no dependence on any special influence emanating from another. My first experiments on this point [i.e., self-hypnosis] were instituted in the presence of some friends on the 1st May, 1843, and following days. **I believe they were the first experiments of the kind which had ever been tried, and they have succeeded in every case in which I have so operated.**

With due attention to the points above referred to, and with that practice which is requisite to insure adroitness in experimenting in any department of art or science, and with an honest desire to view every fact having no bias to uphold some previous prejudice or opinion, I have no doubt that the facts and observations set forth in this treatise will soon be very generally confirmed. A perusal of the cases recorded in the second part will, I trust, render the importance of the subject sufficiently apparent to stimulate inquiry; and I hope it may be gratifying to others to read, as it is to me to be able to record, that the prediction I had ventured to make [at the end of the book], as to the probability of hypnotism proving a cure for tetanus and hydrophobia, has already been happily realised in respect to the former intractable and generally fatal disease. After this treatise had been in the press the following case occurred, and its importance must be my apology for giving a brief detail of it here:–

Master J. B., thirteen years of age, was suddenly attacked with chilliness and pain all over his body, on the evening of 30th of last March. I was called to attend him the following day, when I considered he had got a febrile attack from cold, and prescribed accordingly. Next day, however, it had assumed a very different aspect. I now found I had got a severe case of opisthotonos [a severe spasm of the back muscles] to deal with. The head and pelvis were rigidly drawn back, the body forming an arch, and the greatest force could not succeed in straightening it, or bringing the head forward. Whilst the spasm never relaxed entirely, it frequently became much aggravated, when the head was so much drawn back as to seriously impede respiration. The legs were also sometimes flexed spasmodically. The effect of the spasm in obstructing the respiration, and hurrying the circulation, was very great, and seemed to place the patient in great jeopardy. The pulse was never less than 150, but during the paroxysm was considerably increased. It was evident I had got a most formidable case to contend with, and that no time ought to be lost. I therefore determined to try the power of hypnotism, well knowing how generally such cases end fatally under ordinary treatment. He was quite sensible, and the only difficulty in getting him to comply with my instructions, arose from the recurrence of the severe spasmodic attacks. In a very few minutes, however, I succeeded in reducing the spasm so that his head could be carried forward to the perpendicular, his breathing was relieved, his pulse considerably diminished, and I left him in a state of comparative comfort. In about two and a half hours after, I visited him again, accompanied by my friend Dr. Cochrane. The spasms had recurred, but by no means with the same violence. Dr. Cochrane had no difficulty in recognising the disease, but did not believe any means could save such a case. He had never seen a patient hypnotised till that afternoon, and watched my experiment with much interest and attention. He seemed much and agreeably surprised by the extraordinary influence which an agency so apparently simple exerted over such a case. The pupil was speedily dilated, as if under the influence of belladonna; the muscular spasm relaxed, and in a few minutes he was calmly asleep. Having ordered three calomel powders to be given at intervals, we left him comfortably asleep. Next day there was still spasm of the muscles, but by no means so severe. Whilst I determined to follow up the hypnotic treatment, which had been so far successful, I considered it would be highly imprudent to trust *wholly* to that in the treatment of such a case. As I consider such cases are generally attended with inflammation of the medulla oblongata, and upper part of the spinal cord, I bled him, and ordered the calomel to be continued. The same plan was persevered in, hypnotising him occasionally for some days, administering calomel till the gums were slightly affected, cold lotion to the head, and the antiphlogistic regimen till I considered all risk of inflammatory action past, when he was treated more generously, and I am gratified to say he is now quite well.

I feel confident that without the aid of hypnotism this patient would have died. I sincerely wish it may prove equally successful in other cases of the kind, and also in that hitherto fatal disease, hydrophobia. **My anxiety to see it fairly tried in the latter disease induces me to offer my gratuitous services in any case of that disease occurring within a few hours' journey of Manchester.**

I consider it necessary to explain that my reason for having inserted some cases attested by the patients and others is that most unwarrantable interferences have been resorted to by several medical men, in order to misrepresent some of them. In one instance, in order to obtain an *attested erroneous* document, the case was READ to *the patient and others present,* THE VERY REVERSE OF WHAT WAS WRITTEN. However extraordinary such conduct may appear, the fact of its occurrence was *publicly proved, and borne testimony to by the patient and other parties present on the occasion when the document was obtained.*

Introduction

General Remarks

It was my intention to have published my "Practical Essay on the Curative Agency of Neuro-Hypnotism", exactly as delivered at the conversazione [a medical lecture and discussion] given, to the members of the British Association in Manchester, on the 29th June, 1842. By so doing, and by appending foot notes, comprising the data on which my views were grounded, it would have conveyed a pretty clear knowledge of the subject, and of the manner in which it had been treated. It has since been suggested, however, that it might readily be incorporated with the short "Elementary Treatise on Neuro-Hypnology", which I originally intended to publish, and which I am earnestly solicited to do, by letters from professional gentlemen from all quarters. I now, therefore, submit my views to the public in the following condensed form. I shall aim at brevity and perspicuity; and my great object will be to teach others all I know of the modes of inducing the phenomena, and their application in the cure of diseases, and to invite my professional brethren to labour in the same field of inquiry, feeling assured, that the cause of science and humanity must thereby be promoted.

It was with this conviction I offered my "Practical Essay on the Curative Agency of Neuro-Hypnotism", to the medical section of the British Association.

In November, 1841, I was led to investigate the pretensions of animal magnetism, or Mesmerism, as a complete sceptic, from an anxiety to discover the source of fallacy in certain phenomena I had heard were exhibited at M. Lafontaine's conversazioni. The result was that I made some discoveries which appeared to elucidate certain of the phenomena, and rendered them interesting, both in a speculative and practical point of view. I considered it a most favourable opportunity for having additional light thrown upon this subject, to offer a paper to the medical section of the British Association, which was about to meet in Manchester. Gentlemen of scientific attainments might thus have had an opportunity of investigating it, and eliciting the truth, unbiased by local or personal prejudice. I hoped to learn something from others, on certain points which were extremely mysterious to me, as to the cause of some remarkable phenomena. I accordingly intimated my intention to the secretaries, by letter, on 18th May and on the morning of Wednesday, the 22nd June, 1842, sent the paper I proposed reading for the consideration of the committee, intimating also, by letter, my intention to produce before them as many of the patients as possible, whose cases were referred to in proof of the curative agency of Neuro-Hypnotism, so that they might have an opportunity of ascertaining, for themselves, the real facts of the cases, uninfluenced by any bias or partiality that I might exhibit as the discoverer and adapter of this new mode of treatment. The committee of the medical section, however, were pleased to decline entertaining the subject.

Many of the most eminent and influential members of the Association, however, had already witnessed and investigated my experiments in private, and expressed themselves highly gratified and interested with them. In compliance with the repeated desire of these gentlemen, and many other eminent members of the Association to whom I could not possibly afford time to exhibit my experiments in private, and who were anxious to have an opportunity afforded them of seeing, hearing, and judging of the phenomena for themselves, **I gave a gratuitous conversazione, when I read the "Rejected Essay", and exhibited the experiments in a public room, to which all the members of the Association had been respectfully invited.** The interest with which the subject was viewed by the members of the Association generally, was sufficiently testified by the number and high respectability of those who attended on that occasion; in reference to which the chairman requested the reporters to put on record, "that he had been in the habit for many years of attending public meetings, and he had never in his life seen a more unmixed, a more entirely respectable assembly in Manchester." It was also manifested by their passing a vote of thanks at the conclusion of the conversazione, for my having afforded an opportunity to the members of the British Association of witnessing my experiments, to which they had previously borne testimony as having been "highly successful".

On that occasion I stated, there were certain phenomena, which I could readily induce by particular manipulations, whilst I candidly confessed myself unable to explain the *modus operandi* by which they were induced. **I referred particularly to the extraordinary rapidity with which dormant functions, and a state of cataleptiform rigidity, may be changed to the extreme opposite condition, by a simple waft of wind, either from the lips, a pair of bellows, or by any other mechanical means.** I solicited information on these points, both privately and publicly, from all the eminently scientific gentlemen who honoured me with their company during the meetings of the British Association in this town; but no one ventured to express a decided opinion as to the causes of these remarkable phenomena. I now beg to assure every reader of this treatise, that I shall esteem it a great favour to be enlightened on points which I confess are, at present, still above my comprehension.

Why Hypnotism has been Separated from Animal Magnetism

It will be observed, for reasons adduced, **I have now entirely separated Hypnotism from Animal Magnetism**. I consider it to be merely a simple, speedy, and certain mode of throwing the nervous system into a new condition, which may be rendered eminently available in the cure of certain disorders. I trust, therefore, it may be investigated quite independently of any bias, either for or against the subject, as connected with Mesmerism; and only by the facts which can be adduced.

How Far Considered useful in the Cure of Disease

I feel quite confident we have acquired in this process a valuable addition to our curative means; but **I repudiate the idea of holding it up as a universal remedy**; nor do I even pretend to understand, as yet, the *whole range of diseases* in which it may be useful. Time and experience alone can determine this question, as is the case with all other new remedies.

Its Powers on the Animal Functions

When we consider that in this process we have acquired the power of **raising sensibility to the most extraordinary degree, and also of depressing it far below the torpor of natural sleep**[98]; and that from the latter condition, any or all of the senses may be raised to the exalted state of sensibility referred to, almost *with the rapidity of thought*, by so simple an agency as a puff of air directed against the respective parts; and that we can also raise and depress the force and frequency of the circulation, locally or generally, in a most extraordinary degree, it must be evident we have thus an important power to act with. **Whether these extraordinary physical effects are produced through the imagination chiefly, or by other means, it appears to me quite certain, that the imagination has never been so much under our control, or capable of being made to act in the same beneficial and uniform manner, by any other mode of management hitherto known.**

Certain Erroneous Beliefs Refuted

That we really have acquired in this process a valuable addition to our curative means, which enables us speedily to put an end to many diseases which resisted ordinary treatment, I think will be satisfactorily manifested by the cases which I have recorded. Many of these cases have been seen by other medical men, and are so remarkable, so self-evident to every candid and intelligent mind, that it is impossible, with any show of propriety, to deny them. Most unwarrantable and novel attempts have been made, not only to extinguish the farther prosecution of Hypnotism, but also to misrepresent all I had either said or done on the subject, and thus damage me, as well as Hypnotism, in public estimation. I am in possession of a mass of documentary evidence in proof of this, to an extent which could scarcely be credited. But I shall not trouble my readers with details of all that has been done in order to prejudice my patients against me.

Opinions and Practice of Bertrand and Abbé Faria, Mr. Brooks, Dr. Prichard

As regards general principles, it has even been attempted, by garbled statements, to set forth such gross misrepresentations as could only be credited by parties totally ignorant of the subject. **Thus it was alleged, that my mode of hypnotising was no novelty; on the contrary, that it was an unacknowledged plagiarism, and that it was the opinion and practice of Bertrand and the Abbé Faria.** Now, so far as I have been able to comprehend the meaning of Bertrand, which Colquhoun observes, "it is rather difficult to comprehend", he adheres "to the theory of imagination, and imagination alone", (Colquhoun's *Introduction*, p. 94). At p. 34, vol. iv, of the *Encyclopaedia of Practical Medicine*, [1833] Dr. [James Cowles] Prichard says of Bertrand, that he "comes at last to the conclusion, that all the results of these operations are brought about through the influence of the mind;" that is, through the influence of the imagination of the patients acting on themselves. Bertrand also supports this opinion by the manner in which the Abbé Faria performed magnetization. His plan was this: "He placed the patient in an arm-chair, and after telling him to shut his eyes, and collect himself, suddenly pronounced, in a strong voice and imperative tone, the word "*dormez*", which generally produced on the individual an impression sufficiently strong to give a slight shock, and occasion warmth, transpiration, and sometimes somnambulism." Had his success by this method been as general as mine, would he have used the word "*sometimes*" on this occasion?[99] It is farther added, "If the first attempt failed, he tried the experiment a second, third, and even a fourth time, after which he declared the individual incapable of entering into the state of lucid sleep." Whilst it is doubted that his success was equal to what he represented it, still Bertrand states, in reference to the Abbé Faria, that it was incontestable, "that he very often succeeded". Now, is this not sufficient proof, that his success was by no means so general as mine? And who does not see, on perusing my directions for hypnotising,[100] that our methods are very different?

---

[98] *Vide* Experiments [Chapter 4]
[99] *Vide* [Chapter 1]
[100] For proof of this, see [Chapter 1]

It is farther added, "The complete identity of the phenomena thus produced by a method which operated confessedly through the imagination, with those which display themselves under the ordinary treatment of the magnetizers, affords a strong reason for concluding that the results in other instances depend upon a similar principle." It is still farther added, that M. Bertrand denies the necessity of strong intense volitions of the operator being necessary to produce the result. He declared, "that in trials made by himself, precisely the same results followed, whether he WILLED to produce them or not, provided that the patient was *inwardly persuaded that the whole ritual was duly observed*". Can any farther remarks be required to prove that Bertrand referred the result entirely to the effect of imagination? And can anyone who has attended to what I have given as my opinion, say that this either was, or is my opinion? Certainly quite the contrary. The parties referred to, therefore, have only proved their belief of how easy it is, by garbled statements, to misrepresent the truth, when submitting such remarks to those ignorant of the subject, or who are blinded by prejudice.

The following remarks by Mr. H. Brookes, a celebrated lecturer on animal magnetism, will illustrate this point rather better than the individuals referred to. On hearing that **I had changed my original opinion about *identity* [of hypnotism and Mesmerism], he writes thus: "I am very glad you have at length found reason to change your original opinion as to the identity of your phenomena with those of Mesmerism. From the very first I freely admitted the value and importance of your discovery, but I could not admit that identity, and I blamed you for insisting upon it so hastily, and using such hard words against the animal magnetists, because they could not agree with you. I thought, and still think, you did wrong in that, and that you certainly did yourself injustice, for in fact you are the original discoverer of *a new agency*, and not of a mere modification of an old one."**

But when so much had been said of Bertrand, with the hope of making it appear that I had either been ignorant of, or copied his views without due acknowledgment, which is evidently erroneous, why not have quoted him also to prove I was wrong in attributing curative effects as resulting from these operations? Let us hear what M. Bertrand says on this point. He "declares, that it is difficult to imagine with what facility the practisers of the art succeed in relieving the most severe affections of the nervous system. Attacks of epilepsy, in particular, are rendered considerably less frequent and severe by their method skilfully employed; which displays in so remarkable a manner the influence of moral impressions on the physical state of the constitution." After such declarations in favour of the *curative power* of Mesmerism, had M. Bertrand's method of inducing the condition been as generally and speedily successful as mine, will anyone believe that it would not have been brought more generally into practice ere now? Mr. Mayo, one of our best authorities, in a letter to me on this subject states distinctly that the great reason for its not being more generally introduced into practice, was the tediousness of the processes for inducing the condition, and the uncertainty, after all the time and trouble devoted to the manipulation, of producing any result whatever. He concludes his observations on this subject, by the remark, "*It took up too much time*." And Dr. Prichard, author of the article referred to in the *Encyclopaedia of Practical Medicine*, adds, "On the whole, when we consider the degree of suffering occasioned by disorders of the class over which magnetism exerts an influence, through the medium of the imagination, and the little efficacy which ordinary remedies possess, of alleviating or counteracting them, it is much to be wished that this art, notwithstanding the problematical nature of the theories connected with it, were better known to us in actual practice."

Its Moral Influence

I am aware great prejudice has been raised against Mesmerism, from the idea that it might be turned to immoral purposes. In respect to the Neuro-Hypnotic state, induced by the method explained in this treatise, I am quite certain that *it* deserves no such censure. I have proved by experiments, both in public and in private, that **during the state of excitement, the judgment is sufficiently active to make the patients, if possible, even *more* fastidious as regards propriety of conduct, than in the waking condition;** and from the state of rigidity and insensibility, they can be roused to a state of mobility, and exalted sensibility, either by being rudely handled, or even by a breath of air. Nor is it requisite this should be done by the person who put them into the Hypnotic state. It will follow equally from the manipulations of anyone else, or a current of air impinging against the body, from any mechanical contrivance whatever. And, finally, the state cannot be induced, in any stage, unless with the knowledge and consent of the party operated on. This is more than can be said respecting a great number of our most valuable medicines, for there are many which we are in the daily habit of using, with the best advantage in the relief and cure of disease, which may be, and have been rendered most potent for the furtherance of the ends of the vicious and cruel; and which can be administered *without the knowledge of the intended victim*. It ought never to be lost sight of, that there is the *use* and *abuse* of every thing in nature. It is the *use*, and only the *judicious use* of Hypnotism, which I advocate.

Should be used by Professional Men Only

It is well-known that I have never made any secret of my modes of operating, as they have not only been exhibited and explained publicly, but also privately, to any professional gentleman, who wished for farther information on the subject. Encouraged by the confidence which flows from a consciousness of the honesty and integrity of my purpose, and a thorough conviction of the reality and value of this as a means of cure, I have persevered, in defiance of much, and, as I think, unwarrantable and capricious opposition.

In now unfolding to the medical profession generally – to whose notice, and kind consideration, this treatise is more particularly presented – my views on what I conceive to be a very important, powerful, and extraordinary agent in the healing art, I beg at once distinctly to be understood, as repudiating the idea of its being, or ever becoming, a universal remedy. On the contrary, I feel quite assured it will require all the acumen and experience of medical men, to decide in what cases it would be safe and proper to have recourse to such a mean; and I have always deprecated, in the strongest terms, any attempts at its use amongst unprofessional persons, for the sake of curiosity, or even for a nobler and more benevolent object – the relief of the infirm; because I am satisfied it ought to be left in the hands of professional men, and of them only. I have myself met with some cases in which I considered it unsafe to apply it at all; and with other cases in which it would have been most hazardous to have carried the operation so far as the patients urged me to do.[101]

In now submitting my opinions and practice to the profession in the following treatise, I consider myself as having discharged an imperative duty to them, and to the cause of humanity. In future, I intend to go on quietly and patiently, prosecuting the subject in the course of my practice, and shall leave others to adopt or reject it, as they shall find consistent with their own convictions.

Definition of Terms
As it is of the utmost importance, in discussing any subject, to have a correct knowledge of the meaning attached to peculiar terms made use of, I shall now give a few definitions, and explain my reasons for adopting the terms selected.

Neurypnology is derived from the Greek words νευρον, nerve [*neuron*]; υπνος, sleep [*hypnos*]; λογος, a discourse [*logos*]; and means the *rationale*, or *doctrine* of *nervous* sleep, which I define to be, "a peculiar condition of the nervous system, into which it can be thrown by artificial contrivance": or thus, "a peculiar condition of the nervous system, induced by a fixed and abstracted attention of the mental and visual eye, on one object, not of an exciting nature".

By the term "Neuro-Hypnotism", then, is to be understood "nervous sleep"; and, for the sake of brevity, suppressing the prefix "Neuro," by the terms:–

Hypnotic		The state or condition of *nervous* sleep.
Hypnotise		To induce *nervous* sleep.
Hypnotised	Will be understood,	One who has been put into the state of *nervous* sleep.
Hypnotism		*Nervous* sleep.
Dehypnotise		To restore from the state or condition of *nervous* sleep.
Dehypnotised		Restored from the state or condition of *nervous* sleep.
Hypnotist		One who practises Neuro-Hypnotism.

Whenever, therefore, any of these terms are used in the following pages, I beg to be understood as alluding to the discovery I have made of certain peculiar phenomena derived and elicited by my mode of operating; and of which, to prevent misconception, and intermingling with other theories and practices on the nervous system, I have thought it best to give the foregoing designation.

I regret, as many of my readers may do, the inconvenient length of the name; but, as most of our professional terms, and nearly all those of a doctrinal meaning, have a Greek origin, I considered it most in accordance with good taste, not to deviate from an established usage. To obviate this in some degree, I have struck out two letters from the original orthography, which was Neuro-Hypnology.

---

[101] The circumstances which render my operations dangerous, the symptoms which indicate danger, and the mode of acting when they occur, to remove them, are pointed out [at the end of Chapter 3].

PART I:
The Theory & Practice of Hypnotism

Chapter 1:
The Discovery of Hypnotism

Introductory Remarks
Having in the introduction presented a cursory view of certain points, and given a few explanatory remarks, I shall now proceed to a more particular and detailed consideration of the subject. I shall explain the course I have pursued in prosecuting my investigation; the phenomena which I discovered to result from the manipulations I had recourse to; the inferences I was consequently led to deduce from them; the method I now recommend for inducing the hypnotic condition, for applying it in the cure of various disorders, and the result of my experience, as to the efficacy of hypnotism as a curative agent.

By the impression which hypnotism induces on the nervous system, we acquire a power of rapidly curing many **functional disorders**, most intractable, or altogether incurable, by ordinary remedies, and also many of those distressing affections which, as in most cases they evince no pathological change of structure, have been presumed to depend on some peculiar condition of the nervous system, and have therefore, by universal consent, been denominated *"nervous complaints";* and as I felt satisfied it was not dependent on any special agency or emanation, passing from the body of the operator to that of the patient, as the animal magnetizers allege is the case by their process, I considered it desirable, for the sake of preventing misconception, to adopt new terms, as explained in the introduction.

Circumstances which Directed to the Investigation
I was led to discover the mode I now adopt with so much success for inducing this artificial condition of the nervous system, by a course of experiments instituted with the view to determine the cause of Mesmeric phenomena. From all I had read and heard of Mesmerism, (such as, the phenomena being capable of being excited in so few, and these few individuals in a state of disease, or naturally of a delicate constitution, or peculiarly susceptible temperament, and from the phenomena, when induced, being said to be so exaggerated, or of such an extraordinary nature) I was fully inclined to join with those who considered the whole to be a system of collusion or delusion, or of excited imagination, sympathy, or imitation.

A Real Phenomenon observed
The first exhibition of the kind I ever had an opportunity of attending, was one of M. Lafontaine's conversazione, on the 13th November, 1841. That night I saw nothing to diminish, but rather to confirm, my previous prejudices. At the next conversazione, six nights afterwards [19th November], *one* fact, the inability of a patient to *open his eyelids,* arrested my attention. I considered that to be a *real phenomenon,* and was anxious to discover the physiological cause of it. Next night, I watched this case when again operated on, with intense interest, and before the termination of the experiment, felt assured I had discovered its cause, but considered it prudent not to announce my opinion publicly, until I had had an opportunity of testing its accuracy, by experiments and observation in private.

Experiments Instituted to Prove the Cause of it
In two days afterwards [22nd November], I developed my views to my friend Captain [Thomas] Brown [a fellow Wernerian and respected natural historian], as I had also previously done to four other friends; and in his presence, and that of my family, and another friend, the same evening, I instituted a series of experiments to prove the correctness of my theory, namely, that the **continued fixed stare, by paralysing nervous centres in the eyes and their appendages**[102]**, and destroying the equilibrium of the nervous system, thus produced the phenomenon referred to.** The experiments were varied so as to convince all present, that they fully bore out the correctness of my theoretical views.

My first object was to prove, that the inability of the patient to open his eyes was caused by paralysing the levator muscles of the eyelids, through their continued action during the protracted fixed stare, and thus rendering it *physically* impossible for him to open them.[103] With the view of proving this, I requested Mr. Walker, a young gentleman present, to sit down, and maintain a fixed **stare at the top of a wine bottle**, placed so much above him as to produce a considerable strain on the eyes and eyelids, to enable him to maintain a steady view of the object. **In three minutes his eyelids closed, a gush of tears ran down his cheeks, his head drooped, his face was slightly convulsed, he gave a groan, and instantly fell into profound sleep, the respiration becoming slow, deep and sibilant [i.e., slightly wheezing or snoring], the right hand and arm being agitated by slight convulsive movements**

---

[102] By this expression I mean the state of exhaustion which follows too long continued, or too intense action, of any organ or function.
[103] Attempts have been made to prove, that I got this idea from a person who publicly maintained that the patient referred to *could* have opened his eyes *if he liked;* to this the patient having replied, "I have tried all I could and cannot"; the individual referred to, in support of his opinion, alleged, that the inability *was only imaginary;* that he "could easily believe that a man may stand with his back to a wall, and may really believe that he has no power to move from the wall". It is therefore clear this individual attributed the phenomena to a *mental,* whilst I attributed it to a *physical* cause.

[subsequently termed "hypnic jerks"]. At the end of four minutes I considered it necessary, for his safety, to put an end to the experiment.

This experiment not only proved what I expected, but also, by calling my attention to the **spasmodic state of the muscles of the face and arm**, the **peculiar state of the respiration**, and the condition of the mind, as evinced on rousing the patient, tended to prove to my mind I had got the key to the solution of Mesmerism. The **agitation and alarm of this gentleman,** on being roused, very much astonished **Mrs. Braid.** She expressed herself greatly surprised at his being so much alarmed about nothing, as she had watched the whole time, and never saw me near him, or touching him in any way whatever.[104] I proposed that she should be the next subject operated on, to which she readily consented, assuring all present that she would not be so easily alarmed as the gentleman referred to. I requested her to sit down, and gaze on the ornament of a china sugar basin, placed at the same angle to the eyes as the bottle in the former experiment. In **two minutes** the **expression of the face was very much changed**; at the end of two minutes and a half the **eyelids closed convulsively**; the **mouth was distorted**; she give a **deep sigh**, the **bosom heaved**, she **fell back**, and was evidently passing into an **hysteric paroxysm** [Braid possibly means a panic attack], to prevent which I instantly aroused her; on counting **the pulse** I found it had mounted up to **180 strokes a minute**.

In order to prove my position still more clearly, I called up one of my men-servants, who knew nothing of Mesmerism, and gave him such directions as were calculated to impress his mind with the idea, that his fixed attention was merely for the purpose of watching a chemical experiment in the preparation of some medicine, and being familiar with such he could feel no alarm. In **two minutes and a half** his **eyelids closed stoutly with a vibrating motion**, his **chin fell on his breast**, he gave a **deep sigh**, and instantly was in a profound sleep, **breathing loudly**. All the persons present burst into a fit of laughter, but still he was not interrupted by us. In about one minute after his profound sleep I roused him, and pretended to chide him for being so careless, said he ought to be ashamed of himself for not being able to attend to my instructions for three minutes without falling asleep, and ordered him down stairs. In a short time **I recalled this young man, and desired him to sit down once more, but to be careful not to go to sleep again**, as on the former occasion. He sat down with this intention, but in the expiration of two minutes and a half his eyelids closed, and exactly the same phenomena as in the former experiment ensued.

I again tried the experiment by causing Mr. Walker to gaze on a different object from that used in the first experiments, but still, as I anticipated, the phenomena were the same. **I also tried him *à la Fontaine,* with the thumbs and eyes**, and likewise **by gazing on my eyes without contact**, and still the effects were the same, as I fully expected.

Opinions and Conclusions Drawn From Them

I now stated that I considered the experiments fully proved my theory; and expressed my entire conviction that **the phenomena of Mesmerism were to be accounted for on the principle of a derangement of the state of the cerebrospinal centres, and of the circulatory, and respiratory, and muscular systems, induced, as I have explained, by a fixed stare, absolute repose of body, fixed attention, and suppressed respiration, concomitant with that fixity of attention;** that the whole depended on the physical and psychical condition of the patient, arising from the causes referred to, and not at all on the volition, or passes of the operator, throwing out a magnetic fluid, or exciting into activity some mystical universal fluid medium. I farther added, that having thus produced the *primary* phenomena, I had no doubt but the others would follow as a matter of course, time being allowed for their gradual and successive development.[105]

Reasons for Separating Hypnotism from Mesmerism

For a considerable time I was of opinion that the phenomena induced by my mode of operating and that of the Mesmerisers, were identical; and, so far as I have yet personally seen, I still consider the condition of the nervous system induced by both modes to be at least analogous. It appeared to me

---

[104] [Though this is rare, certain subjects are known to experience feelings of spontaneous panic or acute anxiety during hypnosis and deep relaxation.]

[105] It has been asserted, for the mere purpose of proving the contrary, that I had claimed being the first to discover that *contact* was *not* necessary, and that a magnetic fluid was not required to produce the phenomena of Mesmerism. I never made any such claim, but illustrated these facts by the most simple and conclusive experiments probably which were ever adduced for that purpose. In one of my lectures, I gave a history of Mesmerism, including Mesmer's attempt to Mesmerise trees in Dr. Franklin's garden, to prove to the Commission of 1784, that the patients would become affected when they went under the Mesmerised trees, from the magnetic fluid passing from the trees to the patients. This was proof sufficient, that even *Mesmer* did not hold that *contact* was necessary. I farther stated the fact, that the experiment was a failure, as the patient became affected, *not* under the *Mesmerised,* but under *the unMesmerised* trees, which led the Commission to infer, that the phenomena resulted from imagination, and not from the influence of a magnetic fluid. Here, then, we had two theories, neither of which considered contact necessary. Surely no one could suppose that I wished to lay claim to these facts as discoveries of my own, seeing I gave the dates when the occurrence took place, which was many years before I was born.

Moreover, I explained at the same lecture the different modes of Mesmerising, by passes at a *distance,* and by pointing the fingers at the eyes and forehead, adopted by others, long before I made any experiments on the subject; and at subsequent lectures, from observing the graceful attitudes some patients assumed during the hypnotic state, and the ease with which they could maintain any given position, by becoming cataleptiformly fixed in it, I hazarded the opinion, that it may have been to hypnotism the Grecians were indebted for their fine statuary; and the Fakirs for their power of performing their remarkable feats. I also expressed my belief, that the rapt state of religious enthusiasts, such as that of the monks of Mount Athos, arose from the same cause, although none of the parties might have understood the true principle by which they were produced.

that the fixation of the mind and eyes was attained occasionally during the monotonous movements of the Mesmerisers, and thus they succeeded sometimes, and as it were, by chance; whereas, by my insisting on the eyes being fixed in the most favourable position, and the mind thus riveted to one idea, as the *primary and imperative conditions,* **my success was consequently general and the effects intense, while theirs was feeble and uncertain.** However, from what the Mesmerisers state as to effects which they can produce in certain cases, there seem to be differences sufficient to warrant the conclusion that they ought to be considered as distinct agencies; and for the following reasons. The Mesmerisers positively assert that they can produce certain [paranormal] effects, which I have never been able to produce by my mode, although I have tried to do so.[106] Now, I do not consider it fair or proper to impugn the statements of others in this matter, who are known to be men of talent and observation, and of undoubted credit in *other* matters, merely because *I* have not *personally* witnessed the phenomena, or been able to produce them myself, either by my own mode or theirs. With my present means of knowledge I am willing to admit that certain phenomena to which I refer *have* been induced by others, but still I think most of them may be explained in a different and more natural way than that of the Mesmerisers. When I shall have personally had evidence of the special influence and its effects to which they lay claim, I shall not be backward in bearing testimony to the fact.

Hypnotism More Generally Successful than Animal Magnetism

However, the greatest and most important difference is this, that **they can succeed so seldom, and I so generally**, in inducing the phenomena which we both profess thus to effect. Granting, therefore, to the Mesmerisers the full credit of being able to produce certain wonderful phenomena which I have not been able to produce by my plan, still it follows, that mine is superior to theirs in as far as *general applicability and practical utility are concerned.* Mine has also this advantage, that **I am quite certain no one can be affected by it, in any stage of the process, unless by the free will and consent of the patient**, which is at once sufficient to exonerate the practice from the imputations of being capable of being converted to immoral purposes, which has been so much insisted on to the prejudice of animal magnetism. This has arisen from **the Mesmerisers asserting that they have the power of overmastering patients irresistibly, even whilst at a distance, by mere volition and secret passes.**

Mr. Herbert Mayo's Testimony on This Point

I am fully borne out by the opinion of that eminent physiologist, Mr. Herbert Mayo [Professor of Physiology & Anatomy at King's College, London], **in my view of the subject, that my plan is "the best, the shortest, and surest for getting the sleep", and throwing the nervous system, by artificial contrivance, into a new condition, which may be rendered available in the healing art.** At a private conversazione, which I gave to the profession in London on the 1st of March, 1842, he examined and tested my patients most carefully, submitted himself to be operated on by me both publicly and privately, and was so searching and inquisitive in his investigations as to call forth the animadversions of a medical gentleman present, who thought he was not giving me fair play; but which he has assured me proceeded from an anxious desire to know the truth, not being biased by having any peculiar views of his own to bring forward; and because he considered the subject most important, both in a speculative and practical point of view. [Herbert Mayo published an article entitled 'On Mr. Braid's experiments', in *The Medical Times*, vol. vi, 1842, p. 11.]

Proofs of this Referred to

Whatever I advance, therefore, in the following remarks, I wish to be distinctly understood as strictly in reference to my own mode of operating, and distinct from that of all others. The latter I shall merely refer to in as far as is necessary to point out certain sources of fallacy by which the phenomena of the one may be confounded with those of the other.

In proof of the general success of my mode of operating, I need only name, that at one of my public lectures in Manchester, **fourteen male adults, in good health, all strangers to me, stood up at once, and ten of them became decidedly hypnotised [71%]**. At Rochdale I conducted the experiments for a friend, and hypnotised twenty strangers in one night. At a private conversazione to the profession in London, on the 1st of March, 1842, **eighteen adults, most of them entire strangers to me, sat down at once, and in ten minutes sixteen of them were decidedly hypnotised [89%]**. Mr. Herbert Mayo tested some of these patients, and satisfied himself of the reality of the phenomena. On another occasion **I took thirty-two children into a room, none of whom had either seen or heard of hypnotism or Mesmerism. I made them stand up three times, and in ten or twelve minutes had the whole thirty-two hypnotised, maintaining their arms extended while in the hypnotic condition, and this at mid-day.** In making this statement, I do not mean to say they were in the *ulterior* stage, or

---

[106] The effects I allude to are such as, telling the time on a watch held behind the head, or placed on the pit of the stomach; reading closed letters, or a shut book; perceiving what is doing miles off; having the power of perceiving the nature and cure of the diseases of others, although uneducated in medical science; Mesmerising patients at miles' distance, without the knowledge or belief in the patient that any such operation is intended.

state of *torpor* but that they were in the *primary* stage, or that of *excitement*, from which experience has taught me confidently to rely that the torpid and rigid state will certainly follow, by merely affording time for the phenomena to develop themselves. In the *Stockport Chronicle* of 4th February, 1842, there is a report of a lecture delivered in that town a few days before. A dozen male patients were made to stand up at once, and treated according to my method, six of them became hypnotised [50%], and two of them so deeply, as to cause the lecturer very considerable trouble to rouse them. With one named "Charlie", all the usual means, including buffeting and frictions before a fire, did not succeed in restoring speech until he had been made to swallow nearly half a tumbler glass of *neat gin*.

Different Modes by which it can be Induced

I consider this important as being the testimony of *an enemy*. It can take place also in the dark, as well as by day or by gas light; when the eyes are bandaged, as when they are uncovered, by merely keeping the eyes fixed, the body in a state of absolute rest, and **the mind abstracted from all other considerations. In cases of children, and those of weak intellect, or of restless and excitable minds, whom I could not manage so as to make them comply with these simple rules, I have always been foiled, although most anxious to succeed. This I consider a strong proof of the correctness of my views. By arresting the attention, and fixing the eyes, it is also successful with brute animals.**

Can only be Expected to Succeed by Complying with the Whole Conditions Required

This general success of my plan, both with man and brute animals, I consider sufficient to prove it proceeds from a law in the animal economy [i.e., an innate physiological mechanism]. The exceptions to success are so few as to lead to the conclusion that they arise from a non-compliance with the conditions. It is, however, unquestionable, that there exists great difference in the susceptibility of different individuals, some becoming rapidly and intensely affected, others slowly and feebly so. I am aware that some say they have tried my mode, and failed to produce the phenomena. The reason, I presume, is simply this. They will not believe the necessity of complying with the WHOLE of the conditions I have distinctly insisted on. But, in all fairness, if they do not comply with the WHOLE conditions, they have no right to expect the promised results, nor to be disappointed because they fail. If the patient and operator comply in *all* respects as I direct, success is almost certain; but, on the contrary, he is almost equally certain to fail if *all* the conditions are not *strictly* complied with.

When we consider the great difficulty to some persons of abstracting their minds, and the greater difficulty of ensuring that patients operated on in a public room shall be able to abstract their minds entirely from the circumstances with which they are surrounded, and from other considerations concentrate their ideas entirely on the subject in hand, and the equally great difficulty of securing absolute quiet where a large number of people are assembled, and **the extreme quickness of hearing when patients are passing into the hypnotic state, which makes them liable to be roused by the slightest noise**, it must be evident, that a public lecture-room is by no means a favourable place for operating on patients for the first time.

Prosecuting the investigation, as I have been doing, by experiments and observations, I have, as might be expected, had occasion to modify and alter some of my views and manipulations; but still the principle remains the same.

Chapter 2:
On The Hypnotic Induction Process

Mode of Hypnotising
I now proceed to detail the mode which I practise for inducing the phenomena. Take any bright object (I generally use my lancet case) between the thumb and fore and middle fingers of the left hand; hold it from about eight to fifteen inches from the eyes, at such position above the forehead as may be necessary to produce the greatest possible strain upon the eyes and eyelids, and enable the patient to maintain a steady fixed stare at the object.[107]

Circumstances Necessary to be Complied with
The patient must be made to understand that he is to keep the eyes steadily fixed on the object, and the mind riveted on the idea of that one object. It will be observed, that owing to the consensual adjustment of the eyes, the pupils will be at first contracted: they will shortly begin to dilate, and after they have done so to a considerable extent, and have assumed a wavy motion, if the fore and middle fingers of the right hand, extended and a little separated, are carried from the object towards the eyes, most probably the eyelids will close involuntarily, with a vibratory motion. If this is not the case, or the patient allows the *eyeballs to move,* desire him to begin anew, giving him to understand that he is to allow the eyelids to close when the fingers are again carried towards the eyes, but that the eyeballs *must be kept fixed, in the same position, and the mind riveted to the one idea of the object held above the eyes.* It will generally be found, that the eyelids close with a *vibratory* motion, or become spasmodically closed. After ten or fifteen seconds have elapsed, by gently elevating the arms and legs, it will be found that the patient has a disposition to retain them in the situation in which they have been placed, if *he is intensely affected.*

Peculiar Phenomena which Follow; Excitement first, and Afterwards Depression of Function
If this is not the case, **in a soft tone of voice desire him to retain the limbs in the extended position**, and thus the **pulse will speedily become greatly accelerated,** and **the limbs, in process of time, will become quite rigid and involuntarily fixed.** It will also be found, that all the organs of special sense, excepting sight, including heat and cold, and muscular motion, or resistance, and certain mental faculties, are **at** *first* prodigiously *exalted,* such as happens with regard to the primary effects of opium, wine, and spirits. After a certain point, however, this exaltation of function is followed by a state of depression, far greater than the torpor of *natural* sleep.[108]

How These May be Made to Alternate with Each Other
From the state of the most profound torpor of the organs of special sense, and tonic rigidity of the muscles, there may, at this stage, instantly be restored to the opposite condition of extreme mobility and exalted sensibility, by directing a current of air against the organ or organs we wish to excite to action, or the muscles we wish to render limber, and which had been in the cataleptiform state. By mere repose the senses will speedily merge into the original condition again. The *modus operandi* of the current of air producing such extraordinary effects, I acknowledge myself quite unable to explain, but I have no difficulty in producing and reproducing the effects by the same means, whether performed by myself or others, and whether the current of air is from the lips, from a pair of bellows, or by the motion of the hand, or any inanimate object. The extent and abruptness of these transitions [see Chapter 4] are so extraordinary, that they must be seen before the possibility is believed.

Extraordinary Influence of a Current of air during Hypnotism
An abrupt blow, or pressure over the rigid muscle, will de-hypnotise a rigid part; but, I have found pressing the nose will not restore smell, unless very gentle and continued, nor will pressing a handkerchief against the ear restore hearing when the ear has become torpid, nor will *gentle* friction over the skin restore sensibility to the dormant skin, or mobility to the rigid muscles underneath, (unless so gentle as to be titillation, properly so

---

[107] At an early period of my investigations, I caused the patients to look at a cork bound on the forehead. This was a very efficient plan with those who had the power of converging the eyes so as to keep them *both steadily* directed on the object. I very soon found, however, that there were many who could not keep *both* eyes steadily fixed on so near an object, and that the result was, that such patients did not become hypnotised. To obviate this, I caused them to look at a more distant point, which, although scarcely so rapid and intense in its effects, succeeds more generally than the other, and is therefore what I now adopt and recommend.

[108] I wish to direct especial attention to this circumstance, as from overlooking the fact of the first stage of this artificial hypnotism being one of excitement, with the possession of consciousness and docility, many imagine they are not affected, whilst the acceleration of pulse, peculiar expression of countenance, and other characteristic symptoms, prove the existence of the condition beyond the possibility of a doubt, to all who understand the subject. I consider it very imprudent to carry it to the ulterior stage, or that of torpor, at a first trial. Moreover, there is great difference in the susceptibility to the neuro-hypnotic impression, some arriving at the state of rigidity and insensibility in a few minutes, whilst others may readily pass into the primary stage, but can scarcely be brought into the ulterior, or rigid and torpid state. It is also most important to note, that many instances of remarkable and permanent cures have occurred, where it has never been carried beyond the state of consciousness.

called) and yet a slight puff of wind will *instantly* rouse the whole to abnormal sensibility and mobility: a fact which has perplexed and puzzled me exceedingly.

Reasons for Certain Modifications of Original modes of Operating
At first I required the patients **to look at an object until the eyelids closed of themselves, involuntarily**. I found, however, that in many cases this was followed by **pain in the globes of the eyes**, and slight inflammation of the conjunctival membrane. In order to avoid this, **I now close the eyelids, when the impression on the pupil already referred to has taken place, because I find that the *beneficial* phenomena follow this method, provided the eyeballs are kept fixed, and thus, too, the unpleasant feelings in the globes of the eyes will be prevented. Were the object to produce astonishment in the person operated on, by finding himself unable to open his eyes, the former method is the better; as the eyes once closed it is generally impossible for him to open them; whereas they may be opened for a considerable time after being closed in the other mode I now recommend.** However, for curative purposes, I prefer the plan which leaves no pain in the globes of the eyes.

Hypnotism Proceeds from a Law of the Animal Economy
In fine, from a careful analysis of the whole of my experiments, which have been very numerous, I have been led to the following conclusion:– **That it is a law in the animal economy, that by a continued fixation of the mental and visual eye, on any object which is not of itself of an exciting nature, with absolute repose of body, and general quietude, they become wearied; and, provided the patients rather favour than resist the feeling of stupor of which they will soon experience the tendency to creep upon them, during such experiments, a state of somnolency is induced, accompanied with that condition of the brain and nervous system generally, which renders the patient liable to be affected, according to the mode of manipulating, so as to exhibit the hypnotic phenomena. As the experiment succeeds with the blind, I consider it not so much the optic, as the sentient, motor, and sympathetic nerves, and the mind through which the impression is made.** I feel so thoroughly convinced that it is a law of the animal economy that such effects should follow such condition of mind and body, that I hesitated not to give it as my deliberate opinion, that this is a *fact* which cannot be controverted. As to the *modus operandi* we may never be able to account for that in a manner so as to satisfy all objections; but neither can we tell why the law of gravitation should act as experience has taught us it *does* act. Still, as our ignorance of the cause of gravitation acting as it is known to do, does not prevent us profiting by an accumulation of the facts known as to its results, so ought not our ignorance of the *whole* laws of the hypnotic state to prevent our studying it practically, and applying it beneficially, when we have the power of doing so.

Arises from the Physical and Psychical Condition of the Patient
I feel confident that the phenomena are induced solely by an impression made on the nervous centres, by the physical and psychical condition of the patient, irrespective of any agency proceeding from, or excited into action by another – as **anyone can hypnotise himself by attending strictly to the simple rules I lay down**; and the following is a striking example of the fact, which was communicated to me and two other gentlemen, by a most respectable teacher.

Example for Proof
He found that a number of his pupils had been in the habit of hypnotising themselves, and he had ordered them to discontinue the practice. However, one day he ascertained a girl had hypnotised herself by looking at the wall, and that her companions had put a pen in her hand, with which she had written the word "Manchester"; and she held the pen very firmly – in fact the fingers were cataleptiformly rigid. He spoke to her in a gentle tone of voice, and called her. She arose and advanced towards him, and when awoke, was not aware he had called her, or of what had passed.

Exhibits no Appreciable Electric or Magnetic Change
I have also had the state of the patient tested before, during, and after being hypnotised, to ascertain if there was any alteration in the magnetic or electric condition, but although tested by excellent instruments, and with great care, no appreciable difference could be detected. Patients have been hypnotised whilst positively, and also whilst negatively, electrified, without any appreciable difference in the phenomena; so that they appear to be excited independently of electric or magnetic charge.

Two Patients may Hypnotise each other by Contact
I have also repeatedly made two patients hypnotise each other, at the same time, by personal contact. How could this be reconciled with the theory of a special influence transmitted being the cause of the phenomena, *plus* and *minus* being equally efficient?

Phenomena arise Spontaneously in Course of Disease
It is also well-known, that occasionally the phenomena arise spontaneously in the course of disease.

Mr. Wakley's Admission on this Point
It is now admitted even by [Thomas Wakley] the editor of *The Lancet*, one of the greatest opponents of Mesmerism, in the leading article of 4th February, 1843, that the phenomena "are wonderful only to those who are unacquainted with the aspects of disease"; and "that we continually see patients labouring under hysteria, and analogous forms of nervous disease, falling suddenly into various states of stupor, trance, and convulsion, without *any* assignable cause".

Mr. H. Mayo's Testimony as to the Effects of Hypnotism
When it is acknowledged that such effects as those named, may spring from such slight influences as to be said to arise *"without any assignable cause"*, can it be wondered at that important changes may be induced by acting on the nervous system in the way I have adopted, of which Mr. Herbert Mayo (whose competence to give an opinion on *any* physiological subject no one will question, and who himself publicly submitted to be operated on by me) observed, in the course of our correspondence, that it induces "a feeling of stupor, which anyone may observe has a disposition to creep upon him, when he tries your experiment of looking fixedly at an object as you direct". I thought it desirable, therefore, to adopt the name I did, for the reasons explained in the introduction.

Effects of Different Positions of the Eyes
A patient may be hypnotised by keeping the eyes fixed in *any* direction. It occurs most *slowly* and *feebly* when the eyes are directed straight forward, and most *rapidly* and *intensely* when they can be maintained in the position of a **double internal and upward squint.**[109]

Consensual Adjustment of Eyes; Effects on Size of Pupil
It is now pretty generally known, that during the effort to look at a very near object, there is produced, according to the direction of the object, a double internal squint, or double internal and downward or upward squint, and the pupils are thereby powerfully contracted. I am not aware, however, that it has been recorded, that by directing the eyes loosely, upwards or downwards, to the right or to the left, as if looking at a very distant object, the pupils become very much *dilated*, irrespective of the quantity of light passing to the retina; so that in this manner we can contract or dilate the pupil at will. To those who consider the movement of the iris as the mere effect of irritability, I may observe, in that view, the former position increases, the latter diminishes, the irritability. I may farther remark, if the eyes are much *strained* in ANY direction, I think the pupils will be found to contract as a consequence.

Power of Habit and Imagination
It is important to remark, that the oftener patients are hypnotised, from association of ideas and habit, the more susceptible they become; and in this way they are liable to be affected *entirely through the imagination*. Thus, if they consider or imagine there is something doing, although they do not see it, from which they are to be affected, they *will become affected;* but, on the contrary, the most expert hypnotist in the world may exert all his endeavours in vain, if the party does not expect it, and mentally and bodily comply, and thus yield to it.

Docility of Patients, and Exalted Sensibility, and their Effects
It is this very circumstance, coupled with the extreme docility and mobility of the patients, and extended range and extreme quickness of action, at a certain stage, of the ordinary functions of the organs of sense, including heat and cold, and muscular motion, the tendency of the patients in this state to approach to, or recede from, impressions, according as their intensity or quality is agreeable or the contrary, which I consider

---

[109] It is not a little amusing to find anyone try to distort so greatly, by garbled statements, the plain meaning of an author, as to make it appear that a writer of some articles on Animal Magnetism, in the *Medical Gazette* in 1838, was well acquainted with my mode of operating. He observes at page 856, "On the majority of persons no influence whatever is exhibited". How does this coincide with the general success of my mode as stated at page 24? "On those least affected a number of anomalous slight symptoms are produced". He then describes those "feelings of heat and cold, and those of creeping and trembling", which, he adds, "are only the usual imaginary feelings which most persons have if their attention be strongly directed to any particular part of the body, more especially if (as is generally the case with magnetic patients) something is expected to occur". Such are the symptoms attributed by this writer to "attention", but are these the symptoms or phenomena induced by Hypnotism, as stated in Chapter 4? Or is there the slightest similarity in the cause? In this author's view it is the result of "attention strongly directed to *different parts of the body"*, whereas mine is by attention riveted to something *without* the body. The best mode of gathering the opinion of an author appears to me to be that of his summing up at the conclusion of his subject. Now, at page 1037, the subject is concluded by the following observations: "This, then, is our case. Every credible effect of magnetism has occurred, and every incredible is *said* to have occurred in cases where no magnetic influence has been exerted, but in all which excited imagination, irritation, or some powerful mental impression, has operated: where the mind has been alone acted on, magnetic effects have been produced without magnetic manipulations: where magnetic manipulations have been employed, unknown, and therefore without the assistance of the mind, no result has ever been produced." Now, can anything more be required than this, to prove that this writer, as well as Bertrand, adheres to the theory of imagination? Such was the impression left on my mind by reading these papers when they were published; and, together with Wakley's experiments, determined me to consider the whole as a system of collusion or illusion, or of excited imagination, sympathy, or imitation. I therefore abandoned the subject as unworthy of further investigation, until I attended the conversazione of Lafontaine, where I saw one fact, the inability of a patient to open his eyelids, which arrested my attention; I felt convinced it was not to be attributed to any of the causes referred to, and I therefore instituted experiments to determine the question; and exhibited the results to the public in a few days after.

has misled so many, and induced the animal magnetizers to imagine they could produce their effects on patients at a distance, through mere volition and secret passes.[110]

Patient Hypnotised Whilst Operating on Another
It would be difficult to adduce a more striking example than the following of the fact, that the phenomena are produced by the fixation of the mind and eyes, and general repose of the patient, and not from imagination, or the look or will of another. After my lecture at the Hanover Square Rooms, London, on the 1st of March, 1842, a gentleman told Mr. Walker, who was along with me, that he was most anxious to see me, that I might try whether I could hypnotise him. He said both himself and friends were anxious he should be affected, but that neither Lafontaine nor others who had tried him, could succeed. Mr. Walker said, "If that is what you want, as Mr. Braid is engaged otherwise, sit down, and I will hypnotise you myself in a minute." When I went into the room I observed what was going on, **the gentleman sitting staring at Mr. Walker's finger,** who was standing a little to the right of the patient, with his eyes fixed steadily on those of the latter. I passed on, and attended to something else, and when I returned a little after, found Mr. Walker standing in the same position *fast asleep, his arm and finger in a state of cataleptiform rigidity,* and the patient wide awake, and staring at the finger all the while.

Mode of Resisting Influence
After I had roused Mr. Walker, the gentleman observed, "This is really very strange, that no one can Mesmerise *me;* I must have extraordinary powers of resistance." I requested him to stay a little, and I would try what I could do for him when all was quiet. In three minutes I had him asleep, and in a little more quite rigid. The following reasons may be assigned for my success after Mr. Walker had so signally failed. He tried it whilst there were several people in the room, who were moving about and talking; I took care not to commence till all was quiet – Mr. Walker had not taken the precaution to make the patient direct his eyes in the best possible manner, but I was careful that he should do so. Moreover, although Mr. Walker had not succeeded in putting him into the somnolent condition, he had, no doubt partially affected him, and the influence had not entirely passed off when I began my operation. Two days after, Mr. Walker accompanied me when I called on one of the most celebrated Mesmerisers in Europe, who, during our conversazione, stated, that a glance of the eye was quite enough, in many cases, to produce the effects. During our conversazione, I presume, he had determined to surprise both Mr. Walker and myself, by keeping his large intellectual eyes fixed on Mr. Walker. The latter, however, suspecting what was intended, and knowing my opinion as to the mode of *resisting* the influence of *such fascination,* kept his eyes moving, and his mind roaming, and thus frustrated the volition of one of the most energetic minds, and the glances and fascination of one of the finest pair of eyes imaginable for such a purpose. I must remark, that Mr. Walker was once magnetized by M. Lafontaine, after having been several times operated on by me, a circumstance which of course would render him more susceptible to the influence of the animal magnetizers' modes of operating, according to their own theory. Had Mr. Walker believed in the power, I know he would have become affected, even supposing the gentleman referred to had no such intention – and I am not prepared to say he had. Mr. Walker, however, firmly believed he was trying to Mesmerise him by the fascination referred to; but, relying on my opinion, and acting accordingly, he escaped. **In order to show the efficacy of my simple plan, in a short time after, in the presence of the same gentleman, I requested Mr. Walker to hypnotise himself. By simply fixing his eyes and mind this was accomplished in about a minute.**

---

[110] [See appendix (originally a lengthy footnote) entitled 'Excerpts from Medical Times Article'.]

Chapter 3:
On Hypnotism & Natural Sleep

Phenomena of Natural Sleep, Dreaming, and Somnambulism Contrasted
I consider it unnecessary, in this treatise, to enter into a *detailed* account of the ordinary phenomena of sleep, dreaming, and somnambulism, as contrasted with the waking state. Suffice it to say, the waking condition is that of mental and bodily activity, during which we are enabled to hold communion with the external world, by perceiving the ordinary impressions of appropriate stimuli through the organs of special sense, and of exercising the power of voluntary motion, and the mental functions generally. The state of *profound* sleep is exactly the *reverse* of this – a state of absolute unconsciousness of all that is going on around, and suspension of voluntary motion, and intellectual activity. In as far as regards the organs of special sense, and voluntary motion, and a temporary suspension of the mental energies, **it is the emblem of death.**

Between these extreme points there are *gradual* transitions, so that there are all possible varieties of condition imaginable, from the highest state of mental and bodily activity, to absolute torpor of both. There are two conditions, however, to which I may *briefly* advert – that of **dreaming** and of **somnambulism**. In the former, there are some of the mental and bodily functions in a state of partial activity, but, from the sensations arising from external stimuli being perceived very imperfectly, erroneous impressions are conveyed to the mind; and, as happens in some cases of insanity, the power of controlling the current of thought being absent, one idea excites another, until the most incongruous combinations are produced in many instances. Somnambulism, properly so called, is a state still more nearly allied to the waking condition than dreaming. The mental functions are more awake, a more just estimate of external impressions can be formed, and there is the power of voluntary motion present in a remarkable degree. Persons in this state are thus capable of being directed by those around, into certain trains of thought and action. The principal difference between the natural somnambulists and those who become so through hypnotising, in the manner pointed out in this treatise, is the greater tendency of the latter [hypnotic somnambulists] to lapse into a state of *profound* sleep, unless prevented by being roused and directed by those present. Natural somnambulists seem to be impelled to certain trains of action by *internal* impulses; but, so far as I have seen, the artificial somnambulists have an inclination to remain at absolute rest, unless excited to action by some impression from without. In compliance with such excitement, however, they evince great acuteness and docility. There is also another remarkable difference. **It is stated, that although natural somnambulists cannot remember, when awake, what they were engaged in when asleep, they have a vivid recollection of it when in that state again; but I have found no parallel to *this* in the somnambulism induced by hypnotism.** [Braid subsequently *retracts* this view, e.g., in *The Physiology of Fascination* (1855), having found that hypnotic amnesia can frequently be *removed* by re-hypnotising the subject.]

By this I mean that they cannot explain what happened during the former somnambulistic state, but they may approximate to the words and actions which had formerly manifested themselves, provided they are placed under exactly similar circumstances. For the extent to which peculiar manifestations may be brought out by manipulating the head and face, at a certain stage of hypnotism, see Chapter 6, where examples are given of **memory as regarded events which happened during the *waking* condition**, whilst they seemed to have no recollection of what happened during a former state of hypnotism.

Causes of Common Sleep
As to the causes of common sleep, I may remark, that, by the exercise of the mental operations, and the impressions conveyed through the organs of special sense, muscular effort, and the discharge of other animal functions, the brain becomes exhausted, and ceases to be affected by ordinary stimuli, and lapses into that dormant state we call sleep. During this condition it becomes recruited, and fitted for again receiving its wonted impressions through the organs of sense, and of holding intercourse with external nature, and exercising those powers of voluntary motion and mental function peculiar to the waking condition.

Of Dreaming
It will be generally admitted, that the most refreshing, and therefore the *most natural sleep,* accompanies that condition or languor which follows the *moderate* exercise or fatigue of *all* the bodily and mental functions, rather than an undue exercise of *one* or *more* to the neglect of the others. **It is long since it was observed that inordinate attention to one subject caused *dreaming,* instead of *sound sleep.***

Effects of Variety and Monotony Compared
It will also be found that the absolute length of time during which any function may be exercised, depends very much on the *continuity* of its exertion, or its alternation with that of other functions; thus the mind may become confused and bewildered by continuing one particular study for a length of time, but may be able to

return to it with energy and advantage, and prosecute the subject longer on the whole, by varying it with study of a different nature; moreover, bodily disease, and even insanity, frequently arises from following the mind to be occupied inordinately by one particular object or pursuit, whether that may be religion, politics, avarice, schemes of ambition, or any other passion, emotion, or object of unvaried contemplation.

Changes Alleged to Take Place in the Structure of the Brain by Exertion
In like manner, continued and over-intense muscular effort very soon exhausts the power of the muscles so exercised or over-exerted; and by keeping the eyes steadily and constantly exercised by gazing on a coloured spot, they soon cease to be able to discern the boundaries of the respective colours[111], and ultimately seem scarcely to be capable of distinguishing the spot at all. The same might be proved of the other senses. In fine, *alternate action and repose is the law of animated nature.*[112]

Cause of Hypnotism
It is on this very principle, of over-exerting the attention, by *keeping it riveted to one subject or idea which is not of itself of an exciting nature,* and, over-exercising one set of muscles, and the state of the strained eyes, with the suppressed respiration, and general repose, which attend such experiments, which excites in the brain and whole nervous system that peculiar state which I call Hypnotism, or nervous sleep. The most striking proofs that it is different from common sleep, are the extraordinary effects produced by it. In deep abstraction of mind, it is well-known, the individual becomes unconscious of surrounding objects, and in some cases, even of severe bodily infliction. During hypnotism, or nervous sleep, the functions in action seem to be so *intensely* active, as must in a great measure rob the others of that degree of nervous energy necessary for exciting their sensibility. This alone may account for much of the dullness of common feeling during the abnormal quickness and extended range of action of certain other functions.[113]

M'Nish's article on "Reverie" compared with Mr. Braid's theory of Hypnotism
The untoward result referred to in the note above [the young man, Charlie, who could not be roused from hypnotic catalepsy], I have no doubt, was the effect of permitting the experiment to be carried too far. No such consequence has ever followed in any of my operations, and for this reason, that I have always watched each case with close attention, and aroused the patient the moment I saw the slightest symptom of danger. I shall, therefore, now point out the symptoms of danger, with the mode of arousing patients, and thus preventing mischief which might ensue from want of due caution in the operator.

Mode of Arousing Patients from the State of Hypnotism
Whenever I observe the breathing very much oppressed, the face greatly flushed, the rigidity excessive, or the action of the heart very quick and tumultuous [perhaps signs of anxiety], I instantly arouse the patient, which I have always readily and speedily succeeded in doing by a clap of the hands, an abrupt shock on the arm or leg by striking them sharply with the flat hand, pressure and friction over the eyelids, and by a current of air wafted against the face. I have never failed by these means to restore my patients very speedily.

I feel convinced hypnotism is not only a valuable, but also a perfectly safe remedy for many complaints, if judiciously used; still it ought not to be trifled with by ignorant persons for the mere sake of gratifying idle curiosity. **In all cases of apoplectic tendency [Braid may mean stroke or neurological seizure], or where there is aneurysm, or serious organic disease of the heart, it ought not to be resorted to, excepting with the precaution, that it may be in the mode calculated to depress the force and frequency of the heart's action [rather than the cataleptic state of nervous arousal].**

---

[111] Müller.
[112] [See appendix (originally a lengthy footnote) 'On Exercise & Sleep (Müller)'.]
[113] [See appendix (originally a lengthy footnote) 'On Reverie'.]

Chapter 4:
On the Nature & Phenomena of Hypnotism

Phenomena of Common Sleep
In passing into common sleep objects are perceived more and more faintly, the eyelids close, and remain quiescent, and all the other organs of special sense become gradually blunted, and cease to convey their usual impressions to the brain, the limbs become flaccid from cessation of muscular tone and action, the pulse and respiration become slower, the pupils are turned upwards and inwards, and are *contracted*. (Müller).

Of Hypnotism
In the hypnotic state, induced with the view of exhibiting what I call the hypnotic phenomena, vision becomes more and more imperfect, the eyelids are closed, but have, for a considerable time a *vibratory motion,* (in some few they are forcibly closed, as by spasm of the orbiculares) the organs of special sense, particularly of smell, touch, and hearing, heat and cold, and resistance, are greatly *exalted,* and afterwards become blunted, in a degree far beyond the torpor of natural sleep; the pupils are turned upwards and inwards, but, contrary to what happens in *natural* sleep, they are greatly *dilated,* and highly insensible to light; after a length of time the pupils become contracted, whilst the eyes are still insensible to light. The pulse and respiration are, at first, slower than is natural, but immediately on calling muscles into action, a tendency to cataleptiform rigidity is assumed, with rapid pulse, and oppressed and quick breathing. The limbs are thus maintained in a state of tonic *rigidity* for any length of time I have yet thought it prudent to try, instead of that state of flaccidity induced by common sleep; and the most remarkable circumstance is this; that there seems to be no corresponding state of muscular exhaustion from such action.[114]

In passing into natural sleep, anything held in the hand is soon allowed to drop from our grasp, but, in the artificial sleep now referred to, it will be held more firmly than before falling asleep. This is *a very remarkable difference.*

Power of Locomotion and Accurate Balancing of Themselves
The power of balancing themselves is so great that I have never seen one of these hypnotic somnambulists fall. The same is noted of natural somnambulists. This is a remarkable fact, and would appear to occur in this way, that they acquire the centre of gravity, as if by instinct, in the *most natural, and therefore, in the most graceful manner,* and if allowed to remain in this position, they speedily become cataleptiformly and immovably fixed.

Tendency to Dance on Hearing Appropriate Music; Grace Displayed under its Influence
From observing these two facts, and the general tendency and taste for dancing displayed by most patients on hearing lively music during hypnotism, the peculiarly graceful and appropriate movement of many when thus excited, and the varied and elegant postures they may be made to assume by slight currents of air, and the faculty of retaining any position with so much ease, I have hazarded the opinion, that the Greeks may have been indebted to hypnotism for the perfection of their sculpture, and the Fakirs for their wonderful feats of suspending their bodies by a leg or an arm.[115]

Effects Analogous to Nitrous Oxide in Some
It thus clearly appears that it differs from common sleep in many respects, **that there is first a state of excitement as with opium, and wine, and spirits, and afterwards a state of corresponding deep depression or torpor.**

In the case of two patients, symptoms very much the same as those produced in them by the laughing gas, were produced twice on each patient, and the only time I know of their having been

---

[114] The average of a great number of experiments gives me the following results: The rise in the pulse from mere muscular effort, to enable patients to keep their legs and arms extended for five minutes, is about 20 per cent [*c.* 86 bpm]. When in the state of hypnotism it is upwards of 100 per cent [*c.* 144 bpm]. By arousing all the senses, and the head and neck, it will speedily fall to 40 per cent, [*c.* 101 bpm] (that is, twice what it was when so tested in the natural condition) and by rendering the whole muscles limber, whilst the patient is in the state of hypnotism the pulse very speedily falls to, or even below, the condition it was before the experiment.

[115] It has been suggested to me, that it can scarcely be doubted that the Bacchanalians, who had no feeling of wounds, ("*non sentit vulnera Moenas*" – Ovid) and whose condition was a stupor different from common sleep, ("*Exsomnis stupet Oevias*" – Horace) were in the hypnotic condition or nervous sleep, and therein excited to dance by music; and that, as uneducated maid-servants, when under the full influence of that state of nerve, move with the grace and peculiar action of the most accomplished dancers of pantomimic ballet, there is reason to believe, not merely that the perfect grace exhibited in the attitudes represented in ancient sculpture and painting, was derived from studying the Bacchanalian and other mystic dancers, but that the movements used by stage-dancers, in our days, have been transmitted to us by continued imitation, through Italy, from the dancers in the Greek mysteries. No person can see girls of humble education, under the influence of music while in the nervous sleep, without perceiving, that those individuals, if awake, could not move with the elegance they exhibit under that influence. The reason of such grace probably is that it arises from the simple and pure effects of nature to balance the body perfectly in all its complicated movements while the power of sight is suspended.

hypnotised. One lost the power of speech for two hours, as happened also after the gas. Both these patients had hypnotised themselves.

In what it Differs from this and Intoxication from Wine and Spirits; Analogous to conium

There is a remarkable difference between the hypnotic condition, and that induced by the nitrous oxide. In the latter there is great, almost irresistible inclination to *general muscular effort,* as well as laughter; in the former there seems to be no inclination to *any* bodily effort, unless excited by *impressions from without.* When the latter are used, there is a remarkable difference again in the power of locomotion and accurate balancing of themselves, when contrasted with the condition of intoxication from wine or spirits, where the limbs become partially paralysed, whilst the judgment remains pretty clear and acute. The state of muscular quiescence, with acute hearing, and dreamy, glowing imagination, approximates it somewhat to the condition induced by conium [poison hemlock].

Effects of Monotonous Impressions on any of the Senses

During the course of last spring some lectures were delivered in this town to prove that the *Mesmeric phenomena* might be induced by an "undue continuance or repetition of the same sensible impression on any of the senses". Immediately after the first lecture I instituted experiments according to this plan, but very soon ascertained, that the sleep induced by this mode of operating, *unless through the eye,* was nothing more than NATURAL or common sleep, *excepting in patients who had had the impressibility stamped on them, by having been previously Mesmerised or hypnotised.* The lecturer concluded his course by stating his opinion, that he knew no sleep but natural or common sleep; and by representing that he considered the effects produced by the different modes to be the same.[116]

Power of Habit and Expectation

I believe most, if not all the patients this gentleman exhibited at his lectures had been previously Mesmerised or hypnotised, which, if I am correct in this supposition, from the circumstances already referred to, (see [Introduction] and note hereto appended) would completely nullify the importance of his *apparent* results. However, I have never heard of his having *operated successfully, and exhibited the phenomena on numbers of patients taken indiscriminately from a mixed audience, who had never been operated on before;* or produced curative results such as I have so repeatedly done. I therefore consider it a fair inference, that until the same phenomena are produced by his method in cases of persons which have *never* been hypnotised or Mesmerised, nothing is proved beyond the fact *which I have so often urged,* namely, **the power of imagination, sympathy, and habit, in producing the expected effects ON THOSE PREVIOUSLY IMPRESSED.**[117]

All the Phenomena Consecutive

From overlooking another important fact which I have repeatedly explained, that **all the phenomena are consecutive, that is, first increased sensibility, mobility, and docility, and afterwards a subsidence into insensibility and cataleptiform rigidity**, this gentleman, by mistaking and exhibiting the *primary* phenomena for the *secondary,* seems to have managed to deceive both himself and some others who are satisfied to look at such matters loosely. *This, however, is confounding things which are in themselves essentially different.* I beg especial attention to the note below.[118]

Power of Hypnotism to Cure Intractable Diseases and Disorders

Of all the circumstances connected with the artificial sleep which I induce, nothing so strongly marks the difference between it and *natural* sleep as **the wonderful power the former evinces in curing many diseases of long standing, and which had resisted natural sleep**, and every known agency, for years, e.g. patients who have been **born deaf and dumb**, of various ages, up to 32 years, had continued without the power of hearing sound until the time they were operated on by me, and yet they were enabled to do so by being kept **in the hypnotic state for eight, ten, or twelve minutes**, and have had their hearing still farther improved by a repetition of similar operations. Now, supposing these patients to have spent six hours out of twenty-four in sleep, many of them had had four, five, six, or eight years of *continuous* sleep, but still awoke as they lay down, incapable of hearing sound, and yet they had some degree of it communicated to them by a few *minutes* of Hypnotism. Can any stronger proof be wanted, or adduced, than this, that it is very different from *common* sleep? A lady, 54 years of age, had been suffering for 16 years from incipient

---

[116] [See appendix (originally a lengthy footnote) 'On Monotony Inducing Sleep'.]
[117] A very decided proof of this was exhibited at one of my lectures, where, as may be seen from the report of it, twenty-two who had been operated on before, laid hold of different parts of each other's persons or dresses, and by concentrating their attention to that act, and anticipating the effect, they all became hypnotised in about a minute. After another lecture, in the ante-room, sixteen who had been hypnotised formerly, stood up in the same manner, and also *one* who *had never been hypnotised.* In about a minute all were affected *excepting the latter.* I then operated on him alone in my usual way, and in two or three minutes he was very decidedly affected. Suffice it to say, I have varied my experiments in every possible form, and clearly proved the power of imagination *over those previously impressed,* as the patients have become hypnotised or not by the same appliance, according to the result which they previously expected. This readily accounts for the result of Mr. Wakley's experiments with the Okeys.
[118] [See appendix (originally a lengthy footnote) entitled 'Some Hypnotic Experiments & Observations'.]

amaurosis [loss of sight from disease affecting the optic nerve]. According to the same ratio, she must have had four years of sleep, but instead of improving she was every month getting worse, and when she called on me, could with difficulty read two words of the largest heading of a newspaper. After *eight minutes,* hypnotic sleep, however, she could read the other words, and in three minutes more, the whole of the smaller heading, soon after a smaller sized type, and the same afternoon, with the aid of her glasses, read the 118th Psalm, 29 verses, in the small diamond *Polyglot Bible*, which for years had been a sealed book to her. There has also been a most remarkable improvement in this lady's general health since she was hypnotised. Is there any individual who can fail to see, in this case, something different from common sleep? Another lady, 44 years of age, had required glasses 22 years, to enable her to see to sew, read, or write. She had thus five years and a half of sleep, but the sight was still getting worse, so that, before being hypnotised, she could not distinguish the capitals in the advertising columns of a newspaper. After being hypnotised, however, she could, in a few minutes, see to read the large and second heading of the newspaper, and next day, to make herself a blond cap, threading her needle without the aid of glasses. This lady's daughter, who had been compelled to use glasses for two years, was enabled to dispense with them, after being *once* hypnotised. It is also important to note, that all these three, as well as many others, were agreeably surprised by **improvement of *memory* after being hypnotised**. The memory of one was so bad that she was often forced to go upstairs several times before she could remember what she went for, and could scarcely carry on a conversation; but all this remnant of a slight paralytic affection is gone, by the same operations which roused the optic nerves, and restored the sight. Now, with such cases as these, who can doubt that there is a real difference in the state of the brain and nervous system generally, during the hypnotic sleep, from that which occurs in common sleep? The same might be urged from various other diseases cured or relieved by this process, but I shall only briefly refer to a few.

In the second part of this treatise, where the cases are recorded, will be found many examples of the curative power of hypnotism, equally remarkable with those to which I have just referred: such as **Tic Douloureux; Nervous headache; Spinal irritation; Neuralgia of the heart; Palpitation and intermittent action of the heart; Epilepsy; Rheumatism; Paralysis Distortions and tonic spasm**, etc.

Miss Collins' Case and Miss E. Atkinson's

I shall here give a few particulars of a case which shows in a most remarkable degree the difference of this and common sleep, or that induced by opium and the whole range of medicines of that class. Miss Collins, of Newark, Nottinghamshire, had a spasmodic seizure during the night, by which her head was bound firmly to her left shoulder. The most energetic and well directed means, under a most talented physician, and aided by the opinion of Sir Benjamin Brodie [a distinguished surgeon], had been tried, as far as known remedies could be carried (amongst other means, narcotics, in as large doses as were compatible with the safety of the patient), and although she was carefully watched by night and by day, there had never been the slightest relaxation of the spasm, which had continued nearly six months. When I first examined her, no force I was capable of exerting could succeed in separating the head and shoulder in the slightest degree. Experience led me to hope, however, that I might be able to do so after she was hypnotised. Having requested all present, excepting the patient, her father, and her physician, to retire, I hypnotised her, and in three minutes from commencing the operation, with the most perfect ease to myself, and without the slightest pain to the patient, her head was inclined in the opposite direction, and in two minutes more she was roused, and was quite straight. I visited this patient only three times, after which she returned home. Shortly afterwards, she had a nervous twitching of the head, and on one occasion it was again drawn to her shoulder. Dr. Chawner, however, hypnotised her as he had seen me do, and put it right immediately; and she is now (about twelve months after she was hypnotised) in perfect health, "her head quite straight, and she has perfect control over the muscles of the neck". (See cases).

Miss E. Atkinson had been unable to speak above a whisper for four years and a half, notwithstanding every known remedy had been perseveringly adopted, under able practitioners. After the ninth hypnotic operation she could speak aloud without effort, and has continued quite well ever since – now about nine months. (See case at length, Part II.)

The extraordinary effects of a few minutes' hypnotism, manifested in such cases (so very different from what we realise by the application of ordinary means) may appear startling to those unacquainted with the remarkable powers of this process. I have been recommended, on this account, to conceal the fact of the rapidity and extent of the changes induced, as many may consider the thing *impossible,* and thus be led to reject the *less* startling, although *not more* true, reports of its beneficial action in other cases. In recording the cases, however, I have considered it my duty to record *facts as I found them,* and to make no compromise for the sake of accommodating them to the preconceived notions or prejudices of others.

It may be proper to add, however, that I have afforded opportunities to many eminent professional and scientific gentlemen to see the patients, and investigate for themselves the real state of these respective cases; and to them I can confidently appeal as to the accuracy and fidelity of the reports of most of the cases recorded in this treatise.[119]

Extent to Which it may be Expected to be Useful

After such evidence as this, no one can reasonably doubt that there is a remarkable difference between hypnotism and natural sleep, and that it is a valuable addition to our therapeutic means.

How these extraordinary effects are produced, it may be impossible absolutely to decide. One thing, however, I am certain of, that, in this condition, besides the peculiar impression directly made on the nervous centres, by which the mind is for the time "thrown out of gear", and which enables us, in a remarkable manner, to localize or concentrate the nervous energy, or sensorial power, to any particular point or function, instead of the more equal distribution which exists in the ordinary condition, we have also an extraordinary power of acting on the capillaries, and of increasing and diminishing the force and frequency of the circulation, locally and generally.[120] This can be done in a most remarkable degree, both as regards the extent and rapidity of these changes.[121] And, moreover, changes from absolute insensibility to the most exalted sensibility, may be effected at a certain stage, almost with the rapidity of thought, as exemplified [earlier in this chapter]. On the whole, I consider it is of great importance to have acquired a knowledge of how these effects can be produced and generally applied, and turned to advantage in the cure of disease, although we should never ascertain the real proximate cause, or principle through which we produce our effects. Who can tell how, or why, quinine and arsenic cure intermittent fever? They are, nevertheless, well-known to do so, and are prescribed accordingly.

Whilst I feel assured from personal experience, and the testimony of professional friends, on whose judgment and candour I can implicitly rely, that in this we have acquired an important curative agency for a *certain class* of diseases, I desire it to be distinctly understood, as already stated, that I by no means wish to hold it up as a universal remedy. I believe it is capable of doing great good, if judiciously applied. Diseases evince totally different pathological conditions, and the treatment ought to be varied accordingly. **We have, therefore, no right to expect to find a universal remedy either in *this*, or *any other*, method of treatment.**

---

[119] [It is evident that Braid did exactly this throughout his career, as there are many independent reports of his demonstrations.]

[120] By this I mean that anyone examining the pulse by the radial artery, whilst the patient has his arms in the cataleptiform condition, and held at right angles with his body, (and when, of course, the circulation can only be influenced by the state of rigidity or flaccidity of the muscles) it will be found feeble or contracted, but the moment the rigidity of the muscles is reduced, by blowing on or fanning them, the pulse will become much more developed. This, of course, which may be done without the patient being conscious of the experiment, is totally different from what may be displayed as a trick, by a person voluntarily compressing the axillary and brachial arteries, by drawing his arms firmly against his side. The former is independent of volition, the latter is entirely voluntary, and a mere trick.

[121] The first time I ever had an opportunity of examining a patient minutely, or of feeling the pulse of one, under the Mesmeric influence, was on the 19th November, 1841. I was much struck with the state of the pulse at the wrist – so small and rapid as, combined with the state of tremor, or slight subsultus [convulsive twitching] in the arm, rendered it impossible to count it accurately at the wrist. This circumstance induced me to reckon the velocity of the pulse by the carotid artery, as will be found recorded in the *Manchester Guardian* of the 24th of that month. I adduced this as the cause of the discrepancy between the numeration of the pulse by others and myself, that I had counted it *by the carotid artery*, and considered it impossible for anyone to reckon it correctly by the radial artery in such a case. The injected state of the conjunctival membrane of the eye, and the whole capillary system in the neck, head, and face, was so apparent, as Dr. [Thomas] Radford [a respected obstetric physician from Manchester] very correctly stated, that no one near the patient could fail to observe it: this, together with the cold hands and contracted pulse at the wrist, led me to infer, that the rigid state of the cataleptiform muscles, opposed the free transmission of the blood through the extremities, and would thus cause increased action in the heart and determination to the brain and spinal cord, as resulted from the ingenious experiments of my late friend Dr. Kellie, for speedily terminating the cold stage of ague, by putting a tourniquet round one of the extremities.

Chapter 5:
On Hypnotic Sleep Therapy

Reasons for Delivering Public Lectures on Hypnotism
When I had ascertained that Hypnotism was important as a curative power, and that the prejudices existing against it in the public mind, as to its having an immoral tendency, were erroneous; and the idea, that it was calculated to sap the foundation of the Christian creed, by suggesting that the Gospel miracles might have been wrought by this agency, was quite unfounded and absurd, I felt it to be a duty I owed to the cause of humanity, and my profession, to use my best endeavours to remove those fallacies, so that the profession generally might be at liberty to prosecute the inquiry, and apply it practically, without hazarding their personal and professional interest, by prosecuting it in opposition to popular prejudice. It appeared to me there was no mode so likely to insure this happy consummation as delivering lectures on the subject to mixed audiences. The public could thus have demonstrative proof of its practical utility; and, when it was **proved to proceed from a law of the animal economy, and that the patient could only be affected in accordance with his own free will and consent, and not, as the animal magnetizers contend, through the irresistible power of volitions and passes of the Mesmerisers, which might be done in secret and at a distance**, the ground of charge as to my agency having an immoral tendency, must at once fall to the ground. I have reason to believe my labours have not been altogether unsuccessful, in removing the popular prejudices; and I hope that the more liberal of my professional brethren, now that they know my true motives of action, in giving lectures to mixed audiences, instead of confining them to the profession only, and especially as I made no secret of my modes of operating, will be inclined to approve rather than blame me, for the course I have taken in this respect.

Mode of Procuring Refreshing Sleep, With Low Pulse and General Flaccidity of Muscle
From some peculiar views, I was led to make experiments, by which I hoped to obtain natural or refreshing sleep, and the results were quite satisfactory. **I have thus succeeded in making a patient, who, when operated upon in the usual way, was highly susceptible, and disposed to become strongly cataleptic, with rapid pulse and oppressed breathing, remain in a sound sleep for upwards of three hours, with all the muscles flaccid, and the pulse and respiration slower than natural, when operated on in this manner. All this difference arises from the simple circumstance of the position into which the eyes are placed during the operation, namely, closing the eyelids, and bringing the eyes loosely upwards, as if looking at an object at a great distance, the eye-balls being turned up only gently, so as to cause dilatation of the pupil, as already explained; and the limbs placed so as to relax the muscles as much as possible, and thus prevent acceleration of the pulse.**

I was led to the adoption of this method from the following train of reasoning. If, as I inferred was the case, the spasmodic tendency was reflected to the muscular system generally, from the semi-paralysed state of the branches of the third pair of nerves during the continued fixed stare and straining of the eyes, I thought, were I to insure all the other concomitant requirements for procuring hypnotism, I ought to procure refreshing sleep, without rigidity of muscle or quickened circulation. By closing the eyelids, the first could be obtained, and by turning the eyes up loosely, which dilates the pupils, the other would also be attained; I therefore tried the experiment, which, as already noted, proved most successful.

Efficacy of This Plan
I think the plan I have just pointed out is quite as simple, and I feel assured it will prove as efficacious in procuring "sleep at will" as that of Gardener, lately published by Dr. Binns. I may add, that I publicly stated my plan at my lectures in 1842, which was at least five or six months prior to the publication of Dr. Binns's work. I had also done the same at my lectures in Liverpool, about six weeks before that last period.

Mr. Barrallier, an intelligent surgeon, of Milford, who investigated the subject of Hypnotism with much zeal and success, and published some interesting experiments on the subject in The Medical Times, also referred to the case of a gentleman in that town, whom he had heard of as having been in the habit of procuring sleep immediately "by keeping his eyes fixed" for a few minutes in one direction. Until he adopted this method he scarcely slept at all. For various modes of procuring sleep see [Chapter 4] of this treatise.

In reference to my original theory, Dr. Binns, at page 372, calls in question the justice of my allegation, that during Hypnotism, natural or artificial, there should be any imperfect arterialisation of the blood, notwithstanding the suppressed or modified respiration and circulation. He has adduced no arguments, however, to convince me to the contrary; and I again repent my conviction, that such condition of the blood does exist, and is a cause of ordinary sleep; and that the still more intense state of torpor, which is a certain state of Neuro-Hypnotism, results from a still less perfectly purified blood; and, on the other hand, that the dreamy and exalted states arise from different degrees of stimulating properties of the blood, from being more highly arterialised at various stages, together with the velocity of circulation, and pressure or tension on the brain during the cataleptiform state.

Chapter 6:
On Muscular Suggestion & Phreno-Hypnotism

Introductory Remarks
I have no doubt that some of the views already advanced, and the facts on which they are grounded, have appeared startling to many of my readers, and I feel assured the subject to be discussed in the following chapter must be still more so; namely, that during hypnotism, we acquire the power, through the nerves of common sensation [i.e., the sense of touch], of rousing any sentiment, feeling, passion, or emotion, and any mental manifestation, according to our mode of manipulating the patient. This is what has been designated phreno-magnetism by the discoverers of these curious phenomena, but which, in accordance with my nomenclature, I shall designate phreno-hypnotism. It appears with this, as with many other discoveries that similar investigations were going forward at the same time in England and America, while the discoverers were without the knowledge of each other's views or proceedings, and that the results of their experiments led all parties to form analogous conclusions.

Relation between Mind and Matter Illustrated to Disprove Materialism
It must be evident to everyone who reflects deeply and dispassionately on the subject, that if we really can thus acquire such power as to rouse into great activity any faculty or propensity, whilst we diminish the activity of antagonist faculties, we must thereby acquire an important power for meliorating the moral, intellectual, and physical condition of man. I shall have no difficulty in adducing sufficient proof, that the human mind *can* be so developed and acted on through the bodily organs; but, before entering into a detail of the modes of doing so, I shall endeavour to remove a prejudice against the discussion of this subject, which has arisen from the unhappy circumstance that some of those who promulgated this doctrine have professed a belief in materialism. Such an avowal was indeed calculated to excite, not the prejudices, but the sound principles, of Christian society in general against the reception or dispassionate consideration of the facts on which it rested. For my own part, I can see nothing in the subject to warrant such conclusions as the materialists have avowed; and truth is not to be rejected, because misguided men attempt to build upon it a hollow and unseemly superstructure.[122]

The following are my views of the relation which subsists betwixt mind and matter:— **I look upon the brain simply as the *organ* of the mind**, and the bodily organs as the instruments for upholding the integrity of the bodily frame, and for acquiring and extending its communion with external nature in our present state of existence. **That the mind acts on matter, and is acted on *by* matter, according to the quality and quantity, and relative disposition of cerebral development.** This, however, does not imply, that mind is a *mere attribute of matter.*[123] My thinking and willing, and acting, so as to influence the mental and bodily condition of another, surely does not destroy our separate individuality? As well might we say, that the refined compositions of a Mozart or Beethoven, which were conveyed to the ears of their delighted auditors through different instruments, were created by the thought and will of the instruments.

It appears to me quite clear, that the musician might conceive, and compose, and record every idea, whilst others could have no conception of their nature or merits, unless communicated through an appropriate instrument or instruments. The musician and instrument, therefore, are distinct in their nature, as **the soul and the bodily organs are essentially distinct from each other.**[124]

I shall endeavour to illustrate my views by the following simile. Suppose the instrument is good, and well fitted for expressing musical composition, it is evident, that it will better convey the beauties of the composition, than if represented by a bad or indifferent instrument; and will also afford more delight, and satisfaction, and encouragement to the farther exertions of the composer, than if performed on a bad instrument. Just so the mind furnished with a well developed brain. Supposing the musical instrument is

---

[122] [As a Christian, Braid was sensitive to the accusation of "materialism", which implied atheism to the Victorians, as his subsequent dispute with J.C. Colquhoun proves.]

[123] "A few sounds acting on the tympanum of the ear, or a few black and small figures scribbled on a piece of white paper (see Mr. Renuell's pamphlet) have been known to knock a man down as effectively as a sledge hammer, and to deprive him not only of vision, but even of life. Here, then, we have instances of mind acting upon matter, and I by no means affirm that matter does not also act upon mind; for to those who advocate the intimate connection between body and mind, these reciprocities of action are easily reconcilable; but this will be an insuperable difficulty to those who affirm the identity of mind and body." Again, "This intimate union between body and mind is, in fact, analogous to all that we see, and feel, and comprehend. Thus, we observe that the material stimuli of alcohol, or of opium, act upon the mind through the body, and that the moral stimuli of love, or of anger, act upon the body through the mind: these are reciprocities of action that establish the principle of connection between the two, but are fatal to that of an identity." – "Does not every passion of the mind act directly, primarily, and, as it were, *per se* upon the body, with greater or with lesser influence in proportion to their force? Does not the activity belong on this occasion to the mind, and the mere passiveness to the body? Does not the quickened circulation *follow* the anger, the start the surprise, and the swoon the sorrow? Do not these instances, and a thousand others, clearly convince us that priority of action *here* belongs to the mind, and not to the body? And those who deny this, are reduced to the ridiculous absurdity of attempting to prove that a man is frightened because he runs away, not that he runs away because he is frightened, and that the motion produces the terror, not the terror the motion." – Colton's *Lacon*. The same author also urges the argument effectively by an appeal to the fact of mania being so frequently produced by *moral* [i.e., psychological] causes, and the success which has attended the treatment of the insane by strict attention to *moral* [i.e., psychotherapeutic] management.

[124] [Braid here defends a philosophical commitment to "Cartesian dualism" and "psycho-physical interactionism." This metaphysical theory of mind is intimately linked to Christian theology and has been aggressively disputed by many 20th century philosophers of psychology, especially the behaviourists.]

very perfect in *some* parts, but very imperfect in others, it is evident, that the musician can afford more pleasure to others, as well as more satisfaction to himself, by playing on the more perfect parts. Then, supposing the parts played on are capable of becoming improved, *by being so exercised,* (which is the case with several instruments, as the violin,) it is clear, that there will be greater and greater inducement for the musician to confine himself to the better parts of the instrument, and thus, by concentrating his whole energies to these points, he will more and more enamour himself, as well as his auditors, by the perfection of his performances.

This is exactly what I conceive takes place in reference to the brain, supposing different parts to be appropriated as the instruments for the manifestation of different mental functions. Every part of the human frame is continually undergoing the process of waste and repair – that is to say, the molecular particles of the various organs are continually changing, and *moderate* exercise tends to *increased development and power,* whilst *inaction* has the opposite tendency. This no one will deny. The analogy, therefore, is complete. The soul or mind, by being exercised judiciously in a particular direction, strengthens some peculiar organ, and acquires precision from habit, which gives a tendency to perseverance in the same course of action; and, by refraining from certain practices, the corresponding organs become feeble, and thus exercise a less powerful influence on the mind. **Thus we can account for the power of habit, both physical and mental, each tending to strengthen the other by correct training; and it is on this principle that we can hope to meliorate the condition of the vicious members of society, by separating them from bad companions and practices, and encouraging them in the exercise of virtuous habits.**

Armstrong, Colton, Brown, Abercrombie, Stewart, Plato[125]

Moreover, the mind of the musician may conceive and excite into activity the corresponding organs of the brain; these may react on his corporeal organs, and excite into activity the silent lyre; all these links of intercommunication may be perfected, without conveying any corresponding feeling or emotion to the minds of others, unless they are provided with appropriate recipient organs (musical ears) for conveying to their brains certain vibrations, and thus inducing in corresponding parts of their brains such condition as may awaken in their minds certain associations of ideas, and manifest the peculiar emotions which arise from them. It is not enough that we have *part* of this concatenation complete; the whole must be complete, or the results cannot be perfect.[126]

The same arguments might be enforced in respect to the painter, and sculptor, and orator, but it appears to my mind so evident by what has already been advanced, that I forbear extending my illustrations, conceiving them to be unnecessary. I therefore conclude that the soul and the brain are essentially quite distinct, and stand much in the same relation to each other as the musician and musical instrument.

Another powerful argument of the mind being an independent essence, is the fact, that amidst the continued changes which we know are going on in the physical frame, we still recognise personal identity; and the remembrance of occurrences, even of early life, after every particle of the body has been changed several times, is reconcilable with the idea of the original mind merely having exchanged and renovated the substance of its dwelling-place; but how can we suppose that each particle had, in retiring, transferred its quantum of knowledge to the particle of matter which was to supply its place?

Colton's remark seems very just when he says – "Many causes are now conspiring to increase the trunk of infidelity, but materialism is the main root of them all." I have therefore endeavoured and I hope, by what has already been said, with some success, to prove, that the belief in the brain being the organ of the mind, leads only to the admission of the necessity of certain conditions of matter, in order to make the varied conditions of mind manifest to ourselves and other beings with which we are surrounded during the present state of our existence. The charge against the doctrine of phrenology, therefore, as leading to a belief in materialism, is altogether unfounded; for phrenology merely professes to appropriate to *separate portions* of the brain the *execution of special functions* or *manifestations,* which are generally admitted, without hesitation, to result from its functions as a single organ. I might therefore at once dismiss the subject, leaving the doctrines of the existence of a God, and the immortality of the soul, to the defence of many able writers on that department of mental philosophy. However, as it appears to me that an argument of considerable strength, in support of both these doctrines, may be drawn from the doctrines of phrenology, or the allocation of special functions to particular portions of the brain, I think it may not be out of place for me very briefly to advert to these topics.

The concurrent notions and practices of all nations, savage as well as civilized, clearly indicate their inward belief in a superintendent power who rules the destinies of man and of nations, as verified by their varied forms of worship. Phrenology, as illustrated by Hypnotism, does more – it proves that there is a particular portion of the brain which the mind may use as an organ destined for the especial purpose of adoration; and, as nothing has been made in vain, or without a final cause, we may safely infer that such an organ would never have been made had it not been intended to be exercised; and how could it have been

---

[125] [It is notable that Dugald Stewart, Thomas Brown, and John Abercrombie were all Scottish philosophers associated with the academic tradition known as the "Scottish school of Common Sense".]
[126] [See appendix (originally a lengthy footnote) 'On psycho-physical dualism'.]

exercised worthily had there been no suitable object of adoration? The very fact, therefore, of the existence of such a special organ having been ascertained, stamps the folly of the Atheist; and, as we have proved that mind is not necessarily a mere attribute of organized matter, but a distinct essence, we cannot suppose it to be more perishable than matter; and as it is an acknowledged fact, that matter, so far as we can apprehend, is essentially indestructible, analogy would lead us to infer, that the mind, the more important part of man, will not be less imperishable; and, consequently, the most rational conclusion to which we can arrive is, that the soul is immortal.

> There is mind, then, as well as matter, or rather, if there be a difference of the degrees of evidence, there is mind, more surely than there is matter; and if at death not a single atom of the body perishes, but that which we term dissolution, decay, putrefaction, is only a change of the relative positions of those atoms, which in themselves continue to exist with all the qualities which they before possessed, there is surely no reason, from this mere change of place of the atoms that formed the body to infer, with respect to the independent mind, any other change than that of its mere relation to those separate atoms. The continued subsistence of everything corporeal cannot, at least, be regarded as indicative of the annihilation of the other substance, but must, on the contrary, as far as the mere analogy of the body is of any weight, be regarded as a presumption in favour of the continued subsistence of the mind, when there is nothing around it which has perished, and nothing even which has perished, in the whole material universe, since the universe itself was called into being. – Dr. Thomas Brown.

> The mind remembers, conceives, combines, and reasons; it loves, it fears, and hopes in the total absence of any impression from without, that can influence, in the smallest degree, these emotions; and we have the fullest conviction that it would continue to exercise the same functions in undiminished activity, though all material things were at once annihilated. – [John] Abercrombie [a Scottish physician and philosopher].

Mr. [Dugald] Stewart also says,

> Of all the truths we know the existence of mind is the most certain. Even the system of Berkeley concerning the non-existence of matter, is far more conceivable, than that nothing but matter exists in the universe.

Plato also wrote thus,

> The body being compounded, is dissolved by death; the soul, being simple, passes into another life, incapable of corruption.

That accomplished physician and metaphysician, Dr. Abercrombie, after relating the effects on memory of diseases and disorders of the brain, with, in many instances, serious organic lesion, concludes thus,

> One thing, however, is certain, that they give no countenance to the doctrine of materialism, which some have presumptuously deduced from a very partial view of the influence of cerebral disease upon the manifestations of mind. They show us, indeed, in a very striking manner, the mind holding intercourse with the external world through the medium of the brain and nervous system; and, by certain diseases of these organs, they show this intercourse impaired or suspended; but they show nothing more. In particular, they warrant nothing in any degree analogous to those partial deductions which form the basis of materialism. On the contrary, they show us the brain injured and diseased to an extraordinary extent, without the mental functions being affected in any sensible degree.

This power no doubt arises from each hemisphere having corresponding organs, and consequently when only *one* is diseased, the other may be adequate to the manifestation of the mental phenomena.

> They show us farther, the manifestations of mind obscured for a time, and yet reviving in all their original vigour almost in the very moment of dissolution. Finally, their exhibit to us the mind, cut off from all intercourse with the external world, recalling its old impressions, even of things long forgotten, and exercising its powers on those which had long ceased to exist, in a manner totally irreconcilable with any idea we can form of a material function." *On the Intellectual Powers,* pp. 154, 155.

General Conclusion, That Mind or Life is the Cause of Organism

In addition to what I have already advanced in refutation of the doctrine of materialism, I beg to submit what appears to me much more probable than that mental manifestations are the result of mere organism – namely, that organism is the result of mind, or the principle of life influencing or directing organism in accordance with what may be its especial wants and desires. We know that every seed of a plant has a principle of life imparted to it by the great first cause of all, by which, when sown in congenial soil, it will exert its powers, and appropriate to itself materials from the soil, to form an organism in accordance with its peculiar wants and nature; and that, having passed through certain conditions, and formed other kindred seed or germs to propagate its kind under a return of favouring circumstances, the plant dies, and is resolved into its original elements. Man and animals also possess similar faculties for propagating and multiplying their species; and to me it appears far more probable, that the peculiar organism. of each variety results from the vivifying or intelligent principle we call life or mind (and no one denies the existence of the former, although we know nothing of its essence or mode of operation,) directing and determining appropriate formation, than that the mere accidental union of particles of matter, in definite quantity and form, should be the *cause* of mental phenomena.[127] It is true we can here only speak of analogies, but the analogy in favour of this proposition seems far more natural and probable than the other. Is it not, for example, *a priori,* as probable, on viewing a well planned factory, fitted up with what is called self-acting machinery, for us to suppose that the whole should have been planned, and the machinery constructed, in accordance with the intelligent designs of a skilful artist, as that the brute matter, of which the whole is constructed, came into its particular forms and arrangements of its own accord, or by accident, and thus produced the intelligence of the superintending possessor? The higher and more perfect the original force, or life, or spirit, originally imparted into each species, the more complex and extensive should we expect to find the corresponding organism, to adapt it for the suitable performance of its more varied functions; and it therefore was necessary for man to have that superiority, even in the form and functions of his hands, in which he so much surpasses that of all other animals, to fit him for the execution of the more extended range of operations, which his superior endowments and cerebral organism fitted him to devise.

In this view of the subject, (and it appears to me, after consulting the various opinions of our ablest authorities on life and organization, to be the most satisfactory conclusion I could arrive at,) every plant or animal, however minute, may have a particular vital or directing principle originally imparted to it, and still sustained in its power by the great Creator, without the necessity of according to each an immortal existence and responsibility. Nor is there any thing irreconcilable in the supposition that man, with higher original powers, and more perfect organism, fitting him to use these appropriately, and who is the highest link in the chain, in this world, between inorganic matter and the Supreme Being, should be constituted a responsible agent, and exist hereafter, whilst those creatures with less expansive faculties, both of life and organization, may be exempted from such ultimate responsibility, and may *not* be immortal.

This is only analogous to what we see in respect to a commanding officer and his men, the *former only* being responsible for imprudent enterprises, the latter being considered merely as instruments in his hands.

Power of Conscience

I shall close these remarks on the immortality of the soul by a quotation from that excellent work, Abercrombie's "On the Intellectual Powers."

> This momentous truth rests on a species of evidence altogether different, which addresses itself to the moral constitution of man. It is found in those principles of his nature by which he feels upon his spirit the awe of a God, and looks forward to the future with anxiety or with hope, - by which he knows to distinguish truth from falsehood, and evil from good, and has forced upon him the conviction that he is a moral and responsible being. This is the power of conscience, that monitor within, which raises its voice in the breast of every man, a witness for his Creator. He who resigns himself to its guidance, and he who repels its warnings, are both compelled to acknowledge its power; and whether the good man rejoices in the prospect of immortality, or the victim of remorse withers beneath an influence unseen by human eye, and shrinks from the anticipation of a reckoning to come, each has forced upon him a conviction, such as argument never gave, that the being which is essentially himself is distinct from any function of the body, and will survive in undiminished vigour when the body shall have fallen into decay. There is thus, in the consciousness of every man, a deep impression of continued existence. The casuist [i.e., an ethical sophist] may reason against it till he bewilder himself in his own sophistries; but a voice within gives the lie to his vain speculations, and pleads with authority for a life which is to come. The sincere and humble inquirer cherishes the impression, while he seeks for farther light on a subject so momentous, and he thus receives, with absolute conviction, the truth which beams upon him from the revelation of God, that the mysterious part of his being, which thinks, and wills, and reasons, shall indeed survive the wreck of its mortal tenement, and is destined for immortality.[128]

The Passions, how Excited

It must be obvious to all, that every variety of passion and emotion can be excited in the mind by music; but how does this arise? Simply by the different effects produced by the varied degrees of velocity, force, quality, and combinations of the oscillations of the air acting on the auditory nerves, these again communicated to the brain, and this acting on the mind and body, creating corresponding mental and bodily manifestations. Everyone must have observed the remarkable effects evinced by these means on the physiognomy [i.e., the facial expression], and the more critically observant must have noticed, that in

---

[127] "The original identity of structure of the germ of the most various organic beings, constituted, as it always is, of a cell, with a nucleus, seems to prove, that the cause of the variety of classes, families, genera, and species of animals and plants developed from the germ, resides not in the structure or chemical property of the germ, but in the idea or spirit, implanted in it at its creation." (Müller, p. 1339.).

[128] To those who wish to pursue the subject farther, I beg to refer to Dr. Samuel Clarke on the *Being and Attributes of God*, pp. 70-15; Jackson on *Matter and Mind*, pp. 41-47, 51; Warburton's *Divine Legation*, vol. I, book 3d; Drew's *Essay on the Immortality of the Soul*; and Ramsay's *Principles*, pp. 233-5; also Brougham and Bakewell, where they will find it ably argued as far as Natural Theology can avail; but the sacred volume contains a lucidity and sanction beyond all we can adduce from mere human ingenuity, and I therefore conclude by referring to it, as "life and immortality are clearly brought to light through the Gospel".

susceptible individuals there is also a very marked change in the state of the respiration and general posture of the body. They must also have experienced, in themselves and others, how prone we are to assume a sympathetic condition, both of mind and body, from those with whom we associate, or during a temporary interview [i.e., to imitate or role-model others]. These physical changes seem to result from a mental influence imparted through the eyes and ears, and then reflected from within, through the respiratory, facial, and spinal nerves, on the external form and features. **Now such being the case, is there any great improbability, that by calling the muscles of expression into action during the hypnotic state, by titillating certain nerves, that the impression of the feeling with which such external manifestation is generally associated should be reflected on the brain, and excite in the mind the particular passion or emotion?** [Braid later calls this "muscular suggestion" in his *Observations on Trance* (1850).] **I think it is highly probable this is the true cause of the phrenological manifestations during the hypnotic condition; and as it is the peculiar feature of this condition, that the whole energies of the soul should be concentrated on the emotion excited, the manifestation, of course, becomes very decided. I presume the different points pressed on, through the stimulus given to various fasciculi [i.e., bundles] of nerves, call into action certain combinations of muscles of expression in the face and general frame, and also influence the organs of respiration, and thus the mind is influenced, *indirectly,* through the organs of common sensation [i.e., touch] and the sympathetic, as sneezing is excited in some by too strong a light irritating the optic nerves. Two patients who are highly intelligent, and remain partially conscious, and who acknowledge they did all in their power to resist the influence excited by manipulating the head, state, that the first feeling was a drawing of the muscles of the face, and affection of the breathing, which was followed by an irresistible impulse to act as they did, but why they could not tell.**

In this view of the subject it would resolve itself into the laws of sympathy [a reference to the Scottish philosophers, Adam Smith and Dugald Stewart], and the question then is, where are the external or superficial points of the sympathies located? Experience must decide this, and in the peculiar condition induced by hypnotism, according to my own experience, this can be more readily and certainly determined than in the normal state. These points having been ascertained, we can then determine how and where to act according to our particular object; and it can be of no real importance where the cerebral points or special organs may be posited.

As to the real locations of the sympathetic points, by stimulating which we produce peculiar manifestations, they appear to me not to be quite accurately the same in all heads, but, on the whole, pretty near the centres of the organs as mapped out on heads generally approved by phrenologists, and I have had decided proof that some relation subsists betwixt the size and function, as in general there is more energy displayed when there is large development, and the negative when it is defective. Thus, a patient with large combativeness or destructiveness, when excited during hypnotism, will display great violence and disposition to attack others, whereas, where they are defective, they will shrink and express a fear that someone is quarrelling, or angry with them.

If the solution of the cause of these remarkable phenomena now given should not be deemed correct, the only other which occurs to my mind as at all satisfactory, is this, that the different fasciculi of sentient nerves excite *directly* the *corresponding points* of the brain, and these again the physical manifestations. We know by what musical combinations and movements we can excite the different passions; we know also that this arises from some peculiar impression communicated to the brain through the *portio mollis* of the seventh pair of nerves [i.e., the facial nerves]; and whether this is conveyed to it as a single organ only, or as a combination of organs, it is clear that, as the origin of the *seventh* is *more remote* from the brain than the origin of the *fifth,* there must, consequently, be at least as great difficulty in accounting for such results being excited through the different branches of the *seventh* as through those of the *fifth* pair.

Dr. Elliotson's Opinion as to the Efficacy or Non-Efficacy of Volition

The animal magnetizers do not now [as they originally did] contend for *their volitions* being necessary. Dr. Elliotson distinctly states, in a published letter, dated 11th September, 1842, that he had "never produced any effect by mere willing"; and adds,

> I have never seen reason to believe, (and I have made innumerable comparative experiments upon the point,) that I have heightened the effect of my processes by exerting the strongest will, or lessened them by thinking intentionally of other things, and endeavouring to bestow no more attention upon what I was about than was just necessary to carry on the process. So far from willing, I have at first had no idea of what would be the effect of my processes; in exciting the *cerebral organs,* the effect ensues as well in my female patient though the manipulator be a sceptic, and may therefore be presumed not to wish the proper result to ensue and though I stood aside, and do not know what organ he has in view. I have never excited them by the mere will; I have excited them with my fingers just as well when thinking of other matters with my friends, and momentarily forgetting what I was about, etc.

The Doctor also denies his belief in the phrenological results arising from *sympathy with the state of the operator's brain*. I feel convinced that he is right in these sentiments, and believe that **the same degree of mechanical pressure or stimulus to the integuments of the cranium [i.e., to the scalp], from an inanimate substance, when the patient is in the proper stage of the Mesmeric condition, will produce the same manifestation as the personal touch of either sceptic or believer in animal magnetism.** Thus, touching them with a **knobbed glass rod, three feet long**, has produced the phenomena with my patients as certainly as personal contact, so that if there is any thing of *vital* magnetism in it, it is subject to different laws from that of *ordinary* magnetism or electricity.

Mere pointing I have myself found sufficient to excite the manifestations in several patients, after previous excitement of the organs, but this arises from feeling, as I know the sensibility of the skin in those cases enables them to feel *without actual contact.*

The following experiment seems to me to prove clearly that the manifestations were entirely attributable to the **mechanical pressure operating on an excited state of the nervous system**. I placed **a cork endways over the organ of veneration, and bound it in that position by a bandage passing under the chin.** I now hypnotised the patient, and observed the effect, which was precisely the same, for some time, as when no such appliance was used; after a minute and a half had elapsed, an altered expression of countenance took place, and a movement of the arms and hands, which latter became clasped as in adoration, and the patient now arose from the seat and knelt down as if engaged in prayer. On moving the cork forwards, active benevolence was manifested, and on being pushed back, veneration again manifested itself. I have repeatedly tried similar experiments with this, and other patients, with the like results, including other organs. It is clear there was no mechanical pressure to direct the movement *downwards,* because there was pressure *upwards* also and had there been any preconceived notion in the patient's mind to excite to such action, it ought to have been manifested *immediately on passing into the sleep.* None of the patients had the slightest notion of what was my object in making such experiments, and none of them saw the others operated on. At [the end of this chapter], it will be observed, **pressure by their own fingers produced similar manifestations, even whilst their minds were expecting some other results.**

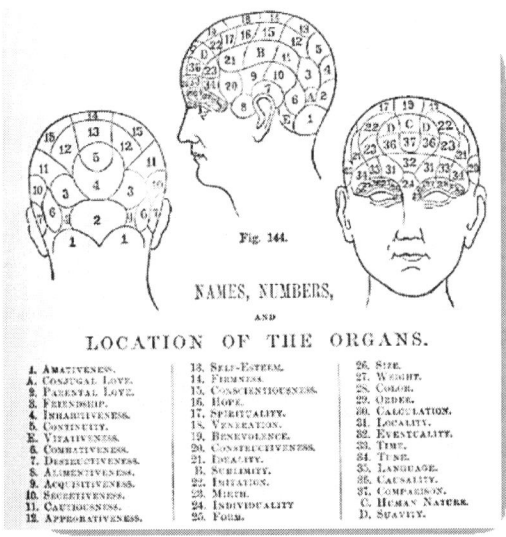

Figure 4 Example of a 19th century phrenological chart, showing organology.

Modes of Dividing the Brain
Whilst it is generally agreed that the brain admits of being divided into regions for the animal propensities, moral sentiments, and intellectual faculties, it has not been at all possible to prove satisfactorily the exact position and size of each organ, as noted by the phrenologists. Granting that there is a distinct organ or point in the brain for each faculty, which I think is highly probable, still there must ever be insuperable difficulty in thus accurately determining character, even supposing we knew the exact position and size of each organ, because much must depend upon the state of perfection of structure, and activity of the point or organ, as well as its absolute size. Thus, a person with a large eye may have defective sight, whilst a person with a small eye may see clearly and distinctly, the greater perfection of structure, and activity of the optic nerves, more than compensating for mere deficiency of size. So it is with the brain, a part may be abnormally large, and the faculty dull, from want of power or activity, or perfection of organic structure; and the reverse may obtain, a small development, with high activity, may render its function predominant.

Causes of Phrenology Being Imperfect
It is from a want of such knowledge as this that phrenology must ever prove imperfect, even granting the localities to be correctly ascertained and established. However, **when we have ascertained the points where, by acting in any peculiar manner, we can excite into activity particular sympathetic *physical and mental* associations, whilst the other faculties are put into a state of quiescence, it appears to me to be a matter of far greater importance, and a subject still more curious, than any thing ever brought forward by phrenologists. It is far more available for practical purposes too.** Phrenologists could at best only pretend to tell the *natural tendencies* of an individual, and direct that he should be educated in accordance with a specific plan, as has hitherto been done independently of phrenology, from watching the natural dispositions and habits of different individuals, by encouraging and directing their studies in such and such a direction; but here, *in addition* to this, we have the power of giving a decided impulse in any particular direction. It ought not to be overlooked, that this does not deprive us of any of our *former* available modes of instruction and morality, but it promises to prove a powerful auxiliary for expediting and ensuring the success of those means. It therefore follows, that it becomes the duty of every well-wisher to his species to investigate this matter, and determine how far it *is generally* applicable. It is still more the duty of the medical faculty to do so, because, should farther experience determine this question in the affirmative, it is reasonable to expect it may be turned to the best account in the cure of disease, by applying our *remedies locally,* to the cutaneous points which have been ascertained to be the centres of the morbid concatenation. Thus, leeching and sedatives, *etc.*, might be applied to such points when there was excitement of the corresponding functions, and *vice versa,* with the reasonable hope of success; and if this method cannot be effective, **we can be pretty certain of success through hypnotism, by exciting the morbidly low faculty where there is depression, and the antagonist organ where there has been excitement.** In this manner I have no doubt but hypnotism may prove of incalculable advantage in the treatment of many cases of insanity, and nervous affections tending to induce that disease.

Objections to Phreno-Hypnotism
I am quite aware some will be ready to start an objection to my views, by stating that the scalp, where many or most of these demonstrations have been manifested, is not highly sensitive, that it is not extensively supplied with sentient nerves, and that they all arise from the fifth pair, and do not pass directly through the skull to the subjacent points of the brain. This, however, does not prove that the terminal branches may not ultimately have a special influence on such points, notwithstanding their circuitous course to arrive there. I beg to remind such individuals that we are by no means sufficiently acquainted with the laws and distribution of the nervous system, to be able to prescribe rules as to *how* it *ought* and *must* act. Who does not know, that until the discoveries of our illustrious countryman, Sir Charles Bell, the same nerve was considered to give both sense and motion? And when he propounded that the true cause of its double functions was because of its having *double* roots, was not this announcement scouted for some time, and then, when proved to be true, were not attempts made to rob Sir Charles Bell of the honour of the discovery? There seems to be great reason to conclude that the distribution of the nerves of the scalp will ultimately be found far more intricate and beautifully arranged than at present we have any conception of.

Mode of Connection between the Brain and Body
I shall now proceed to state my views as to the mode in which different parts of the brain are associated with different parts of the body. I have long quite agreed with those physiologists who consider that the *vis nervosa* [nervous current] is something circulated in tubes, that the primitive nerve-tubes do not anastomose [branch into each other], but only run parallel with others, remaining distinct and isolated throughout their course, and that consequently the "cerebral extremity of each fibre is connected with the peripheral extremity of a single nervous fibre only, and that this peripheral extremity is in relation with only one point of the brain or spinal cord: so that, corresponding to the many millions of primitive fibres which are given off to peripheral parts of the body, there are the same number of peripheral points of the body represented on the brain. The sensation of a single point evidently depends on the impression being conveyed by means of a single fibre to a single point of the sensorium." (Müller.) It is from the same cause that we can regulate simple or associated movements of distinct members.

From all these considerations it appears quite reasonable to suppose, and [the] analogy, as respects distinct organs being appropriated for other special functions, warrants the inference, that different parts of the brain may have special functions to perform, both as regards mind and matter; and that, when such points are excited into inordinate activity, the manifestations will become correspondingly more conspicuous, and *vice versa.*

We know from experience that the various passions and emotions can be excited through the organ of hearing either by music or oratory, through the eyes by painting or sculpture, and likewise, though less extensively and efficiently, through common sensation [i.e., touch], and there seems to me to be nothing, *a priori* to militate against the probability, that this may be effected to a much greater extent than has yet been done, provided we can only discover the peculiar mode of exciting certain portions of the brain. If the views already advanced, that every point of the body supplied by primitive nervous fibres has a distinct corresponding point in the brain, it is clear, that by titillating each peripheral point, we shall excite its corresponding central point; and from what shall be found detailed in experiments recorded, it appears highly probable that the respective parts of the brain corresponding to *every* part of the body, may be excited into activity though certain sympathetic points in the integuments of the head and neck, and if so, we may also excite into activity the whole of those actions, mental and muscular, which are associated with each portion of the cerebrum. In this case Smellie's supposition would be completely realised in man. He expresses himself thus:–

> I can conceive a superior being so thoroughly acquainted with the human frame, so perfectly skilled in the connection and mutual dependence which subsist between our intellect and our sensitive organs, as to be able, by titillating in various modes and directions, particular combinations of nerves, or particular branches of any single nerve, to excite in the mind what idea he may think proper. I can likewise conceive the possibility of suggesting any particular idea, or species of ideas, by affecting the nerves in the same manner as these ideas affect them when excited by any other cause.

This confident aspiration seems to be now in a great measure realised, by certain modes of manipulating patients during the hypnotic condition, of which I shall now adduce a few illustrations.

First Attempts at Phrenologizing During Hypnotism Were Failures

My first attempt to excite the phreno-hypnotic phenomena was in the month of April, 1842, in the lecture-room at Liverpool, but it did not succeed. I then tried the experiment repeatedly in private, putting the patients to sleep by contact as well as in my usual way, but still could not succeed. I was anxious to try it fairly, and therefore applied to Mr. [Henry] Brookes, through the kindness of Dr. Birt Davies of Birmingham, for information as to the mode Mr. Brookes had practised so successfully, and which was most politely communicated to me by both these gentlemen. I tried this mode with several patients, both in my usual plan and that of the animal magnetizers, but was still unsuccessful. I now abandoned it as a hopeless task, presuming the cases which had proved successful with others must have been *lusus naturae* [a freak of nature], or that the operators had deceived themselves, the patients having been led to answer, and give the manifestations they did, from the nature of the leading questions proposed, and might afterwards remember what passed at previous operations, and answer accordingly; whilst, like natural somnambulists, they might not remember, when awake, what had passed during their sleep.

Succeeded by Operating Differently

Last December I was induced to make another attempt, from reading a report of Mr. Spencer T. Hall's two first lectures on the subject, at Sheffield: and it was remarkable, that the very first patient I tried in that way exhibited several of the manifestations. [Spencer T. Hall founded the *Phreno-Magnet*, a journal on phrenology and Mesmerism.] However, I was led to refer the result to a totally different cause from what he and the other animal magnetizers did. **I concluded it arose from the different degrees of sensibility of different parts of the integuments, conveying correspondingly varied impressions when similarly impressed, and exciting different ideas in the mind, and thus calling up old associations; and that when similarly impressed the same ideas might again present themselves to the mind.** I considered this far more probable than that the brain was affected by any transmission from the operator to the brain directly through the skull; and to prove this, **tried the effect of pressure over parts which had *no cerebral substance directly subjacent*, and the results confirmed my expectations.** Thus, pressure on the apex of the *mastoid process* [behind the ear], and the *ossa nasi* [in the nose], and the *chin* were as certainly followed by particular manifestations, as pressure on different parts of the cranium was followed by others. **I also very soon ascertained that the same points of the cranium, when thus excited, did not excite the *same ideas* or emotions to the minds of *different* patients, which I considered ought to have been the case, according to the views of the staunch phrenologists. I have since discovered the cause of this, namely, *not having operated* at the *proper* stage of the hypnotic condition.**

Cases Illustrative

I shall now adduce a few examples. [**Case I.**] On one subject, after being in the hypnotic condition for a few minutes, by applying gentle pressure over the *ossa nasi,* immoderate laughter was immediately excited, and ceased as abruptly on removing the contact. The abruptness of these transitions, especially from immoderate laughter to the extreme gravity and vacancy of expression peculiar to the hypnotic state, was quite ludicrous, and almost beyond belief. Supposing she were singing the most grave tune and solemn words, the moment **the nose was touched** in this manner, by anyone, she was irresistibly thrown into this merry mood, but would join in the tune again with the utmost gravity the moment the contact ceased. **Rubbing the same part, or pinching up the skin over it, seemed to produce no effect whatever.** On applying pressure to this patient's chin there was an immediate catch in the breathing, with sighing and sobbing, which would subside on removing the point of contact. By touching both nose and chin at the same time there was the most ludicrous combination of laughing and crying, each struggling for the mastery, as we sometimes see in hysteric attacks. Both would cease immediately on removing the contact. Friction or pinching the skin on the chin had no effect of producing such phenomena, in short, no part of this patient which I tested seemed capable of being excited by friction or pinching the integuments, excepting around the orbits [of the eyes], which produced spectra [Braid seems to mean illusory colours, i.e., 'phosphenes', as below], although less perfectly so than by simple pressure against the bone. This patient, being always pressed over the phrenologists' organ of time, always expressed her desire "to write" – a letter – to her mother or her brother; over their organ of tune, "to sing"; between this and wit, "to be judicious"; the boundary between wit and causality, "to be clever"; causality, "to have knowledge"; in the centre of the forehead, to have "a certain perception of learning"; below this the phrenologists' eventuality, "to be skilful"; the points of the head occupied by veneration and benevolence were sometimes indicated by the desire "to be virtuous," or "to be honourable"; most frequently, when the point touched was over benevolence, the answer was, "to be honourable", and when over the other point, "to be virtuous", when both points were touched at the same time, it was, "to be honourable and virtuous", and the same answer was always given when these points were touched *combined with No. 1, or amativeness* [i.e., agreement]. When the latter was touched alone, the answer always was "to be commended"; when approximating the mastoid process, or over that process, a remarkable placidity, or expression of delight, came over the countenance, and the desire was for "complacency", which, when hypnotised, she defined, "to be civil", but when awake she seemed at a loss to know what the word meant On touching "combativeness" the placidity of countenance was speedily exchanged for the opposite expression; but on pressure being made immediately above the ears, the most ferocious aspect of countenance was assumed, the breath being suppressed almost to suffocation, the face becoming flushed, with grinding of the teeth; and when the arms were not rigid, the most vigorous efforts at inflicting violence on all who were within her reach, as several gentlemen can attest to their personal knowledge and sorrow. **On pressure being applied to the root of the nose, the idea of seeing different forms, and figures, and colours, seemed to be excited in the mind, more vividly when certain points were thus excited, but it could be excited by pressing the integuments against the *under*, as well as *upper* edge of the orbit, with this difference, that the objects seen, or rather spectra excited, were then generally of a painful and distressing character, whereas they were generally of a bright, and glowing, or cheerful description when excited by acting on the upper margin of the orbit. I should observe, that care was taken, in all these experiments, *not to press against the globe of the eye.*** Thus far the phenomena were pretty uniform in this patient, the answers having been generally very much the same when impressed *exactly in the same way, on the same points, and under similar circumstances in all other respects.* Thus, the last day I had all opportunity of testing this patient, I went over the different points four times with scarcely the slightest variation in the answers, as can be testified by several gentlemen who were present; and they were again repeated two or three times the same evening with like results. This patient was operated on the previous day in presence of several professional and scientific gentlemen, when several answers were given different. More than one being operating on that occasion, and the manner and degree of touching the parts being different, might be the cause of the varied results. **I am satisfied this patient knew nothing of phrenology; and that she remembered nothing of what she said, or was done to her during these operations.**

Case II. In this patient *friction* would *excite*, whilst pressure had *no effect* in calling forth manifestations. In this case, friction over the *ossa nasi* excited the desire for "something to smell", generally aromatic vinegar or Eau de Cologne; over the chin, for something to eat; over the tendon of orbicularis, a tendency to laugh; close upon the root of the nose, friction excited spectra, and around the orbit, in like manner, the same or different spectra, differing to the *degrees of* pressure and friction applied; over the organ of tune, "to sing"; over the back part of the base of the head, expressed herself "very happy and comfortable"; over combativeness and destructiveness, a quarrelsome disposition, as manifested in word, look, and action. The other parts tried were less certain or decided in this patient.

Case III. In this patient, friction excited the desire "to waltz", when applied over the organ of tune, and the desire "to walk", when applied to the organ of wit, as mapped by the phrenologists, and in like manner, "to sing" when veneration was the point affected. Spectra, also, when the integuments were rubbed against the margin of the orbits. Although not corresponding with the phrenological charts, nor with what occurred in the others, similar answers were given when the same points were similarly excited.

Case IV. When asked what she would like, when manipulated as the others referred to, almost always answered, "nothing at all", excepting over the most sensitive parts of the cranium, when her answer was, "leeches to my head".

Case V. Very much the same as the last.

I think the cases referred to support my position, that the different results arise from the circumstance of different parts of the integuments having different degrees of sensibility, and thus

exciting different ideas in the mind when the same quality and intensity of stimulus is applied to each part in succession. There can be no doubt but the point under which the phrenologists have posited "combativeness and destructiveness", is the most highly sensitive of any part of the cranium, and is always accompanied with symptoms of the patients feeling pain, and, as a matter of course, they will offer resistance, and attempt to free themselves from the offending cause; and so of the rest, according to their respective impressibilities.[129]

A Child Operates Successfully

After the above remarks had been written, and my work set to the press, I met with the following most interesting case:– I was informed that a child, five years and a half old, who had been present when I exhibited experiments on [Case] No. I. the same evening had proposed to operate on her nurse. The nurse had no objection to indulge the girl, never supposing any effect could take place. However, it appeared she speedily closed her eyes, when the child, imitating what she saw me do, placed a finger on her forehead, and asked what she would like, when the patient answered, "to dance"; on trying another point, the answer was, "to sing", and the two then had a song together, after which the juvenile experimenter roused the patient in the same manner she had seen me do.

Details of the Case

The above circumstance being related to me the following day, I felt curious to ascertain whether there might not be some mistake, as there had been no third party present, and it depended entirely on the statement of the child, which induced me, when visiting the family the day after, to request permission to test the patient. This was readily granted; and, to my astonishment, she manifested the phenomena in a degree far beyond any case I had tried; indeed, she did so, with a degree of perfection which baffles description.

However frequently she was tried, the same expression of countenance, the same condition of the respiration, and similar postures of the body have been evinced, when the same points were pressed. Indeed, so highly susceptible was she that after a few trials, when I pointed a finger or glass rod over the part, **without contact**, similar manifestations resulted, only in a less rapid and more modified degree. **I also found by trying [Case] No. II.** *at an earlier stage,* **that her susceptibility was almost equal to the present case.** The following are a few of the more striking manifestations: pressure on the chin was followed by movement of the jaws, lips, and tongue, with the desire to eat; on the lower part of the nose, "to smell"; insertion of tendon of the orbicularis, immoderate laughter, which, on being asked why she laughed, the answer indicated, it was from a sense of the ludicrousness being excited; over time, "to dance"; tune, "to sing", with pressure on the eye at the same time, she did sing part of a song; over the back of the head, [Case] No. I. she shuddered and retreated, under the impression that someone was about to take liberties with her, the same feeling of delicacy was also manifested *when any other part of the body was touched excepting the head and face;* over apex of mastoid process, the desire to shake hands and be friendly; the former, with [Case] No. IV., or adhesiveness, she would lean to, or clasp anyone near her; combativeness, the reverse; destructiveness, (it was very small,) she was distressed from the notion that someone *was quarrelling with her;* philoprogenitiveness, she always said, "hark, the poor child is crying!"; secretiveness and caution, she would tell nothing; benevolence, "to travel"; veneration, she knelt down in the most solemn manner and prayed; combined with hope and expression of ecstasy united with devotion; over the eyebrows, spectra of all forms and colours, gay and glowing, and when below the eye, the notion of the sea, a ship, and people about to be drowned; at a farther trial, other manifestations come out equally, or even more strikingly, according to the accuracy with which the corresponding points were touched. In particular, I must note what happened the first time I touched imitation, which was entirely accidental, and whilst, besides a relation of my own, there was present a gentleman whose literary and scientific attainments, and philosophic turn of mind, as well as high standing in society, render him an ornament of our country, beside imitating everything done or said in English, she imitated correctly French, Italian, Spanish, German, Latin and Greek; every word was spoken with the utmost precision, and has been done several times since before many professional and scientific gentlemen, and ladies, who can bear testimony to the extraordinary fidelity of pronunciation and emphasis. I need scarcely add she could not do so when tested after being awakened. Many other patients I have since made do the same, one a girl of only twelve years of age.

Other Successful Cases

On Mr. [Spencer T.] Hall's arrival in Manchester, previous to his first lecture, I had the pleasure of seeing him at my house, when I exhibited my experiments on his and another patient, with which he seemed much gratified. I also afforded him an opportunity of seeing them again next day. After I had them in the hypnotic condition, I requested him to manipulate their heads, which he did more minutely than I had done, and consequently brought out additional manifestations. I was on the alert to all he did and said, for I was

---

[129] [Braid's initial experiments on phrenology, therefore, show quite inconsistent results, and suggest that the effects probably depend upon other factors being present. Two results were positive, two negative, and one somewhat ambiguous. This clearly does not make him a supporter of phrenology, as was sometimes claimed.]

determined he should not have an opportunity *of prompting in any way,* and most assuredly, by exciting acquisitiveness, he very soon led the patient to steal a silver snuff-box from a gentleman present, and it was most striking the anxiety with which she returned it, on Mr. Hall removing the point of contact to conscientiousness; the movement of the arm was *changed instantly,* as if automatically. I had never tried to excite either of these two points. The other manifestations, which I had previously seen developed, were precisely the same under his manipulations as my own. I made several attempts to excite the organ of benevolence, but without effect, until one day I accidentally placed my finger so low as I should have considered to be the middle of comparison, as marked on the busts, when she instantly evinced the emotion in the most active manner, saying, "poor creature, poor creature", and not content, as many are, with *mere words* of compassion, she anxiously presented us with all the money in her pocket. I should not omit to add, that this patient is *quite* unconscious of all she or others do or say whilst in this state, and did not know the location of a single [phrenological] organ.

It would only be an unnecessary waste of time to detail at length all the cases I have had since of similar manifestations, varying in degree according to the original constitution and habit of mind of each patient, the variety is the most striking proof of the reality of the phenomena. **There are some patients who have a sort of indistinct recollection of what had passed, as if it had been a dream; two in particular, who observed they had an indistinct notion of what they were doing, but felt irresistibly impelled, as it were, to do certain things, even whilst they thought complying with the predominant inclination would make them very ridiculous.** This, I presume, referred to imitation and comicality, and such like humorous faculties, which they displayed in a very remarkable degree, these patients are highly respectable and intelligent, and manifested the phenomena quite as prominently as the patient last named, that of veneration and hope, also filial affection, in a manner baffling description. Each knew only one phrenological organ.

That I might be the better certified that all was reality, I also got a relation of my own to submit to the operation, and it was quite conclusive. She has a slight recollection of *some* things which were said and done, but of other seems quite oblivious.

Proper Time for Operating
I had also the opportunity of verifying the truthfulness of these various and interesting phenomena through the kindness of Mrs. Col. ——, who submitted to be operated on by me in the presence of her husband, as also the Major; the Captain and Surgeon of the regiment; also a high dignitary of the church, and who is also an eminently scientific gentleman; Mr. Gardom, surgeon, and other professional gentlemen; Mr. Aspinal Turner, and a number of others, both ladies and gentlemen. In about three minutes after she was asleep, I placed two fingers over the point named veneration, instantly the aspect of her countenance changed; in a little, she slowly, and solemnly, and majestically arose from her chair, advanced towards the table in the middle of the room, and softly sank on her knees, and exhibited such a picture of devout adoration as can never be forgotten by any who had the gratification to witness it. She was tested with a number of other faculties, when the corresponding manifestations were equally striking and characteristic. When awakened, this lady was quite unconscious of all which had happened.

Here, then, we have the testimony of a lady of the highest respectability and intelligence, and energy of mind, corroborating, both in word and action, and look, the reality of the phenomena as exhibited by others, and that in the presence of most respectable and intelligent witnesses, who can bear testimony that there was nothing said or done to direct her in the important manifestations. This lady had been hypnotised by me once before, for a few minutes, at a private conversazione the week before, when she sat down fully convinced she could NOT be affected, but was soon made to acknowledge the power of hypnotism, and now she was a valuable evidence to the more novel investigation as to how far phrenological manifestations could be developed during hypnotism.[130] I have now realised these phenomena very prominently **with forty-five patients, most of whom, I am quite certain, knew nothing of phrenology, some of them not even what the word meant**; and the smallness of the points to which the contact must be made to elicit the manifestations correctly, especially the subdivisions by Mr. Hall, is such as to render collusion most improbable. I was also **careful to avoid prompting, by putting leading questions**. I have also succeeded partially with others; and several of my friends have also been successful with a few other cases. **I attended Mr. Hall's public lectures, and the very first experiment he tried, on February 24th, 1843, convinced me, that the reason why I had not sooner obtained the manifestations more generally was, because I had allowed my patients to pass into the *supersentient* state before testing them. I was aware of the difference in the state of the circulation through the brain in the state in which my patients were, and what it must be in the state in which his were during his operations, and conjectured, that by trying my patients in *that* condition, I might get manifestations which I had failed to do at former trials; and**

---

[130] A report having been circulated, no doubt with the view of neutralizing the interest attaching to the case, that this lady was a phrenologist, I called to inquire whether there was any ground for such a report. Mrs. S. herself assured me it was quite erroneous, for it was a subject she had never paid any attention to, and one she was quite ignorant of. Wishing to be very circumstantially correct in the statement, she added, "I have understood the organ of music is somewhere about the forehead"; when requested to place her finger on the organ, she was quite wrong, so that *she did not know a single organ.* I mentioned this circumstance, in her presence, at another conversazione, when she most distinctly declared the facts here recorded, to be strictly correct.

the very first cases I tried proved this conjecture to be correct. For example, [Case] No. II., already referred to, exhibited a number of additional phenomena beautifully; and cases IV. and V. [which previously failed to respond] in like manner, came out beautifully. From this single observation on Mr. Hall's mode, or rather *time,* of operating, I have been enabled to arrive at a mode of operating which, I believe, by putting patients into the hypnotic condition my own way, there will be no great difficulty in manifesting some of the phenomena in most cases. There are some patients, however, who will evince them much more prominently than others, and the power of habit seems evident in most, being more readily operated on after a few trials. Some, however, seem as perfect as possible at the first trial.

I have also tried several private friends, on whose intelligence, honour, and integrity, I could rely, and also children, and have found the evidence so satisfactory, that I am quite certain as to the reality of the phenomena; but as to my theoretical views, I wish them to be considered as mere conjectures, thrown out for the purpose of exciting others to think, and investigate this curious and most important subject.

Case of an Officer in 1758

I shall conclude this article by calling attention of my readers to the coincidence which appears to subsist betwixt the phenomena now referred to, and **the mode of exciting dreaming, in some patients, by whispering in their ears.** I shall illustrate that by reference to a case recorded in one of Dr. Abercrombie's valuable works, on the authority of the late Dr. Gregory. It is that of the case of an officer in the expedition to Louisburgh in 1758. His brother officers were in the habit of amusing themselves at his expense. They could produce any kind of dream they chose, especially if done by one with whose voice he was familiar. Thus, at one time, they conducted him through the whole process of a quarrel, ending in a duel; and when it was supposed the parties met, a pistol was put in his hand, which he fired, and was awakened by its report. On another occasion, being asleep in the locker of the cabin, he was made to believe that he had fallen overboard, and was told to save himself by swimming, when they told him to dive for his life, as a shark was pursuing him, which he attempted so energetically, that he threw himself from the locker, by which he bruised himself severely. Again, after the landing of the army, he was found one day asleep in his tent, and apparently much annoyed with the noise of the cannonading then going on briskly. He was made to believe he was engaged with the enemy, when he expressed much fear, and betrayed a wish to run away. They remonstrated against this cowardice, whilst they increased his alarm by imitating the groans of the wounded; and when he inquired who was killed, which he often did, they named his particular friends. At last he was told that the man next to him in the line had fallen, when he instantly sprang from his sleep, and relieved from his fears, by falling over the tent ropes. It is added, that after these experiments, he had not distinct recollection of his dreams, but only a confused feeling of oppression or fatigue; and used to say to his friends, that he was sure they had been playing him some tricks.

Inferences as to Its Curative Powers

I shall add one illustration of the probability of benefit accruing to society from this subject being prosecuted with zeal and due consideration. A highly scientific friend, who had honoured me with his presence at a private conversazione, called two days thereafter, and stated that from reflecting on what I had said and exhibited the day before as to the mode of exciting certain points or functions of the brain through acting on certain points of the scalp and face, it appeared to him most reasonable to expect that by applying *such* points, we might most readily afford relief to disorder of the corresponding internal organs. I told him I was so thoroughly induced to act accordingly; and that the day before I had been visiting an insane patient, who entertained the horrible idea, that she must murder everybody she knew, and then murder herself also; that on placing my hand upon the organ of combativeness and destructiveness, in a few seconds, she gave a violent shudder, and seemed greatly excited, and becoming perfectly furious. On examining these parts, I found the integuments [i.e., skin] quite red. I ordered leeches, and cold lotion afterwards, but next day she remained equally violent, and the pulse between 140 and 150 [i.e., racing], which it had been for some time, notwithstanding medicines had been given to depress it. I now made an incision an inch and a half long through the integuments, and down to the bone, and in twelve hours after found her much calmer, and the pulse down to 100, and it remained there for several days. There was no such loss of blood as could have acted constitutionally on the heart directly by the quantity effused. On again rising, Belladonna plasters were applied – these not having the desired effect, recourse was again had to scarification behind both ears, and with great success, as in a few days she was so calm as not to require the strait jacket, and for two months has been sullen but harmless.

At another conversazione, the same gentleman requested me to excite philoprogenitiveness, which I did, and he then asked me to combine destructiveness along with it. I told him the faculty would not be developed, because the organ was so small in this patient as to make her always imagine someone was quarrelling with her. Still he wished me to try, which I did, and the result was that she immediately seemed distressed about someone being angry with the children. Two days after, I was informed that the object of the request was to prove that such would be the case, as he had whispered to a professional gentleman present, before the answer was elicited, and no one else in the room knew this remark. Two days after, on a slip of paper handed to me by the same gentleman, he had noted, that if I would excite the same organs in another patient, whose destructiveness was more prominent, I would find she would be angry with the children, and wish to punish or send them away, and assuredly it proved so. He also added, that this is the combination of morbid excitement which he conjectured, and I think with great justice, is the cause of parents murdering their own children during a fit of insanity. An example of more acute, beautiful, and successful induction than this could scarcely be conceived possible; and it is highly gratifying to know that the opinions of a gentleman of such talents and attainments coincides so much with my general views on this subject.

Opinions of La Roy Sunderland, and Mr. Hall
The doctrine propounded by the Rev. La Roy Sunderland, and Mr. Spencer T. Hall, and others, seems to be this, that there is a separate organ in the brain for every mental faculty, emotion, propensity, desire, and action, mental or corporeal; that every positive organ has also its negative organ proximate; and that by certain manipulations during the Mesmeric state, these organs may be stimulated into activity singly or combined, and thus caused to manifest the corresponding faculty by thought, word, and action. They do not deny the correctness of the outlines as given by former phrenologists; on the contrary, they bear positive testimony to their general correctness. However, they subdivide each of the former faculties, which we may designate the pure faculties, into groups of distinct organs, for the specific manifestation of special faculties, the tendencies to which were naturally included in the simple or primitive general organ; and they allege they can thus give such a special or characteristic direction to the feeling as to entitle it to be considered as the manifestation of a distinct organ or faculty.

It occurs to me, that this might be much simplified, by considering, that on the central point of the general organs, we stimulate fasciculi of nerves connected with a general manifestation, for example, benevolence; but that, as we approach the surrounding organs, we partially excite proximate faculties, from some of their corresponding peripheral sentient nerves co-mingling with those of the other faculty, and thus engender a mixed manifestation; just as we find the intercourse between neighbouring countries modifies the national character which peculiarly belongs to each nation. Thus, in one direction, benevolence (by which I illustrate my position) will be blended with comparison, or excited through the influence of association respecting someone we have known, or from supposing what might be our feelings were we placed in such and such circumstances; in another direction, it will be influenced more or less by the tendency to imitate the benevolent acts of others, and, as we approach veneration, it will partake more of a religious and moral obligation in reference to the Deity. If I am right in this conjecture, of course there will be every possible shade of manifestation as we approach nearer to the adjoining organ. I am not acquainted with the mapping of the head either by La Roy Sunderland or Mr. Hall; but, if the original compartments are to be so divided and subdivided, according to the mere varieties of manifestation during the hypnotic state, I feel assured, that each of their *subdivisions* may be again *divided,* as a shade of difference will be manifested by every possible change in the point of contact.

I had much pleasure in witnessing Mr. Hall's experiments, and bore public testimony to the reality of the general phenomena. This I could have done from the mere circumstance of carefully watching the peculiar expression of countenance, and state of the respiration, induced by every move of the point of contact. The shades of difference were so minute that collusion was all but impossible. Moreover, I had personal experience of the reality of the leading phenomena in a number of my own patients, with parties who know nothing of phrenology, and whose respectability and known character placed them above the possibility of being suspected as acting a part, either for the purpose of gratifying or deceiving others. **Whilst I readily bear testimony to the reality of the phenomena, and I saw nothing in Mr. Hall to lead me to suppose he wished to deceive anyone, it is due to the cause of truth for me to state, that the varieties which I observed in his phenomena and those occurring in my own patients, I consider were the mere results of the different manipulations used, and not of any such *special* influence as he and other animal magnetizers allege.**

Presumed Cause of Phenomena Called Cross Magnetism
In reference to the phenomena which were designated "cross-magnetizing", and which appeared most distressing to the patients, as well as to the operator, (fortunately no such effects have occurred in my patients,) I think they may be explained thus: it seems probable, part may be the result of imagination, or an accidental circumstance **exciting the opposing classes of muscles into action** at the same time. This may also be caused by **exciting two antagonistic emotions**, such as one requiring the energetic action of the muscles of inspiration, and the other the muscles of expiration, the consequence of which is, very speedily to throw the patient into a state of partial asphyxia; and the result must be, a great difficulty in restoring the patient from the deleterious influence of insufficiently decarbonated blood circulating through the brain. Such I consider was the case with the patient I saw create so much trouble to Mr. Hall on the evening of the 24th February, 1843, in the lecture-room of the Athenaeum, Manchester.

Return Stolen Property to Proper Owners and Proper Place by Smell and Touch

Having heard Mr. Hall state, that patients who had stolen anything would always seek out the persons from whom it had been taken, and restore it to them after conscientiousness was excited, and that they would find out the rightful owner, whatever part of the room he had removed to, I was curious to prove this. My first object was to ascertain whether it was a fact, which I very soon did with my own patients, and my next objective was to ascertain *by what means they accomplished this,* and **I readily determined it was *by means of smell* and *touch.*** The first thing they did, on rousing conscientiousness, was to look thoughtful, then they began sniffing, and traced out the parties robbed, and restored it to them. When asked, "What are you doing?" the answer was, "I am giving back something which I had stolen." On being asked, "How do you know the person?" (having gone to the opposite side of the room,) the answer was, "I smell them, or him." Every time the experiment was tried, the result was the same and the answer the same, as was obvious to everyone in the room. Another patient did the same *when the sense of smell was acute,* but when I tried the experiment with the *sense of smell dulled,* the stolen article was *merely laid down,* without giving it to the proper person. There was thus both positive and negative proof of exalted smell being the cause of them restoring to the proper party; and feeling directs them as to place. I have found this done with the same promptitude and certainty when six, eight, or twelve faculties had been roused and manifested before conscientiousness was excited. I have found this same in all I have tried; only some will throw the article down as if horror-struck.

Power of Hearing Faint Sounds

The movement of the jaws also, and various other movements in imitation of the operator, I have ascertained arise from their remarkable power of hearing *extremely faint sounds,* and the most curious point is this, that they seem to have the power of discerning such *faint sounds,* when they seem not to be affected by *very loud* sounds. It is also the same with feeling. They will in some states be insensible to pricking, pinching, or maiming, but so highly sensible to a breath of air, or the tickling of a feather, that they may be instantly roused by the latter means, when the former would have no such influence. Probably this is the cause of the remarkable effects of a current of air, its rousing cutaneous sensibility, directing the nervous influences to the skin, and withdrawing it from rigid muscles, thus reducing the cataleptiform state, and permitting the blood and *vis nervosa* to flow in their usual manner. The latter change being induced gradually, may probably be the cause of the feeling which is described as that of needles and pins running into the extremities, and producing a twitching, when gently pressing on the extremity with the finger, *etc.* as already noticed.

Additional Cases

In concluding this chapter, I am well aware the statements it contains must appear startling, and almost beyond belief, to many of my readers. Some may be disposed to think I have been deceived; and because many of the manifestations *might* be simulated, I know it has been alleged, that the patients of those who have been exhibited publicly, were either deceiving the operator, or that both patients and operators were engaged in a shameful system of collusion. In respect to my own patients, I have endeavoured to take every possible precaution that they should *not* deceive me, and with this view **have invited the most sceptical persons I know, both in the profession and out of it, to have it *rigorously* tested**, and the result has been my entire conviction as to the reality of the phenomena in my *own* patients, and I am ready to believe others to be as candid as myself. Because much *might* be simulated, and parties have been avowedly trained and exhibited to prove the dexterity of teachers and pupils in a system of avowed collusion, that it might thereby be inferred the patients exhibited by other lecturers were impostors, is a most illogical mode of deciding such a question; there ought to be positive proof of the justice of such imputation, before so assailing anyone, when there is so much proof to the contrary, as has been furnished by the concurrent testimony of so many experimenters who have met with such susceptible subjects. Surely it would not be fair to infer, that because some are trained as dexterous thieves, there can, therefore, be no such thing as an honest man in the world?

Opposite Faculties can be Excited at the Same Time by Acting on the Opposite Hemispheres

The question to be decided here is not what patients can be trained to do in violation to nature's laws; that is, by giving them some stronger motive of action, by artificial means, than the impulse arising from natural feeling. What might be achieved in this way I know not, as I have not tried such experiments connected with this branch of the subject. It is well-known, however, that so long ago as December, 1841, I particularly pointed out the remarkable docility of patients during Hypnotism, which made them most anxious to comply with every proper request or supposed wish of others. I have, therefore, no more doubt that they might be trained to manifest, during Hypnotism, opposite tendencies, in accordance with conventional arrangements, than that during their waking moments they could be taught to do so, and **thus call black white and white black, night day and day night, and such like, in respect to every custom, word, or action.** The proper question to be determined seems to me to be this:– Can the passions, and emotions, and intellectual faculties, be excited during Hypnotism simply by contact or friction over certain sympathetic points of the head and face, without previous knowledge of phrenology, training, or whispering, or such leading questions as must naturally excite in the mind such passions, emotions, or mental and bodily manifestations? My own experience warrants me to answer in the affirmative, and I shall give a few additional cases in illustration of the data from which I have come to this conclusion.

Two patients, healthy, strong servant girls, entirely ignorant of phrenology, neither of whom has ever seen an experiment, and one was so sceptical, as to wish to try and convince me *she could not be hypnotised at all,* were operated on separately. At first trial, I succeeded in hypnotising both, and in developing a great number of the leading organs, such as the desire to eat, benevolence, friendship, pity, attachment, self-esteem, love of approbation, imitation, (when they readily spoke five languages correctly,) stealing under acquisitiveness, and under conscientiousness restoring to the proper person and place what was stolen; eventuality most remarkable: this was tried twice or thrice in each, when they could tell correctly the events of the previous day while the organ was excited, whereas they could not tell a single circumstance before it was stimulated; and a number of others, such as forms, figures, and colours, by exciting the corresponding points. These experiments were tried before several friends, who were astonished with the result, several of the most remarkable manifestations being evinced without a single word being spoken by anyone. They were not tried at the same time, and neither saw nor knew of the other.

Mr. T., a gentleman of forty-five years of age, who was ignorant of phrenology, and had never seen a hypnotic experiment, was hypnotised without expecting any experiment of the kind to be tried. On touching "benevolence" the manifestation was so powerful as to compel me quickly to desist; "self-esteem", very decidedly; "ideality", very decidedly, combined with "tune and language", he sang when the latter were pressed on, but instantly stopped when the pressure was removed, and resumed as readily on renewing the contact, exactly at the same note and word where he left off. Also, the usual spectra when the region of the orbit was pressed on. When aroused, he was quite unconscious of all which had happened. He has been tried three times, with the same results, only that additional manifestations came out. His friends, who were present, can testify he had no signal given to lead him to do so. His wife, also, who had never seen anything of the kind before, was operated on, when a great many manifestations came out most decidedly. Their daughter, who had seen nothing of this, was now called into the room, and operated on, and exhibited a great many manifestations, and all this by the mere effect of pressure and gentle friction on the integuments. None of the three remembered any of what had happened. W.T., a boy, had been magnetized, and exhibited a few manifestations. He was again tried in public, but without success. I was requested to try him, when a number of manifestations came out at once beautifully – under benevolence, he took off his coat to give to some distressed person, and after a number of other manifestations had been educed, on being awakened he seemed very much surprised to find his coat off.

John W., twenty-two years of age, had been magnetized publicly, with the hope of eliciting the phrenological manifestations, but he became so stolid that it was quite a failure. I was afterwards requested to try him, in my way, in the presence of a number of gentlemen, when I at once succeeded in exciting several; pity was so characteristic, that there could be no difficulty or doubt upon the subject, as it was not only exhibited by his features and sobbing, but by the tears which ran over his face in torrents. On trying to excite imitation, on the right side, no effect was produced, which I suspected to be the result of an injury he had sustained, which had destroyed the integuments, and also caused exfoliation of the outer table of the skull. I therefore tried in the opposite side of the cranium, when the faculty was manifested beautifully. This seems a good corroboration of my theory, that it arises from the peculiar condition of the nerves of the scalp. On farther trials many more came out without any cause beyond simple excitation of the integuments by pressure and friction. Not only may such general manifestations be thus excited, but, what is far more curious, by exciting *antagonist* points in the *opposite hemispheres* of the brain, the patients may be made to exhibit correspondingly opposite feelings in the different sides of the body. If the antagonist faculties are excited on the *same* side, there will be exhibited only the *stronger of the two*. These "opposite influences on the two sides", as Dr. Elliotson has well remarked, "are the most astonishing and beautiful experiments that all physiology affords"; and are also the most beautiful examples of the correctness of Mr. Mayo's fifteenth aphorism, at page 28 of his *Nervous System and its Functions*, where he says, "Each lateral half of a vertebral animal is separately vitalized. Or the preservation of consciousness in one half is independent of its preservation in the other." It is true that vivisections have proved this, but neither so beautifully or humanely as in the experiments I now refer to, and those already recorded at [chapter 4] of this treatise. Miss S., a lady who had never seen a phrenohypnotic experiment, and knew nothing of phrenology, exhibited at first trial a great number of the leading manifestations, and at a second and third, these opposite ones in a remarkable manner. Under friendship and adhesiveness, she embraced a female friend in the most affectionate manner, and on destructiveness being excited *on the opposite side of the head,* she rushed forward with great impetuosity to repel some imaginary adversary, whilst, with her other arm and hand, she contrived to shield her friend. Had I not laid hold of her, she would most certainly have rushed through the window. On being roused she was quite oblivious of all she had done. Mrs. C. another equally ignorant of the subject, displayed the same phenomena. The effect of music in exciting to ecstasy, elegance of movement, and graceful dancing, was most remarkable. Remembered nothing.

Miss ——, entirely ignorant of the subject, and had never seen an experiment of the kind, and expected only to be *attempted* to be hypnotised, but whilst she wished to be tried, she had expressed to the friend who introduced her, that she could not be made to sleep. [Braid seems to have made a long series of hypnotic experiments by stimulating different phrenological points in turn.] She exhibited veneration solemnly, with hope, glowing devotion, and with ideality and language, overwhelming ecstasy, expression her happiness and prospect of entering into heaven; "self-esteem", the most conceited prude; "firmness" most decided; "adhesiveness and friendship", and this on one side, and "combativeness and destructiveness" on the other at pleasure; "imitation" in perfection, speaking correctly every language tried, "benevolence" extremely marked, to the effusion of tears; "acquisitiveness, conscientiousness, eventuality, the desire to eat , to smell, spectra", etc., etc. She was quite unconscious of all that had happened, and the friend who brought her to me knows she had no prompting. She has been tried once since with the same results.

Some parties, who were excellent critics, after seeing the latter and two others operated on, and expressing their utter astonishment with the accurate and natural manner in which every passion and emotion was manifested, expressed a strong desire to see someone operated on for the first time. I offered to operate on any of three young ladies whom they had introduced to me that afternoon, and whom I had not known previously; indeed, one was a stranger in town, from the south of England, who knew nothing of hypnotism or phrenology, and had no faith in either, notwithstanding what she had just seen. She, Miss S., sat down an entire sceptic, but in a few minutes was not only most decidedly hypnotised, but also one of the most beautiful and decided examples which could possibly have been met with of the phrenological sway during hypnotism, simply by stimulating the nerves of the scalp and face. The moment "veneration" was touched, her features assumed the peculiar expression of that feeling, the hands were clasped, she sank on her knees in the attitude of the most devout adoration; combined with "hope", the features were illuminated, and beamed with a feeling of ecstasy, the hands being unclasped and moved about in the utmost delight; and when "ideality" was added, the ecstasy was so extreme as scarcely to be supportable. On changing the point of contact to "firmness", she instantly arose, and stood with an attitude of defiance; "self-esteem", flounced about with the utmost self-importance; the "love of approbation" was painted to the greatest perfection; "irritation" imitated accurately everything done or spoken in any language; "friendship and adhesiveness", clasped hold of me; and by stimulating "combativeness" on the opposite side of the head, along with the other, she struck out with the arm of the side on which combativeness had been touched, but held me fast, as if to protect me, with the other. Under "benevolence", she seemed much affected, and distributed her property to the imaginary distressed objects her fancy had painted; under "acquisitiveness" she stole, and under "conscientiousness" she restored; "tune", the desire for music, and sang beautifully, a waltz being played, she danced with a grace and elegance surpassing all which any of us ever witnessed. Eventuality was also most remarkable; the desire to eat, to smell, was also excited; also form, figures, colours, etc., philoprogenitiveness admirable. All this was done at first trial, with an entire stranger, and the lady's immediate friends, as well as others present, can bear testimony that there was not the slightest prompting either by one or other, and when awakened she was quite unconscious of all which had happened. This lady has been twice operated on since, when all these manifestations, and many others, were exhibited in the most perfect manner, as can be certified by Sir Thomas Arbuthnot [a distinguished military general], Major Wilbraham, Colonel Wemyss, the Rev. Mr. P., and another high dignitary of the church, and the patient's family and friends; and that when under "number" she wrote down a sum, and under "constructiveness and ideality", she drew a very good sketch of a cottage, putting in doors and windows correctly. The uncle of the latter subject was so much astonished and gratified with what he had seen, that he begged I would try one of his daughters. I hypnotised the eldest, and all the manifestations came out quite as decidedly as in her cousin. Under "adhesiveness and friendship", she clasped me, and on stimulating the organ of "combativeness" on the opposite side of the head, with the arm of that side she struck two gentlemen (whom she imagined were about to attack me), in such a manner as nearly laid one on the floor, whilst with the other arm she held me in the most friendly manner. Under "benevolence", she seemed quite overwhelmed with compassion; "acquisitiveness", stole greedily all she could lay her hands on, which was retained, whilst I excited many other manifestations, but the moment my fingers touched "conscientiousness", she threw all she had stolen on the floor, as if horror-stricken, and burst into a flood of tears; on being asked, "Why do you cry?", she said, with the utmost agony, "I have done what was wrong, I have done what was wrong." I now excited "imitation and ideality", and had her laughing and dancing in an instant. On exciting form and ideality, she seemed alarmed, and when asked what she saw, she answered, "The [Devil]." "What colour is he?" "Black." On pressing the eyebrow, and repeating the question, the answer was, "red," and the whole body instantly became rigid, and the face the most complete picture of horror which could be imagined. "Destructiveness", which is largely developed, being touched, she struck her father such a blow on the chest as nearly laid him on the floor; had I not endeavoured to restrain her, he must have sustained serious injury, Having now excited veneration, hope, ideality, and language, we had the most striking example imaginable of extreme ecstasy, and on being aroused, she was quite unconscious of all that had happened, excepting that she had heard music, and had been dancing. Her philoprogenitiveness was admirable.[131]

At a conversazione a few days after, in the presence of Lady S., Sir Thomas Arbuthnot, Colonel Arbuthnot, Major Wilbraham, John Frederick Foster, Esq., Chairman of the Quarter Sessions, D. Maude, Esq., stipendiary magistrate, and many others, both gentlemen and ladies, after exhibiting the phenomena on those who had been previously tested, there was a wish expressed to see someone operated on *for the first time.* I offered to try anyone present, and a lady at length consented, whom I never saw before that day, nor since. She exhibited all the usual phenomena very decidedly. Under "acquisitiveness", she stole two handkerchiefs from ladies, and a ring from Mr. Foster's finger. After several manifestations had been exhibited, the moment I touched "conscientiousness", she seemed distressed, and set off and searched out the proper parties to whom to restore the respective articles. They had changed places, but she found them out, and gave back the handkerchiefs to their owners, and also put the ring on the very finger of Mr. Foster from which she had taken it. She was a strict Methodist, who had never danced in her life, and who, if awake, would have considered it a sin to dance.[132] However, under the excitement of suitable music, she cut a very good figure at waltzing. When awakened, she remembered nothing of all which had happened.

Miss L., a lady of twenty-one years of age, very accomplished, and with great energy of mind, braved me to try to hypnotise her. She felt assured I could not do so. However, she was very soon under the influence, and gave twenty manifestations in the most decided manner. Under friendship and adhesiveness, and destructiveness on the opposite side, she protected me, and struck her own mother. She knew only one organ, and was inclined to scoff at hypnotism and still more so at phreno-hypnotism. Under form and ideality she wrote very nicely, without the use of her eyes, but by no means equal to what she does when awake. When awakened she seemed surprised when told what had happened. She remembered me touching her head, wondered what I was doing it for, said she felt different impulses arise when I was manipulating different parts, but did not know why, nor could she remember what she had done.

A married lady, Mrs. E., and the mother of a family, would not believe anyone could be so affected. After seeing one patient done, she still felt assured *she*, at least, could not be so operated on. I desired her to try, and she at once exhibited upwards of twenty manifestations in the most distinct manner, some of them very strikingly. Under benevolence she shed tears, drew out her purse, and gave half-a-crown "to the poor creatures". She also exhibited the opposite tendencies at the same time, as already described.

Miss R., a young lady of twenty-two years of age, very well educated, and intelligent, wished to be tried, because she was decidedly sceptical. It so happened that every manifestation tried came out beautifully and prominently, although, when aroused, she admitted she remembered everything she had done, and added, that she had resisted to the utmost of her power doing anything, but felt irresistible impulses come over her to act in the way she did, as I touched certain points, but why it was she could not tell. She declared it was not from any association with what ought to be the case, as she was ignorant of the organs, but added, that **she first felt a drawing in the muscles of the face, and then the breathing became affected, and with this the peculiar impulse followed.** On another occasion, with the eyes bandaged, she had a pencil put in her right hand, when a number of organs were excited, but she showed no evidence of any desire to use the pencil till "constructiveness and ideality" were excited. The moment this was done, however, she scrambled till she got some paper, and began drawing, and made a very tolerable profile. When "acquisitiveness" was excited, she stole a ring off Mr. Foster's finger, who, while I was exciting various manifestations, left the room. The moment I touched "conscientiousness", she set off in search of Mr. Foster, walked round the room the very way he went, then left that room, crossed the lobby into the front parlour, and having made a gyration in this room she came out and went into a back parlour, where she found Mr. Foster, and put the ring on the very finger from whence she took it. She evidently traced him through the air by smell, as she followed the exact track he had taken, for he had first gone into the front parlour. Had it been by clairvoyance, she of course ought to have gone to him direct, and by the shortest way. Such facts are almost past belief, but here they are as they happened, and there could not have been more competent individuals, than those present, to detect any mistake or deception, namely, Mr. Foster, Mr. Brandt, and Mr. Lloyd, barristers; Mr. Langton, Mr. Bagshaw, Mr. Schwabe, and many others, both gentlemen and ladies.

---

[131] There were a dozen present on this occasion, of whom Mr. [John M.] Vandenhoff [a successful English actor] was one. Being well-known as an accomplished artist, I requested him to watch all he saw with the most critical attention, and to tell me whether the passions were painted naturally or the contrary. After witnessing the first case with evident delight and surprise, he made the following observation:– "If this is acting, it is the most perfect acting I have ever seen. In acting, we aim at being natural, but there is generally some point in which we fail; but here I see nature's language in every point." Similar expressions followed, in what was seen in the next two cases, and when he witnessed the effects on the two ladies, whose cases have just been recorded, he confessed himself so overpowered, as to be scarcely capable of expressing his feelings of delight and astonishment, but said he should write me on the subject. The following is part of a letter I received from him two days after – "I thank you for your kind invitation to witness a repetition of those experiments which so much delighted me on Saturday last, and with the result of which I was no less gratified than astonished. Never have I seen nature manifesting herself more distinctly – never so beautifully, as in the course of the exhibition on that evening. I believe you know I was a decided sceptic in the Mesmeric influence – and I was something more in relation to its phrenological sway – of which the manifestations while under its mysterious influence, by the two young ladies of my own immediate acquaintance, who had not, who could not have had, any knowledge of the subject prior to their experience on that evening, have perfectly convinced me by their truthfulness. I may take a farther opportunity to dilate more fully upon this interesting and wonderful discovery, the beneficial results of which cannot yet be appreciated, because we know not to what extent they may be carried out."

[132] [Note: this appears to contradict Braid's claim that hypnotic subjects cannot be made to act immorally.]

Miss W., a very intelligent lady, who knew nothing of phrenology, and had never seen a phreno-hypnotic experiment, was operated on. On "benevolence" being excited, she seemed very distressed, and when asked what she was thinking of, said it was of a poor man who had lost his saw and hammer, that he had no money to purchase others with, and his children were starving. Under "veneration and ideality", wished to die, to go to heaven; under combativeness, first looked very angry, then jumped up and gave a blow, which upset the candlestick. On "destructiveness" being excited, (after she had exhibited several other organs,) she shook her fist, then started on her feet, looked furious, and sprang across the room, her arm at full length, similar to a person fencing, and seized hold of a young lady's hand, and nearly transfixed it with her nails.

Mr. Walker, twenty-two years of age, after passing into the hypnotic state, showed no symptoms of susceptibility for some time, but at length he did so in the most perfect manner; namely, benevolence, veneration, firmness, self-esteem, combativeness, destructiveness, acquisitiveness, caution, conscientiousness, imitation in perfection, pity, benevolence with the one side, and destructiveness on the other, eventuality, smell, form, colours, number, ideality, *etc.* This gentleman has seen busts and phreno-hypnotic experiments also, but, excepting two or three, would be puzzled to point out any of the organs correctly when awake. He remembered nothing of what had passed.

Being desirous of ascertaining whether he might not, during hypnotism, remember the organs better than whilst awake, and thus be led to give the manifestations in the manner he did, I tried the following experiment. I explained my intentions to the friends who were to be present, but he was entirely ignorant of them. He had never seen or heard of such experiment having been tried. When I considered him in the proper condition, I requested him to place the point of a finger on different organs, but it was remarkable that he was wrong in every instance, even with respect to the few he knew when awake. Another most interesting fact was discovered, that whilst his mind was directed to the organ I had named, the *true* manifestation of *the point touched* came out *in every instance.* Thus, when requested to point out ideality, he placed the finger over "veneration", and immediately indicated that feeling. When asked what he was thinking about? "I did not go to church yesterday." "What of that?" "It was wrong." When he accidentally pressed on benevolence, the feeling was manifested; firmness in like manner; self-esteem in a powerful degree. On evincing symptoms of uneasiness, I asked what he was thinking of? He replied, "Something hurts my head." The fact was, his arm had become cataleptiform and the points of the fingers were pressed so strongly against the scalp as to be the cause of complaint, but he had no idea of that. His hand having rested on philoprogenitiveness, he began to hush and rock on his chair as if nursing a baby, his motion became more and more violent till I judged it necessary to put a stop to it, by removing his hand. However, I found his arm and neck had both become so rigid, that they were too firmly fixed to permit of being separated by mechanical force, but so soon as this was reduced, by blowing on them, the peculiar manifestation ceased. Every point pressed on by him showed the same tendency to excite its peculiar manifestation. I am quite certain this gentleman acted a candid part, and could not be induced to do otherwise by anyone. Another most interesting fact connected with the latter case, was the circumstance of his having hypnotised himself, excited the different manifestations as stated; and on being requested to rub his eyes, he did so, and thus roused himself from the hypnotic condition. I have tried similar experiments with many other patients, and, with the exception of two, each of whom hit upon one organ, have found none of them could point accurately to the organ named, but in every instance the usual indication of the peculiar organ touched came out. None of these subjects remembered anything of what had happened. Here, then, we have decided proof, that all the phenomena of hypnotising, exciting the phrenological manifestations, and rousing to the waking condition may be accomplished by the personal acts of the patient on himself, as the only influence required to excite him to the necessary movement might be conveyed by an automaton.

A few days ago, one of these patients, who knows no foreign language, when imitation and tune were excited, followed correctly both the music and words of Italian, French, and German songs, which she never heard till they were played and sung by the wife of a learned barrister, who was also present himself, and who, with the Rev. Mr. F. and his lady, can bear testimony to the great accuracy of her performance. Such is the power of Hypnotism.

Besides the **twenty-five cases** here briefly recorded, I have had many more exhibiting the phenomena in the same decided manner, simply by exciting the sympathetic points by contact. **If I am to believe the evidence of my senses, therefore,** *in anything,* **I cannot see how I can doubt the relation which subsists between certain points of the cranium, and the mental manifestations, which are excited by acting on them during Hypnotism. I believe there are very few physiological phenomena which can be more clearly demonstrated, especially at such an early stage of their investigation.** Were it not that I consider it would only be an unnecessary waste of time to prosecute the investigation farther, after the number of most unequivocal cases which have been met with by myself, as well as by other experimentalists here and elsewhere, I feel convinced I might soon increase the number of my own cases to any extent I chose.

With all intelligent and honest experimentalists I anticipate similar results to what happened with Mr. Ebbage, an intelligent surgeon at Leamington. He had been a determined sceptic, and had much annoyed several of our mutual friends by his strong expressions to that effect. However, whilst on a visit at

Manchester lately, at our first interview, I made a convert of him by offering to exhibit the phenomena in his own wife, who had never been so operated on, or even tried the experiment. She soon became decidedly hypnotised, and also exhibited several phrenological manifestations most distinctly. A servant of the family was now called into the room, who had seen no operation of the kind, and did not know what was to be done. She also became decidedly hypnotised, and exhibited several phrenological manifestations most distinctly. Mr. E. now admitted that rational scepticism could not resist such conclusive evidence; and having seen another case or two at my house, of remarkably susceptible subjects, with instructions from me how to operate, be promised to prosecute the inquiry on his return home.

In a letter to me, dated 1st May, 1843, he writes that he had tried the experiments with several; that in some he was unsuccessful, while "in others a perfect state of sleep and unconsciousness was produced at different periods, varying from two to ten minutes. In the case of one lady, who had never seen any thing of the kind before, and, I may add, had not even heard it spoken of as connected with any phrenological developments, the most marked effects were soon produced, resembling very strongly the case you showed me when I was at your house." He farther adds the following judicious remarks:– "I must say the peculiar development shown by the influence of this sleep, if closely and scrutinizingly watched, must open to the mind of any thinking man a wide expanse for speculation as to the truly mysterious means by which the effects of sensation and emotion can be produced."

The above is a good illustration of what may be done, even by a determined but honest sceptic. Mr. E. had only two interviews with me; and if anyone should be less successful in his attempts, it behoves him to inquire, whether his failures are not to be attributed to his unskilful or uncandid performance of the experiments, rather than to inefficiency of the method recommended.

As to those who will not believe the testimony of others without seeing the experiments tried before themselves, on fresh patients, I beg to remark, that the best plan is for them to try patients *fairly* themselves, and they must soon be convinced; only they must be careful to take them at *the proper time,* otherwise they may fail as I did myself at first.

Mode of Operating

The following is the mode of operating:– Put the patient into the hypnotic condition in the usual way, extend his arms for a minute or two, then replace them gently on his lap, and allow him to remain perfectly quiet for a few minutes. Let the points of one or two fingers be now placed on the central point of any of his best developed [phrenological] organs, and press it very gently; if no change of countenance or bodily movement is evinced, use gentle friction, and then in a soft voice ask what he is thinking of, what he would like, or wish to do, or what he sees, as the function of the organ may indicate; and repeat the questions and the pressure, or contact, or friction, over the organ till an answer is elicited. If very stolid, gentle pressure on the eyeballs may be necessary to induce him to speak. If the skin is too sensitive, he may awake, in which case try again, *waiting a little longer* if too stolid, try again beginning the manipulations *sooner*

The operations should be tried again and again with the same patient, varying the time of beginning the manipulations, as it is impossible to tell, *a priori,* the exact moment they should be commenced; and many of the best cases have only succeeded partially, or not at all, at a first or second trial. When this point has been hit upon, however, there will be little difficulty in getting out additional manifestations, and this will be still more evident at each succeeding trial.

Whispering or talking should be carefully avoided by all present, so as to leave nature to manifest herself in her own way, influenced only by the stimulus conveyed through the nerves of touch exciting to automatic muscular action. We all know that during common sleep a person unconsciously changes from an uncomfortable position to one which is agreeable. This is a sort of instinctive action, and, as already explained, **I think it highly probable, that by thus calling into action muscles which are naturally so exerted in manifesting any given emotion or propensity, they may, by reflection, thereby rouse that portion of the brain, the activity of which usually excites the motion. In this case there would be a sort of inversion of the ordinary sequence, what is naturally the consequence becoming the cause of cerebral and mental excitation.** The following hypothesis will illustrate my meaning. **It is easy to imagine, that putting a pen or pencil into the hand might excite in the mind the idea of writing or drawing or that stimulating the *gastrocnemius* [calf muscle], which raises us on our toes, might naturally enough suggest to the mind the idea of dancing, without any other suggestion to that effect than what arises from the attitude and activity of the muscles naturally and necessarily brought into play whilst exercising such functions. However, I would very much doubt the probability of stimulating the muscles of the leg exciting the idea of writing, or that placing a pen or pencil in the hand would excite the idea of dancing, without previous concert and arrangement to that effect. It is upon the same principle, as I imagine, that, during the dreamy state of hypnotism by stimulating the *sterno-mastoid* muscle, which causes an inclination of the head, the idea of friendship and shaking of hands is excited in the mind, and when the *trapezius* is excited at the same time, the greater lateral inclination of the head manifests still greater attachment, or "adhesiveness". Philoprogenitiveness, by calling into action the *recti* and *occipito frontalis* muscles, gives the rocking motion, and hence** the idea of nursing, *etc*.; pressure on the vertex, by calling into action all the muscles requisite to sustain the body in the erect position, excites the idea of unyielding firmness; veneration and benevolence, from giving the tendency to stoop and suppress the breathing, thus create the corresponding feelings. By exciting the muscles of mastication into action, the idea of eating and drinking is roused, and the same may arise from pressing between the chin and under lip, which excites a flow of saliva, and this again the motion of the tongue and jaws, with an inclination to swallow. In like manner, gently pressing the tip of the nose, by exciting inspiration, creates the desire for something to smell at; if the point of contact is the cheek, under the orbits, over the exit of the infra-orbital branch of the fifth pair, the breathing becomes suppressed, and depressing emotions are excited; whereas, *above* the orbit, so as to stimulate the supra-orbital branch of the fifth pair, generally the reverse manifestations are evinced.

Those familiar with Professor Weber's experiments, know that each of those points differs from the other in its degree of sensibility. **It is remarkable that the point marked "eventuality", (and which I have strong grounds for believing is the chief seat of memory,) is in the centre of the forehead, which is one of the most sensitive parts of the scalp, and where pressure applied necessarily excites the corresponding points in *both* hemispheres of the brain at the same time.**

There seems, in fact, to be less matter of wonder in this discovery than some lately brought forward in other departments of physical science; for example, who would have believed, till it was proved, that by looking into a camera-obscura for a few minutes, or even seconds, he might have his likeness accurately and indelibly transferred to a plate of metal, or the still more recent discovery of Professor Moser, that such impressions as he referred to could be effected in the dark?

Concluding Remarks on the Value of Testimony

I shall conclude this article by a quotation, from Dr. Abercrombie, on the value of testimony. He observes:–

> A very small portion of our knowledge of external things is obtained through our own senses; by far the greater part is procured through other men, and this is received by us on the evidence of testimony. While an unbounded credulity is the part of a weak mind, which never thinks nor reasons at all, an unlimited scepticism is the part of a *contracted* mind, which reasons upon imperfect data, or makes its own knowledge and extent of observation the standard and test of probability. *On the Intellectual Powers,* pp. 71, 72.

Chapter 7:
Summary & Conclusion

General Résumé

Before concluding the first part of this treatise, I shall make a short *résumé* of what I consider the points made out by what has been advanced.

1. [Eye-fixation] That the effect of a continued fixation of the mental and visual eye in the manner, and with the concomitant circumstances pointed out, is to throw the nervous system into a new condition, accompanied with a state of somnolence, and a tendency, according to the mode of management, of exciting a variety of phenomena, very different from those we obtain either in ordinary sleep, or during the waking condition.
2. [Hypnotic Stages] That there is at first a state of high excitement of all the organs of special sense, sight excepted, and a great increase of muscular power; and that the senses afterwards become torpid in a much greater degree than what occurs in natural sleep.
3. [Nervous Excitation & Depression] That in this condition we have the power of directing or concentrating nervous energy, raising or depressing it in a remarkable degree, at will, locally or generally.
4. [Heart Rate] That in this state, we have the power of exciting or depressing the force and frequency of the heart's action, and the state of the circulation, locally or generally, in a surprising degree.
5. [Muscular Tone] That whilst in this peculiar condition, we have the power of regulating and controlling muscular tone and energy in a remarkable manner and degree.
6. [General Physiological Effects] That we also thus acquire a power of producing rapid and important changes in the state of the capillary circulation, and of the whole of the secretions and excretions of the body, as proved by the application of chemical tests.
7. [Therapeutic Use] That this power can be beneficially directed to the cure of a variety of diseases which were most intractable, or altogether incurable, by ordinary treatment.
8. [Pain Control] That this agency may be rendered available in moderating or entirely preventing, the pain incident to patients whilst undergoing surgical operations.
9. [Muscular Suggestion] That during hypnotism, by manipulating the cranium and face, we can excite certain mental and bodily manifestations, according to the parts touched.

Many Phenomena Admit of Physical and Chemical Proof

I have obtained analogous results with so many patients, as to make me quite certain of the *reality of the phenomena* referred to, and to warrant me, as I think, to draw these inferences. **Many of the phenomena are of such a nature as to admit of physical and chemical proof**, in respect to which, the patients cannot possibly deceive us; and as regards those phenomena where they *might do* so, I have had the assurance of so many patients, on whose veracity I can implicitly rely, proving the same facts, that there remains not the slightest room for *me* to doubt the correctness of these statements. I have been equally anxious to avoid being myself misled, as I should be not to mislead others; and I would recommend those who have not had an opportunity of watching such phenomena, *in the most critical manner,* or who have not entered on the investigation with candid minds, to suspend their opinions until they have had such opportunity.

Difficulties of Comprehending Many Phenomena

I have no hesitation in saying it is most improbable that any man should form a just estimate in this matter from *mere reading* or *hearsay evidence,* and equally so if he does not approach it with a mind open to honest and fair investigation. The subject itself is so very subtle in its manifestations, so very different from all we are accustomed to meet with in the ordinary condition, that, with the utmost candour and openness for receiving the truth, and the whole truth, it will be found extremely perplexing to follow it out in many of its bearings. How then can it be expected anyone should prosecute the inquiry successfully who enters on it with his mind blinded by indomitable prejudice?[133]

State of the Circulation

As to the proximate cause of the phenomena, I believe the best plan in the present state of our knowledge, is to go on accumulating facts, and their application in the cure of disease, and to theorize at some future period, when we have more ample stores of facts to draw inferences from. **From the first I was of opinion, that much of the excitement and many of the phenomena developed, were attributable to the altered state of the circulation in the brain and spinal cord, and especially to the greater determination of blood to them, and all other parts not compressed by rigid muscles, arising from the difficulty, during the cataleptiform state, of the blood being propelled in due proportion through the rigid**

---

[133] [See appendix (originally a lengthy footnote) 'Debate on Mesmeric Anaesthesia'.]

extremities. I have not yet seen occasion to alter this opinion; but rather to conclude, that the ganglionic, or organic system of nerves, is *also* inordinately stimulated from the same cause, and thus having acquired an undue preponderance induces many of the remarkable phenomena which have been referred to. Whoever examines carefully the injected state of the conjunctival membrane, and of the capillary circulation in the head, face, and neck, the distended state of the jugular veins, the hard bounding throb of the carotid arteries, and the greatly increased frequency of the pulse, during the rigid condition of the limbs, cannot fail to perceive that there is great determination to the head.

Conjectures as to the Cause of the Cataleptiform Condition

Again, when all these symptoms are so speedily changed on reducing the cataleptiform condition of the limbs, how can it be doubted that the rigidity of the limbs, and consequent obstruction to free circulation through them, is the chief cause of the determination to the head and other parts not directly pressed on by rigid muscles?[134]

In conclusion, I beg leave to remark, that the varieties which are met with as regards susceptibility to the hypnotic impression, and the mode and degrees of its action, are only analogous to what we experience in respect to the effects of wine, spirits, opium, the nitrous oxide, and many other agents. They are all well-known to act differently on different individuals, and even on the same individuals at different times, according to the condition of the system; but who calls in question the reality of their effects merely because of that want of uniformity of action?

---

[134] [See appendix (originally a lengthy footnote) 'A Neurological Theory of Hypnotic Catalepsy'.]

PART II:
Sixty-Six Brief Case Studies

Modes of Operating
Having in the former part so far explained the mode of inducing the phenomena, I now proceed to detail the cases in which I have successfully applied this process in the cure of disease. I shall endeavour to explain my modes of operating in different affections, so as to enable others to apply with advantage in their practice, what I have found so eminently useful in my own.

Objects of Operations
When the artificial state of somnolence has been induced in the manner already pointed out, [at the start of Chapter 2], the manipulations must be varied according to the peculiar object we have in view. If the *force* of the circulation in a limb is wished to be diminished, and the *sensibility* also to be *reduced,* call the muscles of that member into activity, leaving the other extremities limber. On the other hand, if the force of the circulation and sensibility are wished to be *increased* in a limb, keep *it* limber, and call the *others* into activity, by elevating and extending them, and the desired result will follow. If *general depression* is wanted, after one or two limbs have been extended for a short time, cautiously reduce them, and leave the whole body limber and quiet. If *general excitement* of the system is wanted, extend the *whole* limbs, causing the patient to call the muscles into strong action, and very speedily they will become rigidly fixed, and the force and frequency of the heart's action, and determination to the brain, as evinced by the action of the carotids, distended jugulars, flushed face, and injected eyes, will speedily become apparent. By applying the ear over the region of the heart, it will be apparent that the force and frequency of the heart's action becomes prodigiously increased in a very short time after extending the limbs. It will also be found, they may be very speedily altered and brought down by reducing the rigidity of the limbs. The difference of rise in the pulse when extending the limbs *during hypnotism,* from what happens in the natural state, is one of the strongest proofs of the patient being in the hypnotic condition.

It has appeared to me, that we have thus the power of subjecting the brain and spinal cord, and whole ganglionic system, to a high state of excitement, as the pulse may speedily be raised to **double its natural velocity, in most cases** [c. 140-150 bpm], and still more speedily reduced to the natural standard again. Its volume and tension may also be equally rapidly increased or diminished. It is therefore naturally to be expected, that the functions must be greatly influenced by such transitions. **Every medical man knows that chronic nervous disorders of the most painful nature may have resisted every known remedy for weeks, or months, or years, but have speedily vanished on the accession of some acute attack.** Now, my views were, in such cases, to induce an intense state of excitement for a *short time,* to be terminated abruptly, with the hope of changing the former action, and thus terminating the disorder; and assuredly, in many instances the most obstinate chronic functional disorder is gone, or greatly meliorated, by a few such operations.

Then, again, by keeping any particular organ awake or active, whilst the others were asleep, I considered there would be a great increase of activity induced, by the whole nervous energy, or sensorial power, being directed to that point; or by keeping all the other organs active, whilst one which had been too active was allowed to remain, in the torpid state, that inordinate activity would be reduced in intensity, and that probably permanently – that the inordinate stimulus, in one case, would remove the susceptibility to lower impressions, which were frequently exciting, or habitually keeping up morbid feeling or action; and **in the other cases, that by suspending the morbid sensibility of a part for a time, and rousing antagonist functions, such condition might be permanently improved.**

Whether I have been right or wrong in my theoretical views, there can be no doubt of the fact that in many instances I have been successful in the application of Hypnotism as a curative agent; and the beneficial results of the operations have been so immediate and decided, as to leave no doubt that they stand in the relation of cause and effect. **However, that much of the success depends on the impression arising from the altered condition of circulation, seems to me to be proved by the fact, that in cases where the sleep was induced *without* the *rise* in the *force and frequency in the heart's action,* by insuring this condition, the beneficial result has instantly followed, where there has been no previous improvement with the *low* pulse.** The following is a remarkable instance of this:– Nodan, deaf mute, twenty-four years of age, was considered never to have heard sound excepting the report of a gun or thunder, when there was succussion [i.e., vibration] of the air sufficient to induce *feeling* rather than hearing, properly so called. The mother told me Mr. Vaughan, head master of the Deaf and Dumb Institution when Nodan was at school, considered any indication of hearing referred to was *feeling,* and not hearing, properly so called. At the first operation there was very little rise of pulse, and afterwards I could not discern he had any sense of hearing whatever. At next trial the pulse was excited, and so remarkable was the effect, that in going home he was so much annoyed with the noise of the carts and carriages, that he would not allow himself to be operated on again for some time. He has only been operated on a few times, and the result is, that although he lives in a back street, he can now hear a band of music coming along the *front* street, and will run out to meet it.

Cases of Sight Improved

I shall first illustrate the efficacy of hypnotism on the various senses, and also on the mental condition. And first, of sight. The mode of operating in chronic cases, is first to induce the sleep, then extend the extremities, and keep the eyes from getting into the torpid state, by fanning them, or passing a current of air over them occasionally. The length of time required to keep such patient in this condition may vary **from six to twelve minutes**, according to the state of the circulation. The following cases will illustrate the affections of the eyes in which I have applied this mode of treatment with advantage.

Case I. Mrs. Roiley applied to me on the 6th April, 1842. She stated she was fifty-four years of age; that for the last sixteen years she had been a great sufferer from an affection of the head, attended with pain in the eyes and weakness of sight; that it was now become so bad, that she could not continue to read for more than a few minutes at a time, even with the aid of glasses. She had undergone the most active treatment under first rate medical men, including bleeding general and local, blistering – on one occasion, she was twice bled with leeches, and had five blisters to her head in one month – and almost every variety of internal medicine which could be suggested for such a case; but still without improving her sight. For years she had required to have her head shaved every few weeks, and cold effusions and spirituous lotions frequently applied to it, to reduce the excessive heat and other uncomfortable feelings. The skin of the palms of the hands was so hard, dry, and irritable, as to render it liable to chap whenever she attempted to open the hands fully. The pain during the day, and general irritability, had rendered it necessary for her to take a composing pill three times in twenty-four hours, for some time; still her rest was so bad as to force her to rise and walk about the room several times during the night; and her memory had become so much impaired, that she often required to go up stairs and then down again several times before she could remember what she went up for. About three years before consulting me, she had a paralytic attack, which deprived her of power of the muscles of the right side of the face for a few days. That such had been the general state of her health before consulting me, and the state of her *sight*, and the result of my operation will be understood by the following document, which is attested by herself and others, who were present when I first operated on her:–

> Mrs. Roiley, (aged 54,) Chapel Street, Salford, formerly of South Windsor Street, Toxteth Park, Liverpool, as Miss Robinson, (four years ago,) has been gradually losing sight since thirty-eight years of age. Called on me for the first time, 6th April, 1842. Could not read the heading of the newspaper, excepting the words, 'Macclesfield Courier'; after being hypnotised for eight minutes, she could distinctly read 'and Herald', and in a few minutes more the whole of the smaller line, 'Congleton Gazette, Stockport Express, and Cheshire Advertiser', also the day, month, and date of the paper. That the above is a correct report, is attested by the patient herself and other three patients, who were present the whole time.
>
> (Signed)
> Alice Roiley.
> M.A. Stowe.
> Ann Stowe.
> Henry Gaggs.

When Mrs. Roiley called on me two days after, she gave me the following report. After leaving my house on the 6th, she was much gratified to find her sight so much improved, which induced her to go and test it by looking at articles displayed in shop windows, and in particular remarked that she had walked up to Mr. Agnew's shop window, and was able to see distinctly the features of a portrait of Sir Robert Peel, and to read under it, "Sir Robert Peel, Bart.", *without* her glasses, neither of which she could have done for long before. She also stated, that after being at home, she took up the small diamond *Polyglot Bible*, and with the aid of her glasses, was agreeably surprised to find she was enabled to read the 118th Psalm, (29 verses,) although this had been, as she expressed it, a sealed book to her for years. The following is the report which was recorded and attested by her on the 12th April, 1842:–

> Mrs. Roiley was able to read a Psalm with the aid of her glasses in the smallest sized Polyglot Bible same afternoon she was first hypnotised. Two days after, (8th April,) was hypnotised a second time. Next day, made a net handkerchief with the aid of her glasses. April 12, has gone on improving, and in my own presence and several others, with the aid of her glasses, read the Polyglot Bible with ease and correctness, which she said, had been a sealed book to her for years before I operated on her.
>
> (Signed)
> Alice Roiley.

M. A. Stowe.
Wm. Halliday.

It is gratifying to be able to add, that the improvement of the sight has been permanent; and not only so, but that the whole painful catalogue of complaints with which she had been afflicted speedily disappeared, namely, pain of the chest, head, and eyes, loss of memory, disturbed sleep, irregularity of the secreting and digestive functions, and instead of the arid skin, regular action of it, so that the palms of the hands, which were so harsh and arid that she could not extend them without lacerating the skin, causing great pain and annoyance, were very soon as soft as a piece of chamois leather.[135] The whole of this improvement was accomplished entirely by this agency, as she had no medicine whatever during her attendance on me; nor has she required any up to this date, 20th February, 1843, when I read this report to her, and when she remarked it was much *under* drawn; that with great truth I might have represented her as having been a greater sufferer.

Mrs. Roiley is a very intelligent person, and one whose Christian profession and principles place her statements above all suspicion. She has been seen by many eminent professional and scientific gentlemen, who can bear testimony that they have had from her own lips the same statements as I have recorded above.

It appears to me that it would be impossible to adduce a more striking proof than this case affords, of the great and undoubted benefit resulting from the application of any remedial measure. The improvement was so remarkable, as to admit of no doubt as to its reality, and so immediate after the hypnotising, as to prove they stood in the relation of cause and effect, no other remedy being in operation; and **whatever may be supposed capable of being achieved through the mere power of imagination, as regards *certain* functions, the sense of *sight* could scarcely be supposed capable of being so much meliorated directly through that influence.**

Case II. is that of Mrs. M. A. Stowe. This lady was present when I first operated on Mrs. Roiley, and was so much gratified by the effects she witnessed in that case, as to induce her to consult me as to the state of her own eyes, and the probability of benefiting them by a similar operation. Mrs. Stowe was forty-four years of age, and had experienced such weakness of sight as to require the aid of glasses for the last twenty-two years, to enable her to sew, read, or write, and, for some years past, she required them to enable her to transact her most ordinary household duties. The following is the statement of her condition, which I noted at the time, and is attested by her own signature, and that of others then present:—

Mrs. Stowe, aged 44, 1, Bank Place, Red Bank, Manchester, has been troubled with weakness of sight for twenty-two years, so as to require glasses to enable her to read or sew. When tested to-day, 8th April, 1842, without her glasses, could not distinguish the large (capital) letters of advertisements in a newspaper, nor large heading of the paper. After being hypnotised for eight minutes, she could distinctly read both the large and small heading, and day, month, and date of the paper.

(Signed)
M. A. Stowe.

She has also been able to sign her name to attest the accuracy of the above statement, before her daughter, and another patient.

(Signed)
Ann Stowe.

10th, Called on me, and informed me she had been able to make herself a blonde cap, and to thread her needle *without* spectacles[136], which she could not do before for twenty-two years. 12th, Continued improving; told one she had been able to write up her accounts *without* glasses.

(Signed)
M.A. Stowe.
Wm. Halliday.
Alice Roiley.
Ann Stowe.

This patient has retained the improvement of her sight. She has also informed me, that she was agreeably surprised, after she left my house, the *first day she was operated on,* to find, as she went along the streets, that she could read the *sign-boards,* which she could not do for years before. She has also named to many others, as well as myself, a very convincing proof of her great improvement in this respect. Before being

---

[135] Very lately, a lady about twenty-five years of age was hypnotised by me. On being roused, she expressed her surprise to find her hands bathed in perspiration, as she observed *she was never known to have the slightest moisture on her hands till that moment.*
[136] I have myself seen her thread a No. 8 needle on several occasions.

operated on by me, on the 8th April, 1842, if she went a-shopping, *without her glasses,* she was sure to make some mistake as to the quality of goods purchased, and have the trouble of going back to have them exchanged, but now she never requires to take her glasses with her, as can be testified by the shop-men where she makes her purchases. Her memory and general health have also been greatly improved by the same operations.

Case III. Miss Stowe, daughter of the former patient, twenty-two years of age, "was under the necessity of reading, and doing any particular work, with the aid of glasses, for the last two years, but has never required them since she was first hypnotised, and can now read the small *Polyglot Bible*". This is attested by her mother, herself, and Mr. William Halliday, and Mrs. Roiley.

The improvement has been permanent, and she has threaded a No. 12 needle in my presence, eight months after I first operated on her.

Case IV. Mr. J. A. Walker, twenty-two years of age, had always had very weak sight, but since being hypnotised has been greatly improved in his sight, as well as in his memory and general health.

Case V [a[137]]. Mrs. C., aged eighty-three, had, from her age, required the use of glasses for many years, to enable her to sew or read. Last August I hypnotised her for deafness, with very decided advantage, and I told her I also expected to improve her sight at the same time. She was very incredulous, but was agreeably surprised to find, that after a *second* operation she was not only able to *hear* much better, but also to sew some flannel, threading her needle *without* her glasses. She had been thus occupied for several hours, when I called to see her, after the second operation.

There have been cases in which I have tried this method without success, but this proves only that we must never expect to obtain possession of a universal remedy. Cases of confirmed amaurosis [blindness due to optic nerve damage], which had resisted every other known remedy, and which were only undertaken by me at the desire of the patients, and sometimes of medical men also, as a forlorn hope, have, as in most cases was suspected might be the result, proved unsuccessful, and, through these, attempts have been most ungenerously and unwarrantably made to throw discredit on the power of hypnotism altogether. It has proved successful in too many instances, however, to be borne down by such paltry and pitiful misrepresentation. I could easily adduce many more successful cases, did I deem it necessary, but shall only give two more.

Case V [b]. Mr. J— has always had imperfect vision, is near-sighted, has strabismus of right eye, and the sight so dull, that it was with great difficulty he could, without glasses, see the large letters (on white paper) in the title page of the *Medical Gazette*. After the first operation he could see better, and after it had been repeated a few times he could, without glasses, read a few words of the leading article of that work, and after a few more operations, could read the type in which the lectures, at the beginning of the work, are printed.

Case VI. Mrs. S., one of my own near relatives, had a severe rheumatic fever in January, 1839. During the course of this disease the left eye became implicated, involving both the internal and external structures of the organ. She had the benefit of the advice of one of the first-rate oculists in Edinburgh. She was under his care till the August following, when he considered farther attendance unnecessary, but gave such instructions as he deemed expedient for her future management of it, and which had been duly attended to till the period when I first saw her, in June, 1842. At that time she came on a visit to my house. The eye was free from pain, but was of no service as an organ of vision. There was an opacity over more than one half of the cornea, sufficient to prevent distinct perception of any object placed opposite the temporal half of the eye, all being seen through a dense haze; and objects placed towards the opposite side were seen very imperfectly, owing to the injury the choroid and retina had sustained in the points on which the images of such objects were reflected. The opacity of the cornea was not only an obstacle to distinct vision, but was also a source of annoyance, from its disfigurement, being obvious even to those at a considerable distance.

Notwithstanding the great advantage I had seen other patients, afflicted with affection of the eyes, derive from hypnotism, it never occurred to me that such a case as that of Mrs. S. was likely to be benefited by such an operation. I had, however, recommended it to her for a severe rheumatic affection of the right shoulder and arm. She had been in my house about three months before she could make up her mind to undergo the operation, but at length, the violence of the pain impelled her to try it, or anything else I should recommend. I of course hypnotised her, which immediately relieved her pain so much, that after the first operation, she could move the arm freely. The operation was repeated the following day, with complete relief as regarded the arm; and to the surprise and delight of the patient, myself, and others present, she found her *sight* so much improved as to be able to see everything in the room, and to name different flowers, and distinguish their colours, whilst the right eye was shut, which she had not been able to do for more than

---

[137] [Braid seems to have listed two different patients numbered "Case V" by mistake.]

three years and a half previously. I consequently now **repeated the operation daily**, and, in a very short time, had the satisfaction of seeing the cornea so transparent, that it requires close inspection to observe where tiny opacity remains. Neither external nor internal means were used during this improvement, nothing but the hypnotising was had recourse to; and during the three months I had an opportunity of watching it prior to these operations, there was no visible change in the condition of the organ. I should observe, that after the first operation, there was considerable smarting in the eye, which continued all night, and, in a less degree, after future operations, which, no doubt, roused the absorbents, and effected the removal of the opacity of the cornea. Stimulating the optic nerve to greater activity, however, must have been the chief cause of the very rapid improvement, which enabled her to see objects after the second operation. I should remark, that the sight, with regard to objects seen from the temporal side of the eye, is much more distinct than from the nasal side, owing to the retina and choroid having sustained irreparable damage during the inflammatory stage at the commencement of the attack in 1839.

Case VII. Mr. Holditch, thirty-nine years of age, had been partially paralytic for ten years, which came on some time after a fall. Shortly after the fall, he experienced an attack of double vision, which went off after bleeding, blistering, and the usual treatment, but was followed by paralysis of the lower limbs, which induced him to consult me on the 18th February, 1843. See Case XXVII [further on this section]. He was very much surprised, when I told him he had defective vision of the right eye, said he was not aware of it, *and would not believe that I was not mistaken, till I tested him,* when he found he could barely see the capitals of the words, "Medical Gazette", as heading of the leading article of that work, whilst he could read the ordinary size print of the page with the other eye. After being hypnotised, I tested him in the same position, and with the same degree of light, and he could then read the *same sized print with it,* and it has continued so ever since. He could also walk across the room without crutch or stick, which he could not do before, at which he was very much surprised, as he was quite conscious the whole time, and therefore could not believe any good could have resulted to him from what was done, till he had the positive evidence of it in being able to see and walk.

Here, then, we have seen three cases of improved vision consequent on hypnotising for other affections, and where, consequently, **the improvement could not at all be attributable to imagination, but to the altered condition in the capillary circulation and distribution of the *vis nervosa*.** In cases of active inflammation of the eyes, either external or internal, I have never tried hypnotism. By the mode calculated to excite the circulation, of course it would be quite inadmissible; and it could only be speculation for me to hazard an opinion as to its probable result by the other mode.

Hearing

The extraordinary excitement of the auditory organ, which I had observed in the course of my early experiments, and the fact that **hearing was the last sense to disappear during this artificial sleep**, (unless we except that of the sensibility to a current of air,) led me to anticipate most satisfactory results from this process in the treatment of deafness, arising from torpor of the auditory nerves. I consequently tried it in such cases, and where there has not been destruction, or irreparable organic injury to the auditory apparatus, I can confidently say, I know of no means equal to hypnotism, for benefiting such cases. Of course, it cannot suit *all* cases, but I am satisfied it will succeed in a numerous class of cases, and in some which bid defiance to all other known modes of treatment.

I am enabled to state this confidently, not only from my own personal success, but also from that of others who have fairly tried it. One professional friend, Mr. Gardom, introduced to me two patients whom he had improved so much by hypnotism only, that they were enabled to hear the sermons of their respective pastors, which they could not do before, in consequence of which one of them had to leave her favourite minister, and go to another church; but, after being hypnotised, has been able to hear so much better, that she has been thus induced to return to her *former* pastor.

Deaf and Dumb

The great success which I had experienced from hypnotism, in improving those who were deaf through disease, led me to hope it might be of service to some of those who were born deaf and dumb, and I therefore tried it in such cases with a considerable degree of success, ultimately with a success beyond my most sanguine expectations. **In consequence of what had been done and exhibited at my lectures, the medical profession of Liverpool, to their credit be it recorded, recommended to the governors of the Deaf and Dumb Institution there, to permit an experimental trial to be made at their Institution.** The governors refused their assent to this *within the walls of the Institution,* but agreed to permit a trial to be made with such out-door pupils as could be induced to submit to it elsewhere, the consent of the parents having been obtained. In consequence of this, a committee of the governors and the medical faculty was appointed to superintend the said investigation, and I was invited to go over and conduct the experiments in their presence, and it was proposed a report of the results should be published in the medical journals, at the termination of our labours. The difficulty of getting the pupils and their parents to attend, induced us to abandon the proceedings after two trials had been made, so that it would be quite inconsistent with the conditions stipulated, at the commencement of said investigation, to publish any report of the result of this *partial* investigation. However, I think I cannot better illustrate the extent of my expectations, in reference to such cases, than by transcribing an extract from my address to the said committee, prior to commencing our experimental trial.

> Hitherto, these patients have been considered beyond the pale of human aid, so decidedly have they resisted all means tried for their relief; and the morbid condition of the organs, as ascertained by dissection, was sufficient to warrant the inference that it was *improbable* any remedy could ever be discovered for such cases. Fully aware of this pathological difficulty, I was nevertheless inclined to try the effect of neuro-hypnotism with congenital deaf mutes, knowing it could be done with perfect safety, and without pain or inconvenience to the patients. Moreover, from having witnessed its extraordinary power of rousing the excitability of the auditory nerves, I entertained the hope that it might thus be capable of exciting *some* degree of hearing, from the increased sensibility of the nerves compensating for the imperfection of the organ. I was not, and am not even now, so visionary, as to expect *perfection of function,* when there is great imperfection of the organ. Perfection of organization and function must be co-existent; at least the function cannot be *perfectly* performed when the organization is *much* impaired. The result of my first trial was beyond my most sanguine expectations, which induced me to persevere, and the result has been, that I have scarcely met with a case of congenital deaf mute, where I have not succeeded in making the patient hear in some degree. Many may never hear so well as to make it available to holding conversation by its aid; but still it is most interesting in a physiological point of view, to know the fact, that by this means the imperfect organ can be roused to *any* degree of sensibility to sound, as even this must tend to the improvement of the general functions of the brain, rather than being entirely deprived of one source of its appropriate stimuli. I have no doubt, moreover, that many cases will, by this means, be restored to such degree of hearing as will be available for colloquial intercourse in society, which never could have been accomplished by any other means hitherto tried. If my success with the cases assembled here is at all equal to what it has been with others elsewhere, I think it cannot be otherwise than gratifying to you to find that our art has acquired a new and important power in this agency. I must not, however, omit to add, that many cases may show no improvement at a *first or second trial,* and yet be very satisfactory after a few trials. According to my experience, there is much greater chance of benefiting *congenital* deaf mutes, than those who have become so from disease or accident, *to the extent of total loss of hearing.*
>
> In testing patients as to their power of hearing, I consider it quite necessary to adopt a different plan for those who are *congenital* deaf mutes, from what we do with those who have known what perfect hearing was at some former period of their lives. It is quite true that the latter class may be unable to hear a musical box, or the tick of a watch, when held at a little distance from the ears, but can hear it when pressed *against* the ear, or the mastoid process, or greater conducting power of the bony structure. There are patients of this class, however, who declare they have no sense of sound when so tested, because their previous knowledge of the sense enables them to distinguish betwixt *hearing, properly* so called, and *common feeling.* In testing *congenital* deaf mutes, from their want of this previous knowledge, they will all signify they hear if any sonorous or vibrating body is pressed against the ear. This, however, I do not consider we have any proof of being *hearing,* but *feeling;* because they had no previous knowledge to direct them as to the peculiar sensation of *correct hearing;* and they will give the same indication if the sonorous body is placed on any other solid part of the body, according to its respective degree of sensibility. In applying tests to *congenital* deaf mutes, therefore, I consider they have no sense of hearing, if they cannot hear the sound of a musical box *held close to,* but *not touching* the ears, or any other sonorous body whose vibrations do not excite such oscillation in the air as is sufficient to be recognised by *common feeling* [i.e., the sense of touch]. It ought also to be borne in mind that the *common* feeling of the deaf and blind is generally much more acute than in those who have not been deprived of those senses. At all events we cannot err in taking this as our standard, because, if those who did not hear on the application of such a test *before* the operation, do not hear it also *after* the operation, we shall consider there is no improvement; and if those who hear it at a certain distance *before* the operation, cannot after the operation hear it at a greater distance, it must also be considered no improvement has been made. But if the former can, *after* the operation, hear *without* the *box touching* the ear, and the latter can hear at a *greater* distance, then of course we are entitled to say an improvement has resulted from the operation.

These extracts should be sufficient to explain what the extent of my expectations were as to meliorating the condition of *congenital* deaf and dumb patients, the principles upon which these expectations were based, and my mode of testing the original and subsequent condition of such patients. The following cases will prove that my anticipations have been so far realised in one case to an extent I never calculated on. **The mode of operating is, hypnotise the patient, extend the limbs, and gently fan the ears.**

Case VIII. The case of Nodan has already been referred to at [the start of this section], and I shall therefore merely add here, that he was twenty-four years old, was never considered to have had the power of hearing, properly so called, according to the opinion of the head master of the Deaf and Dumb Institution, where he was a pupil; that after the first operation I satisfied myself he *had no sense of hearing,* but after the second, which I carried still farther, he *could* hear, and was so annoyed by the noise of the carts and carriages when going home, after that operation, that he could not be induced to call on me again for some time. He has been operated on only a few times, and has been so much improved, that although he lives in a back street, he can now hear a band of music coming along the front street, and will go out to meet it. I lately tested him, and found he could hear in his room on the second floor a gentle knock on the bottom stair. His improvement, therefore, has been both decided and permanent, and is entirely attributable to hypnotism, as no other means were adopted in his case.

Case IX.

Mr. John Wright, Pendleton, nineteen years of age. Congenital deaf mute. Was four years at the asylum under Mr. Vaughan. Never heard sound. On testing, could not discern the tick of a watch pressed against the ears, nor a musical box, *unless when pressed* against the ears, which was evidently *feeling, and not hearing,* as he evinced the same expressions when it was applied to the shoulder, chest, or back of the hand. After being hypnotised for eight minutes, he could hear the musical box held *more than an inch from* the *left* ear, but not at all with the *right,* if not pressed against it, which was of course only feeling. Certified as correct by the father of the patient.

(Signed)
John Wright.
Manchester, *8th April,* 1842.

After writing the above statement, he was again tested, and could hear the box *half an inch from the right ear*

(Signed)
John Wright.

Mr. Curtis' Remarks

The latter fact, of hearing better after being roused than at the very moment they are roused, occurs in cases generally. This patient attended daily for a short time, and made considerable progress in the power of hearing, but **like too many others he had not patience to persevere**, which his father, who is a very respectable and intelligent man, wished him to do. Unfortunately the deaf and dumb are not aware of the *extent of their privation,* or of the real advantage they would obtain by persevering, and their expectation, and that of their friends, in most cases seems to be, that the moment they have the power of *hearing* restored in some degree, they should, as by a miracle, also be immediately inspired with the gift of tongues, and be able to speak and understand language without study, toil, or trouble. This has been so well expressed by John Harrison Curtis, Esq. that I shall quote a paragraph from his pen on the subject.

> Kramer condemns the cases recorded as cures by Itard, Deleau, and others, because, when published, the patients had not acquired a facility of speech equal to that evinced by other people of the same age; forgetting, that when the deafness has been cured, the individual is placed precisely in the position of a child that has to acquire the faculty of speech, and not infrequently the power of thought; while, at the same time, if he have approached the age of puberty, he has to contend with false impressions created by the erroneous perceptions which affected him while unable, from his infirmity, to impart his feelings and ideas to his fellow-creatures; in fact, he is placed in the same position in regard to hearing as Cheselden's patient was with respect to vision. The organ, when the cophosis [total deafness] is removed, requires to be carefully educated to perceive, understand, and distinguish the variety of sounds which will impinge upon the auditory nerve, a task requiring much time for its accomplishment. The cure of congenital deafness, consequently, may be effected, and yet rendered effete [i.e., ineffectual], for want of this necessary subsequent education.

After remarking that many cases of deaf dumbness arise from disease, and are only partially deaf, he added,

> Many of these cases admit of amelioration, some of cure; and I hold, that wherever there is a chance only of doing good, it ought not to be neglected; it may certainly raise hopes which may be nullified hereafter, but not in the patient, who cannot comprehend the motives of the proceeding; nor would the friends be much annoyed thereat, if the surgeon has performed his duty properly, by showing, that although there is a chance of success, it is after all only a chance. (...) It does not occasion a loss of valuable time, worthy to be put in competition with the prospect of restoring even one individual to the enjoyment of the society and converse of his fellows. (...) Many would be rendered (by proper treatment) useful members of society, who, under the present system, remain hopeless objects of commiseration as long as they live."

Mr. Curtis farther adds, "I perfectly agree with Dr. Williams, who says, a cure ought always to be attempted, and that at the earliest moment at which deafness is detected; and children so affected should mix with others not deaf, and no symbolical education should take place until all chances of cure are gone." *Medical Gazette,* 23rd September, 1842.

These remarks are so judicious and important as to require no comment by way of enforcing them on any intelligent and candid reader.

The following case having been the cause of much controversy I shall give it in detail. Before operating on the boy, in the presence of the gentleman who brought him to me, I asked the lad, in writing, if he ever heard, to which he returned answer, (also in writing,) "No." I then proceeded to operate on him, and the following is a report of his case from my note-book.

James Shelmerdine's Case
Case X.

James Shelmerdine, Mr. Barker's, 83 High Street, Manchester, aged fourteen years and a half, was born deaf and dumb, and educated at the Manchester Deaf and Dumb Asylum, and came out last June, in consequence of his age. 4th January, 1842, I subjected him to the Mesmeric influence, by causing him look at my glass rod, and in thirteen minutes aroused him by a clap of the hands, when he could hear the tick of my watch applied to the right ear, but only very slightly so when applied to the left. Could hear me speak loudly, but could not tell what I said to him. This took place in presence of his master, who brought him to me, and now attests the correctness of the above. The boy has other two brothers deaf and dumb.

(Signed)
Matthew Barker.[138]

5th January. Again subjected him to the operation. In twelve minutes he could hear my watch at nine inches from right ear, and at six from left.

7th January. Called upon me, and could hear with the right ear at four and a half inches, and one inch from left ear. After being hypnotised for ten minutes, he could hear the watch at seven inches from right, and at four inches from left ear.

17th January. After operation could hear six and a half inches with *left*, and seven and a half with *right*.

20th. Could, after being roused, hear my watch at seven and a half inches from left ear, and at nine inches from right.

The boy was now tested by competent judges, and pronounced capable of imitating articulate sound *without seeing the motion of the lips.* To render this the more certain he was tried with a word requiring no motion of the lips and spoken near his ear, which he distinctly imitated.

I now commenced to teach him to speak a few simple words, and he got on very well; and that he could do so very satisfactorily, I considered there was ample proof by what he accomplished at my lectures. There were some who could not believe he could have been born entirely deaf and dumb, when they heard how well he imitated articulate sounds when the motions of the lips were concealed. This was particularly and warmly disputed at a lecture I gave at Liverpool, on the 1st of April, 1842. The boy was asked, without my knowledge, by Mr. Rhind, head master of the Deaf and Dumb Institution of Liverpool, if he ever heard before being operated on by me, to which he answered, "No." Next day, in the presence of several friends, I again questioned him in writing as to his original condition, when he gave the following answers, which he certified by his signature as being correct. Fortunately, this document, by the merest accident, (having been written on the back of a letter belonging to another gentleman,) has been preserved, and I shall here transcribe it *verbatim.*

"Could you ever hear before I operated on you?" – "No."
"How did the master of the school teach you to say, papa, mamma?" – "Few days."
"*How* did he do it?" – "Ba, be, bi, bo, bu."
"Did the master ask you to watch the motions of his lips?" – "Yes."
"Did he try to teach you to speak by applying his mouth to your ear?" – "No."
"Did you ever say what you did to me before?" – "No."
"Did you ever read it, so far as you remember?" – "No."

(Signed)
James Shelmerdine.

Hitherto the boy had only been taught single words. The last two questions refer to part of the "Lord's Prayer", in English which I had been teaching him to speak by *means of hearing;* and although he speedily made a good attempt at repeating part of it, the effect was so different from that of the mode adopted at school, or that conveyed to his mind through the organ of sight, when reading it, as he must have been accustomed to do, *that he did not know what it was I had been teaching him to speak* Could a stronger proof than this be adduced that the boy did not learn to speak by *hearing* before he was under my treatment?

I also, on the same day, taught this boy to repeat part of the Lord's Prayer in Latin, to do away with all ground of cavil as to what he *might* have learned at the Institution; and at my next lecture at Liverpool, the week after, he was heard to be able to repeat it when spoken to him in a moderate tone of voice whilst the motions of the lips were concealed, and that taking the words in *any* order, so that there would be no ground of mistake as to his *hearing* what he repeated.

Mr. Bingham's Testimony

Various surmises having now got out, that this boy, James Shelmerdine, *might* have had, or *must* have had, the sense of hearing originally, and that his present condition could not possibly be the result of hypnotism. I addressed a letter to Mr. Bingham, who was head master of the Asylum during the five years this boy was at

---

[138] Mr. Barker was not the boy's master, but employed some of his friends, as was afterwards explained to me.

school, requesting him to favour me with information as to James Shelmerdine's real condition up to the time when he left school. The following is his reply, and I may add, I am not personally acquainted with Mr. Bingham. After describing the partial hearing of this boy, which varied greatly, Mr. Bingham adds:–

> I never considered his hearing sufficient to distinguish one sound from another in conversation, and consequently, never attempted to teach him to speak in any other way than that which I use with all children born deaf. If hypnotism, or Mesmerism, has enabled him to imitate the sounds you wished to communicate to him without his observing the lips, I do not hesitate to say that you have achieved that which I never could have expected; and, under such circumstances, I think every encouragement ought to be given to your plan. You would greatly oblige me by saying if this has been accomplished, as *the boy was quite incapable of distinguishing one word from another when he left me, if spoken behind his back.*

Fortunately I had no difficulty in satisfactorily substantiating this, for, besides having been so repeatedly proved in the public lecture-room, here and elsewhere, he had also been tested before a number of the most distinguished members of the British Association last June, and, more recently, before a dozen witnesses, including the present head master of the Deaf and Dumb Institution of this town. I instituted this investigation in consequence of some gross attempts which had been made to misrepresent my conduct in reference to this case. The following is an extract from the report of his condition on the 25th July last, (1842,) and is attested by Mr. A. Patterson, head master of our Deaf and Dumb School, and twelve more witnesses:–

> James Shelmerdine was examined at Mr. Braid's before the undersigned, in reference to his hearing, and he readily repeated part of the Lord's Prayer, both in English and Latin, both backwards and forwards, after Mr. Braid repeating the words in a moderate tone of voice, without being able to see the movement of the lips.

I had not seen the boy for about a month before this investigation, and I would ask, did he not here manifest a decided improvement from the state he was in when he left school, when, as borne testimony to by Mr. Bingham, "he was quite incapable of distinguishing one word from another", if spoken so that he could not see the motion of the lips? And I am quite certain this was his condition *immediately after the first operation.* As has been already stated, he could not then distinguish one word from another, however loudly spoken close to his ear.

After communicating these statements of what the boy *could* do, as recorded at the investigation on the 25th July, Mr. Bingham favoured me with a second letter, from which I make the following extract:–

> James Shelmerdine's performance in repeating the Lord's Prayer, in Latin and English, when the motions of the lips were concealed from him, is a convincing proof that he must have benefited greatly by it (hypnotism,) as he could not distinguish one sound from another by oral communication.

The following fact also proves the great improvement in the boy's hearing. One afternoon he was in my hall, when a lady was playing the piano, and singing, in a room upstairs. He seemed so much pleased with the music that I gave him permission to go and hear it. He instantly went upstairs, and into the drawing-room by himself, and seemed quite delighted with the sound of the music, as several who saw him can testify. This, I am quite certain, he could not have done for some time after he came under my care.

In fine, I feel confident, that had this boy persevered with the operations and been taken pains with by his parents, to teach him to speak, and understand the meaning of what he spoke, he would, long ere now, have been able to hold oral communication with others with less trouble, and in a more moderate tone of voice than we must resort to with many whom we meet with, who have become hard of hearing from age or disease. It is, however, so much more trouble, at first, for the friends to teach them language, than to hold intercourse with them by signs, that they will not bestow it, and the patients, from not knowing the extent of their privation, can be less expected to exert themselves for acquiring the good they know not; and therefore, I feel assured there will never be much achieved for the *poor* in this way, unless within the walls of some public institution; but, that there are many who might be permanently benefited in such situations I have no doubt. In the paper by Mr. Curtis, to which I have already referred, he writes thus in reference to the pathological condition of the organ in those born deaf and dumb:–

> I am of the same opinion as Braid in this respect, that structural disease does not occasion more than one case in five, leaving, consequently, many cases in which medical assistance may prove of service; and I do not acknowledge that the "weakness of the nerve, approaching to paralysis, or an actual paralysis of the nerve," which Dr. Kramer assumes to exist in those cases where congenital cophosis is present, and no structural derangement, must necessarily be as incurable as structural deficiency. We are not apt to abandon incipient palsy of a nerve of sense or motion, in other parts of the system, without an attempt at relief; and I see no reason why the unfortunate being afflicted with deaf dumbness, should be surrendered to his fate, without a well directed attempt being previously made to redeem him therefrom.

This, together with the statement of his experience, ought to encourage farther trials, and especially now that we have got a new and more powerful agent to operate with than any hitherto brought into operation in such cases. The results of the following case have far more than realised my most sanguine expectations. It clearly proves, that persons with perfect organization may have been deaf and dumb from birth, and continue so merely for want of a sufficient stimulus to set the machinery in motion.

In consequence of the remarkable improvement; if hearing, through hypnotism, evinced in the case of Mrs. C., (Case IV already recorded,) I was asked to give my opinion as to the probability of a similar operation benefiting a girl who had been deaf and dumb from birth, and who was sister to a servant in the family I was then visiting. I told them what my experience had been in respect to such cases, and it was accordingly arranged that I should see the patient, and try what could be done for her, the following day.

S. Taylor – Sense of Smell
Case Xa. 9th August, 1843. The girl, Sarah Taylor, was nine and a half years of age, very small for her age, and very stupid looking. The following is the history of the case, as stated by father, mother, and elder sister. She was a seven months' child, remarkably small, the head large for the size of the body, and soft, ("like a bladder full of water",) and it was long before they expected to be able to rear the child. As she grew up they were much annoyed with her not speaking, and by her paying no attention to what was said to her. At last they found that this was not obstinacy, to which it had been at first attributed. They now came to the painful conviction that she was deaf and dumb. The father has assured myself, and many others, that in his anxiety to obtain proof of her having any degree of hearing, he has "often stood behind her, and shouted (as he expressed himself) till he was hoarse again", without her evincing any sign of hearing; and that when she was out of sight they were in continual terror she would be run over by carts or carriages, as she could not hear their approach. The testimony of the mother and sister was to the same effect, that they never could make her hear, or pay any attention by calling her, when her back was towards them. In such position they could only make her observe them by touching her. They all agree, also, in stating, that she never could speak so as to be understood, till after being operated on by me, excepting two or three words – father, mother, sister, which she had learned from watching the motions of their lips. I regret not having had her tested by a musical box before I operated on her; but I am quite certain, that after the first operation she could not distinguish one word from another; and I afterwards had the best possible proof of her never having heard for any useful purpose, as she was quite ignorant of the name *of any part of her own body, or of any person, place, or thing,* as is well-known to many who saw her after I had operated on her. After the third and fourth operation I could manage to make her speak a few simple words, and also to make a tolerable attempt at following me when singing the musical scale.

Ten days after the fourth trial, she was tested and proved able to do this before **fifty or sixty highly respectable witnesses**, including many professional gentlemen. For months past she has been attending the Scotch Session School, and is making very good progress in learning, and I have no doubt, will prove to be a clever girl; she hears so correctly now, as not only to be able to imitate speaking, but also singing. Mr. E. Taylor, Gresham Professor of Music, lately afforded a number of my professional and scientific friends a good proof of this, as he composed an extemporary tune which she and two other patients sang correctly, whilst in the state of neuro-hypnotic sleep. She could have done the same whilst awake, and **hundreds have witnessed her speak and sing, both when asleep and when awake.**

It is curious, that in some who have a very incorrect musical ear, so that they could not be taught to sing the most simple air correctly when awake, can nevertheless be made to do so, when in this peculiar sleep. This was remarkably exemplified in a young lady, whom I wished to be taught a simple air which she might sing by way of exemplification, at some lectures I was to give at a distance, but it could not be accomplished; she could not follow in tune more than a note or two together; but when asleep, she can sing any air correctly which I have tried her with. Still, when awake, she cannot do so. For an example of the same sort during natural somnambulism, see pages 296-298, and 309, of Dr. Abercrombie's work *On the Intellectual Powers*. Of one it is noted, "She often sang, both sacred and common pieces, incomparably better, Dr. Dyce affirms, than she could do in the waking state." Of the other, "She was, when awake, a dull awkward girl, very dull in receiving any kind of instruction, though much care was bestowed upon her, and, in point of intellect, she was much inferior to the other servants of the family. In particular, she showed no kind of turn for music, and she did not appear to have any recollection of what passed during her sleep." During somnambulism, she sang beautifully, and exhibited great intellectual powers.

I shall conclude this department by recording the following case from my note book. The inability of this patient to sing *in tune* may have been partly owing to a defect in the organ of hearing, and partly to a state of nervousness affecting the vocal organs. The experiment was undertaken merely to gratify the particular desire of the patient, as at that time I had had no similar case, and was not prepared to say, whether it was likely or not to be successful. However, I felt assured it would do him no harm, and made the trial accordingly, and assuredly nothing could have proved more successful or more gratifying than the result.

Case XI. 7th July, 1842, I was consulted by Alexander M'Roberts, twenty-nine years of age, residing with Mr. Hannay, of 42, Thomas Street, Manchester. He said, he had never been able to join in tune, although he had frequently attempted to do so. After being hypnotised for some time, (about ten minutes,) I roused him, and desired him to walk into the dining-room, and after hypnotising him once more, a friend played the organ, and I directed (or led) him to sing the scale, beginning with D, as he could not sing C, owing to the natural pitch of his voice. He very soon managed to sing the scale quite correctly, upwards and then downwards. I now roused him, and made him sing it when awake, which he did remarkably well. I now tried him with the first part of "Robin Adair", which he followed in correct tune several times. This took place in presence of Mr. James Reynolds, Mr. Daniels, Mr. James Braid, my nephew, and myself. In the evening of that day, after being again hypnotised, he sang the first part of "Robin Adair" very correctly several times, and also Pleyel's "German Hymn", and the old "Hundred Psalm", quite correctly. Pleyel's "German Hymn" he never heard before. This took place in presence of four gentlemen.

His inability to sing prior to these operations was borne testimony to by several of his friends, one of whom had a good knowledge of music, but despaired of ever seeing M'Roberts able to sing, and he was exceedingly surprised at the result. This patient was operated on several times afterwards, and when I last saw him, could sing a considerable number of tunes, and follow any simple air with ease and correctness.

The next sense I shall refer to is that of smell. Having put the patient into the hypnotic state, he ought to be kept in it a longer or shorter time, according to the object had in view. If to excite or quicken the sense, the limbs should be extended and a gentle current of air should be passed against the nostrils occasionally; but if to diminish the sense, this ought not to be done.

Case XII. is an interesting example of restoration of the sense of smell by hypnotising. A young lady was subjected to this operation for a different complaint. On being aroused, and after I left the room, she made inquiries as to the cause of the great noise she heard in the house, and expressed her surprise at the noisy manner in which the various duties of the apartment where she was were performed. They assured her there was nothing going on in the room where she was, different from what was usually the case, nor was there any thing to account for the noise she complained of, and they therefore held her complaints to be only imaginary. She persisted they were real. The fact was, she had been for a length of time dull of hearing, and the improvement of this sense consequent on the hypnotising, had so quickened the faculty as to account for the difference she experienced. Moreover, she had for a considerable time previously lost the sense of smell, and it was now ascertained *that this sense had also been restored, through the same operation.* Another patient who had lost the sense of smell for nine years, had it restored after being twice hypnotised. For a beautiful illustration of the extent to which this sense is aroused during the hypnotic sleep, see footnote, extracted from a report of my conversazione to the Members of the British Association, as recorded by the *Manchester Times*.[139]

Touch and Resistance
The next senses I shall refer to, are touch and resistance; under which I shall adduce examples of the beneficial results of this agency, in the cure of abnormal exaltation or depression of these functions. There are few diseases more striking in their manifestations, or more important in their character and tendency, than those included in this class, namely, paralysis of sense or motion, or both; or the reverse, exalted feeling, and tonic or clonic spasm.

Tic, Paralysis of Sense and Motion, Cured
Tic douloureux [trigeminal neuralgia] is well-known to be one of the most agonizing affections to which the human frame is liable. It may arise from a functional disorder of the nervous system, of a local or more general character, or from an organic cause. The symptoms are much the same in both varieties, but the chances of effecting a cure are very different. In the former variety, a cure may be effected, and by no means I know, so speedily and certainly as by hypnotism; but in the latter, the chances of success are very different, either from this or any other known remedy. I have repeatedly applied it in the one case, without any apparent effect, either good or bad, but, in the other, with the most immediate and striking advantage. I give a few cases in illustration of this success in functional disorder.

Case XIII. W. M'Leod had been suffering for two months from a violent attack of tic of the head and face, which had resisted the treatment prescribed by his surgeon. He had been taking carbonate of iron in ample quantity. After eleven minutes' hypnotism, he was aroused quite free from pain, and it never returned in the same degree of violence, and by a few repetitions of the same process, he was completely cured, and has remained well for about a year. The general state of his health required the aid of other means, but the violence of the tic was overcome before he took a single dose of medicine from me.

Case XIV. A young lady was suffering from a most violent attack of tic douloureux, so much so, that I heard her screams before entering the house. The paroxysms came on so frequently that she was roused before I could succeed in hypnotising her at first trial. I now administered thirty drops of laudanum, in a little water, sprinkled some over the poultice on her face, and instantly commenced hypnotising her again. In five

---
[139] [See appendix (originally a lengthy footnote).]

minutes she seemed to be in a comfortable sleep, the features perfectly placid, the respiration calm, not a muscle seemed to move during the time I remained in the room, (which was a quarter of an hour,) whereas she had a violent paroxysm every three minutes previously, contorting her whole body, and when I examined her, after having been down stairs a considerable time, she was lying in exactly the same posture as when I left her, with the same appearance of placid sleep. When I called next morning I was told she had slept for five hours and a half, and had had no return of tic after awaking. As she was in the somnolent state, and the paroxysms of pain suspended *within five minutes,* it is quite clear this could not be due to the few drops of laudanum, as they could not have been adequate to arrest such a violent complaint, at all events, not in the course of five minutes.[140]

Case XV. Miss —— had been suffering severely from tic for several weeks, and had several teeth extracted without relief. During a violent paroxysm, I succeeded in hypnotising her, and when aroused, it was quite gone, and has never returned.

In the affection to which these cases belong, there is frequently such irritability of the skin, that a slight touch over the affected nerve is quite sufficient to excite a paroxysm of pain. I shall now adduce some cases illustrative of the *opposite* condition, when there was deficiency or entire loss of feeling; and which have nevertheless been greatly benefited, or entirely cured by hypnotism. The following case is illustrative of its successful application where there was paralysis both of sense and motion.

Case XVI. Mrs. Slater, thirty-three years of age, in the autumn of 1841, had suffered a good deal during her pregnancy, and in December of that year was delivered of a seven months' child. From this period, her legs, which had been very weak for some time previously became very much worse, and in a short time she lost all voluntary power over them, together with loss of natural feeling. She had been under the care of three professional gentlemen, but as she became worse instead of better, notwithstanding the means used, the case had been considered hopeless, and left to itself, for some time previous to my being consulted, which was on the 22nd April, 1842. I found she had not only lost feeling and voluntary motion of her legs and feet, but that the knees were rigidly flexed, the heels drawn up, the toes flexed, and the feet incurvated, and fixed in the position of slight club foot (varus). She had not menstruated since her confinement, but there was no other function as regarded the secretions or excretions, which appeared to be at fault. Her speech was imperfect and her memory impaired. I hypnotised her, and endeavoured, whilst in that condition, to regulate the morbid action of the muscles, and malposition of the feet and legs. In five minutes I roused her, when she thanked God *she now felt she had feet, could feel the floor with them, and could move her toes.* I now raised her on her feet, and with the assistance of her husband supporting her by the one arm, and myself by the other, she went across the room and back again to the sofa, moving her legs and supporting half the weight of her body on them. I operated on her again the same evening, after which she was able to support herself standing with the soles of her feet on the floor. She required merely to be steadied by placing the points of the fingers of one of my hands against her back. Before being operated on, the heels were drawn up, and the feet twisted so that she could only have touched the floor with a small portion of the outer edge of the feet, near the root of the little toes. I hypnotised her in the same manner daily for some time with increasing improvement, so that in a week she was able to walk into her shop alone, merely requiring to steady herself by the wall, and in two weeks more she could walk into it *without any assistance whatever.* Two months from my first seeing her, she went to Liverpool, and was able to walk several miles in a day. She could walk from the middle of the town where she lodged, to the pier head and back, and from her lodgings to Everton and back, all in the same day, which was several miles partly on very steep acclivities. She had no relapse, and has continued well ever since.

In a very few days after I first operated on this patient, the catamenial discharge appeared for the first time since her confinement. She had no internal medicine, nor external application whatever to her legs for several days after I first saw her. Her extraordinary improvement, therefore, resulted entirely from the

---

[140] The following is the statement of the above case, attested by Mr. Mallard, druggist, who had been called to visit this patient before my arrival, which I give because of some very unwarrantable interference by other medical men:—

"I was present with Miss G. when Mr. Braid visited her, in consequence of a violent pain in the face, coming on in severe paroxysms, as occur in tic douloureux. I had applied poultices, and had other means in readiness, but owing to the violence of the pain, Mr. Braid, the usual medical attendant of the family, was sent for. Her screams were heard in my house, during the paroxysms, and they recurred about every minute, and lasted nearly a minute and a half, as nearly as I can recollect. Mr. B. had an opportunity of hearing her on coming into the house; and shortly after being in her bedroom she had a second attack. Mr. B. now tried to hypnotise her in his usual way, but she was roused by the violence of the pain. He now gave her a few drops in water, and sprinkled a few over the poultice, and applied it to the cheek again, and immediately repeated his operation, after which she seemed to be in a sound sleep, and gave no farther indication of pain in less than five minutes. Mr. Braid, as well as myself, remained a considerable time, at least three quarters of an hour, and both left convinced she was comfortably asleep, and next morning I heard she had passed a good night, having slept about five and a half hours, and that the tic had not returned since we left. Every word of this has been carefully read and considered before being signed.

(Signed)
A.T. Mullard.
21st June, 1842."

effects of the operations. After I had attended her some days, she required some simple aperient [mild laxative] medicine, and I afterwards prescribed a diuretic, which I hoped might expedite the cure. The feeling and power of her legs and feet were greatly restored, her speech perfect, and her memory much improved, before she had a single dose of medicine from me. Her improvement therefore was strictly the result of hypnotism only.

The extraordinary effects manifested in this case, as well as in many others, after a few minutes' operation – so different from what is realised in the application of ordinary means – may appear startling to those unacquainted with the powers of hypnotism. On this account, I have been advised to conceal the facts, as many may consider it *impossible,* and reject the *less* startling, although *not more true* reports of its beneficial action in other cases. In recording cases, however, I consider it my duty to report *facts as I have found them,* and to make no compromise for the sake of accommodating them to the preconceived notions or prejudices of anyone.

Case XVII. Samuel Evans, forty-five years of age, had suffered much from pain in the spine, and also been afflicted with impaired feeling as well as power of the superior extremities for four years. He suffered also occasionally in the head, for which he had undergone every variety of treatment usual in such cases, under many medical men, myself included, but with so little success that he had not been able to dress himself for five years:– he could not lift the left arm, and natural feeling was almost entirely gone from it. The right arm was also affected, but in a less degree, when he applied to me on the 25th April, 1842. I hypnotised him and he was so fully satisfied with the improvement he experienced, as to induce him to come to Manchester to be operated on daily. In a very short time his improvement, both as regarded strength and feeling, was most decided, as he could lift a heavy chair with the worst arm and could feel a small object such as a pin, which could not have been distinguished by him with that hand when I first saw him. The pain in his back was also speedily much relieved. He was exhibited at my conversazione to the British Association, 29th June, 1842, in this improved state, and has made still farther progress since, although not yet able to follow his usual avocation. I should not omit to add, that this patient was under my own care for some time in 1841, when, although he derived benefit from the means used, he was not nearly so much or so rapidly relieved, as by my present mode of treatment by hypnotism.

Case XVIII. Mr. —— fifty-eight years of age, consulted me in consequence of a paralytic affection of two and a half years' standing. Stated by his friends that he had had an apoplectic seizure two years and a half before, which was at first accompanied with total loss of consciousness, and of sense and motion of the right side for six weeks. He then gradually recovered, so as to be able to walk a little in the course of four or five months. When he called on me 3rd June, 1842, his gait was very feeble and insecure, always advancing the right side foremost, his arm had always been supported in a sling, he could raise it with an effort as high as the breast, had not the power of opening the hand, the thumb was much and rigidly flexed. Had little or no feeling in that hand. After being hypnotised for five minutes, feeling was restored, he could open the hand and grasp much firmer, and *raise it to his forehead.* His speech, which had been very imperfect, was also much improved. This patient was operated on for some time with partial improvement, so that he could manage his arm without a sling, and the feeling continued improved, and there was also slight improvement in his gait, but I was of the opinion, that there was organic mischief in the brain which would prevent a perfect restoration, and therefore discontinued farther trials.

Case XIX. Miss Sarah Mellor had been under my care for nine months, for an affection of the lower part of the spine, accompanied with pain and weakness of the lower limbs, and with contraction of the knees, so that she had been unable to stand or walk without crutches during that period. I had used every means usually adopted in such cases, but instead of improving, she was getting worse in every respect, till I tried hypnotism, the satisfactory results of which were too immediate and apparent to admit of the slightest doubt of its great value on this occasion. The following is a statement attested by the patient:–

> I had suffered severe pain in my ankles, with contraction of the knees, and pain at the bottom of my back, so that I had been unable to walk without a pair of crutches for nine months. During this period, I had taken medicines internally, used liniments to the legs and spine, been leeched and blistered over the lower part of the spine, but still, instead of improving, I was getting worse, both as regarded the pain and contraction, so that I was becoming quite deformed, from the legs being bent on the thighs, and they on the body. I was thus about nine or ten inches less in stature than formerly, and than I am now. About the beginning of last March (1842) I came to Mr. Braid, who had prescribed the other means to me without benefit, when he said he would try his *new method* with me. After being hypnotised *three times,* I was able to walk from my lodgings to the house of a friend who lived a few houses distant in the same street WITHOUT MY CRUTCHES, and in two days after, from that house to Mr. Braid's WITHOUT CRUTCHES. I was operated on almost daily for three weeks, when I returned home, and at that time I was able to walk *half a mile without crutches.* After being at home five weeks, I returned to Manchester, and have been attended by Mr. Braid for two months, and always found myself better after the operations. I took no medicine during my first stay in Manchester; and on this occasion having only done so when required for a violent cold on two occasions, from imprudent exposure. Since I came to

Manchester last, one day I walked to Grosvenor Street, Piccadilly, and back again to my lodgings in Lower Mosley Street, fully a mile and a half, without inconvenience; on another occasion to Hulme and back again, *fully two miles. I was quite sensible, and could hear all that was said or done during all the operations.*

(Signed)
Sarah Ann Mellor.
Jane Livesey, Witness.
C. Wilson, Witness.
Manchester, 12th July, 1842.

This patient was exhibited at my conversazione 29th June, 1842. After returning home, she had the misfortune to get entangled by one of the feet in a cart rut, in a lane, which threw her back, but having returned and been hypnotised, I was enabled to send her home much improved, and when she called on me lately, she continued so.

Case XX. Mrs. J. twenty-nine years of age, requested my attendance, 17th February, 1842. Had been attacked in the autumn of 1840, with slight degree of weakness of left side, and difficulty of speech, neither of which had ever been entirely removed. Three months after, she was delivered of a still-born child, and had been affected with convulsions ten days prior to delivery, for which she seemed to have been treated in the usual manner. In about a month after delivery, 31st January, 1841, she had an apoplectic attack, attended with total loss of consciousness, and paralysis of the left side, for which her medical attendant had prescribed the usual treatment. I was called to attend her on the 17th February, and continued to do so for five weeks, when, as there was no particular improvement manifested, she passed into other hands, and after being under treatment with them for ten weeks, without improving, she was sent into the country, where she remained for about thirteen months, when she was brought back to town to be placed under my care, 15th June, 1842. The following was her condition at this period. Her mouth very much drawn to the right side; her speech very imperfect; and her mind confused. The left hand and arm were quite powerless, and rigidly fixed to the side, the hand clenched, the fingers and thumb being rigidly and permanently flexed. The left leg very rigid, the heel drawn up, and the foot twisted so that it could only approach the ground by resting on the outer edge near the root of the little toe; she could move this leg a little, but had never been able to stand, or walk a step, or support any weight on it. I hypnotised her, though owing to her mind being so confused, I experienced considerable difficulty in getting her to attend to the necessary instructions for producing the condition. However, I at length succeeded, and after the first operation – I kept her in the hypnotic state for ten minutes – she could hold her mouth much straighter, could move the fingers a little, and lift the hand and arm four inches, and, with the assistance of her mother-in-law and myself supporting her by the arms, she was able to support half the weight of her body in walking across the room and back again. Her speech was also improved, and she evinced less confusion of mind. Next day I found the improvement was permanent, and hypnotised her again with advantage. On 17th, found her improved, and still more so after being again operated on. She could now, on merely steadying herself by laying hold of her mother-in-law's shoulder, stand supporting herself on the left leg, when the right foot was lifted clear from the floor. Her speech was still more improved, and mind more collected, so that I had very little difficulty in hypnotising her now.

She was operated on daily, with advantage, till the end of that month, and the results shown to some of the most eminent professional and scientific gentlemen in this town. During the next two months she was operated on at times only, being so much better. In a few weeks she could walk to the door, steadying herself against the wall, and in a few weeks was able to walk into the street with the aid of a crutch. She had no medicine during this attendance. I only saw her occasionally now, and on the 11th September, when I had not seen her for nine days before, whilst taking her usual airing in the street, she was seized with apoplexy, from which she died within sixteen hours. On inspection, the whole of the superior and anterior lobes of the right side of the brain were found to be in a state of atrophy; only a thin layer, and that in a state of *ramolissement* [softening], covering the ventricle, which was filled with serum, as was also the space between the *pia mater* and *arachnoid* [two of the membranes enclosing the brain], to make up the space vacated by the wasting of the cerebral substance. There was no effusion of blood. It is not at all surprising that such a case should have resisted former treatment, or proved fatal at last; but it seems surprising that, with such a state of brain, hypnotism should have had the power of producing so much improvement as it did.

Case XXI. 14th June, 1842, Mr. Thomas Morris, forty-two years of age, consulted me. He had had a paralytic stroke fifteen years previously, which deprived him entirely of the use of the right leg, and rendered the left weak and numb. In six weeks was able to walk a little, but never recovered entirely, being always weak and lame. Fifteen months ago had a second attack, with total loss of consciousness for a week, and also complete loss of voluntary power of the *whole body.* For several weeks required the urine to be drawn off by catheter. He has lately had the urine passing involuntarily sometimes, at other times voided with great difficulty. He has never regained the power of his legs so as to enable him to stand or walk without assistance; and has been, for the last six months, growing worse. The arms very weak, being unable to raise the right higher than the head, and even that accomplished with great difficulty. Speech also very imperfect, and his ideas so confused that he could make himself understood with great difficulty. Hypnotised him for five minutes, when he could speak much better; could raise his arm and hold an umbrella perpendicularly, or horizontally, with his body, with perfect ease, and could walk across the room WITHOUT ASSISTANCE, *for the first time since last seizure.*

(Signed)
Thomas Morris.

Witnessed by,
John Shipley
  Duncan Street, Strangeways.
C.C. Morris.
John W. Pacey.
James Braid, Junior.

15th, had the pleasure of finding the improvement noted above was permanent, and also, that *he had been able to retain his urine and void it at pleasure,* whereas it had been passing *involuntarily,* both by night and day, *immediately before being* hypnotised. He was again hypnotised today with additional advantage. 17th, found him still better, having been able to walk in the street with *one stick* for the first time for *last five years.* Repeated the operation. 18th, still better, so that, with the aid of his two sticks, he had walked into Ducie Street by himself. Operation repeated.

This patient went on improving, and on the 29th June was exhibited at my conversazione. His speech was greatly better immediately after *first* operation, and his ideas seemed more vivid and clear. He was also able to sign his name, and which he did very well, for the first time since his last seizure. Nor should I omit to add, that he had regained power over the rectum, which he had not previously; and in about ten days he had got sufficient power of his hands to enable him to work. After he was considerably recovered he had the misfortune to fall, and injured the lower part of the back very much, which impaired the recently acquired power of the legs. They are somewhat better, but not nearly so well as they were a few weeks after he had been under my care. His arms, however, still retain their increased power, as I saw him lately lift a bedroom chair with the right arm, and hold it up nearly at full arm's length; and the mind keeps pretty clear, much more so than before being hypnotised, notwithstanding he has had a severe attack of bowel complaint, from which he has been liable to suffer occasionally.

It would be difficult to adduce a more striking proof than the above, of the extraordinary power of hypnotism, there having been so many points at fault, all of which were immediately meliorated, and some of them permanently so.

Case XXII. Mr. John W., 21 years of age, called to consult me, 18th April, 1842, for a paralytic state of the left side of the face, of thirteen days' standing. He had no power of the muscles of the left side of the face, consequently the mouth was drawn to the right, and he had no power of closing the left eyelid. In ten minutes after being hypnotised, and friction used, he could open and close the eyelid with facility, and had the power of retracting his mouth to the left of the mesial plane.

Case XXIII. 11th July, I was consulted by Samuel Edwards, who had been unable to work for six weeks, in consequence of a paralytic state of the extensor muscles of the wrist, and a semi-paralytic state of the flexor and extensor muscles of the fingers. He had injured the arm by a heavy lift, and by a blow about two years before. The paralytic state came on suddenly about six weeks previously to my seeing him, accompanied by a tingling or prickling feeling in the fingers. I hypnotised him, calling into action the weak and entirely paralytic muscles in the best way I could. In consequence of this, he acquired the power of flexing and extending the wrist, when the arm was held horizontally with the ulna downwards, and of grasping pretty firmly with the fingers, immediately after the first operation, which he could not do before, as witnessed by several highly respectable individuals who were present the whole time. On the evening of the following day, he was able to milk a cow with this hand, and when he called on me two days after, I found him greatly improved. I operated on him again with additional advantage, and found him able to grasp so firmly that he could hold a single finger fast enough to enable him to be thus pulled from his seat without losing his hold. He had undergone various treatments, including blistering, under two surgeons before I saw him.

17th July, 1842, he called on me, and had still greater power of the hand. After being again hypnotised, he could readily lift the one side of a heavy library table with the hand, which was quite powerless when I first saw him six days before. He stated, he had been able to work with it constantly from the time I saw him, on the 14th.

31st, he called on me, stated he had been improving. Was hypnotised once more. August 7th, he called on me, and the first thing he did was to hold out his arm at full length, and show me he could bend and extend the wrist, whilst the arm was in the state of pronation. He had been able to do so for some days.

Had been able to milk *five* cows the day previous. Hypnotised him again, after which he had still more power. He has not required to call on me since, being nine months ago. This patient must have continued well, as I have heard nothing more of him, which I was to do if he had any relapse.

I could easily multiply cases of successful practice in the treatment of paralysis by hypnotism, were it not for occupying too much space, I shall, therefore, condense a few.

Case XXIV. A gentleman, sixty years of age, had a paralytic stroke two years and a half before consulting me, which deprived him entirely of the use of the right arm, and enfeebled the right side and leg. When he called on me, he walked very feebly, could scarcely close the fingers and thumb, and could not extend them fully. He could with great difficulty raise the hand as high as the pit of the stomach, the pupil of the right eye was considerably larger than the left, and not quite circular; speech very imperfect. After being hypnotised for five minutes, he was able to open and close the hand freely, and to raise the hand above the head, and pass it to the back of the head, and he could also walk and speak much better. Pulse regular – before operation, his pulse was very irregular. When he called on me next morning, I found the improvement had been permanent. I hypnotised him once more with advantage, and again on the two following days; seven weeks afterwards he called on me, when I found the improvement was permanent. He could speak and walk much better, could raise the arm, and move the fingers and hand freely, could pass the hand above and over the head, and take off his hat with it. The right pupil also was quite circular now, and nearly the same size as the other.

Case XXV. 4th June, 1842, Mr. J.H., sixty-seven years of age, had a paralytic strike, nineteen months previously which deprived him entirely of speech, and of motion of right leg and arm; when he called on me, his speech was very imperfect, his hearing dull, and he had very little power in closing the hand, could raise the hand to the mouth, said he could sometimes raise it a little higher, but never so high as his head. After being hypnotised for five minutes, he could speak and hear much better, could grasp much stronger, and would raise the hand a *foot above the head,* and put his coat on without assistance, passing it over his head. His walking was also much firmer. He seemed greatly pleased with being able to put his coat on, as it was the first time since his seizure. He was also able to sign his name for the first time, to attest the accuracy of my report of his case, which he did before two witnesses who had been present during the operation. He called on me twice after this, the last time two weeks from his first visit, when I found the improvement was permanent.

Case XXVI. Thomas Johnstone, thirty-six years of age, had a paralytic seizure 13th February, 1842, which deprived him of feeling and motion of left arm and hand. Had partially recovered motion so as to be able occasionally to move the fingers a little, and to raise the arm nearly to the horizontal position, but frequently was suddenly struck with pain and total loss of power of the arm, and hand, and fingers, for four or five hours after. Had been struck in this way just before I saw him, and he was quite powerless, as above described, or rather the arm was spasmodically fixed to the side; had been under medical treatment ever since his first seizure. 4th May, 1842, hypnotised him for four minutes, after which he could move the fingers, hand, and arm freely, elevating it above his head, across his body in either direction, and could retain it in any situation he was asked. The feeling, however, was still very imperfect. 5th May, called on me to go to my lecture, when he had the complete control of the hand, arm, and fingers. He was hypnotised in the lecture-room the same night, and in four days after, the feeling, as well as power, was restored to it. 26th, called on me again, and has perfect voluntary power of the arm, as well as natural feeling and heat of the member. Attested as correct by the patient.

    (Signed by proxy to which the patient affixed his mark.)
    Thomas Johnstone.
    Witnessed by John Harding.

I have also a copy of a certificate of his condition from the physician who attended him immediately before he consulted me. On the 10th January, 1843, his father informed me that his son had requested him to call on me, and say he was in America, and had remained well ever since I saw him, and, that he wished his father to express how grateful he felt for the benefit he had derived from my operations. I shall only give one more case illustrative of this class.

Case XXVII. Mr. H., thirty-nine years of age, had been partially paralytic of the inferior extremities [i.e., the legs] for ten years, which came on some time after a fall, accompanied with double vision. The latter disappeared under treatment, but the former increased. When he called on me, 18th February, 1843, he was walking with a crutch and stick, and with the assistance of both myself and a servant, it was with great difficulty he could ascend the few steps at my door. After the first operation, he could walk across the room and back again, without *either crutch or stick,* and after being operated on next day, he was able to mount twenty-eight steps to his bedroom without his crutch, and has done so ever since. In ten days, I was agreeably surprised to see him on the fourth bench of the lecture-room of the Manchester Athenaeum, to which he had ascended eighty-one steps, with the aid of a stick in one hand.

This patient had not been aware, until I called his attention to the fact, that he had very defective vision of the right eye, and was surprised to find on testing this, that when the left eye was closed, he could with difficulty see the large heading of the header of the *Medical Gazette*, whereas he could read the ordinary sized print of that article with the left. After being operated on, he could read the small print of the leader with the right eye also, at which he felt greatly surprised, as well as at the increased power of his legs, **because, as he had been conscious all the time of the operation, he could not believe I had done anything to him, till he found on trial he had been so much benefited in both functions.**

Here, then, we have the beneficial results most unequivocally ensuing even when the patient imagined no effect could have been induced. The improvement in the sight has remained permanent, and he also improved in the power of his limbs, till he had the misfortune to fall, whilst carelessly looking at something when walking on the street one day.

In confirmation of the efficacy of a few minutes of hypnotism, in curing many cases of paralysis, I may refer to the reports of the Liverpool papers, as to what took place at my lectures in that town in April, 1842. There were hundreds who witnessed the effects when I publicly operated on such patients, who were entire strangers to me. Cases where the patients had been for years powerless of limbs, so that they could not unlock the clenched hands, nor raise the arm to the chin, even with the aid of the other arm, have been enabled in eight or ten minutes, to open the hand, and lift the arm above the head. My intelligent friend, Mr. Gordon, lately informed me, he had treated a paralytic case most successfully by hypnotism.

Case XXVII^A. Mrs. E., thirty-seven years of age, had a paralytic affection when thirteen months old, which deprived her entirely of the use of the right leg, which has never been recovered. At seven years of age, she had a second attack, which deprived her also of the use of the right arm, which was recovered after nine months' professional attention to it. At fifteen years of age she had a third attack, which drew her face, and deprived her of speech for some time, but was recovered from; and she had no farther attack of the sort till 8th January, 1842 (being twenty-two years from former attack). The latter attack enfeebled the right arm, and completely paralysed the whole of the left side.

Being of full habit, she was bled from the arm, had active cathartics, leeches, and blisters. In six days there was improvement to this extent, that the right hand could be raised as high as the shoulder, the left arm could be moved feebly, and the hand closed feebly and slowly. When sitting on a chair, the left leg could be moved with great difficulty, so as to raise the heel from the ground. I hypnotised her, and in five or six minutes she could raise her right hand and arm *above her head,* could move the left arm freely, and grasp firmly, and could raise the left leg so as to place the heel eighteen inches from the ground. Next day she was able to walk across the floor with her one crutch. A pain in the knee induced her to avoid walking afterwards, but in three weeks she could walk quite cleverly as before the last attack.

The other cases were all in the chronic state, of long standing, and had resisted all ordinary means, and the restorative powers of nature and time, and yet we have seen what extraordinary powers can be exerted, and effects produced, in such cases by hypnotism. The latter proves its superior efficacy, to other means, in more recent cases.

Miss E. Atkinson's Case, Voice Recovered
Case XXVIII. I shall conclude the subject of paralysis with the following most interesting case. The subject of it was Miss Atkinson, a middle-aged and very intelligent lady, and I shall give the case as recorded by herself in a letter she was so obliging as to furnish me with, for the purpose of publication in this work.

> Letter From Miss E. Atkinson,
> (of the Priory, Lincoln.)
> "Mosley Arms, Manchester.
> Monday, 4th July, 1842.
>
> Dear Sir,
>
> I have very great pleasure in furnishing you with a statement of my case, I beg you will make whatever use of it you think proper, and most sincerely do I wish that it may lead others suffering from disorders on the nerves, to seek relief from the same source, and with the same success.
>
> In January, 1838, I was attacked with cold and influenza, accompanied by a violent cough, on the 9th of this month. Ten or twelve days after the first attack, without any previous warning, my voice left me instantaneously, and I could not utter a sound louder than the faintest whisper. For three weeks I had no medical advice, hoping daily, from my ignorance of the nature of the complaint, that my voice would return; but

being disappointed, and feeling my health and strength declining, consulted Mr. Howitt, an experienced and eminent surgeon in Lincoln, who immediately requested I would confine myself to my own lodging-room which was to be kept at a regular temperature. He prescribed such medicines as my case required, and ordered blisters to my throat and chest, which were kept open, until I became so completely debilitated that it was considered necessary to discontinue them. Towards the latter end of April my health was considerably improved, and I was allowed to leave my room though my voice was still merely a feeble whisper. Shortly afterwards, I paid a visit to a sister in York, whose family surgeon, Mr. Caleb Williams, a man in extensive practice, prescribed for me, and took great interest in my case. Soon after my return to Lincoln, I consulted Mr. Joseph Swan, 6, Tavistock Square, London, who entirely approved of the treatment I had undergone, and prescribed such additional remedies and medicines as he thought would be beneficial. Since then he has continued to visit me whenever he has been in the country. Galvanism has been tried without producing any effect; electro-magnetism also, by a scientific friend (not a medical man). I have frequently conversed with several other professional gentlemen, who have also taken a great interest in my case. They all agree in opinion that the attack was paralysis of the organs of voice, without disease; and that the treatment I have undergone has been most judicious; in fact, that every thing has been done for me the medical profession could suggest. Every one of them has told me, that when my health and strength returned, there was every reason to believe I should recover my voice. I remained in a very weak and delicate state for some time, but have now been in perfect health for more than twelve months, yet without having the power of speaking above a whisper.

I considered the recovery of my voice hopeless, until hearing of the many cures you had performed by hypnotism, I was induced to state my case to you, and request your opinion as to the probability of this system benefiting one. Your reply was, *"If,* as seems to be the opinion of most of the professional gentlemen consulted, your loss of voice is owing to *exhaustion* of the *nervous energy* of *the vocal nerves,* and not *to positive destruction of any portion of them,* I consider my mode of operating is likely to be very speedily successful. On the other hand, if there is positive destruction of the nervous substance, *with loss of continuity of the principal trunks of the nerves,* it will alter the chances very materially. However, as this cannot be positively known without trial, and as the extraordinary power we possess of rousing nervous energy may be sufficient to enable the function to be restored with a state of nerve which could not be of service under any other agency, I should decidedly give it as my opinion that it ought to be tried, as no risk can attach to the trial, and a week or two at most, will be all the time required for giving it a fair trial." This raised my hopes; I came to Manchester on Tuesday the 28th of June. You operated on me twice that evening, and twice each succeeding day [i.e, 8 times], but without producing any change on my voice until Saturday, July 2nd, when, on rousing me from the hypnotic state, I spoke aloud without the slightest effort. My voice was then weak; you have continued to operate on me until now, Monday morning, (4th July,) and my voice is fully restored to its original strength, with the power to vary its tone at will [after *c.* 14 sessions]. Thus has hypnotism given me back the power to make myself understood by those to whom I address myself, of which I had been deprived for the last four and a half years. I have not suffered the slightest pain or inconvenience while submitting to the operations nor any unpleasant effects afterwards; neither did I ever once lose consciousness of all that was passing around me.

With heartfelt humble thanks to our heavenly Father for this and every blessing, particularly for the hitherto unknown power bestowed on man; and with deep gratitude to you for your kind attentive care while so skilfully and successfully using this power for the restoration of my voice, I beg you to believe me, dear sir, yours very respectfully, and greatly obliged,

Elizabeth Atkinson.

It is but justice to the professional gentlemen who had been consulted in this case prior to application being made to me, to say, that I consider they had treated the case most judiciously, according to our previous experience in such cases; and it must be interesting to them to find that in this agency our art has acquired a new and efficient resource for such cases.

This case is interesting in many points of view. The circumstance of the patient having been operated on twice each day successively, that is, *eight* times, without any visible improvement for I had her tested before and after *each* operation – and being able to speak aloud, without effort, on being roused from the hypnotic condition on the *fifth* day, is **sufficient proof that the improvement was *not the effect of imagination,* but of the physical condition induced by carrying the operation farther. Any effect to have been anticipated from mere mental emotion we should have expected to have been greatest at first, and to have become less and less as the party became familiar with such operations.** Here, however, it was quite the reverse. I found, on testing the patient on the 2nd of July, *immediately before being operated on,* that no improvement had been effected from the former operations, (she had been operated on eight times,) and therefore resolved to carry it farther that time; and the result was, as noted above, that on being aroused she spoke aloud without effort. **It is also important, as corroborating the statement of many others who have been cured of various obstinate complaints by hypnotism, that they *could hear quite distinctly, and retained consciousness the whole time,* of all that was going on around them. In some cases, however, it is necessary to carry it to the ulterior stage, or that of *insensibility*.**

On the 19th October, 1842, [*c.* 15 weeks later] I had the pleasure of receiving a letter from Miss E. Atkinson, from which I make the following extract, in proof of the *permanency* of the cure. "You will be glad to hear that I have retained my voice without any intermission, since I left you. The only difference is, that it has become stronger; and my health is in every respect perfectly good." I had also the pleasure of hearing from a friend, a few days ago, that she still continues well, and it is now nine months and a half since her voice was restored.

I doubt not there may be some who, on reading the cases I have recorded in this treatise, will be disposed to appeal to the well-known fact, that various complaints have been suddenly cured by mere mental emotion, hoping thus to throw discredit on the curative powers of hypnotism. Whilst I grant the premises, I deny the justness of the inference. That I may meet the subject fairly, I shall now quote some of the most remarkable cases of the sort which have been recorded.

> Dr. Gregory was accustomed to relate the case of a naval officer, who had been for some time laid up in his cabin, and entirely unable to move, from a violent attack of gout, when notice was brought to him that the vessel was on fire; in a few minutes he was on deck, and the most active man in the ship. Cases of a still more astonishing kind are on record. A woman, mentioned by Diemerbroeck, who had been many years paralytic, recovered the use of her limbs when she was very much terrified during a thunder-storm, and was making violent efforts to escape from a chamber in which she had been left alone. A man, affected in the same manner, recovered as suddenly when his house was on fire; and another, who had been ill for six years, recovered the use of his paralytic limbs during a violent paroxysm of anger. Abercrombie *On the Intellectual Powers,* pp. 398-9.

To these might have been added the influence of the sight of a tooth key or forceps, or even the approach to the house of a dentist, in curing toothache.

Now, what are the legitimate conclusions to be drawn from the history of such cases? **Is it not simply this, that such results are possible, and that they can be effected by different means? Now as it is apparent that analogous results can be induced by hypnotism, I would ask is hypnotism not quite as convenient and desirable a remedy as setting a ship on fire, raising a thunderstorm, converting the patient's house into a bonfire, or exciting him into "a violent paroxysm of anger"?**

Again, of those who talk so much about the power of imagination, I would ask, what is it? **How does imagination act to produce such extraordinary and contradictory results? For example, the mental emotions of joy and sorrow, love and hatred, fear and courage, benevolence and anger, may** *all* **arise either from** *real,* **or from** *imaginary causes only,* **and may seriously affect the physical frame. In many instances these different and opposite emotions have proved almost instantly fatal; in other instances equally sanative. How is this achieved? Are not the whole of the emotions accompanied by remarkable physical changes, in respect to the respiration and circulation as well as sensation? Are they not highly excited in one class, and depressed in the other? And may not this act as the proximate cause in effecting the permanently beneficial results during hypnotism? As already explained, analogous physical results can be produced by hypnotism; and it is no valid reason why we should not profit by it in the treatment of disease, that we cannot positively decide as to its** *modus operandi.* **It seems quite evident that we have acquired, in hypnotism, a more ready and certain control over the physical manifestations referred to, and which can be turned to useful purposes, than by any mode of acting on the imagination only, which has hitherto been devised.**

Rheumatism, Ten Cases

Rheumatism is another affection, for the relief of which I have found hypnotism a most valuable remedy. I have met with some cases of rheumatism, however, which have resisted this, as they had every other method tried; and others, where it afforded only *temporary* relief; but I am warranted in saying, that I have, on the whole, seen far more success, more rapid and decided relief, follow this mode of treatment, than any other. It has been chiefly in chronic cases in which I have tried it. **In its application, I first induce the somnolent state, and then call into action the different muscles which I consider directly affected, or which, by being so called into action, are calculated to change the capillary circulation and nervous sensibility of the part implicated.** The patient must be retained in such position a longer or shorter time, according to circumstances. The following cases will illustrate the effects of this mode of treatment:–

Case XXIX. Joseph Barnet, near Hope Inn, Heaton Norris, Stockport, sixty-two years of age, called to consult me on the 10th December, 1841, for a severe rheumatic affection of the back, hip, and leg, of thirteen years' standing, which had been so severe, that he had not been able to earn a day's wages during that period. He had been equally a stranger to comfort by day, as to refreshing sleep by night. He came to me leaning feebly over his stick, suffering anguish at every step, or movement of his body. He was treated at the commencement of his complaint by a surgeon; but feeling no relief, like many others similarly afflicted, he had recourse to all sort of nostrums [quack remedies], and also to hot salt water baths. I hypnotised him, placing him in such attitudes as his particular case required, and in fifteen minutes aroused him, when he was able to bend his body freely, and not only to walk, but even to run. He called on me in a few days after, when he stated he had slept comfortably, and been perfectly easy from the time he left me till the night before. I hypnotised him again with advantage, and a few more times sufficed to restore him entirely. This patient was seen, and bore testimony to these facts, at two of my lectures. After one of them, from being too late for the coach, he walked home, a distance of six miles. This was by no means judicious, but proves incontestably his great improvement.

I was not at that time so well aware, as I have been since, of the great power of hypnotism in such cases, and therefore ordered him some medicine after the first operations; but from observing that the relief immediately followed the operation *before taking medicine,* and that the pain returned in some degree the night *before next visit,* and when, had there been benefit resulting *from the medicine, it ought to have been diminished after using it,* and that relief was again afforded during the hypnotism, I felt convinced the medicine *had no share in the improvement,* and therefore discontinued it, and trusted entirely to hypnotism. In the beginning of January, 1842, when this patient called on me, he was so well, that I told him no farther operations would be necessary for the present, but added that should he have any relapse, if he called on me again, I would hypnotise him, without charge, of which offer he promised to avail himself.

At my lecture on the 17th December, 1841, several questions were put which elicited the following answers:– "Do you mean to say you were never so well as you are now?" "Yes; I never earned two shillings during all that time. This last winter I was worse than ever." "Did you walk, sir, before ever you left my surgery, without taking any medicine?" – "I did, and ran too." See *Manchester Guardian,* 1st January, 1842.

I heard nothing farther of this patient for about seven months, and therefore, after the offer I had made him at last visit, had every reason to conclude he had remained well. However, it appears he had a relapse shortly after he left me, and his family, upon whose exertions he depended, being out of work, he could not afford to pay the railway charge for coming to see me again. His relapse having been laid hold of, and construed into a charge against me as having falsely represented his case, I was induced to call on the patient, accompanied by two friends, when he furnished us with the following document:–

> Joseph Barnet, Providence Street, Heaton Norris, had suffered from a severe rheumatic affection prior to last December, when he applied to Mr. Braid. He was first under the care of Mr. ——, Higher Hillgate, who bled, blistered, and prescribed medicines for him; but the complaint remained unabated. From this period, took various medicines, and other means recommended to him by those who had been similarly afflicted, and who considered he would be benefited by such means as had relieved them, but received no relief. After that applied to Mr. —— of Manchester, from whom he considered he derived benefit for a fortnight but the pain returning, he went to Liverpool to the water baths, where he remained as long as money lasted, but without being relieved.
>
> From this time tried various means as recommended by different parties. During the whole of this period, he had never been able to earn a day's wages. When he applied to Mr. Braid in December last, (1841,) had been suffering extreme pain in every movement of the body; in short, he had walked nearly double, supported on a stick. He was operated on by Mr. Braid, and in a quarter of an hour he was roused, and found himself able to walk and run. At first, Mr. Braid walked him about by the hand, and afterwards made him run without any assistance whatever, as his wife and others present can testify. The case as stated by Mr. Braid in his lectures in my (his) presence was perfectly correct, as I (he) bore testimony to at the time. Owing to being unable to pay the expenses of the railway, he did not return to Mr. Braid, when he had a recurrence of the pain. He had never informed Mr. Braid, that he had had a recurrence of the pain, and never saw him afterwards until the evening of the 26th June, 1842.
>
> (Signed)
> Joseph Barnet. (his mark)
> J.A. Walker.
> Thomas Brown.
> Harait Brooks.
> (Daughter of J. Barnet.)

Case XXX. 11th January, 1840. Mrs. B, forty-eight years of age. Catamenia ceased last spring. She has suffered from a severe rheumatic affection for the last three months, and been confined for the last two months to her bedroom. The legs, arms, neck, and head, were excessively painful, so that the slightest movement was attended with great agony. She was quite alarmed at my taking hold of her arm to feel the pulse. When in bed could not turn over, nor bear the slightest touch. 11th January, 1842, hypnotised her, and roused her in ten minutes, when she was quite free from pain, being able to walk, stoop, and move the arms, wrists, and fingers, with perfect freedom. 12th, had slept comfortably all night; had been able to lie on her side, which she could not do before for three months; could rise from the chair, and move legs and arms without pain. There was, however, a soreness or uneasy feeling, although not amounting to pain, in some parts of the limbs. Hypnotised her for eight minutes, when she felt less of the numbness, and followed me down stairs, and ascended them again, without taking hold of the banister, and taking the steps regularly and cleverly with both feet alternately. 14th, found her down stairs enjoying herself with her father, husband, and friends, almost quite well. Hypnotised her again, and also in a day or two after, and she had no recurrence of the rheumatism, although a degree of stiffness of the limbs remained. She had no medicine from me till the rheumatism was gone, when she had some for a different complaint. This patient was seen at my house seven months after by about sixty friends, including several professional gentlemen, when the above statement was read in her presence, and confirmed by her as correct to that time; and as I have heard no intimation, I feel assured she has not had a relapse.

Case XXXI. Mrs. S. has been already referred to; case VI. She had suffered much from rheumatism for many years, and had never been entirely free of it, notwithstanding she had undergone much treatment. After first operation she was much relieved, and after a few more was entirely free from pain. It has recurred occasionally since, but has always been removed by one or two more operations of the same sort, and which are neither painful, nor in any way unpleasant.

Case XXXII. Another rheumatic case of a patient fifty-three years old, of seven years' standing, where sleep had not only been courted by exhausted nature, but also by the most powerful doses of narcotic drugs; on one occasion 400 drops of laudanum had been taken in *two hours;* still the pains continued, and yet, by *fifteen minutes* of hypnotic sleep, procured by the simple agency I recommend, this patient was relieved of his agonizing pains. In this case, from my knowledge of the eminence of the professional gentleman who had prescribed for him, I feel assured every known remedy had been resorted to, but without effect, and yet this agency succeeded in a few minutes. This patient had suffered severely for seven years; was first hypnotised 10th February, 1842, and again on the 17th and 19th. He seemed as nearly as possible entirely free from pain, and had suffered very little after the first operation, less than at any previous period during the seven years he had been a rheumatic subject. I have lately heard he had a relapse some time after I last saw him; but no reasonable person could expect three operations should have sufficed to eradicate such an obstinate complaint permanently; most probably a repetition of the process would.

Case XXXIII. Mr. John Thomas, 155, Deansgate, consulted me at the end of April, 1842, for a severe rheumatic affection of the loins, and right hip and leg, which had continued for two weeks. Had a rheumatic fever two years before, which confined him to bed for sixteen days, and to his room for a week longer; and he did not get rid of the pains for three months after he was able to go out, although he tried Buxton and Matlock baths, and also the medicated and sulphur baths in Manchester. When he called on me, (April, 1842,) I hypnotised him, and when roused he was almost entirely free from pain, and never required a repetition of the operation. He had no medicine. On the 28th July, he called on me to say he had continued quite well in every respect from the time he was hypnotised, and attested the same, and the correctness of the above statement, by appending his name to it in my case-book, and he has also been seen by many professional and other friends who can bear testimony to the same effect; he continued well when I saw him lately.

Case XXXIV. Master J. Lancashire, 12 years of age, was brought to me in September, 1842, he was suffering from a violent rheumatic affection of the legs, back, and chest, so that he required to be carried into my house. After being hypnotised, he was so much relieved is to be able to walk about the room freely, and to walk to his cab without assistance. Next day he called, and was hypnotised again, and left my house quite free from pain, and has kept so well as never to require another operation. He had no medicine, either externally or internally. His mother and he called some time after to inform me he had remained quite well, when they both attested the correctness of the above statement of his case.

Case XXXV. Mrs. P., a lady upwards of fifty years of age, had suffered so severely from rheumatism that she had not enjoyed a sound night's sleep for seven months. External and internal means, which had been beneficial in a former similar attack, had been tried without effect, before I was sent for to visit her. She was suffering excruciating pain in one leg, particularly about the knee joint. When I proposed to relieve her by hypnotism she repudiated the idea, told me she had no faith in it, and felt assured in her own mind such an operation could be of no use to her. I told her I cared little for her want of faith in the remedy, provided she would submit to be operated on as I should direct. She at last consented, and in the presence of her three daughters was hypnotised. In eight minutes she was aroused, and was quite free from pain; wished to know what I had done to her; said she felt assured hypnotising her could not have relieved her. To this I replied by asking where her pain was felt now. She answered she felt no pain, but persisted she was sure I had done nothing to take it away. The manner in which she could walk and move her limbs was sufficient proof the pain was gone, notwithstanding her scepticism about the agency. When I called next day, I was informed by her family *she had slept comfortably all night,* and had gone out, being quite well. Two days after, I called again, and was informed by her that she had been overtaken in a shower, and had over-exerted herself on that occasion, and had had a return of the pain, although not so bad as at first. I hypnotised her again with complete relief, and she has never required a repetition of the operation since, so that she has now enjoyed a release from her old enemy for eleven months, in defiance of her scepticism. **Here, then, we have a very decided proof that it was not imagination; in short, that it was a physical and not a mental change which effected the cure.**

Case XXXVI. Mr. Hampson, another rheumatic case, I was called to 16th May, 1842. The patient was a powerful young man, twenty-three years of age; had suffered severely for three weeks, the last two been entirely confined to bed, unable to move his legs, or to feed himself; for two weeks had not known what it was to have ten minutes continuous sleep, from the violence of the pain, and spasmodic twitching of the limbs rousing him, his left hand, fingers, and wrist were so swollen and painful, that he was quite alarmed at my attempting to feel his pulse. After being hypnotised for five minutes whilst in the recumbent posture, I had his arms extended, and he was now roused and able to move the wrist and fingers with comparative ease. I now hypnotised him once more, and operated on his legs. In *six minutes* he was able to get on his feet, walk round the bed and back again and get into bed and lie down *without assistance*. Next morning I found him up and dressed, and able to walk very comfortably. He had slept well through the night. I hypnotised him again. Next night he slept uninterruptedly, and in the morning felt nothing of his pains excepting in the left shoulder; but this was quite well by the next day. He had no medicine except a mild aperient [laxative].

The cases adduced I consider sufficient to prove this to be a valuable agency in the treatment of *chronic* rheumatism. I shall now adduce the results of its application in two cases of *acute* rheumatism.

Case XXXVII. Mr. G., a literary gentleman, consulted me last winter. I found him complaining of severe pain in the right arm and hand; one point, the size of a crown piece, on the outer edge of the arm, a little below the elbow joint, was exquisitely painful. He was enveloped in double clothing, but, notwithstanding, was quite starved and chilly with *cutis anserina* [goose bumps], pulse 120 strokes a minute. I told him I considered it was the commencement of an attack of rheumatic fever, and I should wish to try whether it could be cut short by hypnotising him. He had never been operated on in this way before, but readily assented. In six minutes I had him bathed in perspiration, and his pain greatly relieved. He was now ordered to bed, to take a mixture with *vinum colchici* [wine of colchicum root, a herb used to treat rheumatism]. Next morning I found him much freer from pain, it had never been severe since the operation the day before, the skin comfortable, and his pulse only 80. To remain in bed and continue his medicine. Next day the pulse was 70 [i.e., returned to normal], and no complaint of pain, and the following day, he was able to go out and attend to his business. No relapse.

Case XXXVIII. Mrs. B., the mother of a numerous family, had a severe attack of rheumatic fever, affecting different joints in succession, and also violent pain in her head. I proposed she should be brought out of bed and hypnotised. The pain of her knees, feet, and ankles, was so severe that she could not stretch her legs, nor attempt to support herself, in the least degree, upon them. She had therefore to be carried from the bed to the chair where she was to be hypnotised. In five minutes she was roused, the headache gone, and the pain in her legs and feet so much relieved that she was able to walk to bed, requiring only to be slightly supported by the arm. The pains never returned with the same degree of severity. She was hypnotised a few times more, and always with benefit. Of course I prescribed such medicines as I considered necessary to improve the state of the secretions, so as to put as speedy a termination to the attack as possible, but there could be no doubt that hypnotism contributed very much to meliorate her suffering, and also in bringing the attack to a more speedy termination, than would have been the case had I trusted to the effects of medicine only.

Irregular Muscular Action
The following cases can perhaps scarcely be introduced in any other place with more propriety than the present. They are cases of painful affection of the members, arising from irregular action of the muscles, consequent on mechanical injury.

Case XXXIX. Mr. J.J. consulted me on the 6th November, 1842. He stated he had a fall from a horse five months previously, when he sustained severe injury of the left hip and thigh. He was confined to bed for two weeks, under medical treatment, supposing the parts to be only bruised and sprained. He then began to move about with crutches, but with great pain; and a consultation being held, it was considered there was dislocation of the hip joint, but the attempts made to reduce it failed. At the end of nine weeks from the accident, another surgeon, forty miles off, was sent for, who confirmed the opinion that there was dislocation of the hip joint, and he succeeded in reducing it. The patient was now confined to bed for two weeks, and, on rising, was able to move about with the aid of a stick, but without crutches. However, he was still very lame, and in much pain. When he called on me, which was on the 6th November, 1842, he was not suffering much pain, but was extremely lame. The knee was a little advanced forwards, and the toes considerably everted. In attempting to walk without the aid and support of his stick, the body was thrown so much to the left at every step, as if the leg were considerably shorter, that with other circumstances coupled with this, led me to suspect fracture of the neck of the femur within the capsular ligament. A minute examination satisfied me this was not the case; and I now considered the affection was one of irregular action of the whole muscles of the hip and thigh, some being atrophied and semi-paralysed, and others inordinately tense. With this view I believed I should be able to rectify the irregular distribution of nervous and muscular energy by hypnotism, an opinion the correctness of which was quickly verified. Having hypnotised the patient, and placed the leg in that position calculated to restore the functions according to the view I had taken, in about six minutes he was roused, and was agreeably surprised with such a remarkable improvement. Next morning he was again operated on, and was then almost entirely free from lameness, and entirely free from pain, so that he asked my opinion whether I considered it at all necessary for him to take his stick in going through the town on some business. He called on me the three following days, after which he went home, equally gratified as myself with the result of our operations. He had no internal medicine, nor external application, whilst under my care. He attested the accuracy of the above report before leaving; and, as I have not heard from him since, have reason to believe he continues well.

This patient was seen by several gentlemen, some of them members of the profession, who can bear testimony to the correctness of these statements, as they had an opportunity of hearing the whole from the patient himself.

Case XL. Mr. J.H., sixty-eight years of age, called to consult me on the 8th November, 1842, relative to a painful state of his left shoulder, the consequence of a blow he had sustained two months previously. He had been under the care of two eminent professional gentlemen from the time he received the injury till within a few days before I saw him. There was a wasting of the muscles about the shoulder, great pain in moving the arm, and it was so weak that he had not been able even to button his coat with it. After being hypnotised the first time he could use it, raising it above his head, and moving it in any direction with ease and freedom. After being operated on next day he had still more power. The following day he felt a little pain behind the shoulder, under the scapula, which was entirely removed by being once more hypnotised, and calling the affected muscles into action. On Saturday, the 11th November, 1842, he left me, quite well, to return home to attend to his business. Both this patient and his son attested the correctness of the above report in my casebook.

Case XLI. J.W., fifteen years of age, had a severe injury of the hip, which was followed by suppuration between the *trochanter* and *ischium*, where there was a fistulous opening; the leg was flexed and perfectly useless, being supported by a sling passed over his shoulders, whilst he supported himself very feebly on two crutches, his health having suffered greatly during his affliction. He stated that he had just left a public institution, where he was given to understand no hopes were entertained of his recovery. I hypnotised him, and during that condition regulated the malposition of the limb, stretching the contracted muscles, and strengthening others, by exciting into action those which had been weakened by being overstretched and enfeebled by inaction. The result was, that on being aroused he could straighten his leg, and walked (using his crutches of course) with the sole of his foot resting on the floor. He was operated on daily with the most marked improvement both as regarded his leg and his general health. In three weeks he could walk with one crutch, in two weeks more threw that aside, and walked with a stick, and shortly after could walk without that aid, and is now well, excepting a little weakness of the ankle joint. He had no internal medicine from me, and no external application, excepting one box of ointment, the discharge having entirely ceased within a week of his being under my care.

Headache
I shall now advert to the remarkable power of this agency in speedily overcoming nervous headache. I have so many examples of this, sometimes two or three fresh cases in a day, that it is almost useless to instance individual cases. However, I shall give a few.

Case XLII. Mrs. B., the mother of a family, has been constantly annoyed with headache and maziness [i.e., confusion and disorientation], for the last two or three years, varying in intensity at different times, but never entirely free from it. Consulted me, 22nd January, 1842, for the above complaints, and also stated that she was subject to attacks of epilepsy. I hypnotised her, and in five or six minutes aroused her, when she was quite free from headache. She was hypnotised almost daily for some time, and remained quite free from headache, five weeks after she was first operated on, and had much less of the mazy feeling, and no fit for two months. She appeared so much better as to be taken notice of by all her friends.

Case XLIII. Miss B., daughter of the above, was brought to me on the 23rd January, 1843, in consequence of the improvement her mother had experienced from the operation. She had suffered severely from headache for six months, so much so, as frequently to cause her cry and shed tears, and was never entirely free from it for that period. I hypnotised her, and in five or six minutes roused her quite free from headache or any other ache. She was operated on almost daily for some time, and has had no return of the headache to this time, – four months – and has had her appetite much improved, and looks very much better. She had no medicine.

Case XLIV. Miss S., on the 25th January, 1843, was suffering from a most violent headache, and had been so all day. She could scarcely open her eyes or see when they were open, and seemed quite prostrated. I hypnotised her, and in five minutes she was aroused quite well, and has had no return of it at the end of ten days.

Case XLV. Miss A., twenty years of age, had suffered severely from headache from childhood, and never knew what it was to be entirely free from that complaint, but frequently had it so severely as to incapacitate her for any exertion, and almost to deprive her of sight. She also had constant uneasiness at stomach, sometimes amounting to severe pain, and when the attacks of headache were at the worst, the pain at stomach was also much aggravated, and a severe attack of vomiting generally terminated the violence of these paroxysms. In April, 1842, I hypnotised her, and from that period she has been almost entirely free from both headache and stomach complaint. At the end of fifty-four weeks, I had the pleasure of hearing from herself, as I had previously from her mother, that she scarcely had suffered from headache at all since the operation, and never severely, or even in the slightest degree for one hour at a time.

Case XLVI. Mrs. T. had been suffering from severe pain of the head for more than two weeks, without intermission either by night or day when aggravated by a cough. For the last two days, the pain of the side had been most distressing. The pulse was rapid, the cough frequent and severe, and the pain in the side so acute as to prevent free expansion of the chest as in ordinary respiration. I found there was considerable spinal tenderness on pressing betwixt the shoulder blades. I hypnotised her, and in five minutes, when aroused, she was quite free from headache, the pain in the side so much relieved, that she could move her body freely, and take a moderate breath with very little inconvenience. Next day I found she had no return of the headache, and very little of the pain in the side. She was again hypnotised with advantage, which I repeated daily, and in six days the pain of the side was quite gone, the pain of the head had never returned, the cough was gone, the spinal tenderness which disappeared at first operation had never returned after the first operation, and the patient was now quite convalescent. She had no medicine but some pectoral mixture to moderate the cough.

Spinal Irritation
I shall now refer to spinal irritation, which is well-known to be the source of much suffering, not merely in the course of the spinal column, but also, from its influence on the origins of sentient nerves, on distant parts of the body. I have already referred to this in cases XVI and XIX, where there was loss of feeling and motion in one case, and pain of the legs with contraction in the other. Where the affection does not depend on active inflammation, I hesitate not to say, that the pain of the spine, and other painful affections dependent on the state of the spinal nerves which arise therefrom, may be relieved more speedily, and certainly, and effectively, by hypnotism, than by any means I have either tried, read, or heard of. I shall give an example or two.

Case XLVII. Miss C. had suffered for years from spinal irritation and headache, the pain extending round the chest, so that deep breathing or free motion of the chest could not be tolerated. I tried every variety of treatment, but in vain, and at last despaired of benefiting her, and, from the extreme difficulty of breathing, suspected it must end in pulmonary consumption. I now tried hypnotism, which immediately succeeded in relieving the whole catalogue of painful symptoms, and she was speedily restored to perfect health, and has continued so ever since.

Case XLVIII. Miss —— had suffered much from spinal irritation for years, and had undergone much severe treatment. Had been restored to health and strength under my treatment, but was again threatened with a relapse. I hypnotised her, and when roused, the spinal tenderness was gone. A few more operations made a most marked improvement, and she continued well for some months. She had a recurrence of the complaint, when hypnotism was again had recourse to, with immediate and decided advantage.

I could easily multiply cases of this sort, were it not for swelling the volume unnecessarily. I shall therefore pass on to cases of irregular or spasmodic action of the muscles. I have found it decidedly useful in several cases of chorea; and also in cases of nervous stammer.

Epilepsy
In epilepsy it also frequently proves highly useful, but there are some varieties of this complaint over which it has no control. These I presume are such cases as depend on organic causes, and which are found to resist every known remedy. It is however well-known that many cases which were supposed to have been of this class have worn themselves out, or time and the efforts of nature have effected some organic change. Whether hypnotism if persevered in, might have a tendency to expedite the favourable result in such cases, I am not prepared to say, but think it highly probable it might do so. **I feel quite confident, however, that in cases which are amenable to treatment, this will be found one of the most speedy and certain remedies. Of all the complaints for which Mesmerism has been lauded as beneficial, there are none so conspicuous as epilepsy**, as has already been referred to in the introduction. As the effects of

hypnotism are so nearly allied to Mesmerism it would be superfluous for me to detail a number of cases. I shall therefore give only a few.

Case XLIX. A girl who had been liable to six or eight fits in twenty-four hours, had only one the day after she was first hypnotised, none for next five days, and was shortly quite well.

Case L. John Barker, aged nineteen years, applied to me in August, 1842, for epileptic fits. He had first been seized with them when four or five years of age, at first every week or fortnight, but as he got older, became more frequent, so that, for some months previous to applying to me, he had had as many as three fits a-week – had been under treatment at a public institution for two months before calling on me, and had a great variety of treatment, but derived no benefit, and was then told by the attendant, that he must never expect to get rid of them. He was subjected to my usual hypnotic operation for such cases, was operated on ten times altogether, and has had but one fit since he was operated on; and that was the day after first operation. He had no medicine from me excepting three aperient powders. He has now been free of the fits for upwards of nine months.

Case LI. Mrs. B., the mother of a family, had been subject to epilepsy for seven years, and notwithstanding every variety of treatment, allopathic and homeopathic, she had an attack at least once a month. From the time she was hypnotised she had no fit for four months, and has had none since.

Case LII. Miss B., had been subject to fits for nearly two years, latterly had as many as five and six a day; consulted me the end of December, 1842; was hypnotised seven times, and had no return of the fits for four months, when she had one, and in two weeks after a second.

Spinal Curvature
Hypnotism may be applied with great success in the treatment of various distortions, arising from weakness of certain muscles, or inordinate power or contraction of their antagonists; and I feel convinced, that by this means, we may rectify many of those cases which have hitherto been treated by section of the tendons or muscles. **The success which I have already had, by this means, of treating lateral curvature of the spine, warrants me to speak very confidently on the subject, in most cases.** *I feel convinced there are very few recent cases which may not be speedily cured by hypnotism, without either pain or inconvenience to the patient.* Patience and perseverance will of course be necessary where the disease has been of long standing, and though in such cases the cure may not be perfect, the patient may be greatly improved by hypnotism.

The method of treating such cases is, first to induce the sleep, and then to call such muscles into action as are calculated to bring the body into the most natural position. By bringing these muscles into play during this condition they acquire increased power, and ultimately are permanently strengthened. As one side of the chest is enlarged, and the other collapsed, I endeavour to restrain the enlarged side, by applying compression to it during the sleep, whilst the patient is directed to take deep inspirations, so as to expand the *opposite* side. I also endeavour to make the patient stand in a position *the very reverse of that which I consider to have been the chief cause of the curvature.* As already remarked, I feel convinced this method will prove very speedily successful, more decidedly so than any other mode of treatment I know of, and *especially in such cases as are accompanied with spinal irritation.*

Case LIII. The following is a case of its remarkable success with a young lady, fourteen years of age, who had had the advice of some of the most eminent members of the profession in the provinces, and also in Dublin and London. She was first observed to become malformed when four years old, when brought to me on the 12th September, 1842, her chin rested on her breast, and there was no power of raising it, from the weakness of the *recti* muscles of the back, and contraction of the *sterno-cleido-mastoid* muscles. The dorsal part of the spine and shoulders were thrown backwards, the lumbar vertebrae and pelvis were thrown forwards, so that the deformity was very great, and the vigour of the mind, as well as of the body, was greatly impaired. She had no medicine nor external application, but was hypnotised night and morning, and treated in the manner referred to, and the result was, that in six weeks she could hold herself so much better, that when the outline was taken, it was found that her spine was three inches nearer the perpendicular than when I first saw her. During this period, no mechanical means had been used, nor throughout any part of the time she was under my care were any resorted to, with the exception of a support for the chin, by way of remembrance [an *aide-mémoire*], till the habit of attention was acquired of supporting the head by mere muscular effort, which she now had the full power of doing. Nor should I omit to add, there was also a great improvement in the mental faculties.

Neuralgia, and Palpitation of the Heart

Neuralgic pain in the heart and palpitation, I have also found to be relieved, or entirely cured, by neuro-hypnotism, more certainly and speedily, than by any other means. The following are examples:–

Case LIV. Miss Tomlinson, sixteen years of age, I have already referred to. She had suffered severely from painful affection of the heart, with palpitation, which had resisted all treatment, and she had been prescribed for by eminent professional men, both physicians and surgeons. After being twice hypnotised, the affection of the heart disappeared, and has never returned but once, when it was immediately removed by hypnotism. It is now seventeen months since she was first operated on, and she is in perfect health.

Case LV. Miss Stowe, twenty-two years of age. I have already referred to her as one of the cases in which sight was remarkably improved by hypnotism. She had also suffered most severely from palpitation of the heart, accompanied with difficulty of breathing and dropsy, and various other symptoms which led the medical attendants, one of them an eminent physician, to pronounce the case hopeless, considering there was serious organic disease of the heart. After being twice hypnotised, all symptoms of affection of the heart disappeared, (sufficient proof it had been only functional derangement,) and she was speedily in the enjoyment of perfect health, and has been so now for the last twelve months, and that from hypnotism only. This patient had leucorrhoeal [genital] discharge, which had resisted every remedy for years, and was so offensive as to cause suspicion she had malignant uterine disease. It was completely gone in a week, after being first hypnotised. She had no medicine excepting a simple aperient pill occasionally. I should add, her hearing, as well as sight, was very much improved by it.

Case LVI. Mr. —— had suffered severely from pain in the heart and palpitation. He was hypnotised with decided relief, and a second operation completely restored him, and he has kept well for the last eight months.

Case LVII. Miss —— had suffered much from palpitation of the heart, so that she could not ascend an easy stair without bringing on the most violent palpitation. I tested this before operating on her. After being operated on, caused her to ascend the same flight of steps, which produced no palpitation, and she has never required the operation to be repeated.

Case LVIII. A young man had suffered much from valvular disease of the heart and palpitation and difficulty of breathing for four years, the consequence of a rheumatic fever. He could not walk more than twenty or thirty paces without being forced to stand or sit down. After being hypnotised for a short time he could manage to walk upwards of a mile at a stretch. In this case there was so much organic disease as precluded the hope of a perfect cure, but no means could have achieved for him what hypnotism did, and in such a short time too.

Surgical Operations without Pain

When considering the power of hypnotism in blunting morbid feeling, I may advert to its power of relieving, or entirely preventing, the pain incident to patients undergoing surgical operations. I am quite satisfied that hypnotism is capable of throwing a patient into that state in which he shall be **entirely unconscious of the pain of a surgical operation**, or of greatly moderating it, according to the time allowed and mode of management resorted to. Thus, **I have myself extracted teeth from six patients under this influence without pain, and to some others with so little pain, that they did not know a tooth had been extracted**; and a professional friend, Mr. Gardom, has operated in my way lately, and extracted a very firm tooth without the patient evincing any symptom of feeling pain during the operation; and when roused, was quite unconscious of such an operation having been performed. He has extracted a second for this patient, and one for another, without their being conscious of the operation. **To insure this, however, I consider that, in the majority of instances, it is quite necessary the patient should not, when he sits down, know or imagine the operation is to be performed at that *time*, otherwise the distraction of the mind, from this cause, may render it impossible for him to become hypnotised deeply enough to render him *altogether insensible to pain*.** The following case will illustrate this view.

Case LIX. Mr. Walker called on me, stating he had been suffering from a violent toothache; said he was anxious to have the tooth extracted, but that he suffered so much pain from the operation, on former occasions, that he could not make up his mind to submit to it, unless when hypnotised. **He had been frequently hypnotised, and was highly susceptible of the influence. I told him I should be most happy to try, but that unless he could restrain his mind from dwelling *on* the *operation*, I might not be able to succeed in extracting the tooth, *entirely without pain*.** He sat down, and speedily became hypnotised, but I could not produce rigidity of the extremities, nor *insensibility to pinching*, which in general were so readily induced in him. I therefore roused him, and told him the fact. **He stated he went on as usual to a *certain point*, but then began to think, "now he will be putting the instrument in my mouth", after which the hypnotic effects went no farther. The pain was gone, and he left. In the evening he again called on me, when I tried him once more with the same results. **I now aroused him, told him it could not be done with him reduced to a state of *total insensibility,* and that I should therefore extract it now that he was awake. I now extracted the tooth. He was conscious of my laying hold of it, but had felt so little pain that he could not believe the tooth had been extracted. Nor would he believe it till he had the tooth put into his hand.** I now requested him to be hypnotised once more, when he became *highly rigid and insensible, in a shorter time than I had ever seen him before.* **From this, and other cases, I infer, that if it is intended to perform a surgical operation *entirely without pain,* whilst in the hypnotic condition, the patient's consent should be obtained for it to be done *sometime,* but he ought on no account to know *when* it is to be done, otherwise, in most cases, it would foil the attempt.**

However, that patients may be operated on with greatly less pain even when in the *first* ["partial" or "conscious"] degree of hypnotism, and whilst expecting an operation, is quite certain, from the result of the case of Mrs. ——, related below which I now refer to as Case LX. I have also performed other operations under similar circumstances, and with similar results, namely, with *greatly diminished* pain, although not *entirely without pain.*

Case LX. A lady had abscess connected with disease of the orbital process of the frontal bone, had the matter discharged by small puncture, the wound closed by first intention and again opened, as required, by the lancet. She experienced so much pain on each occasion as to induce me to hypnotise her, after which she made no complaint, although I dared not carry it far owing to the state of the brain. On one occasion I was anxious to ascertain how she would feel by operating *without hypnotising,* when the result was so distressing, as to induce me always in future to hypnotise her, before such operations, and then all went on well.

Case LXI. An adult with worst variety of *Talipes varus* [club foot], of both feet, had the first operated on in the usual way, and the other whilst in the primary state of hypnotism. The present case and future advantage, in respect to the latter operation, was most remarkable. **I have operated on upwards of three hundred club feet now, and am warranted in saying I never had so satisfactory a result as in the one now referred to.**

Diseases of the Skin
In cases of dyspepsia [indigestion] it is of the greatest service. Most patients feel the appetite greatly increased by being hypnotised, and that the digestion is more vigorous than before being operated on. All complaints, therefore, immediately connected with, or dependent on, indigestion, may be expected to be benefited by hypnotism. It is well-known, many cutaneous diseases are of this class; and the following will illustrate the remarkable power exercised by hypnotism on this symptom, as well as several others associated with it.

Case LXII. Mrs. O., thirty-three years of age, the mother of a family, had been very nervous for fifteen years, with tremor of the arms, was easily alarmed, much disturbed by distressing dreams, and required being aroused several times every night from severe attacks of nightmare. She had also suffered severely from an inveterate eczema of the chest and mamma, and integuments of the abdomen, which, for five months, had resisted every remedy, both external and internal, under highly respectable medical men. The fingers of one hand were also affected with impetigo. She consulted me 31st August, 1842, when she was hypnotised, and was aroused greatly relieved from the distressing feelings of the head, and general nervousness. Her husband assured me, that on walking out with her same evening, had he not seen her, he could not have believed it was his wife who had hold of his arm, so much was the tremor of her arm improved, and she slept soundly all night without being troubled either by dreams or nightmare. She was hypnotised daily, and in a few days she was quite well, both as regarded her general health, and the obstinate skin disease; and as she had no medicine nor external application, there could be no disputing that it resulted entirely from the influence of hypnotism. She has been well nearly ten months.

Case LXIII. J.C., aged forty, had been severely afflicted for eighteen months with *impetigo sparsa,* extending from a little below the knee to near the toes. He had also severe pain in the ankle joint, so that he had been disabled for work for eighteen months. I hypnotised him, when he could walk better after first operation, without his stick, than he could do immediately before with it. In a few days the improvement was very remarkable, and within a week the disease of the skin was nearly well, and very little pain in the joint. He was hypnotised almost daily till the end of the month, had no medicine, and no dressing but a little spermaceti ointment to prevent the cloth surrounding his leg from adhering to the sore; and the skin disease being now quite well, and very little pain in the ankle joint, in a few days after he was enabled to resume his work. He had undergone much treatment, under both public and private practitioners, but was becoming worse instead of better. The immediate improvement in the appearance of the cutaneous disease, as well as feelings of the patients in the two last cases, were too obvious to admit of a doubt as to the remarkable powers of hypnotism.

Locked Jaw [Tetanus]
The next cases I shall refer to are those of permanent contraction or tonic spasm. The following are interesting examples of this form of disorder, and the success of hypnotism in the treatment of them.

Case LXIV. Mr. J.O. twenty-one years of age, called on me 1st October, 1842, complaining of a pain in the left temple, a continual noise in the left ear, with occasional shoots of pain, and the hearing of that ear very imperfect. He complained also of inability to open the mouth so as to enable him to take his food comfortably, and that mastication caused great pain, so that he frequently felt compelled to decline taking his meals. Complaints had been coming on since previous Easter, and were becoming worse, notwithstanding he had been under the care of two medical men up to the day before he called on me. That day, 10th October, 1842, he could not eat breakfast but, with great difficulty, and had been compelled to take rice and milk for dinner for two days, as he could eat nothing solid. I found he could not permit the mouth to be opened more than half an inch without great pain and difficulty, and besides the dullness of hearing already referred to, I found he had also very imperfect sight of the left eye, which I tested very accurately. He had not been aware of this until I called his attention to it. I hypnotised him for about eight minutes, during which I was enabled to open the mouth till the front teeth were nearly two inches asunder, and he experienced no inconvenience from me doing so. On being aroused, all the pain in the temple was gone; he could himself separate the teeth one inch and three quarters, as accurately measured, in presence of four very intelligent gentlemen who had been present during the operation; and he could move the jaws with the most perfect freedom and without pain. The hearing was also much better, and the sight of the left eye also most remarkably improved. 2nd October, called on him again, when he stated he had been enabled to eat a good supper after he left me the night before, and to take his breakfast and dinner with perfect comfort to himself; that his hearing was much better; and the sight of both eyes as nearly as possible equal. He had had no pain in the temple since he was operated on, unless when the mouth was opened to the utmost extent, and even then it was trifling. He could now open the mouth to nearly one inch and three quarters, before being operated on today, and after the operation, to the extent of two inches, that is, the front teeth were two inches apart.

This patient called on me a few days after to be operated on a third time, and retained the improvement noted above. He was to call again if he had any relapse, but as he has not done so, I conclude he continues quite well, and it is now nearly seven months since I last saw him.

Tonic Spasm
I shall now refer to other cases of spasmodic affection, which are most interesting, as they afford us strong grounds to hope that Tetanus, Hydrophobia [i.e., rabies], and other analogous affections, may be arrested and cured by this agency.

Case LXV. A girl was seized with violent tonic spasm of the right hand and arm, and side of the face. A respectable surgeon was consulted, who ordered a blister to the nape of the neck, medicine, fomentation, and liniments to the parts affected. The symptoms became more urgent, and they sent for the surgeon again, but as he was out, and as they were much alarmed, I was consulted. The blister had been applied, but the medicines had not been used as directed. I found the hand so firmly clenched that it was impossible to open it, the arm so rigid it could not be moved; but, knowing the efficacy of my new remedy, I hypnotised her, and in two minutes, with the most perfect ease, I unlocked the hand, and removed the other spasmodic contractions, and she was instantly quite well, and has continued so ever since, now more than a year.

I shall only record one additional case, and a more remarkable or satisfactory one I think could scarcely be adduced. **I give the case as correctly recorded by the patient's father, in a letter he sent for my approval, previous to having it sent to be recorded in some periodical.** I preferred having its publication postponed, and now give it precisely in his own words.

Miss Collins
Case LXVI. Miss Collins of Newark.
> My daughter, 16 years of age, had been afflicted for six months with a rigid contraction of the muscles on the left side of the neck, to so great a degree, that it would have been impossible to insert an ordinary card between the ear and shoulder, so close was their contact; and consequently she was rapidly becoming malformed. She had had the best advice to be procured in the country, and I had taken her to London with a written statement of the treatment previously employed, and had the opinion of Sir Benjamin Brodie, who approved of what had been done, but gave no hope of speedy relief.
>
> In consequence of seeing a report of a lecture given on the subject by Mr. Braid, surgeon, St. Peter's Square, Manchester, and a letter written to that gentleman by Mr. [Herbert] Mayo of London, I went with her, by the advice of Dr. Chawner, who indeed accompanied us, and placed her under the care of Mr. Braid on

Thursday evening, the 24th March last, (1842). In less than a minute after that gentleman began to fix her attention, she was in a Mesmeric (neuro-hypnotic) slumber, and in another minute was partially cataleptic. Mr. Braid then, without awaking her, and consequently without giving her any pain, placed her head upright, which I firmly believe could not, by any possibility, have been done five minutes before, without disruption of the muscles, or the infliction of some serious injury, and I am thankful to say, it not only continues straight, but she has the perfect control over the muscles of the neck. A nervous motion of the head, to which she had been subject after her return from Manchester, has entirely ceased, and she is at present in excellent health. It is necessary to remark, that at Dr. Chawner's recommendation she was frequently watched while asleep, but not the slightest relaxation was observed in the contracted muscles.

Many respectable persons can bear testimony to the statements herein made.

(Signed)
James Collins.
Newark, 11th May, 1842.

Concluding Remarks
I have been informed that some very absurd reports have been circulated, even in the metropolis, as to my mode of operating on this patient, namely, that I had exhibited a vast display of gesticulations and hocus pocus, in order to work upon her imagination. SUCH STATEMENTS ARE UTTERLY UNTRUE, **I simply desired her to maintain a steady gaze at my lancet case, held above her eyes in the manner pointed out at [in Chapter 2] of this work, and after the eyes had been closed, and the limbs extended for about two minutes, I placed my left hand on the right side of her neck, and my right hand on the left side of her head, and, by gentle means, gave a new direction to the sensorial and muscular power, and was thus enabled by** *art,* **rather than mechanical force, in less than half a minute, to incline the head from the left to the right of the mesial plane. The muscular contraction being thus excited on the right side of the neck, in muscles which had been inactive for six months previously, was the surest and most natural mode of withdrawing the power from their antagonists, and reducing the spasm of the contracted muscles on the left side. After allowing the patient to remain two minutes supporting her head, now inclined towards the right, by her own muscular efforts, to give them power on the principle already explained, I aroused her in my usual way, by a clap of my hands.** The patient's father, and Dr. Chawner of Newark, were present the whole time, and to them I appeal as to the correctness of this statement, and in refutation of the vile, unfounded calumny above referred to.

After the lapse of a year Mr. Collins was so kind as to write, to inform me his daughter continued in perfect health, with complete control over the muscles of the neck.

I could easily adduce many more interesting cases, but trust those already recorded may be sufficient to prove that hypnotism is an important addition to our curative means, and a power well worthy of the attentive consideration of every enlightened and unprejudiced medical man.

Added Appendices
Appendix:
Letter to *The Medical Times* (26th March 1842) with Comments

[This was a footnote in the original edition of *Neurypnology*, but contains the original letter in its entirety, apart from the introductory comments re-inserted below. It was first published as "Animal Magnetism", *The Medical Times*, 26th March, 1842, vol. V., p. 308.]

In *The Medical Times* of 26th March, 1842, I published a letter on this subject, from which I make the following extracts:–

> [Sir, – According to [my] promise, I send you a report of my last lecture, which is both copious and very correct, and is quite at your service. Several important facts are referred to, both as to the causes of certain phenomena and practical result of this agency when applied as I recommend.]
>
> The supposed power of seeing with other parts of the body than the eyes, I consider is a misnomer, so far as I have yet personally witnessed. It is quite certain, however, that some patients can tell the shape of what is held at an inch and a half from the skin, on the back of the neck, crown of the head, arm, or hand, or other parts of the body, but it is from *feeling* they do so; the extremely exalted sensibility of the skin enabling them to discern the shape of the object so presented, from its tendency to emit or absorb caloric. This, however, is not *sight,* but *feeling.*
>
> In like manner I have satisfied myself and others, that patients are drawn, or induced to obey the motions of the operator, not from any peculiar inherent magnetic power in him, but from their exalted state of feeling enabling them to discern the currents of air, which they advance to, or retire from, according to their direction. This I clearly proved to be the case today, and that a patient could feel and obey, the motion of a glass funnel passed through the air at a distance of *fifteen feet.*
>
> To remove all sources of fallacy as to the extent of influence exercised by the patient herself, independently of any personal or mental influence on my part, whilst I was otherwise engaged, my daughter requested the patient to go into a room by herself, and, when alone, try whether she could hypnotise herself. In a short time, I was told the patient was found fast asleep in my drawing-room. I went to her, bandaged her eyes, and then, with the glass funnel, (which I used to avoid the chance of electric or magnetic influence being passed from my person to that of the patient) elevated, or drew up her arms, and then her whole body. I now retired fifteen feet from her, and found every time I drew the funnel *towards me,* she approached nearer, but when it was forced sharply from me, she invariably retired; and if it was moved laterally, she moved to the right or left accordingly. I now continued drawing the funnel so as to keep up the currents towards the door, and in this way, her arms being extended, and eyes bandaged, she followed me downstairs and up again, a flight of twenty-two steps, with the peculiar characteristic caution of the somnambulist. After arriving at the top of the stair, I allowed her to stand a little, and again began the drawing motion. She evidently felt the motion, and attempted to come, but could not. I now endeavoured to lead her by the hand, but found that *the legs had become cataleptiform, so that she could not move.* I now carried her into the drawing-room, and, after she was seated on a chair, awoke her. She was quite unconscious of what had happened, and could not be made to believe she had been down stairs – she said she was quite sure she could have done no such thing without falling – and to this moment believes we were only hoaxing her by saying she had had such a ramble.
>
> I had repeatedly performed this experiment with this patient and others before, with the same result in all respects but walking up and down stairs; and proved their readiness to be drawn by others equally as myself when in that state; so that I consider it quite evident to any unprejudiced person, that a patient can hypnotise himself independently of any personal influence of another; and that it is by extreme sensibility of the skin, and docility of the patients, that they are drawn after an operator, rather than by magnetic attraction; and that the power of discriminating objects held near the skin in different parts of the body, is the result of *feeling,* and *not of sight.*
>
> The moment I witnessed the attempts of a celebrated professor, *to draw a patient,* I formed my opinion of the cause – that it arose from currents of air produced by his hand, together with the extreme sensibility of the skin, and docility of the patients when in that state; and my experiments have clearly proved this, *some patients acknowledging the fact.*
>
> It may be interesting to remark, that whilst passing up and down stairs the door bell rang, which produced such a tremor through the whole frame as nearly caused the patient's fall – a fact quite in accordance with the effect of any abrupt noise on NATURAL somnambulists.

It is owing to this extreme sensibility of the skin during hypnotism, that patients may walk through a room blindfolded, without running against the furniture – the difference of temperature, or rather degree of conducting power of objects, and the resistance of the air directing them.

I have frequently illustrated this with very sensitive patients in the most beautiful and satisfactory manner, thus:– By throwing any fragrant and agreeable scent on a bare table the patients will approach, anxious to smell it, but are repelled before they come quite close to the cold table. Place a handkerchief on the table, on which place the scent, and now the patient will approach close to it, and revel in its fragrance. Remove the handkerchief, and the attractive and repulsive movements will again ensue.

This was beautifully illustrated at a private conversazione at my house lately, in the presence of several medical and other eminently scientific gentlemen. Two patients were hypnotised, when one became so enamoured of the scent of a gentleman's snuff-box as to follow him round the room. He then laid the box about eighteen inches from the edge of an uncovered table, when she advanced, her arms being extended, anxious to reach the box, but when about ten or twelve inches from it, she started back, from perceiving the impression of the cold table at that distance. She now made another attempt to approach the box, being attracted by the fragrance of its contents, but was as speedily repelled by the cold table before she approached it, and now kept bobbing over the box, much in the same manner as I have witnessed in the attempts of a hungry dog to partake of very hot food. The other patient, in passing round the table, also caught the smell of the box, and advanced from another point, and thus both kept bobbing over it, much to the amusement of all present. I now covered the table with a handkerchief, and placed the box on it, when they instantly approached close to it, and seemed to feast on its fragrance; on removing the handkerchief they withdrew, and commenced bobbing over it as at first. The former patient had never seen such experiments, or been tested in this way before.

Appendix
On Exercise & Sleep (Müller)

This subject is beautifully illustrated by Müller, at page 1410, vol. II. (Baly's translation) which I now quote.

> The excitement of the organic processes in the brain which attends an active state of the mind, gradually renders that organ incapable of maintaining the mental action, and thus induces sleep; which is to the brain what bodily fatigue is to other parts of the nervous system. The cessation or remission of mental activity during sleep, in its turn, however, affords an opportunity for the restoration of integrity to the organic conditions of the cerebrum, by which they regain their excitability. The brain, whose action is essential to the manifestation of mind, obeys, in fact, the general law which prevails over all organic phenomena – that the phenomena of life being particular states induced in the organic structures, are attended with changes in the constituent matter of these structures. Hence, the longer the action of the mind is continued, the more incapable does the brain become of supporting that action, and the more imperfectly are the mental processes performed, until at length sensations cease to be perceived, notwithstanding the impressions of external stimuli continue. This is entirely analogous to what frequently occurs during the waking state, in the case of individual sensations.

I must beg leave to take one exception to the correctness of these remarks, and that is, *moderate* exercise, I consider, instead of *exhausting,* seems rather to act as a *salutary stimulus,* and thus *strengthens* both *organ and function.* He then goes on to state, most lucidly and fairly,

> Nor merely the action of the mind, but the long continued exertion of other functions of animal life, such as the senses or muscular actions, induces the same exhaustion of the organic states of the brain, and thereby want of sleep and sleep itself; for these different systems of the body participate in the change which the organic condition of any one of them may undergo. Lastly, impairment of the normal organic state of the brain, by the circulation through it of blood charged with imperfectly assimilated nutriment, as after full meals in which spirituous drinks have been taken, also induces sleep. The narcotic medicaments act still more strongly by the change they produce in the organic composition of the sensorium. Even the increased pressure of the blood upon the brain, produced by the horizontal posture, may become the cause of sleep.

Here then is the opinion of this author in a few words. The exercise of function is attended with a change, deterioration, or wasting of the organic structure at a more rapid rate than can be repaired by the slow, but regular and persistent organic renovation continually going on in the whole system. A cessation of sentient, and mental, and muscular functions, therefore, as happens in sleep, becomes necessary to afford time for the renovation of the deteriorated organic structures of the respective organs, and of the brain in particular, which, in so eminent a degree, sympathizes and participates in the organic changes which have been induced in other organs.

Liebig's views seem confirmatory of this, where he points out the fact, that the chemical principles of those substances which act most energetically on the brain and nerves have a composition analogous to that of the substance of the brain and nerves, as in the case of the vegetable alkaloids. He believes that all the active principles which produce powerfully poisonous or medicinal effects, in minute doses, are compounds of **nitrogen**; and that those compounds, being resolved into their elements, take a share in the formation, or transformation, of brain and nervous matter.

Appendix:
On Reverie

It was certainly presuming very much on the ignorance of others for anyone to attempt so to pervert the meaning of an author, as to twist what M'Nish has written on the article "Reverie", and represent it as the basis of my theory. How does M'Nish define it? He says,

> Reverie proceeds from an unusual quiescence of the brain, and inability of the mind to direct itself strongly to any one point; it is often the prelude of sleep. There is a *defect* in the *attention* which, instead of being fixed on *one* subject, *wanders over a thousand,* and even on these is feebly and ineffectively directed.

Now this, as everyone must own, is the very *reverse* of what is induced by *my plan,* because I *rivet* the *attention to one idea,* and the eyes to *one point,* as the *primary and imperative conditions.* Then, as to another passage,

> That kind of reverie in which the mind is nearly divested of all ideas, and approximates nearly to the state of sleep, I have sometimes experienced while gazing long and intently upon a river. The thoughts seem to glide away, one by one, upon the surface of the stream, till the mind is emptied of them altogether. In this state we see the glassy volume of the water moving past us, and hear its murmur, but lose all power of fixing our attention definitively upon any subject; and either fall asleep, or are aroused by some spontaneous reaction of the mind, or by some appeal to the senses sufficiently strong to startle us from our reverie.

Now, I should have read this passage a thousand times without discovering any analogy between it and my theoretical views. They appear to me to be "wide as the poles asunder". Instead of ridding the mind of ideas "one by one, till the mind is *emptied* of them *altogether",* **I endeavour to rid the mind at *once* of all ideas but one, and to fix *that* one in the mind *even after passing into the hypnotic state.*** This is very different from what happens in the reverie referred to, in which M'Nish confesses the difficulty "of fixing our attention definitively upon *any* subject". Again, so far from a reaction of the mind being sufficient to rouse patients from the hypnotic state, as in the reverie referred to, I can only state, that **I have never seen patients deeply affected come out of it without assistance**; and I heard Lafontaine say, he had been unable to restore the Frenchman who was with him for twelve hours on one occasion, when a surgeon operated on him; and I have read the report of another, who operated on a patient at Stockport, "Charlie", according to my method, and, from having allowed him to go too far, experienced no small difficulty in rousing him, nor could he be restored to speech after much manipulation, and buffeting, and friction, till he had swallowed nearly *half a tumbler glass of neat gin.* To prevent misrepresentation, I shall quote the case as reported in the *Stockport Chronicle* of 4th February, 1842,

> To the final instance the lecturer now drew particular attention. It was that of a young man, recognised by many in the room by the familiar name of "Charlie". He was just entering upon the state of somnolence, and the attention of the audience was directed to the fact, that it was so indicated, by the different members becoming rigid. Presently his eyelids closed, and he became as though apparently under the influence of catalepsy. It was tried to make him sit down, but his whole frame was perfectly rigid, and that object could not therefore be accomplished. He was then laid on the floor, and the usual means, with cold water added, were employed in order to bring him to a state of consciousness. After a time these partially succeeded, his limbs became once more supple, and he was set in a chair, apparently conscious, though his eyelids were not yet open. He was several times requested to open them, and as often made the most vigorous efforts to do so, but was unable; at last they were opened, and it was discovered that the operation had so far influenced the entire functions of his body, that he had for a time lost the power of utterance, the muscles of the throat and tongue still remaining in a state of the most perfect rigidity. In this state, and being affected by a tremor which seized every part of his person, the patient was conducted into an ante-room, and placed before a fire, while the operator continued to rub the parts, in order to excite them to renewed action, and to restore animation. All this, however, had not the desired effect for some time, during which the patient evinced feelings of considerable surprise at his condition; but nevertheless was exceedingly lively, and made several efforts to speak, but could not. At last half a tumbler glass of neat gin was brought, the greater portion of which he drank off, and this partially restored the power of utterance, for he was afterwards able to articulate a little, and asked, though only in a whisper, for his hat; and also requested that some water might be mixed with the remaining portion of the gin. He complained also of a sense of excessive fullness of the stomach; and said, in answer to inquiries, that although not feeling cold, he was yet unable to resist the tremor which had seized him.

Was not this a beautiful illustration of the facility with which patients might be roused from this condition *"by a reaction of the mind"?* Nor was this the only case that evening, in which great difficulty had been experienced in rousing patients from the hypnotic state.

Appendix
On Monotony Inducing Sleep

[In the main body, Braid begins: 'During the course of last spring some lectures were delivered in this town to prove that the *Mesmeric phenomena* might be induced by an "undue continuance or repetition of the same sensible impression on any of the senses". Immediately after the first lecture I instituted experiments according to this plan, but very soon ascertained, that the sleep induced by this mode of operating, *unless through the eye,* was nothing more than NATURAL or common sleep, *excepting in patients who had had the impressibility stamped on them, by having been previously Mesmerised or hypnotised.* The lecturer concluded his course by stating his opinion, that he knew no sleep but natural or common sleep; and by representing that he considered the effects produced by the different modes to be the same.']

This being his belief, there could be no novelty in his views. The following was the language of Cullen, long before he was born,

> If the mind is attached to a single sensation, it is brought very nearly to the state of the total absence of impressions; or, in other words, to the state most closely bordering upon sleep; remove those stimuli which keep it employed, and sleep ensues at any time.

M'Nish also writes,

> Attention to a single sensation has the same effect (of inducing slumber). This has been exemplified in the case of all kinds of monotony, where there is a want of variety to stimulate the ideas, and keep them on the alert.

And again, M'Nish writes,

> **I have often coaxed myself to sleep by internally repeating half a dozen times any well-known rhyme. Whilst doing so the ideas must be strictly directed to this particular theme, and prevented from wandering.**

He then adds, that the great secret is to compel the mind to depart from its favourite train of thought, into which it has a tendency to run, "and address itself solely to the *verbal* repetition of what is substituted in its place"; and farther adds, "the more the mind is brought to turn upon a *single impression,* the more closely it is made to approach to the state of sleep, which is the total absence of all impressions." Willich also, some forty years ago, wrote thus,

> Sleep is promoted by tranquillity of mind, (...) by *gently and uniformly affecting one of the senses;* for instance, by music or reading; and lastly, a gentle external motion of the whole body, as by rocking or sailing.

Counting and repeating a few words have been also long and generally known and resorted to for the purpose of procuring sleep.

Let anyone read attentively the following extract from the *Medical Gazette* of February 24th, 1838, on the power of weak monotonous impressions on the senses having the power of inducing sleep, and many phenomena usually attributed to Mesmerism, and say what merit could be due to a person acquainted with the article referred to, for *recording a note to the same effects some six or eight months thereafter,* and that without having instituted a single experiment to prove the correctness of the hypothesis?

> For the other slight symptoms (others enumerated having been attributed to imagination or emotion of mind) of vapours, drowsiness, and at last natural sleep, no other cause need be sought than the tediousness and ennui of passing the hands for more or less than an hour over the most sensitive parts of the body. This is only an instance of the well-known effect of weak, monotonous impressions on the senses inducing sleep; analogous examples are found in the soothing influence of a body seen slowly vibrating, or of a distant calm scene, or the motions of the waves, or of quivering leaves; or in impressions on the sense of learning by the sound of a waterfall, the rippling of billows, the humming of insects, the low howling of the winds, the voice of a dull reader; or on the nerves of common sensation by *gentle friction of the temple or eyebrow, or any sensitive part of the body;* the rocking of a cradle, any slow and regular motion of the limbs or trunk; all these instances show that the effect of monotonous impressions on the senses is to produce, in most persons, tranquillity, or drowsiness, and ultimately sleep.

Where, then, is the great merit of anyone having recorded a note six or eight months after this was published, that these phenomena were induced by "the undue continuance and repetition of the same sensible impression"?

Appendix:
Some Hypnotic Experiments & Observations

In illustration of this [confusion caused by not attending to differences between stages of hypnotism], I may here state the following remarkable facts, which have been frequently repeated before many most competent witnesses, and of which, therefore, I consider there can be no doubt.

The first symptoms after the induction of the hypnotic state, and extending the limbs, are those of extreme excitement of all the organs of sense, sight excepted. I have ascertained by accurate measurement, that the **hearing is about twelve times more acute** than in the natural condition. Thus a patient who could not hear the tick of a watch beyond three feet when awake, could do so when hypnotised at the distance of thirty-five feet, and walk to it in a direct line, without difficulty or hesitation. Smell is in like manner, wonderfully exalted; one patient has been able to trace a rose through the air when held forty-six feet from her. May this not account for the fact of Dr. Elliotson's patient Okey, discovering the peculiar odour of patients in *articulo mortis* when she said on passing them, "there is Jack"? The tactual sensibility is so great, that the slightest touch is felt, and will call into action corresponding muscles, which will also be found to exert a most inordinate power. The sense of heat, cold, and resistance, are also exalted to that degree, as to enable the patient to feel anything *without actual contact,* in some cases at a considerable distance, (eighteen or twenty inches) if the temperature is very different from that of the body; and some will feel a breath of air from the lips, or the blast of a pair of bellows, at the distance of fifty, or even ninety feet, and bend from it, and, by making a back current, as by waving the hand or a fan, will move in the opposite direction. The patient has a tendency to *approach to, or recede from impressions, according as they are agreeable or disagreeable, either in quality or intensity.* Thus, they will approach to soft sounds, but they will recede from loud sounds, however harmonious. A discord, such as two semi-tones sounded at same time, *however soft,* will cause a sensitive patient to shudder and recede when hypnotised, although ignorant of music, and not at all disagreeably affected by such discord when awake. By allowing a little time to elapse, and the patient to be in a state of quietude, he will lapse into the opposite extreme, of rigidity and torpor of all the senses, so that he will not hear the loudest noise, nor smell the most fragrant or pungent odour; nor feel what is either hot or cold, although not only approximated to, but brought into actual contact with, the skin. He may now be pricked, or pinched, or maimed, without evincing the slightest symptom of pain or sensibility, and the limbs will remain rigidly fixed. At this stage a puff of wind directed against any organ *instantaneously* rouses it to inordinate sensibility, and the rigid muscles to a state of mobility. Thus, the patient may be unconscious of the loudest noise, but by simply causing a current of air to come against the ear, a very moderate noise will *instantly* be heard so *intensely* as to make the patient start and shiver violently, although the whole body had immediately before been rigidly cataleptiform. A rose, valerian, or asafoetida, or strongest *liquor ammonioe,* may have been held close under the nostrils without being perceived, but a puff of wind directed against the nostrils will instantly rouse the sense so much, that supposing the rose had been carried forty-six feet distant, the patient has instantly set off in pursuit of it; and even whilst the eyes were bandaged, reached it as certainly as a dog traces out game; but, as respects valerian or asafoetida, will rush *from* the unpleasant smell, with the greatest haste. The same with the sense of touch.

The remarkable fact that the whole senses may have been in the state of profound torpor, and the body in a state of rigidity, and yet by very gentle pressure over the eyeballs, the patient shall be instantly roused to the waking condition, as regards all the senses, and mobility of the head and neck, in short to all parts supplied by nerves originating above the origin of the fifth pair, and those inosculating with them, and will not be affected by simple mechanical appliance to other organs of sense, is a striking proof that there exists some remarkable connection between the state of the eyes, and condition of the brain and spinal cord during the hypnotic state.

This is also a remarkably good illustration of the propriety of Mr. Mayo's designation of the origin of the fifth pair of nerves, which he styles "the dynamic centre of the nervous system". (*The Nervous System, and its Functions,* p.27).

Another remarkable proof to the same effect is this; supposing the same state of torpor of all the senses, and rigidity of the body and limbs to exist, a puff of air, or gentle pressure against ONE eye will restore sight to *that eye,* and sense and mobility to *one half of the body* – the same side as the eye operated on – but will leave the other eye insensible, and the other half of the body rigid and torpid as before. Neither hearing nor smell, however, are restored in this case to either side. Thus, by one mode of acting through the eye, we reduce the patient to a state of hemiplegia, by the other to that of paraplegia, as regards both sense and motion. In many cases, when the patient has been hypnotised by looking sideways, this gives a tendency to the body to turn round in that direction when asleep.

It seemed puzzling, that by acting on one eye, both sense and motion could be communicated to the *same* side of the body, seeing the motor influence is communicated from the *opposite hemisphere of the brain.* It has occurred to me that the partial decussation of the optic nerves may account for this, and that this partial decussation may be for the express purpose of perfecting the union of sensation and motion through the eyes, "on which we lean as on crutches"; thus enabling us to balance ourselves so much more perfectly than we could otherwise have done.

There is another most remarkable circumstance, that whilst the patient is in the state of torpor and rigidity, we may pass powerful [electric] shocks of the galvanic battery through the arms, so as to cause violent contortions of them, without his evincing the slightest symptom of perceiving the shocks, either by movement of the head or neck, or expression of the countenance. On partially arousing the head and neck, as by gentle pressure on the eyes, or passing a current of air against the face, the same shocks *will* be felt, as evinced by the movements of the head and neck, the contortions of the face, and the whine, moan, or scream of the patient. All this may happen, as I have witnessed innumerable times, and the patient be altogether unconscious of it when roused from the hypnotic condition.

Moreover, whilst the patient is in the condition to be unconscious of the shock passed through the arms whilst a rod is placed in each hand, if one of the rods is applied to any part of the head, or neck, or face, in short, to any part, which is set at liberty by acting on *both eyes,* as formerly referred to, he will instantly manifest symptoms of feeling a shock, though it be much less powerful than that which had failed to produce any sensation or consciousness when passed through both arms. This might readily be accounted for on the principle of the circuit being shortened, and also by one of the rods being nearer the centre of the sensorium; but that it depends on something else is apparent from the following fact. Without moving the rod placed on the neck, head, or face, carry the other rod *from the hand,* to any other part of the head, neck, or face, and all evidence of feeling will disappear, *unless the power of the galvanic current is increased.*

Analogous to this is another most puzzling phenomenon: The brain being in a state of torpor, the limbs rigid, and the skin insensible to pricking, pinching, heat or cold, by gently pressing the point of one or two fingers against the back of the hand, or any other part of the extremity, the rigidity will very speedily give place to mobility, and quivering of the arm, hand, and fingers, and which is greatly increased by pressing another finger against the neck, head, or face. Indeed, in the latter case, the commotion of the whole body is as violent in some patients as from shocks of the galvanic battery. By placing BOTH fingers on any part of the head, face, or neck, the commotion almost, or entirely ceases. By pinching the skin of the hand or arm with one finger, and the skin of the neck or face with the other, no effect is produced. Pressure, made with insulating rods, glass, or sealing wax, is followed by the same phenomena as when done by the points of the fingers. The flat hand applied has very little effect. The pressure being made against both hands, the arms are contorted, and if the head is partially dehypnotised, the patient will complain of pins running into the fingers, especially if one point of contact is the hand, and the other the face or head. These phenomena do not occur whilst the skin remains sensible to pricking or pinching.

Moreover, during the state of cataleptiform rigidity, the circulation becomes greatly accelerated, in many cases it has more than double the natural velocity; and may be brought down to the natural standard, in most cases in less than a minute, by reducing the cataleptiform condition. It is also found, that it may be kept at any intermediate condition between these two extremes, according to the manipulations used; and that the blood is circulated with less *force* (the pulse being always contracted) in the *rigid limbs,* and sent in correspondingly greater quantity and force into those parts which are not directly subjected to the pressure of rigid muscles. It is also important to note, that by acting on both eyes in the manner required to induce the state of paraplegia, as already explained, the force and frequency of the heart's action may be as speedily and perceptibly diminished, as the action of a steam engine by turning off the steam.

By again fixing the eyes, its former force and velocity will be almost as speedily restored, as can be satisfactorily proved to anyone who keeps his ear applied to the chest during these experiments. The amount of change in the pulse, by acting on the two eyes, and thus liberating the organs of special sense, and the head and neck, is about 60 per cent of the actual rise of the pulse when at the maximum above the ordinary velocity of the circulation. We might therefore, I think, *a priori,* infer that in this new condition of the nervous system we have acquired an important power to act with.

N.B. It is to be observed, that owing to the extreme acuteness of hearing during the first stage of hypnotism, it is extremely apt to mislead the operator, or those who do not understand this fact, during operations on the acuteness of the other senses, such as smell, currents of air, and heat and cold. To avoid such mistakes, therefore, it is best to allow the hearing to disappear, by which time all the other senses will have gone to rest, with the exception of the susceptibility to be affected by a current of air. I allow all the senses to become dormant, and then rouse only the one I wish to exhibit in the state of exalted function, when operating carefully.

Appendix
On Psycho-Physical Dualism

Some time after I had written the above, I had the satisfaction to meet with a somewhat analogous illustration from the pen of the late celebrated Dr. John Armstrong, which I now quote from his work on *Fever,* p. 418:–

> It will have been perceived, that I consider insanity as the effect of some disorder in the circulation, whether produced by agencies of a corporeal or mental nature. It might be shown by familiar facts, that the brain is the principal organ through which the operations of the mind are performed; and it does not, as many have supposed, necessarily involve the doctrine of materialism to affirm, that certain disorders of that organ are capable of disturbing those operations. If the most skilful musician in the world were placed before an unstrung or broken instrument, he could not produce the harmony which he was accustomed to do when that instrument was perfect, nay, on the contrary, the sounds would be discordant; and yet it would be manifestly most illogical to conclude, from such an effect, that the powers of the musician were impaired, since they merely appeared to be so from the imperfection of the instrument. Now what the instrument is to the musician, the brain may be to the mind, for ought we know to the contrary; and to pursue the figure, as the musician has an existence distinct from that of the instrument, so the mind may have an existence distinct from that of the brain; for in truth we have no proof whatever of mind being a property dependent upon any arrangement of matter. We perceive, indeed, the properties of matter wonderfully modified in the various things of the universe, which strike our senses with the force of their sublimity or beauty; but in all these we recognise certain radical and common properties, that bear no conceivable relation to those mysterious capacities of thought and of feeling, referable to that something which, to designate and distinguish from matter, we term mind. In this way, I conceive, the common sense of mankind has made the distinction which every where obtains between mind and matter, for it is natural to conclude, that the essence of mind may be distinct from the essence of matter, as the operations of the one are so distinct from the properties of the other. But when we say that mind is immaterial, we only mean, that it has not the properties of matter; for the consciousness which informs us of the operations, does not reveal the abstract nature of mind, neither do the properties reveal the essence of matter. When anyone, therefore, asserts the materiality of mind, he presupposes, that the phenomena of matter clearly show the real cause of mind, which, as they do not, he unphilosophically places his argument on an assumption. And his ground of reasoning is equally gratuitous, when he contends that mind is an attribute of matter, because it is never known to operate but in conjunction with matter, for though this connection is continually displayed, yet we have no direct proof of its being necessary.

In like manner, Mr. Herbert Mayo, in the introduction to his late work on *The Nervous System and its Functions* [1842], writes thus:–

> Life is a force so contrived and used, as to qualify the materials of the inert world for a temporary union with consciousness – a means how mind may enter into such relations with matter, that it may have its being and part in physical nature, and its faculties developed, and its capabilities and tendencies drawn out and proved (for whatever ulterior purpose) in subjection to, and in harmony with, her laws.
>
> As we imagine the Supreme Mind to be ubiquitous, infinite, controlling, but uncontrolled by matter, so in contrast with these attributes we conceive the finite mind to be bound down to place, and to be dependent on a certain arrangement of matter, for its manifestation, each power displayed as the property of a tissue, each agency as the function of an organ.
>
> These views do not lead to materialism. For one cannot disjoin the physiology or the nervous system from mental philosophy, nor investigate the play of its organs without attending to the mind itself. And if equal consideration is given to the two classes of phenomena, it is impossible (so at least it appears to myself) to avoid the conviction, that they are essentially independent the one of the other, and belong to distinct essences; and that the consciousness of personal being, is not a mode of material existence, nor physical impenetrability an attribute of that which feels and thinks.

Appendix:
Debate on Mesmeric Anaesthesia

It would perhaps be difficult to adduce a stronger proof of the extent to which prejudice may overcloud the brightest intellects, and render them incompetent to do justice to the subject they would investigate, than that which was presented at a late meeting of the Medico-Chirurgical Society of London, when a debate took place after the reading of Mr. Ward's case of amputation of the leg during Mesmeric sleep. As I am not an animal magnetizer, nor personally acquainted with any of the parties referred to, any remarks I am about to make are of course uninfluenced either by pique or prejudice.

The operation referred to was said to have taken place in a public hospital; in the presence of medical, and also non-medical witnesses. The patient is alleged to have exhibited no manifestation of feeling pain, as far as his countenance could be taken as a correct index, and there was no movement of the limbs or body; and after the operation he is said to have declared that he did not feel any *pain*, but had heard "a grunching", which it has been inferred was the noise of the sawing of the bone; and it was also admitted he had groaned during the time he was under the operation.

How was this announcement met? First, it was questioned whether the man was not a person of *little* or *no feeling* at *any* time, because *other* patients had been known, whilst wide awake, who were very insensible to pain. But had not the patient, in this case, been declared to have been suffering so much pain from his knee, that he had been unable to sleep, and that his health was so much impaired by his suffering as to render amputation of the leg indispensable? Nay, had it not been set forth, that the pain of his leg had been greatly diminished, and his sleep restored, and his health greatly improved, after he was Mesmerised, *preparatory to the operation,* which he had consented to undergo whilst in that state; and yet, that after he had been asleep, and considered in a fit state for being operated on, the mere movement of the joint, whilst drawing him to the edge of the bed, was followed by so *much pain* as *to awake him.* Was this any proof of his being a person devoid of feeling?

Then it is held, that as he *heard*, as it is presumed he did, the *sawing* of *the bone,* he must have *felt* the *cutting of the skin and soft parts.* It is thus assumed that it is impossible for a person to hear, and be in the state *not to feel inflictions on the limbs at same time.* It is well-known, however, that disease of the trunks of the sentient nerves, or of the spinal cord, may induce such a state, independently of any lesion of the brain. But then, say others, had he *not felt* when the *principal nerve was irritated,* the *other leg* must have been convulsed. This is assuming, that the speakers *fully* knew every law which *has* been known, or *ever shall* be known of the nervous system, in *every possible condition,* which is rather a bold position to assume, and what few who have studied the subject will be disposed to accord even to the gifted individuals referred to. Others assume the non-expression of feeling was a mere matter of stoicism, and the general inference to be deduced from the whole harangues of these parties is, that the whole was a piece of collusion and deception. Had the parties intended collusion and deception, would they have admitted that the patient heard the sawing of the bone, or groaned or moaned during the operation? One gentleman, the learned editor of a medical journal, I think, admitted he was bound to believe the testimony of those who had brought the case forward, but frankly avowed, that for his own part, "he could not have believed it, although he had seen it himself". When a man has attained to this state of prejudice and incredulity, of course, it would be idle to adduce to him either experiment or argument.

I would beg respectfully to ask, had the mind of any of these gentlemen never entertained the possibility of a patient, long accustomed to severe pain, moaning from habit, whilst free from pain at the moment; or even feeling pain, and manifesting the same by sensible signs *during sleep,* and yet being quite unconscious of it when he awoke? Do we never meet with similar results in consequence of accidents, in the course of disease, or as the effects of overdoses of narcotics? That such is the case during the artificial sleep induced by the methods I have pointed out in this treatise, I am quite certain. I am equally certain that the sensibility to pricking, and pinching, and maiming the rigid limbs, is gone, some time *before* hearing disappears. Even a piece of paper may be inserted, and retained under the eyelids, without the slightest inconvenience, not even inducing nictitation [winking of the eyelid]. In short, I am quite certain that a patient may be sufficiently sensible to hearing to enable him to answer questions, whilst unconscious of pricking, pinching, or strong shocks of galvanism passed through the arms, and that even when roused sufficiently to give expression to feeling such inflictions, if allowed to remain quiet a little afterwards, so as to fall into the profound state again, that he may have lost all recollection of such inflictions when roused and fully awake.

From the circumstance of the patient having heard, as it is alleged he did, the sawing of the bone, I am of opinion the operation was commenced sooner than it *should* have been; and I think it very probable that the moaning referred to might have arisen from a slight feeling of pain, but not sufficient to arouse the patient, or to impress him sufficiently to enable him to remember it when awake.

In conclusion, from the numerous opportunities I have enjoyed of witnessing analogous results, in the course of my operations in Neuro-Hypnotism, if I may venture to give an opinion in this matter, I have no hesitation in expressing my thorough conviction that Mr. Topham, Mr. Ward, and the patient, have all spoken and represented the case with the utmost good faith and candour.

To those who wish to stifle investigation, and hold we ought to rest satisfied with the decision of the French Commission, I beg to remark, that a commission of the same learned body was appointed to investigate and to report on Harvey's discovery of the circulation of the blood, and that this most important discovery was rejected by them as a fallacy. Did their decision alter the laws of nature, or prevent the ultimate triumph of our immortal countryman? And when so much in error while investigating the more apparent and demonstrable one of the circulation of the blood, is it not quite as likely that they may have been mistaken in their decision on the still more abstruse and subtle subject of the laws and distribution of the nervous influence?

It is matter of history, in respect to the profession in our own country, that there was not a medical man in England, who had attained forty years of age, who would believe in the truth of Harvey's discovery. Is it to be wondered at, then, that Hypnotism should meet with opposition at the present time?

To conclude these remarks in respect to this operation: the fact that patients have been known, in some few instances, from natural causes which were not understood, to have undergone severe surgical operations without any sense of pain, instead of militating against the truth of the insensibility of the patient whose limb was amputated during the nervous sleep, tends directly to confirm it; for if such a remarkable state can exist from some accidental circumstances not understood, there is no reason why a similar condition may not be induced by artificial means.

Appendix:
A Neurological Theory of Hypnotic Catalepsy

[Braid hypothesises that hypnotic catalepsy differs from normal voluntary muscular contraction in being controlled by the ganglionic system of nerves, i.e., the *autonomic* nervous system. Focused attention and other factors in hypnosis are capable of gradually bringing on a powerful muscular contraction which does not seem to cause fatigue as quickly as voluntary effort.]

In reference to the cataleptiform condition, I beg leave to offer the following remarks *merely by way of conjecture,* and with the hope that they may excite others to direct their attention to the investigation.

Muscular contraction or motion is voluntary or involuntary. The voluntary arises from a mandate of the mind, proceeding from the brain, and effecting contraction or shortening of the muscular fibres; the involuntary, or reflex, from irritation conveyed to the spinal cord, producing a like result, and may be excited by tickling, pricking, or pinching the skin of the extremities of a decapitated or pithed animal [i.e., with a severed spinal cord]. It appears to me, however, that much of the efficiency and tendency to muscular contraction is dependent on another cause, namely, the state of *tone* or *tension* of the muscles when considered to be in a state of quiescence; and this state of tone I consider depends on the ganglionic or organic system of nerves. Supposing, from deficiency of this, the muscular system is relaxed, a morbid tendency to reflex action will be induced, as a musical string will be more easily excited to vibrate if *moderately* tight, than if drawn *very tense*. It will also render muscular effort less efficient and certain, because part of the muscular contraction, which would have been efficient as available force or motion, will be expended in bringing up the muscular structure to that state which ought to have been its *normal condition* of tension or tone. [In other words, if the resting level of muscle tone is too low, more effort will be required to initiate movement.]

On the other hand, supposing the organic system has been extremely active, and rendered the muscular *tone abnormally great,* it will produce the very reverse effect of that just referred to. It will not only offer resistance to reflex motion, but also to *voluntary* motion; and, if carried to a certain extent, may render the parts fixed and rigid, from the ganglionic system overpowering the cerebro-spinal system.

That this is not mere hypothesis seems to me to be in some degree proved, by the result of operations referred to in my paper in the *Edinburgh Medical and Surgical Journal* for October, 1841, where muscles which had been rigidly contracted, and had lost all power of motion, had motion restored by dividing the tendons, and allowing a new portion to grow between the divided ends, thus elongating the muscles; and, in other cases, where there was paralysis *from relaxation,* power was regained by *cutting out a portion of tendon,* bringing the divided ends together, and ensuring their adhesion, and thereby shortening the muscles, and giving them artificially that tone or tension, the want of which I considered was the great cause of the continuance of the paralysis. **It therefore appears to me, that during the hypnotic state there is a complete inversion of the ordinary condition, and that the force of the ganglionic system becomes predominant, instead of being, as in the ordinary condition, only subordinate.** [Muscles therefore being contracted or relaxed due to an involuntary, and effortless, neurological mechanism.]

Another argument in favour of this view is the well-known fact, that all voluntary motion, or reflex muscular action, speedily exhausts the powers, and renders the subject unable to continue such efforts, and fatigued in consequence of them. Voluntary effort also is *strongest at first,* and gradually becomes weaker. The functions of the organic system of nerves, on the contrary, are more equable and persistent in their nature; and, although they may be influenced in some degree as to the activity of their functions, by directing attention in a particular manner – as the secretion of saliva by thinking of food, the secretion of milk by the nurse thinking of her child, *etc.* – still they cannot be said to be under voluntary control in the same direct manner and degree as muscular motion. **The cataleptiform state induced by Hypnotism comes on gradually. For some time voluntary power predominates; but at length the involuntary rigidity, or organic tonicity gains the ascendency; and, although persisted in for a great length of time, is followed by no exhaustion or fatigue; on the contrary, so far as I have carried the experiments, the whole functions seem to be invigorated by the continuance of this condition.**

Appendix:
'Excerpts from Report on British Association Meeting'

[This is an excerpt from a report from the *Manchester Times* on a conversazione with members of the British Association in Manchester which took place on 29th June 1842. Braid seems to say in the Introduction to *Neurypnology* that he delivered a paper entitled "Practical Essay on the Curative Agency of Neuro-Hypnotism", at this event. He also states that he exhibited patients, including Sarah Ann Mellor (Case XIX), Thomas Morris (Case XXI), and Samuel Evans (Case XVII).]

A beautifully contrived experiment was here put in practice by Mr. Clarke, and Mr. Townend, to test the truth of the phenomena. Mr. Braid had drawn their attention to the wonderful exaltation of the sense of smell. A rose had been held before the patient, the scent of which she had followed about the platform in every direction with the most excessive eagerness – now standing on tiptoe to reach it when held aloft, anon bending herself forward with the most graceful ease, till her face came almost in contact with the floor – now darting after it across the platform (notwithstanding that her eyes were bandaged) with unerring aim as to the direction in which it was moved – or throwing herself into the most fantastic attitudes, but always with surprising ease, to catch its fragrance when moved merely round her person in tantalizing play. At length she no longer followed it, and Mr. Braid now explained that the sense of smell had entirely gone, and could only be renewed by a current of air across the nostrils. Mr. Clarke here motioned Mr. Townend to go across the platform, which he did very softly, and Mr. Clarke then threw the rose to him, a distance probably of from four to five yards. Mr. Clarke having thus taken the precaution to guard against the suspicion of collusion or trick, himself passed a current of air, across the nostrils of the patient, so as to again exalt the sensibility of the organ. She now moved forward as though in search of some object that had escaped her, and was advancing in front of the stage, which was not exactly in the direction the rose was thrown, when suddenly her limbs and entire body shook with a tremulous motion, and she stooped slightly, and evinced the utmost terror. Mr. Braid explained that this was occasioned by the rattling of a carriage over the pavement under the window partly, and partly by a feeling of insecurity, arising from the boards on which she stood being limber and yielding considerably to the foot. When the noise of the carriage had ceased, she turned her face about till it pointed in the direction where Mr. Townend stood, when, though he held the rose at a distance of three yards from her, she evidently caught the scent, and darted towards it with unerring precision, and appeared almost to revel with delight in its fragrance. A sudden burst of applause from the audience, quick as thought, dissipated the charm; and she stood aghast, apparently in an agony of terror. Mr. —— laughed, and attempted to convey to a small circle around him the impression that all this was feigned, but the attempt was disregarded. In the very front of the company, and amongst those most narrowly watching the experiments, were the Dean of Manchester, the Rev. C.D. Wray, the Rev. N.W. Gibson, the Rev. H. Ethelston, Colonel Wemyss, and a number of others whom we might mention, including several surgeons, who were capable of forming an opinion of their own, and we heard from several of them expressions at once of surprise at the phenomena, and of conviction that they were real. In fact, it was the conviction of common sense, since it would have been far more wonderful as a piece of trickery than as Mr. Braid accounts for it. Every one must have felt that it was impossible for any person in a natural state to follow a flower about the stage blindfolded, (supposing the patient was awake,) passed about as it was from hand to hand backwards and forwards, with such ease, certainty, and rapidity; but taking Mr. Braid's solution of the difficulty, that the senses are unnaturally exalted, the mystery is at an end. The only thing extraordinary that then remains is that such an agency should not before have been discovered.

"On Neuro-Hypnotism":
Letter to *The Medical Times* (1842)

> Braid wrote this letter on 4th July 1842 and published it in *The Medical Times*, 1842, No. 146, vol. 6, just a few weeks after publishing his pamphlet on *Satanic Agency*, etc. It may be the first time he uses the term hypnotism in a medical publication, although the term had already been employed in defence of his views in the former booklet and probably in his various lectures, and unpublished papers. It was written following a public *conversazione* delivered on 29th June 1842 to members of the British Association, after the same organisation had refused to permit an official presentation of Braid's report on Neuro-Hypnotism.

To the Editor of *The Medical Times*.

Sir,

I send you a copy of the *Manchester Times*, containing a pretty correct and full report of proceedings of the Medical Section of the British Association in reference to an essay I offered to read to them, on the curative agency of neuro-hypnotism, as I practise it.[141] I offered to produce patients, whose cases were referred to that they might have an opportunity of judging facts for themselves, free from all partiality, or bias of me, as an operator. They were pleased to reject the essay as unsuitable, although many of the cases referred to had been speedily cured by this agency, after resisting the best endeavours of what I have no doubt, on the old plan, was orthodox treatment, by the very gentlemen who pronounced the paper explaining this new and successful mode, as unsuitable for their consideration. As I know you are liberal enough to encourage and foster new and particularly useful discoveries, I beg briefly to state to the profession generally, through your pages, two cases which occurred to me last Saturday.

A middle-aged lady [Miss Anne Atkinson, reported subsequently in *Neurypnology*] had a severe catarrhal affection in January, 1838. In ten or twelve days after this attack she entirely lost her voice, so that she could only speak in a whisper, or occasionally in a scream, ever since. She had undergone most judicious treatment, under able medical men, including one of our most distinguished London surgeons. The treatment had embraced galvanism and electro-magnetism. Some time ago she consulted me by letter, being desirous of not undertaking so long a journey unless with the prospect of benefit, and by this time she had given up all hopes of a cure. My answer was this:–

> If, as seems to be the opinion of most of the professional gentlemen consulted, your loss of voice is owing to exhaustion of the nervous energy of the vocal nerves, and not from positive destruction of any portion of them, I consider my mode of operating likely to be very speedily successful. On the other hand, if there is a positive destruction of nervous substance, with loss of continuity of the principal trunk of the nerve, it will alter the chances very materially. However, as this cannot be positively known without trial, and as the extraordinary power we possess of rousing nervous energy may be sufficient to enable the functions to be restored with a state of nerve which could not be of service under any other agency, I should decidedly give it as my opinion that it ought to be tried, as no risk can attach to the trial; and a week or two at most will be all the time required for giving it a fair trial.

In accordance with this advice the patient called on me last Tuesday evening, when she could only speak in a low whisper, as already named. I hypnotised her for a few minutes, but without improvement; again next day and on Thursday and Friday twice, but still unable to speak; after carrying it a little farther on Saturday she could speak pretty well, and by next evening as well as at any period of her life.

Same day, a gentleman sixty-five years of age, who had for a year and a half been blind of right eye and weak in right leg and arm, supervening on a paralytic seizure, consulted me. He could not discern a lighted candle with the right eye. In the presence of his surgeon, his daughter, and two very intelligent friends, who came along with him, he was hypnotised for eight minutes, and when aroused he could not only see light, but discern my fingers with the right eye, could see much better with the left than before the operation, and felt much stronger in his arm and leg. He has been with me again yesterday and to-day, and is still better.

Neither of these patients had this operation carried beyond the first degree [the initial, or "conscious" stage of hypnotism], and were quite conscious all the while.

I would ask, is such an agency as this unsuitable for professional investigation? I am sure you will

---

[141] [Braid's "rejected essay", entitled 'Practical Essay on the Curative Agency of Neuro-Hypnotism'.]

be liberal enough to think otherwise, and by recording these cases, which have occurred since my conversazione to the members of the British Association, who honoured me with their company last Wednesday, you will much oblige me.

I shall send you some additional cases shortly, in the hope that they may induce others to follow out this interesting inquiry, and aid in working out the difficult problem of the *modus operandi* by which the effects are produced.

I am, Sir, your most obedient,

James Braid.

3 St. Peter's Square.
July 4th, 1842.

"The Discovery of Hypnotism":
"Satanic Agency & Mesmerism" Reviewed (1842)

Editor's Preface
Donald Robertson

Dr. McNeile, an Irishman by birth, was one of the most popular Anglican preachers in the country at the time of delivering a scathing attack upon Braid, in which he appears to accuse him of deceiving his patients, and even of doing the work of Satan.

The sermon was given on Sunday 10th April 1842 at St. Jude's Church in Liverpool and reported in the regional newspapers. Braid immediately wrote to McNeile responding to the accusations, but received no reply. He then held a public lecture on April 21st 1842, in response to the sermon, to which he formally invited McNeile, but he did not attend. In fact, McNeile responded by publishing the text of his original sermon in his *Penny Pulpit* review. Frustrated, Braid's hand was forced and he rushed into print on 4th June 1842 with his first publication on hypnotism. Though he had previously penned some short articles, he had this "open letter" printed himself and distributed as a twelve-page booklet.

The following pamphlet was addressed by Braid to McNeile as a defence, equally acerbic in places, against what he saw as an outrageous defamation of his character. McNeile's public attacks were perceived by Braid as posing a serious threat to his professional standing as a surgeon, and of considerable offence to him personally as a Christian, and presumably also to his family. Braid took similar action to defend himself throughout his career, most notably in 1852, responding to a publication by Colquhoun containing apparent insinuations of *atheism*.

In 1955, Dr. F.A. Volgyesi published a copy of the text in *The British Journal of Medical Hypnotism* (vol. 7, no. 1, Autumn 1955). Volgyesi states that Wilhelm Preyer, who published a German edition of Braid's works, had travelled to Britain in 1881 and met with Braid's family, but was unable to locate a copy of this booklet. It seems that the contents were lost until Volgyesi ("under romantic circumstances") stumbled across an original copy of the missing work, and a copy of another rare work by Braid, *The Physiology of Fascination* (1855). Volgyesi states with surprise that, at the time, he was unable to locate *"Satanic Agency and Mesmerism" Reviewed* in several major British Libraries, including the British Library. Two additional copies were finally located in the Library of the Royal Society of Medicine and Manchester Reference Library. However, we undoubtedly owe it to Volgyesi's research that the booklet found its way back into print once again in the 1950s, over a century after Braid had written it.

This document required few changes. Comments and section headings have been added in square brackets. Some of the longer quotations have been indented for readability, and key sections have been set in bold type.

"Satanic Agency and Mesmerism" Reviewed

in a letter to the Rev. H. McNeile, A.M.
of Liverpool
in reply to a Sermon preached by him in St. Jude's Church,
Liverpool, on Sunday April 10th 1842

To the Reverend Hugh McNeile, A.M.

Reverend Sir,

[McNeile Accuses Braid of Satanism & Deceit]

I have read in the newspapers a report of a Sermon on the subject of Mesmerism which you are alleged to have delivered in St. Jude's Church, Liverpool, on the evening of Sunday, the 10th of April last. In that Sermon you are pleased to ascribe the various phenomena exhibited in certain lectures then recently delivered or in course of delivery, in Liverpool, on the subject of animal magnetism and Mesmerism, to Satanic Agency, and to brand the lecturers as necromancers, and with other terms characterised neither by the gentle spirit of that Master whose precepts you profess to inculcate, nor even by the ordinary dictates of gentlemanly courtesy. You are pleased farther, in that Sermon, to refer to myself in the following terms:- "Or the other who is in the town at this time, of whom I have read something, but whose name I forget at this moment" and to include me in the charge of dishonesty which you have preferred against those who refuse to come forward and state the laws of nature by the uniform action of which this thing (Mesmerism) is done; and also as being one of those who confine themselves to experiments in a corner, upon their own servants, or upon females hired for the purpose.

Had you been content with the oral delivery of the Sermon which contained these attacks upon myself, I should have been satisfied with my own reply as given in the lecture delivered by me in Liverpool on the 21st of April; but as you have thought proper to publish that Sermon, without, as it appears to me, the slightest modification of your strictures, notwithstanding the subsequent opportunity which I afforded you of ascertaining their utter groundlessness, I consider that I have no course left for the proper vindication of my professional character, other than that of adopting the same medium for giving publicity to my statements which you have yourself adopted.

Without pausing to inquire into the motives which could have induced you, in this instance, to abandon the sacerdotal office for the discussion of simple physiological questions from your pulpit (in which discussion, I may venture to remark, you have displayed a degree of ignorance of mental as well as medical philosophy which can hardly be credited of any man of education) I proceed at once to the main subject of this letter.

On perusing the report referred to I was inclined to exercise towards your proceeding that charity "which thinketh no evil". I was inclined on that occasion, as I am in all cases, to adopt the most charitable view which could be taken, as to the motives of action which swayed you; and I thereupon addressed you a letter, accompanied by a copy of the *Macclesfield Courier*, containing an ample report of a lecture which I delivered, a few days before in which I explained the nature and causes of the phenomena on physiological and psychological principles, proving, from the uniform success of my mode of operating, that the whole arose from a law of the animal economy which had not hitherto been found out. I referred to what has been done in this respect in the case of strangers, who have presented of themselves to be operated upon, at my lectures; some from mere curiosity – others to test the accuracy of my statements, and many others with the view of benefiting from the application of this new agency to cure diseases from which they have suffered much and long, in defiance of all other remedies which had been tried. I also appealed to the value of this agency from its success incurring such cases; and concluded by respectfully inviting you to attend my next lecture, for which I enclosed a free admission ticket, at which lecture you were to have an opportunity of testing the accuracy of what I have stated. What has been your conduct in this respect? First, you never had the courtesy to acknowledge the receipt of my letter either by note or verbally; nor to acknowledge it by attending the lecture; and finally, the face of all the evidence I had thus adduced, you publish, or suffer to be published, with your sanction, the said Sermon, which contains a number of statements which are utterly untrue, and most offensive and injurious to me as a professional man. There might have been some shadow of excuse for this when you could plead ignorance; but after the documentary evidence with which I had personally furnished you, it is altogether without excuse.

[Braid's Statement on his Original Position]

I shall give an extract or two from this report referred to in proof of this:–

> The various theories at present entertained regarding the phenomena of Mesmerism may be arranged thus:

First, those who believe them to be owing entirely to a system of collusion and delusion; and a great majority of society may be ranked under this head.

Second, those who believe them to be real phenomena, but produced solely by imagination, sympathy and imitation.

Third, the animal magnetists, or those who believe in some magnetic medium set in motion as the exciting cause of the Mesmeric phenomena.

Fourth, those who have adopted my views, that the phenomena are solely attributable to a peculiar physiological state of the brain and spinal cord.

In answer to the first, or those who believe the whole to be a system of collusion and delusion – or in plain terms, a piece of deception – the UNIFORM and general success of the results by my method must be sufficient to prove that the Mesmeric phenomena are not "humbug", [as Braid's colleague Mr. Wilson had said at the lecture of Lafontaine] but real phenomena. In answer to the second I have to state that I by no means deny that imagination, sympathy or imitation, are capable of producing the phenomena; that I believe they do so in many cases, especially in cases where the impressibility has been determined by operating as I direct, and may heighten their effects in others; but my experiments clearly prove that they may be induced and are generally induced in the first instance, independently of any such agency. In answer to the third I have to state that I consider the theory of the animal magnetists as a gratuitous assumption, unsupported by fact and that it is far more reasonable to suppose that an exaltation of function in natural organs of sense is the cause of certain remarkable phenomena and a depression of them the cause of others, than that they arise from a transposition of the senses [i.e., through ESP], or are induced by a silent act of the will of another [i.e. through a kind of telepathic influence]. We know the exercise of the will is not adequate to remove sensibility to pain and hearing in our own bodies; and would it not be passing strange if it could exercise a greater effect on the bodies of others, whilst inoperative in our own?[142]

I shall merely add that my experiments go to prove that it is a law in the animal economy [i.e., a law of human physiology] that by the continued fixation of the mental and visual eye on any object in itself not of an exciting nature, with absolute repose of body and general quietude, they become wearied; and provided the patients rather favour than resist the feeling of stupor which they feel creeping over them during such experiment, a state of somnolency is induced, and that peculiar state of brain, and mobility of the nervous system, which render the patient liable to be directed so as to manifest the Mesmeric phenomena. I consider it not so much the optic as the motor and sympathetic nerves and the mind through which the impression is made. Such is the position I assume; and I feel so thoroughly convinced that it is a law of the animal economy that such effects should follow such conditions of mind and body that I fear not to state as my deliberate opinion that this is a fact which cannot be controverted.

I have already explained my theory to a certain extent, namely that the continued effort of the will to rivet the attention to one idea, exhausts the mind; that the continuance of the same impression on the retina exhausts the optic nerve, and that the constant effort of the muscles of the eyes and eyelids, to maintain the fixed stare quickly exhausts their irritability and tone; that the general quiet of body and suppressed respiration which take place during such operation, tend to diminish the force and frequency of the heart's action; and that the result of the whole is a rapid exhaustion of the sensorium [i.e., sense organs] and the nervous system which is reflected in the heart and lungs; and a feeling of giddiness with light tendency to syncopy [faintness], and a feeling of somnolency [drowsiness] ensue; and thus and then the mind slips out of gear.

I must beg, however, that it be particularly understood that I by no means hold up this agency as a universal remedy. Whoever talks of a universal remedy, I consider must either be a fool or a knave; for as diseases arise from totally opposite pathological conditions, all rational treatment ought to be varied accordingly. I must also warn the ignorant against tampering with such a powerful agency. It is powerful either for good or for evil according as it is managed and judiciously applied. It is capable of rapidly curing many diseases for which, hitherto, we knew no remedy; but none but a professional man, well versed in anatomy, physiology and pathology is competent to apply it with general advantage to the patient, or credit to himself, or the agency he employs. My experiments, moreover, open up to us a field of inquiry equally interesting as regards the government of mind as of matter.[143]

[Braid Defends Himself]

Now, Sir, in the face of all this evidence to the contrary, with what propriety could you publish the following remarks:-

It belongs to philosophers who are honest men and who make any discovery of this kind, to state the uniform action. But this is not done at present; we hear of these experiments, but we hear nothing of a scientific statement of the laws on which they proceed.

---

[142] [Braid refers to an argument repeated elsewhere, that there are obvious limits to the scope of mere willpower alone within one's own body, and therefore that it seems a priori unlikely that a person lacking complete conscious control over their own physiology, should be able to influence the bodies of others, at a distance, by sheer willpower alone.]

[143] [This is perhaps an excerpt from Braid's "rejected essay", entitled 'Practical Essay on the Curative Agency of Neuro-Hypnotism'.]

In this paragraph you would brand me as being dishonest for not stating the nature or uniformity of its action, although I had most unequivocally stated that my mode of operating, from its uniform action, proved it to be a law of the animal economy that certain effects shall follow certain compliances, mentally and bodily. And moreover, in the face of the elaborate details into which I had entered as to the scientific explanation of the laws on which they proceed – you publish your discourse flatly denying I have done any such thing. Is there any proof here that you were actuated by a sense of honesty, truth or justice, in making such an attack upon me, a person who had never done you wrong? I therefore beg leave to ask, does not your conduct, in this instance, savour strongly of being influenced by "*Satanic agency*"?

But I must not omit another important point. You have quoted from *Chambers' Journal*; now, it is rather curious, if you wished to act honestly in this matter, that you should have quoted from the work what would never answer your purpose in respect to [Charles] Lafontaine [the Mesmerist], but should have overlooked the fact that in the same work, they had referred to my having attended his conversazioni, and discovered the cause of the phenomena, and had given lectures and successful courses of experiments, **to prove its true nature to be neither in the operator nor in the Devil, but solely in the individuals operated on keeping their minds and eyes riveted to one idea and in one fixed position**. I may reasonably ask were you ignorant of this when you penned your notable sermon? Or had you taken pains to be correctly informed on the subject? Or was it "Satanic agency" which blinded your bodily eyes that you could not see it; or your mental [eyes] that it might be wilfully dismissed?

[Published Reports of Braid's Hypnotism]

The talented editors of that work introduce the article from which you quote, with the following pertinent remarks:–

> There appears to us to be too great an inclination in the public to regard these phenomena as something out of the common course of nature. Ordinary sleep-walking, catalepsy and some of the diseases of extreme nervousness, are not wonderful – yet they occur every day. Why, then, may not Mesmerism be only an artificial means of bringing on, in susceptible natures, conditions of a like remarkable kind. This we say, without wishing to be understood that we are either believers or disbelievers in animal magnetism and the subject is not yet ripe for either full belief or full rejection. It only appears to us that, in this art, so to call it, laying out of view some of the extraordinary effects attributed to it, there is nothing judging beforehand, more wonderful, than in some conditions of the nervous system with which medical men are familiar. The vulgar disposition to look upon such things as supernatural is one of the causes why sound thinkers and philosophical inquirers are deterred from them. THE MORE REAL KNOWLEDGE THAT ANYONE POSSESSES OF THE NERVOUS SYSTEM THE LESS, WE BELIEVE, will he be disposed TO BE STARTLED BY THE ALLEGED WONDERS OF MESMERISM AS OUT OF THE ORDINARY COURSE OF NATURE. [*Chambers' Journal*]

As these judicious remarks immediately precede the paragraph you quoted, it cannot be supposed you were ignorant of it. Now, if you wished Mesmerism to be fairly tried, why not have given the above quotation? – And if you wished to do justice either to me or the subject, why deny that the laws by which it acted had been attempted to be explained? Is it not distinctly stated in the number of the same work for the 19th February last, that I had done so, where they say – "It is proper, however, to state Mr. Braid's own notion as the physiological cause of both his own and Mesmer's phenomena. It is, briefly, that by an individual keeping up a steady gaze, or fixed stare at an object," etc., after which follows a condensed view of my theory. Now, Sir, was it fair or honest conduct to have promulgated such statements as you have done, in direct opposition to evidence published in the very work from which you quoted; or to have done so at all without taking pains to be correctly informed?

Besides the numerous cases referred to in my letter as having been operated on successfully at Liverpool and elsewhere, on individuals whom I had never seen before, that presented themselves on the platform in the public lecture-room, and which were reported in your own papers, you had an opportunity of observing, in the report of my lectures at Macclesfield, that the five deaf and dumb patients and one paralytic, all adults and who were strangers to me, were operated on successfully as regarded bringing them under the *Hypnotic influence* and that four of the deaf and dumb patients acquired the power of hearing in consequence of the operation; and the patient who had been paralytic of the right leg and arm was enabled to walk much better, and acquired the power of picking up a pin with that hand which she could not do at any time for fifteen years previously. These facts were seen and borne testimony to by the talented editor of the paper, a stranger to me until I met him that evening in the lecture-room; and by individuals who might be known to him, but who were utter strangers to me. It was also particularly remarked that my attention was chiefly devoted to the investigation with the view of rendering it comprehensible and available as a curative agency, and that I explained how any intelligent medical man might apply the agency to the amelioration of suffering humanity. Moreover, various maladies in which it had been eminently useful where other means had failed, were enumerated, in order to induce other professional men to engage in this important investigation.

Now, Sir, with all these facts plainly laid before you, with what propriety could you implicate me in the charge of "refusing to come forward and state the laws of nature" by the uniform action of which this thing is done; or that I was one of those who "confine themselves to experiments in a corner upon their own servants, or upon females hired for this purpose"? **Had I not, moreover, stated the fact that impressed with the importance of the subject, I had, at great personal inconvenience as well as pecuniary sacrifice, gone to London, that my views might be subjected "to a rigid examination" of the most learned men in our profession, to propound to them the laws by which I consider it to act, and above all, to prove to them "the uniformity of its action" and its practical applicability and value as a curative agency, by [my] mode of operating.** I would therefore ask upon what principle, either of honour or candour, were you warranted in implicating me in such charges?

But even supposing the statements which were put forth could not explain the whole of the phenomena in a manner to satisfy all objections, and that various theories were adduced – as has happened on many scientific questions – surely, when beneficial application could be made of the extent of knowledge we had acquired, we ought to be at liberty to do so without being stigmatised from the pulpit as necromancers, or producing our effects by "Satanic Agency", etc. Supposing one hundred passengers start in one of your packets, and twenty or thirty of them become seasick, and the others escape, would it be fair to implicate the captain in the charge of acting by Satanic agency because the whole were not sick, and because according to Mr. McNeile, "if it be in nature, it will operate uniformly and not capriciously"? If it operate capriciously then there is "some mischievous agent at work; 'and we are not ignorant of the devices' of the Devil". Would any man but Mr. McNeile say, that, because the captain gave the signal to heave anchor, to spread the sails, and other "talismanic tokens" for steering the vessel, and because only part of the passengers became sick, he was consequently affecting them through Satanic agency – or that it would alter the matter one whit because medical men could not assign the true cause of this, or why anyone should be so affected? Is it not lamentable that the sacred and important duties of the Sabbath ministration of the pulpit should be so degraded, and perverted to such unworthy purposes?

[Hypnotism Requires the Subject's Compliance]
I also vindicated *Neurohypnotism* against the erroneous prejudices excited against it as having an immoral tendency. **I proved by experiments, both in public and in private, that during the somnambulistic state, whilst consciousness lasts, the patients are more sensitive and fastidious in their feelings of strict propriety than in the neutral condition.** I did not, and do not, claim for it the power of implanting a principle. I do not say it will make a vicious person virtuous; but I am most confident it will not make a virtuous person vicious. On the contrary, I feel assured that a person of habitually correct feelings will, during the somnambulistic condition, whilst consciousness lasts, manifest fully as much delicacy and circumspection of conduct as in the waking state. And again, even supposing the contrary were the case, **I have clearly proved that the animal magnetisers are in error, in supposing they had the power of irresistibly overpowering anyone by mere volition and secret passes. In proof of this I have challenged the whole of them to exert their combined influence to prevent me, by such secret means, from delivering my lectures, in which I was exposing the fallacy of their assumptions; but hitherto I have felt no lethargic influence brought into operation to retard my proceedings.** [This remark is a stroke of genius on Braid's part.] **Moreover, I have proved that no one can be affected at all unless by voluntary compliance,** and consequently **it has no right to be held as an agency which could be converted to immoral purposes as many have supposed**. If anyone would say it may have this tendency because in the state of torpor, insensibility and cataleptiform rigidity, the party is unconscious, immovable, and incapable of self defence, I beg to remind such individuals that the same argument might be urged against the proper use of wine, spirits, or opium, because excess in the use of either might be followed by like results. Had the Mesmerisers' notion been true, that any individual could obtain such irresistible power over others by mere volition and secret passes of the operator, most assuredly it would have been a dangerous agency, and might be used for most improper purposes. And, did I believe any such dangerous power could thus be obtained by one individual over others, I would be as ready to denounce it, as I am now desirous of defending a valuable agency against what I know to be unmerited obloquy [public denunciation]. Of the truth of these statements I shall furnish ample proofs in a small work on the subject which I intend to publish shortly.

[Further Defence of Hypnotism]
I also defended *Neurohypnotism* against the charge of having a tendency to sap the foundation of the Christian creed, by making the Gospel miracles appear as wrought by the agency. I explained, that were the animal magnetisers' views correct, there were a few of the Gospel miracles the importance of which might be invalidated; but, as **I distinctly deny the existence of a magnetic fluid or medium**, according to my views the Gospel miracles are rendered more invulnerable than ever. **I explained also that the phenomena of insensibility at one time, and exalted sensibility at another, were real phenomena, arising from the peculiar condition of the brain and spinal cord at different times.** Now, I would ask any rational man, was there anything in all this like a wish to conceal, or savouring of Satanic agency? As to your remarks about the Estatica [of Caldaro] and Adolorata [of Capriana], I fully explained, and exhibited experiments to prove, that their exhibitions resulted entirely from the individuals hypnotising themselves by their fixed gaze

and deep contemplation. [These are the names of two contemporary Christian mystics residing in Italy.] This I did at one of my early lectures and it has since been done in the *Achill Herald* by someone else; so that your remarks on this subject are not only not original, but bear strong marks of being an *unacknowledged plagiarism*.

[Cases Treated]

As you appeal to Scripture, I have no objection to do so too, and I consider the best plan is to take the Scripture rule, "By their works we shall know them." Now, I shall adduce a few cases in illustration of what I have done and can do, and can teach any intelligent medical man to do, without being a "necromancer", or having any more to do with the devil than yourself, when, in the exercise of your vocation, you are composing and delivering your sermons.

By the aid of this agency I have **extracted teeth** from most sensitive patients without pain; I have performed many other important operations with present ease and future advantage; in a few minutes have **removed rheumatic pains** which had resisted every other remedy, and tortured the patients for months or years – in one case for thirteen years; have completely overcome the pain of a violent **tic-douloureux** [i.e., trigeminal neuralgia] in a few minutes which had tortured the patient for eight weeks before I saw him, in despite of the most approved remedies – and other cases in like manner; have **restored strength and feeling to paralytic limbs** in a few minutes – in one case of a patient twenty-four years of age, and who had been so from birth; have **restored hearing to the deaf – sight to the blind** – smell to those who have been deprived of it; **restored the crooked in proper form – calmed the irritable, and roused the desponding; restored the mind from imbecility to intelligence, and the memory from listlessness and torpor to activity**. Thus, those who could not for years read their Bible, or remember, or profit by, what others read, have been enabled, after a few minutes' hypnotic sleep to do both. Now, I would ask any rational person, was it likely the Devil would have assisted me in doing any such thing? Is it not far more like Satanic agency for him to inspire anyone to become the active agent in preventing a dissemination of what, when properly understood, and applied, is calculated to prove such a vast blessing to mankind?

[Concluding Remarks]

At page 149 you make a strange charge against the medical profession. You there say, "It is a very unsuitable profession for the examination of such a matter as this. If there be anything connected with the spiritual world in it, it is wholly out of the cognisance of those gentlemen, whose whole professional study is connected with this matter." In answer to the sweeping charge and insulting remarks contained in the above extract and what follows, I must tell you they are sufficient to prove that you know very little of medical men, or of their habits and pursuits. I must take leave to tell you that the medical man who has not studied the laws of mind as well as matter, and how they act and react on each other, is very unfit for practising his profession, either with credit to himself or advantage to his patient. Let such individual only attend to these studies, and the advantages will soon become apparent, both to himself and others. But I will go farther, and claim for the honour of the medical profession some of the brightest characters who have appeared to illuminate the dark domain of metaphysical science. Need I do more to prove this than name the fact that [John] Locke, Thomas Brown, and [John] Abercrombie, *etc.*, were medical men [and distinguished academic philosophers]?

I by no means wish to laud Neurohypnology as an universal remedy. But that it is a means, when properly applied, of rapidly curing many diseases which resisted all other known remedies, there can be no doubt; and being a law of the animal economy – and, as such, no doubt implanted for some wise purpose – it is certain to prevail in defiance of all opposition.

I consider the uniformity of its action, as I apply it, is sufficient to prove it to be a law of the animal economy; and after the explanations I have given of it in the public lecture-room, to which I invited you that you might investigate the subject for yourself, where I stated my object was "not to mystify, but to dispel all mystery", it has no right to be stigmatised as an "occult" science or the device of the Devil. I have always understood the Devil to be actively engaged in inflicting disease, blindness and ignorance on mankind. But here we have works the very contrary – the cure of diseases which have resisted all other known remedies, the restoration of sight, hearing and intelligence to the benumbed mind.

In reference to your profession, I may, with great propriety, quote the words you apply to mine – "for which no man has a higher respect in its proper place, and for its proper work, than I have"; but, unless by those who can bring to bear on it more extensive knowledge of the subject, or more candour than you have displayed on this occasion, I must be excused for saying that yours is not a profession which peculiarly fits its disciples for the "examination of such a matter as this". I would, therefore, recommend you to consider Gamaliel's advice, and should you wish to preach another Sermon on the subject, that you should adopt it for your text – "Take heed what you do, for if this work or this counsel be of men, it will come to nought; but if it be of God, ye cannot overthrow it, lest haply ye be found even to fight against God."

3, St. Peter's Square,
Manchester.

4th June, 1842.

"On Braid's Hanover Square Talks":
Report & Letter in *The Medical Times* (1842)

Editor's Preface
Donald Robertson

This is possibly Braid's very earliest publication on hypnotism; his letter was dated March 7th 1842 and published in the March 12th edition of *The Medical Times*. In it he does not use the term "hypnotism", though elsewhere he suggests it was already in use by him at his lectures. The anonymous report which precedes his letter mentions his use of the expression "neuro-hypnology", albeit spelt incorrectly.

Indeed, this is one of Braid's most interesting letters, providing a neat summary of his early theory and practice. It illustrates how, from the outset, Braid's work was independently reported, and publicly examined and endorsed by a wide variety of observers, including some of the most distinguished scientists and physicians of his day. In his first booklet on the subject, published shortly after this letter, a frustrated Braid reminds his critics of the sincere and persistent efforts which he made in order to substantiate his views,

> Had I not, moreover, stated the fact that impressed with the importance of the subject, I had, at great personal inconvenience as well as pecuniary sacrifice, gone to London, that my views might be subjected "to a rigid examination" of the most learned men in our profession, to propound to them the laws by which I consider it to act, and above all, to prove to them "the uniformity of its action" and its practical applicability and value as a curative agency, by [my] mode of operating. (*Satanic Agency, etc.*, 1852)

This journalist's report and Braid's subjoined letter, show the extent to which, with the limited means available to him, Braid attempted to develop his theory in a credible scientific manner. In *Neurypnology* (1843), Braid comments on the role of Dr. Herbert Mayo, one of the most distinguished medical scientists of the period, at the meeting,

> I am fully borne out by the opinion of that eminent physiologist, Mr. Herbert Mayo, in my view of the subject, that my plan is "the best, the shortest, and surest for getting the sleep", and throwing the nervous system, by artificial contrivance, into a new condition, which may be rendered available in the healing art. At a private conversazione, which I gave to the profession in London on the 1st of March, 1842, he examined and tested my patients most carefully, submitted himself to be operated on by me both publicly and privately, and was so searching and inquisitive in his investigations as to call forth the animadversions of a medical gentleman present, who thought he was not giving me fair play; but which he has assured me proceeded from an anxious desire to know the truth, not being biased by having any peculiar views of his own to bring forward; and because he considered the subject most important, both in a speculative and practical point of view.

In his *Electro-Biological Phenomena* (1851) Braid describes a successful public demonstration delivered by him in Manchester, adding,

> I was equally successful in operating upon a number of strangers together at a private conversazione, given to the profession in London, in March 1842, sixteen out of eighteen having passed into the sleep, simply by maintaining a steady fixed stare and fixed act of attention, whilst gazing at the root of a chandelier. Most of these had never been so tried before. I never touched any one of them until their eyelids closed. Mr. Herbert Mayo, the eminent physiologist and surgeon, tested them, and ran a needle from the back to the palm of the hand of one patient without his (the patient) evincing the slightest consciousness of pain, or remembrance of it after awaking.

Dr. Mayo subsequently published his own favourable account entitled 'On Mr. Braid's experiments', in the next volume of The Medical Times for 1852.

[Report by Anonymous Correspondent]

Mr. Braid delivered two very excellent lectures on this subject last week, one on Tuesday the 1st of March, at the Hanover Square Rooms, the other, the following day, at the London Tavern.

The lecturer commenced by giving his audience a detailed explanation of the theory and phenomena of animal magnetism, and entered fully into the subject, illustrating the paper by physiological facts, and several interesting anecdotes. **He prefers the term "neurohypnology[144], or the rationale of nervous sleep," to that of animal magnetism, and thinks that that term is more proper, inasmuch as the effect is produced through the medium of the nervous system.** Several experiments were performed after the lecture.

The first was a young woman, whom Mr. Braid directed to look at her own finger; in two minutes the face became flushed, the woman sighed, and the eyes closed. **She was then requested to sit down, which she did; her arms were raised and also her legs; ammonia was placed under her nose, the galvanic battery applied, pins stuck in the forehead and legs, and without the woman evincing the slightest pain.** The second experiment was upon **two deaf brothers**, one of them was magnetised by looking upwards, and in three minutes the effect was produced. Mr. Braid extended both arms, which remained so for some time; he then clapped his hands, and the boy instantly became de-Mesmerised. The experimenter stated that the hearing was increased twelvefold during the time the patient was under the influence of the magnetising process. The elder brother was then subjected to the same process, and became magnetised in about three or four minutes; **a percussion cap was fired at his ear when in this state, but no effect supervened**. It is a singular thing that [presumably at a different stage in the lecture] the pulse in this boy increased from 84 to 140 [bpm], and Mr. Braid remarked that such was generally the case. [Braid repeatedly makes this observation in his writings, which seems to be verified by the reporter. The induction of rigid catalepsy seems to roughly double the pulse, raising it to a level more typical during intense aerobic exercise.]

The third experiment was upon his own footman [perhaps the young "man-servant" discussed in *Neurypnology*]. In this case he bandaged the man's eyes and in three minutes he was asleep; he was subjected to nearly the same experiments as the preceding. Mr. Braid then recovered him and directed the man to turn his eyes to the side; in a few minutes the eyes closed, and the most curious effect was produced; the man began gradually to turn round, a circumstance by no means uncommon with those who turn the eyes to the side (so the lecturer informed us).[145]

The fourth experiment was upon a young lady, whom Mr. Duncan [who had previously conducted lectures introducing Braid's work to the London audience prior to his arrival] had been in the habit of experimenting on. This was a very interesting case; after being magnetised, several objects were placed before her eyes (which were closed), and she distinctly names each article in succession [an illusory feat, later attributed by Braid to the ability to see through eyelids which are not properly closed]; she then walked about the platform, and knelt and arose at the request of the lecturer.

The last and concluding experiment was upon a young woman, who after going through nearly the same operations, finished by singing "*off, off, says the stranger*", and it really seemed as if she were about to go off.

[Braid's Letter to the Editor]

To the Editor of *The Medical Times*,

Sir,

I feel obliged by the kind note you have sent me stating your intention of honouring me by a report of my lecture. I much regret you could not attend the conversazioni, but I shall furnish you with a brief account of what took place on that occasion. **When I had briefly explained to those present my theoretical views, and the ground on which I had come to such conclusions, I expressed my intention to exhibit the phenomena on some of the subjects I had brought with me; some stranger proposed that it might be still more satisfactory and convincing to all present, were I to operate on a stranger, to which I readily assented, provided anyone present was willing to become the subject of experiment. It was then announced that a person born deaf and dumb was present, and had come with the express desire to be operated on, and would now come forward if I chose to begin with him. I assented, and the patient came forward accordingly. He was totally deaf, was never known to have heard sound at any time in his life, and was thirty-two years of age. In about eight minutes, I evinced to all present**

---
[144] [The article actually says "neuohypnology", an obvious typographical mistake.]
[145] [This phenomenon might be compared to Braid's later observations on "muscular suggestion".]

the most incontestable proof of hearing being restored. I then operated on another stranger successfully, and on a third, who was one of my subjects; the varied phenomena intended, and expressed as meant to be exhibited by said patient, were all demonstrated, to the satisfaction of all present. The next operated on was Herbert Mayo, Esq., so well-known to the profession; afterwards my other subjects were operated on, exhibiting these varied phenomena, both mental and corporeal. As the last experiment of the evening, eighteen were subject to their operation at once, and in ten minutes sixteen of the number [89%] were all in a state of somnolency, and some in the cataleptiform state, with insensibility to pain, as tested both by myself and Mr. Mayo [who seems to have shoved a pin straight through a subject's hand]. The other two did not comply with my injunctions. For the correctness of this statement, I beg to refer you to Dr. [Archibald] Billing [a physician and medical author] and Mr. Herbert Mayo, who tested the patients, and neither of whom I had had the honour of knowing till that evening. [In *Hypnotic Therapeutics*, 1853, Braid adds, that of this group, 'twelve of whom had never been tried before', the sixteen responsive subjects 'went into the condition at same time, by gazing fixedly and abstractedly on the root of a chandelier'.] I should feel obliged by your recording the fact now stated, in addition to what your reporter might see or hear at the public lecture. **In short, the whole of my experiments go to prove, that there is a law of the animal economy [a physiological law] by which a continued fixation of the visual organ, and a constrained attention of the mind to one subject, which is not of itself of an exciting nature; a state of somnolency is induced, with a peculiar mobility of the whole system, which may be directed so as to exhibit the whole or greater part of the Mesmeric phenomena.**

The remarks of your talented correspondent, Mr. Barrallier, relative to Mr. Catlow's experiments, are quite in accordance with my own views. I had made experiments to prove this, and had come to the same conclusion as Mr. Barrallier before I was aware of his experiments, and have confirmed them many times since on different subjects. Mr. C.'s cases on the sense of hearing, touch, taste, smelling, and muscular motion, were nothing beyond natural sleep, at any rate totally different from *Mesmeric* sleep, *unless in those cases where the patients had been repeatedly operated on in my way, or through the eye*. After a certain time, and frequency of being operated on in this way, the brain has an impressibility stamped on it which renders the patient subject to be acted on entirely through the *imagination*, and this is the grand source of the follies which have misled Mr. C. and the animal magnetisers. I feel most confident of this, and shall feel obliged by your publishing this letter to record what I believe to be the fact.

On my return home, I delivered a lecture at Birmingham on Thursday evening, 3rd [March 1842], when I exhibited a series of experiments which were quite conclusive on the subject. I am to deliver another lecture in Manchester next Saturday evening, when I shall exhibit the same, and many more, illustrative of the imagined *transposition* of the senses [i.e., seeing with the stomach, and other supposed paranormal abilities called the "higher phenomena" of Mesmerism], and the magnetic power of attraction, a report of which shall be sent to some of our papers, which I shall correct if any mistakes should appear before I send it.

I beg leave farther to state, that as I have operated successfully on the blind, it is evident it is not the optic nerve so much as the ganglionic or sympathetic systems and motor nerves of the eye, and state of the mind, which influence the system in this extraordinary manner.

I have the honour to be, Sir, your much obliged and obedient servant,

James Braid.

3, St. Peter's Square.
March 7th, 1842.

PS. I may add, that last night I was called to a lady suffering the most agonising Tic Douloureux. In five minutes by my mode of inducing refreshing sleep, I succeeded in putting this patient into comfortable sleep, from which she did not awake till Sunday in the morning, being five and a half hours, and was then quite easy. By what other agency, I now ask, could such an effort have been induced?

Bibliography of James Braid's Writings

The following bibliography was published by Bramwell in his *Hypnotism* (1903). I have included additional information supplied in N.M. Kravis' amended bibliography in 'James Braid's Psychophysiology' (*American Journal of Psychiatry,* 145: 10, October 1988). The original numbering system has been retained, though entries are grouped according to their source.

It should perhaps be emphasised that Braid may well have published *other* articles, letters, etc., which have yet to be discovered. There are also *quite probably* additional reports of Braid's writings and lectures, in the words of others from the same period, which have yet to come to light.

The following are all the books and articles by Braid on the subject of hypnotism which I have been able to trace.

[Books, Pamphlets & Major Works]
1. "Satanic Agency and Mesmerism" Reviewed, in a letter to the Rev. H. McNeile, A.M., in Reply to a Sermon preached him (1842).
2. Neurypnology, or the Rationale of Nervous Sleep, considered in Relation with Animal Magnetism, illustrated by numerous cases of its successful application in the Relief and Cure of Disease (1843).
3. The Power of the Mind over the Body, an Experimental Inquiry into the Nature and Cause of the Phenomena attributed by Baron Reichenbach and others to a "New Imponderable" (1846).
4. Observations on Trance or Human Hybernation (1850).
5. Electro-Biological Phenomena, considered physiologically and psychologically, from the Monthly Journal of Medical Science for June, 1851, with Appendix. [Published in July 1851, according to Braid (1852), as a pamphlet.]
6. Magic, Witchcraft, Animal Magnetism, Hypnotism and Electro-Biology; being a Digest of the latest Views of the Author on these Subjects. Third Edition, greatly enlarged, embracing observations on J. C. Colquhoun's *History of Magnetism* (1852).
7. Hypnotic Therapeutics, Illustrated by Cases, with an Appendix on Table-Turning and Spirit Rapping. [Reprinted from the *Monthly Journal of Medical Science* for July, 1853.]
8. The Physiology of Fascination, and the Critics Criticised (1855). [The second part is a reply to the attacks made in *The Zoist*.]

Articles in *The Medical Times*
10. "Animal Magnetism", 12th March, 1842, vol. V., 1841-42, p. 283.
11. "Animal Magnetism", 26th March, 1842, vol. V., p. 308.
12. "Neuro-Hypnotism." vol. VI., 9th July, 1842, p. 239.
13. "Observations on the Phenomena Phreno-Mesmerism", 11th November 1843, vol. IX., 1843-44, pp. 74-75.
14. "Mr. Braid on Mesmerism", 6th January 1844, vol. IX., p. 203.
15. "Observations on some Mesmeric Phenomena", 13th January, 1844, vol. IX., pp. 224-227.
16. "Observations on Mesmeric and Hypnotic Phenomena", 13th April 1844 & 20th April 1844, vol. X., 1844, pp. 31-32 and 47-49.
17. "Case of Natural Somnambulism and Catalepsy, treated by Hypnotism; with remarks on the Phenomena presented during Spontaneous Somnambulism, as well as that produced by various Artificial Processes", 26th October, 1844, vol. XI., 1844-45, pp. 77-78, 95-96, and 134-135.
18. "Experimental Inquiry whether Hypnotic and Mesmeric Manifestations can be adduced in Proof of Phrenology", 30th November, 1844, vol. XI., p. 181-182.
19. "Magic, Mesmerism, Hypnotism, etc., Historically and Physiologically considered", vol. XI., pp. 201, 224, 270, 296, 399, and 439.
20. "Case of Natural Somnambulism, etc.", 17th May, 1845, vol. XII., 1845, p. 117-119. [Article giving further history of case already reported in 17.]
21. "The Fakirs of India", 30th August, 1845, vol. XII., p. 437-438.
22. "Dr. Elliotson and Mr. Braid", 25th October, 1845, vol. XIII., 1845-46, pp. 99-101, 120-121, and 141-142.
23. "On the Power of the Mind over the Body: an Experimental Inquiry into the Nature and Cause of the Phenomena attributed by Baron Reichenbach and others to a 'New Imponderable'", vol. XIV., 1846, pp. 214, 252, and 273.
24. "Facts and Observations as to the Relative Value of Mesmeric and Hypnotic Coma and Ethereal Narcotism, for the Mitigation or entire Prevention of Pain during Surgical Operations", 13th February, 1847, vol. XV, 1846-47, pp. 381-382; continued vol. XVI., 27th February, 1847, pp. 10-11.

25. "Observations on the Use of Ether for Preventing Pain during Surgical Operations, and the Moral Abuse it is capable of being converted to", vol. XVI., p. 130.
26. "Mr. Braid and Dr. Elliotson", 20th November, 1847, vol. XVII., 1847-48, pp. 106-107.
27. "Mr. Braid and Mr. Wakley", 11th December, 1847, vol. XVII., pp. 163-164.
28. "Observations on Trance or Human Hybernation", vol. XXI., 1850, pp. 351, 401, and 416.
50. "The effect of garlic on the magnetic needle", vol. X., 1844, pp. 98-99.
51. "Physiological explanation of some Mesmeric phenomena", vol. X, 31st August, 1844, pp. 450-452.

In *The Lancet*
29. "Queries respecting the Alleged Voluntary Trance of Fakirs in India", vol. II., 1845, p. 325.
39. "Talipes", vol. I. 1841-42, p. 202.
52. "Mr. Braid on hypnotism", vol. I., 1845; pp. 627-628.

In *The Monthly Journal of Medical Science*
30. "Hypnotic Therapeutics, Illustrated by Cases", vol. VIII., third series, 1853, p. 14.
40. "Entire Absence of Vagina, with Rudimentary State of Uterus, and Remarkable Displacement of Rudimentary Ovaries and Appendages, in a married female, 74 years of age", vol. XVI. (Third Series, vol. vii) 1853, p. 230.

In *The Edinburgh Medical and Surgical Journal*
31. "The Power of the Mind over the Body; an Experimental Inquiry into the Nature and Cause of the Phenomena attributed by Baron Reichenbach and others to a 'New Imponderable'", vol. LXVI., 1846, p. 286.
32. "Facts and Observations as to the relative Value of Mesmeric and Hypnotic Coma, and Ethereal Narcotism, for the Mitigation or entire Prevention of Pain during Surgical Operations", vol. LXVII., 1847, p. 588.
33. "On the Use and Abuse of Anaesthetic Agents, and the best Modes of Rousing Patients who have been too, intensely affected by them", vol. LXX., 1848, p. 486.
41. "Observations on Talipes, Strabismus, Stammering, and Contortion, and the best Methods of removing them", vol. LVI. 1841, p. 338.

[In the Manchester Newspapers]
35. "Account of case of deafness successfully treated by hypnotism", *Manchester Times*, September 1st, 1842.
36. "Analysis of Dr. Carpenter's Lectures on the Physiology of the Nervous System", *Manchester Examiner and Times,* (Part I) Saturday 30th & (Part II) Wednesday 3rd April 1853. [Authored by Braid, according to Bramwell, though I can't see any name attached. -DR].
37. "The Late 'Table-Moving' Experiments at the Athenaeum, Letter to the Editor", *Manchester Examiner and Times*, Wednesday, June 22nd 1853. [Subsequently published as a pamphlet according to Bramwell.]
48. "The Manchester and Salford Sanitary Association", November 15th, 1853, the [*Manchester*] *Examiner & Times*. ["A letter (on the means of improving the air of Manchester and upon the connection between cholera and sewers", writes Bramwell.]
49. "The Manchester Geological & Natural History Societies", *Manchester Courier* of November 26th, 1859. [Bramwell labels this, "a controversial letter".]

In *The London Medical Gazette*, New Series
41. "Lateral Curvature of the Spine – Strabismus", vol. I. 1840-41, p. 445.
43. "Stammering", vol. I. p. 445.
44. "Cure of Stammering", vol. II. 1840-41, p. 116.
45. "On the Operation of Talipes", vol. II. p. 186.
46. "Case of Congenital Talipes varus of a Foot with Ten Toes, with Illustration", 1848.

[Translations of Unpublished Manuscripts]
34. "On the Distinctive Conditions of Natural and Nervous Sleep", Manchester, December 17th, 1845. [A manuscript first published in a German translation in Wilhelm Preyer's *Der Hypnotismus*, 1890.]
38. "A Manuscript on Hypnotism by James Braid", January, 1860. Translated into French by Dr. Jules Simon as an appendix to *Neurypnologie*, and into German by Preyer in *Die Entdeckung des Hypnotismus*.

[Other Publications]
9. "Observations on the Nature and Treatment of Certain Forms of Paralysis", *Association Medical Journal*, 1855; 3:848-855. [The *Association Medical Journal* was renamed the *British Medical Journal* in 1857. Bramwell seems to imply that a version of this article was published as a booklet.]
47. "Arsenic as a Remedy for the Bite of the Tsetse, etc.", *British Medical Journal*, March 13th, 1858. [To which the famous explorer David Livingstone replied (BMJ, 22nd March 1858) thanking Braid for his

observations.]
53. "Letter to the editor", *British Record of Obstetric Medicine & Surgery*, 1849; 2:55-59.

Index:
Abstraction, 9, 11, 21, 22, 24, 26, 27 29, 31, 32, 41, 80, 89, 90, 93, 107, 117, 118, 119, 120, 121, 122, 145, 146, 147, 149, 150, 151, 166, 177, 178, 186, 187, 233, 241, 150, 276, 295
Abercrombie, Dr 303, 341
Amnesic, 32
Anaesthesia, 223, 243
Anderson, Charles, 6, 252, 275
Arbuthnot, 316
Armstrong, 302, 359
Ashburner, Dr 86, 152
Atkinson, Miss E 40, 298, 339
Atkinson, James, 224
Autosuggestion, 148, 159
Azam, Dr Etienne Eugene, 21, 51, 52, 55, 62, 75

Bacon, Francis 17, 171
Bandura, 18
Barber, 3 211
Barnet, Joseph 341, 342
Barralier, M. 300, 376
Beard, Dr George Miller, 21, 52, 75
Beck, Aaron 15, 17
Bell, Sir Charles, 22, 262, 307
Benedikt, Professor 52
Bennet, Dr/Professor J. H. 55, 107, 135, 136, 138, 185, 190
Bernard, Dr Jules 52
Bernard, Prudence 168 170
Bernheim, 3, 11, 35, 40, 52, 53, 54, 55, 56, 59
Bertrand, Dr Alexandre 38, 282, 283
Beswick, Miss 210
Bingham, Mr 330, 331
Binns, Dr 158, 300
Birt-Davies, Dr 308
Blessington, Lady Marguerite 73, 181, 193
Boirac, M 41
Brewster, Sir David 78, 108, 144, 158, 165
Broca, Paul 21, 51, 55, 75
Brodie, Sir Benjamin 144, 298, 350
Brown, John 209
Brown, Thomas 6, 7, 17, 24, 130, 269, 286, 303, 342, 372
Brown-Sequard 55
Braid's Method 8 26, 51, 58, 60
Bramwell 21, 27, 35, 36, 47, 51,56, 58, 59, 60 116

Canton, John 23
Caplin, 182
Carpenter, Professor William 7, 9, 17, 21, 22, 23, 24, 29, 31, 53, 57, 69, 80, 81, 86, 103,

107, 108, 114, 116, 121, 122, 123, 144, 204, 207, 218, 220, 228
Catalepsy, 7, 14, 15, 21, 22, 23, 27, 30, 32, 36, 43, 57, 62, 63, 64, 66, 93, 94, 96, 109, 131, 136, 146, 151, 161, 188, 195, 197, 203, 204, 208, 209, 210, 214, 215, 226, 232, 233, 235, 242, 250, 255, 257, 267, 276, 295, 355, 362, 370, 375
Charcot, 3, 52, 53, 55
Chevreul, Michael Eugene 3, 23, 114
Cheyne, Dr John 197
Chawnes, Dr 298, 350, 351
Clark, Sir Andrew 54
Clark, Sir James, 86, 87,
Clarke, Mr 363
Cochrane, Dr 279
Collins, Miss 298, 350
Colquhoun, James Campbell, 20 42, 125, 126, 128 129, 130, 133, 134, 138, 142, 143, 163, 164, 246 282, 367
Conversazione, 7, 8, 9, 22, 36, 89, 108, 111, 137, 177, 186, 228, 281, 286, 288, 293, 331, 312, 316, 333, 335, 336, 337, 363, 364, 374
Curtis, john Harrison, 329, 331

Darling, Dr 136, 177, 178, 185, 187
Davy, Sir Humphrey 277
Dee, Dr John 73, 181, 193
Delboeuf, Joseph 52
Donaldson, Ann 83
Dyce, Dr 332

Edwards, Samuel 337
Edwards, Dr 207
Elliotson, 3, 36, 44, 81, 86, 97, 109, 110, 161, 162, 252, 256, 263, 305, 315, 357
Erickson, Milton 3, 13
Evans, Samuel 9, 335, 363
Eysenck, Hans 12

Faraday, Professor Michael 77, 109, 111, 160, 240
Faria, Abbe de 3, 10, 38, 41, 282
Forel, Professor 54
Foster, John Frederick 316, 317
Freud, Sigmund 54, 247, 259

Gall, Franz Joseph 24, 256
Gauld, 2
Gordon, Evelyn N 224
Gordon, Mr 349
Gregory, Professor/Dr 83, 85, 90, 107, 131, 132, 137, 136, 152, 158, 164, 185, 231, 233, 312
Grimes, J. Stanley, 20, 22, 55, 68
Gull, Sir William 54
Gurney, Edmund 39

Haddock, Dr 132
Hall, Spencer T. 308, 310, 311, 313
Hannay, Mr 332

Hampson, Mr 343
Haygarth, Dr John 25, 44, 141, 162
Hecker 155, 174
Heidenhain, Rudolph 40, 52
Hell, Fr. Maxamillian 23
Herbert, William (Dean of Manchester) 211
Highfield, M. 51
Hilgard, Porfessor E. R. 3
Hull 3 18
Hulme, James 224, 335
Holditch, Mr 327
Holland, Dr (Sir) Henry 44, 66, 90, 108, 117, 137, 161, 171, 188, 191
Hibernation 20, 63, 129, 159, 197, 207, 209, 215, 217
Hypnosis 3, 7, 9, 13, 20, 25, 28, 30 35, 39, 42, 44, 47, 49, 52, 57, 63, 89, 93, 98, 105, 145, 160, 185, 203, 212, 241, 247, 250, 255, 279, 362

Ideo-motor Theory/response/action 7, 9, 20, 23, 31, 69, 86, 107, 114, 118, 122

James-Lange, Theory of Emotion 22, 70
Jarrod, Dr 208
Jewett, Mr 209
Johnstone, Thomas 338
Jones, Mr 338

Kelly, George 33
Kelly, Edward 72, 181, 193
Kreskin 12

Lafontaine, Charles 7, 12, 20, 36, 50, 62, 64, 260, 281, 286, 293, 355, 369
Lancashire, Master J 343
Lane, Mr 72, 181, 193
Lassaigne, M. 168
Leaf, Dr Walter 41
Liebault 41, 53, 55, 58
Liebig 354
Liegous 53
Lind, Jenny 74, 137, 150, 182, 216
London Tavern, the 8, 375
Luys, Dr Jules Bernard 52

Maix, mlle 234
MacNish 295, 208
Manchester Royal Infirmary 204
Manchester Royal Institute 108, 137
Martineau, Miss Harriet 129
Maude, D 316
Mayo, Dr Herbert 8, 42, 77, 108, 118, 137, 148, 177, 186, 283, 288, 292, 316, 350, 367, 369, 374, 376
McGill, Ormond 12
McNeile, Dr 8, 36, 357, 367, 371
M'Naughton 199
M'Roberts, Alexander 332

Mellor, Miss Sarah 9, 335, 363
Mill, John Stuart 17, 23
Monoideism 9, 11, 17, 21, 24, 30, 41, 51, 55, 57, 60, 69, 114, 122, 125
Moreau, M. 205
Morris, Mr Thomas 9, 335, 363
Myers, Mr Frederick 52, 55

Neilson, Mr 82
Neurypnology 6, 9, 17, 20, 22, 26, 29, 36, 39, 42, 51, 55, 60, 64, 82, 130, 158, 226, 249, 252, 255, 260, 264, 272, 284, 352, 363, 374
Newnham, Mr 42, 105, 174
Noble, Dr Daniel 23, 69, 114
Nowotny, mlle. 233

Odyle 51, 121, 134, 152, 161, 178, 180, 188, 192
Oerstedt 110
Okey, Misses 162, 252, 357

Paris, Abbe 105
Pendleton, Mr John Wright 328
Perkins, Dr Elisha (tractors) 25, 44, 72, 141, 162, 181, 193
Peterson, Dr F 52
Playfair, Dr Lion 209
Plowman, Mr 82
Preyer, William T 367
Prudhoe, Lord 72, 181, 193
Psychosomatic illness 14, 148
Puysegur, de 3

Reichenbach, Baron Von 9, 11, 20, 24, 31, 33, 43, 65, 90, 109, 118, 121, 130, 135, 141, 151, 160, 178, 183, 188, 192, 228, 231, 235, 237, 243
Reid, Thomas 17, 23
Reverie 9, 22, 24, 30, 32, 38, 63, 65, 68, 73, 78, 117, 119, 121, 145, 171, 295, 355
Rider-Waite 56
Rodgers, A 224
Roily, Mrs 324, 326
Romanes, Professor George John 40

Salpetriere 52, 55, 58
Sandby, Rev. G. 82, 109, 222
Sarbin 3 28
Schrenck-Notzing 54
Schuh, Carl 161
Schwabe, Mr 39, 317
Schwabe, Mrs..39
Self-Hypnosis 32, 133, 160, 166, 203, 212, 241, 250, 279
Shaw, Professor 211
Shelmerdine, James 329
Simpson, Mr, 7, 260, 266
Simpson, Professor 45, 104, 136
Singh, Maharajah Ranjit 195, 198, 200
Smee, Mr Alfred 182

Smethurst, Dr 252
Smith, Adam 23, 305
Somnambule 39, 44, 47, 52, 58, 74, 118, 204
Sowler 142, 269
Stage Hypnosis 7, 12, 25
Stevens, Dr William 103, 160
Stewart, Dugald 17, 23, 140, 181, 194, 224, 255, 273, 302, 305
Stone 177, 182, 186, 190
Stowe, Miss M. A. 324
Sunderland, Le Roy 313
Sutton, C. W. 55
Swinton, George 195, 198

Taylor, Sarah 332
Thomas, Mr John 343
Thornhill, Dr 209
Tomlinson, Miss 347
Tourette, Giles de la 52
Townsend, Col. 40, 197
Trance 3, 8, 13, 20, 23, 31, 32, 35, 40, 54, 58, 63, 84, 129, 131, 135, 137, 142, 144, 150, 153, 159, 166, 171, 185, 192, 195, 197, 203, 207, 210, 214, 241, 255, 292, 305
Trevelyan, Sir 196, 200
Tuke, Dr Hack 54
Turner, Mr Aspinall 311
Tyler, Dr 221

Urquhart, Mr. David 205, 214

Velpeau, Professor 51, 62
Volgyesi, Dr F. A. 4, 367

Wade, Sir Claude Martin 195, 198, 200, 207
Walker, Mr 157, 286, 293, 317, 326, 342, 348,
Wakley, Thomas 292
Wemyss, Col. 316, 363
Wilbraham, Major 316'
Wilkinson, Dr. J. J. G. 29, 48, 120, 144, 147, 219
Williamson, Professor William Crawford 7, 60
Willshire, Sir Thomas 269
Wolberg 13
Wolpe 13, 247
Woods, John 208

Zoist, the 21, 50, 81, 84, 87, 109, 114, 222, 252

Breinigsville, PA USA
07 October 2009
225438BV00002B/1/P